Focus on Antibiotics – New Challenges and Steps Forward in Discovery and Development, 2nd Edition

Focus on Antibiotics – New Challenges and Steps Forward in Discovery and Development, 2nd Edition

Guest Editors

Aura Rusu
Valentina Uivarosi

MDPI

Basel • Beijing • Wuhan • Barcelona • Belgrade • Novi Sad • Cluj • Manchester

Guest Editors
Aura Rusu
Pharmaceutical and
Therapeutic Chemistry
George Emil Palade
University of Medicine,
Pharmacy, Science and
Technology of Targu Mures
Targu Mures
Romania

Valentina Uivarosi
General and Inorganic
Chemistry Department
Carol Davila University of
Medicine and Pharmacy
Bucharest
Romania

Editorial Office
MDPI AG
Grosspeteranlage 5
4052 Basel, Switzerland

This is a reprint of the Special Issue, published open access by the journal *Pharmaceutics* (ISSN 1999-4923), freely accessible at: https://www.mdpi.com/journal/pharmaceutics/special_issues/L74WL4NHS0.

For citation purposes, cite each article independently as indicated on the article page online and as indicated below:

Lastname, A.A.; Lastname, B.B. Article Title. *Journal Name* **Year**, *Volume Number*, Page Range.

ISBN 978-3-7258-4028-1 (Hbk)
ISBN 978-3-7258-4027-4 (PDF)
https://doi.org/10.3390/books978-3-7258-4027-4

Contents

About the Editors . . . . **vii**

Preface . . . . **ix**

Aura Rusu, Ioana-Maria Moga, Livia Uncu and Gabriel Hancu
The Role of Five-Membered Heterocycles in the Molecular Structure of Antibacterial Drugs Used in Therapy
Reprinted from: *Pharmaceutics* **2023**, *15*, 2554, https://doi.org/10.3390/pharmaceutics15112554 . **1**

Silvana Alfei, Gian Carlo Schito and Anna Maria Schito
Synthetic Pathways to Non-Psychotropic Phytocannabinoids as Promising Molecules to Develop Novel Antibiotics: A Review
Reprinted from: *Pharmaceutics* **2023**, *15*, 1889, https://doi.org/10.3390/pharmaceutics15071889 . **52**

Md. Amdadul Huq, Md. Aminul Islam Apu, Md. Ashrafudoulla, Md. Mizanur Rahman, Md. Anowar Khasru Parvez, Sri Renukadevi Balusamy, et al.
Bioactive ZnO Nanoparticles: Biosynthesis, Characterization and Potential Antimicrobial Applications
Reprinted from: *Pharmaceutics* **2023**, *15*, 2634, https://doi.org/10.3390/pharmaceutics15112634 . **98**

Syed Mohd Danish Rizvi, Amr Selim Abu Lila, Afrasim Moin, Talib Hussain, Mohammad Amjad Kamal, Hana Sonbol and El-Sayed Khafagy
Antibiotic-Loaded Gold Nanoparticles: A Nano-Arsenal against ESBL Producer-Resistant Pathogens
Reprinted from: *Pharmaceutics* **2023**, *15*, 430, https://doi.org/10.3390/pharmaceutics15020430 . **120**

Arif Jamal Siddiqui, Mitesh Patel, Mohd Adnan, Sadaf Jahan, Juhi Saxena, Mohammed Merae Alshahrani, et al.
Bacteriocin-Nanoconjugates (Bac10307-AgNPs) Biosynthesized from *Lactobacillus acidophilus*-Derived Bacteriocins Exhibit Enhanced and Promising Biological Activities
Reprinted from: *Pharmaceutics* **2023**, *15*, 403, https://doi.org/10.3390/pharmaceutics15020403 . **140**

Cecilia Fiore, Federico Antoniciello, Davide Roncarati, Vincenzo Scarlato, Fabrizia Grepioni and Dario Braga
Levofloxacin and Ciprofloxacin Co-Crystals with Flavonoids: Solid-State Investigation for a Multitarget Strategy against *Helicobacter pylori*
Reprinted from: *Pharmaceutics* **2024**, *16*, 203, https://doi.org/10.3390/pharmaceutics16020203 . **165**

Kseniya Shapovalova, Georgy Zatonsky, Natalia Grammatikova, Ilya Osterman, Elizaveta Razumova, Andrey Shchekotikhin and Anna Tevyashova
Synthesis of 6′′-Modified Kanamycin A Derivatives and Evaluation of Their Antibacterial Properties
Reprinted from: *Pharmaceutics* **2023**, *15*, 1177, https://doi.org/10.3390/pharmaceutics15041177 . **177**

Ahmed I. El-Tantawy, Elshaymaa I. Elmongy, Shimaa M. Elsaeed, Abdel Aleem H. Abdel Aleem, Reem Binsuwaidan, Wael H. Eisa, et al.
Synthesis, Characterization, and Docking Study of Novel Thioureidophosphonate-Incorporated Silver Nanocomposites as Potent Antibacterial Agents
Reprinted from: *Pharmaceutics* **2023**, *15*, 1666, https://doi.org/10.3390/pharmaceutics15061666 . **199**

Hyeju Lee, Byeongkwon Kim, Minju Kim, Seoyeong Yoo, Jinkyeong Lee, Eunha Hwang and Yangmee Kim
Characterization of the Antimicrobial Activities of *Trichoplusia ni* Cecropin A as a High-Potency Therapeutic against Colistin-Resistant *Escherichia coli*
Reprinted from: *Pharmaceutics* **2023**, *15*, 1752, https://doi.org/10.3390/pharmaceutics15061752 . **232**

Natália Vitória Bitencourt, Gabriela Marinho Righetto, Ilana Lopes Baratella Cunha Camargo, Mariana Ortiz de Godoy, Rafael Victorio Carvalho Guido, Glaucius Oliva, et al.
Effects of Dimerization, Dendrimerization, and Chirality in p-BthTX-I Peptide Analogs on the Antibacterial Activity and Enzymatic Inhibition of the SARS-CoV-2 PL^{pro} Protein
Reprinted from: *Pharmaceutics* **2023**, *15*, 436, https://doi.org/10.3390/pharmaceutics15020436 . **254**

About the Editors

Aura Rusu

Aura Rusu is currently a Professor at the Pharmaceutical and Therapeutical Chemistry Department, Faculty of Pharmacy, George Emil Palade University of Medicine, Pharmacy, Science and Technology of Târgu Mureș, Romania.

She has a Degree in Pharmacy (1994); Specialist (primary pharmacist) in Pharmaceutical Laboratory (2003); Trainer of Trainers (2008); PhD in Pharmacy (2013), Master Degree in Quality of Medicine, Food and Environment (2013); Habilitation in Pharmacy (2017); and Coordination of PhD students (2018).

She works mainly in pharmaceutical chemistry, medicinal chemistry, drug design, antibacterial and anticancer agents, metal complexes, drug analysis, capillary electrophoresis, and patient–pharmacist communication.

She was involved in research projects as a director (one) or member (three) and in other institutional projects as a director (one) or member (two), all supported by the George Emil Palade University of Medicine, Pharmacy, Sciences and Technology of Targu Mures, Romania. In addition, she is the author or co-author of 12 books, 2 chapters in books, 78 articles published in international peer-reviewed journals, and over 80 conference presentations.

Valentina Uivarosi

Valentina Uivarosi is currently a Professor of General and Inorganic Chemistry at the University of Medicine and Pharmacy Carol Davila in Bucharest (Faculty of Pharmacy), Romania. She graduated in Pharmacy from the University of Medicine and Pharmacy Carol Davila in 1993 and in Chemistry from the University of Bucharest in 2006. She received her PhD (2004) and Dr. Habil. (2015) degrees in Pharmacy from the University of Medicine and Pharmacy Carol Davila in Bucharest.

Her main research interests focus on the synthesis of metal complexes with biological activity (e.g., antibacterial, anticancer, and antidiabetic activity), DNA binding, protein interaction, cytotoxicity studies, and drug repositioning.

She is the author or co-author of 10 books, 6 chapters in books, 70 articles, 8 patent applications (4 are granted), and over 100 conference presentations and conducted 5 national research grants.

Preface

The design of new antibiotics remains a primary weapon against growing bacterial resistance. This Special Issue "Focus on Antibiotics – New Challenges and Steps Forward in Discovery and Development, 2nd Edition", explores innovative strategies and groundbreaking research to combat antibiotic resistance.

Five-membered heterocycles are essential in many antibacterial drugs, significantly influencing their biological activity. Some phytocannabinoids have shown antibacterial effects against Gram-positive bacteria, including methicillin-resistant *Staphylococcus aureus* (MRSA). Cannabigerol can inhibit MRSA biofilm formation and eradicate mature biofilms. Zinc oxide nanoparticles (ZnONPs) demonstrate activity against multidrug-resistant (MDR) pathogens through different mechanisms. Gold nanoparticles (AuNPs) have shown the potential to enhance the efficacy of antibiotics against MDR strains. Bacteriocin-derived silver nanoparticles (Bac10307-AgNPs) exhibit potent antibacterial activity against *Staphylococcus aureus* and *Pseudomonas aeruginosa*. Levofloxacin and ciprofloxacin were co-crystallised with flavonoids, forming co-crystals. These co-crystals enhance antimicrobial activity, reducing the required amount of fluoroquinolone to achieve the same efficacy against *Helicobacter pylori*. Researchers have synthesized 6′-deoxykanamycin A analogues with additional protonatable groups, improving activity against *Staphylococcus aureus*. Mono- and bis-thioureidophosphonate (MTP and BTP) analogues were used as reducing/capping agents for silver nitrate to create silver nanocomposites (MTP(BTP)/Ag NCs). These nanocomposites demonstrated significant antibacterial activity, particularly against *Pseudomonas aeruginosa* and MRSA, with enhanced antibiofilm activity and antifouling rates. The insect AMP *Tricoplusia ni* cecropin A (*T. ni* cecropin) showed significant antibacterial and antibiofilm activities against colistin-resistant *Escherichia coli*, with low cytotoxicity to mammalian cells. Additionally, *T. ni* cecropin demonstrated antiseptic effects in an endotoxemia mouse model. Peptide [des-Cys^{11},Lys^{12},Lys^{13}-(p-BthTX-I)2K] (p-Bth), an analogue of p-BthTX-I, has shown enhanced antimicrobial activity, stability, and hemolytic activity. Dimerisation and dendrimerization are crucial for its antibacterial activity, with dimers and tetramers effective against Gram-positive and Gram-negative bacteria.

We appreciate the authors' valuable contributions and hope this Special Issue will inspire further antibiotic research. We also thank the reviewers for their time and expertise and the editorial team for supporting this Special Issue. We aim to encourage further antibiotic research and development by highlighting novel therapeutic options and innovative methodologies.

Aura Rusu and Valentina Uivarosi
Guest Editors

pharmaceutics

MDPI

Review

The Role of Five-Membered Heterocycles in the Molecular Structure of Antibacterial Drugs Used in Therapy

Aura Rusu [1,*], Ioana-Maria Moga [1], Livia Uncu [2] and Gabriel Hancu [1]

1 Pharmaceutical and Therapeutic Chemistry Department, Faculty of Pharmacy, George Emil Palade University of Medicine, Pharmacy, Science and Technology of Targu Mures, 540142 Targu Mures, Romania; moga.ioana-maria@stud18.umfst.ro (I.-M.M.); gabriel.hancu@umfst.ro (G.H.)

2 Scientific Center for Drug Research, "Nicolae Testemitanu" State University of Medicine and Pharmacy, 8 Bd. Stefan Cel Mare si Sfant 165, MD-2004 Chisinau, Moldova; livia.uncu@usmf.md

* Correspondence: aura.rusu@umfst.ro

Abstract: Five-membered heterocycles are essential structural components in various antibacterial drugs; the physicochemical properties of a five-membered heterocycle can play a crucial role in determining the biological activity of an antibacterial drug. These properties can affect the drug's activity spectrum, potency, and pharmacokinetic and toxicological properties. Using scientific databases, we identified and discussed the antibacterials used in therapy, containing five-membered heterocycles in their molecular structure. The identified five-membered heterocycles used in antibacterial design contain one to four heteroatoms (nitrogen, oxygen, and sulfur). Antibacterials containing five-membered heterocycles were discussed, highlighting the biological properties imprinted by the targeted heterocycle. In some antibacterials, heterocycles with five atoms are pharmacophores responsible for their specific antibacterial activity. As pharmacophores, these heterocycles help design new medicinal molecules, improving their potency and selectivity and comprehending the structure-activity relationship of antibiotics. Unfortunately, particular heterocycles can also affect the drug's potential toxicity. The review extensively presents the most successful five-atom heterocycles used to design antibacterial essential medicines. Understanding and optimizing the intrinsic characteristics of a five-membered heterocycle can help the development of antibacterial drugs with improved activity, pharmacokinetic profile, and safety.

Keywords: heterocycles; five-membered heterocycles; antibiotics; antibacterials; nitrogen heterocycles; oxygen heterocycles; sulfur heterocycles; biological activity; drug design; drug discovery

Citation: Rusu, A.; Moga, I.-M.; Uncu, L.; Hancu, G. The Role of Five-Membered Heterocycles in the Molecular Structure of Antibacterial Drugs Used in Therapy. *Pharmaceutics* **2023**, *15*, 2554. https://doi.org/10.3390/pharmaceutics15112554

Academic Editor: Tihomir Tomašič

Received: 17 September 2023
Revised: 24 October 2023
Accepted: 26 October 2023
Published: 29 October 2023

1. Introduction

Heterocyclic compounds play a significant role in sustaining life, as they are abundant in nature. The genetic material comprises crucial heterocycles such as purine and pyrimidine bases. Additionally, several heterocycles are structural components of common therapeutic drugs, either obtained by chemical synthesis or naturally occurring [1,2]. The significance of heterocycles in drug design stems from their ability to modify the drug candidate's physicochemical characteristics, biological impacts, pharmacokinetics, and toxicological profile [2]. Numerous recent studies have targeted therapeutic agents the structures of which are based on different heterocycles [3–6]. In the last decade, scientists have successfully synthesized numerous heterocyclic compounds to develop new antibacterials capable of treating infections caused by drug-resistant bacterial strains. Certain five-membered heterocycles containing two or three heteroatoms (e.g. thiazole, benzothiazole, thiazolidinone, triazole, and others) are crucial structural components in various antibacterials [7].

The physicochemical properties imprinted by a five-membered heterocycle are associated with the biological activity of the antibacterial drug (spectrum of activity and potency) and its pharmacokinetic, pharmacologic, and toxicological profiles. Highlighting the relationships between certain five-membered heterocycles in the molecular structure of the antibacterial drugs and their biological properties can be the basis for many other rational design studies for discovering new antibiotics.

1.1. Antibacterials Shortage

In the ongoing fight against bacterial infections, there is an urgent need for new antibacterials. Antibiotic resistance appears inevitable, and pharmaceutical companies consistently demonstrate little interest in financing the research of new antibacterials [8]. New compounds from plants, animals, or bacteria are tested for their antimicrobial properties. Discovering and developing new antibacterials can be scientifically challenging [9].

The lack of antibiotics results from production problems, supply chain disruptions, increased demand, regulatory difficulties, and pharmaceutical companies discontinuing specific drugs. Major pharmaceutical corporations stopped developing antibacterials despite the ongoing need for novel antimicrobial medications. Developing antibacterials can be costly, and the return on investment may not be as attractive as other therapeutic areas. Due to the high costs of clinical trials, new regulatory uncertainty over approval requirements, and a low rate of return, companies have left aside the antibacterial research and development field. The lack of antibiotics might affect patient care. Potential outcomes include more extended hospital stays, a higher risk of complications, poor or delayed treatment for infections, and the development of antibiotic resistance. The antibiotic regulatory pathway is rigorous, which can increase the time and cost of bringing new drugs to market, discouraging pharmaceutical companies from pursuing antibiotic research. The Food and Drug Administration's (FDA) dropping of approval of antibacterials is a reflection of pharmaceutical companies' unwillingness to invest in antibacterial drug development [10,11].

Shortages can affect a wide range of antibiotics, both generic and branded. Addressing the issue of antibiotic resistance requires a multi-pronged approach involving governments, public health organizations, pharmaceutical companies, and the scientific community. Older antibiotics are scarce and have been taken off the market for known or unknown reasons. Many countries do not have access to many older, possibly helpful, and occasionally "forgotten" antibiotics since they were either never released or discontinued. Older antibiotics that have disappeared from use can be revived to minimize this burden [12,13]. The management of antibiotic shortages involves a team of healthcare experts. To promote proper antibiotic use, healthcare professionals must maintain effective patient communication, offer alternative treatments when necessary, and follow antimicrobial stewardship guidelines [14].

1.2. Bacterial Resistance Phenomenon

The rise of antibiotic resistance is a grave and urgent global health concern. The consequences of antibiotic-resistant infections are significant, leading to increased mortality, prolonged illness, higher healthcare costs, and limited treatment options. The gravest issue is the increased bacteria resistance to standard antibiotics, even to last-choice medications such as vancomycin. When these antibiotics become ineffective, limited treatment options remain, and infections can become virtually untreatable. The alarming increase in a problem that affects public health worldwide and necessitates international cooperation is confirmed by the speed with which resistance genes can spread worldwide. The World Health Organization (WHO) identified this phenomenon as a significant health issue in response to the worldwide observation of an alarming increase in the population of multi-drug-resistant strains [15,16]. Unfortunately, antibiotic resistance-related studies are becoming more prevalent every year. Antibiotic-resistant infections significantly burden healthcare systems, with more extended hospital stays, increased use of healthcare resources, and higher costs [17].

Antibiotic resistance has many negative effects: (a) failure to respond to treatment increases the length of illness and the number of deaths; (b) longer hospitalization and illnesses raise the possibility of spreading an infection to more persons in the community; (c) when a first-line antibiotic is no longer effective, the need to switch to second- or third-line antibiotics, which are always more expensive and occasionally more toxic; (d) first-line antibiotic resistance is more likely to develop in low-income countries due to the scarcity of numerous second- and third-line antibiotics; (e) the number of medications available in low-income countries to treat bacterial infections is declining, and the essential drug list does not include all the necessary antibiotics; (f) the advancements of modern medicine are under jeopardy due to antibiotic resistance; chemotherapy, organ transplants, and some procedures become more dangerous without the efficient antibiotics [8].

Fewer new antibiotics are being developed, and the pipeline for innovative antibacterial drugs remains relatively small.

1.3. FDA-Approved Antibiotics Whose Structure Includes Five-Members Heterocycles

Over time, many antibiotics that have been approved for use in therapy contain in their structure a heterocycle with five atoms or even more. In Table 1, we have chronologically summarized the antibiotics approved by the FDA in the last forty years and the essential heterocycles with five atoms in their molecular structure.

Table 1. FDA-approved antibiotics and their essential heterocycles during 1980–2023 [18,19].

FDA Approval Year	Antibiotic Compound	Antibiotic Class (Generation)	Five-Member Heterocycle in the Structure
1980	Cefotaxime	Beta-lactam cephalosporin (2nd generation)	1,3-Thiazole
1981	Cefoperazone	Beta-lactam cephalosporin (3rd generation)	Tetrazole
1981	Cefotiam	Beta-lactam cephalosporin (2nd generation)	1,3-Thiazole, Tetrazole
1982	Ceftriaxone	Beta-lactam cephalosporin (3rd generation)	1,3-Thiazole
1982	Latamoxef/Moxalactam	Beta-lactam, oxacephem cephalosporin (1st generation)	Tetrazole
1983	Cefonicid	Beta-lactam cephalosporin (2nd generation)	Tetrazole
1983	Cefuroxime	Beta-lactam cephalosporin (2nd generation)	Furan
1984	Ceftazidime	Beta-lactam cephalosporin (2nd generation	1,3-Thiazole
1986	Aztreonam	Beta-lactam monobactam	1,3-Thiazole
1987	Cefotetan	Beta-lactam cephalosporin (3rd generation)	Tetrazole
1992	Cefpodoxime proxetil	Beta-lactam cephalosporin (3rd generation)	1,3-Thiazole
1991	Cefuroxime axetil	Beta-lactam cephalosporin (3rd generation)	Furan
1992	Ceftibuten	Beta-lactam cephalosporin (3rd generation)	1,3-Thiazole
1992	Tazobactam	Beta-lactamase inhibitor	1,2,3-Triazole
1993	Cefixime	Beta-lactam cephalosporin (3rd generation)	1,3-Thiazole
1996	Cefepime	Beta-lactam cephalosporin (4th generation)	Pyrrolidine, 1,3-Thiazole
1996	Meropenem	Beta-lactam carbapenem	Pyrrolidine
1997	Cefdinir	Beta-lactam cephalosporin (4th generation)	1,3-Thiazole
2000	Linezolid	Oxazolidinone	1,3-Oxazolidine
2001	Ertapenem	Beta-lactam carbapenem	Pyrrolidine
2001	Telithromycin	Ketolide macrolide	Imidazole
2003	Gemifloxacin	Fluoroquinolone	Pyrrolidine
2009	Ceftobiprole	Beta-lactam cephalosporin (5th generation)	Pyrrolidine
2014	Doripenem	Beta-lactam carbapenem	Pyrrolidine
2014	Finafloxacin	Fluoroquinolone	Pyrrole (in a bicycle)
2014	Tedizolid	Oxazolidinone	1,3-Oxazolidin-2-one, Tetrazole
2018	Eravacycline	Tetracycline	Pyrrolidine
2018	Gemifloxacin	Fluoroquinolone	Pyrrolidine
2019	Imipenem + Cilastatin + Relebactam	Relebactam: beta-lactamase inhibitor	2-Imidazolidinone (in an azabicycle)
2019	Cefidorocol	Beta-lactam cephalosporin (5th generation)	Pyrrolidine, thiazole
2021	Ceftidoren pivoxil	Beta-lactam cephalosporin (5th generation)	Thiazole (2 groups)
2023	Sulbactam + durlobactam	Sulbactam: beta-lactam antibacterial and beta-lactamase inhibitor Durlobactam: beta-lactamase inhibitor	Sulbactam: 1,3-Thiazolidine 1,1-dioxide Durlobactam: 2-Imidazolidinone (in an azabicycle)

1.4. Aim of the Work

The five-membered heterocycles are among the most significant structural components of pharmaceuticals. They are used to optimize potency and selectivity through bioisosterism, pharmacokinetic, and toxicological features by providing numerous options to modify the antibacterials' lipophilicity and solubility. Thus, in this review, we identified the majority of the antibacterial drugs used in therapy, which contain five-membered heterocycles, to better understand the properties that these heterocycles confer to an antibacterial agent. The antibiotics that include a particular five-membered heterocycle belong to structurally different classes with different mechanisms of action. The review addresses the pressing global health challenge of bacterial infections and antibiotic resistance by strategically incorporating five-membered heterocyclic rings into drug molecules. Consequently, our work aims to provide a well-structured collection of helpful information regarding antibacterials containing five-membered heterocycles for the rational design of new antibacterials.

2. Materials and Methods

References were gathered from the Clarivate Analytics, ScienceDirect, PubMed, and Google Books databases, using as the primary keywords the terms "heterocycles", "five-membered heterocycles", "nitrogen heterocycles", "oxygen heterocycles", and "sulfur heterocycles", combined with "antibiotics" or "antibacterials". These keywords were also combined with the name of representative heterocycles, such as "pyrrolidine", "pyrrole", "furan", and so on. Furthermore, other keywords such as "biological activity", "drug design", "drug discovery", and "drug candidates" were combined with the specific name of the five-membered heterocycle. The references were chosen if they contained appropriate details concerning the primary topic of our review. The chemical structures were drawn with Biovia Draw 2022 (https://discover.3ds.com/biovia-draw-academic, accessed on 9 August 2023) [20]. IUPAC names of the compounds were used from the PubChem database (https://pubchem.ncbi.nlm.nih.gov/, accessed on 12 July 2023) [21].

3. Five-Membered Heterocycles Used in the Design of Antibacterial Drugs

Heterocyclic compounds contain at least two distinct atoms (either as ring atoms or as members of the ring) in the ring. The actual ring is referred to as a heterocycle. The total number of ring atoms and the type is crucial since it determines the ring size. Three-membered rings are the minor shape conceivable. The most significant rings in the antibiotic design are heterocycles, with five and six members [22].

The five-membered heterocycles used in antibacterial drug design contain one to four heteroatoms as follows:

- One heteroatom (nitrogen, oxygen, or sulfur);
- Two heteroatoms (oxygen and nitrogen; sulfur and nitrogen atoms);
- Three heteroatoms (three nitrogen atoms, e.g., triazoles, and one sulfur and two nitrogen atoms, e.g., thiadiazoles);
- Four heteroatoms (tetrazoles).

The most common heterocycles with five atoms in the molecular structure of approved antibiotics are presented in Table 2 and are individually addressed in the following sections.

Table 2. The most common heterocycles with five atoms found in the molecular structure of antibacterial agents (HBA—Hydrogen Bond Acceptor Count, HBD—Hydrogen Bond Donor Count, MW—Molecular Weight) [21].

Five-Membered Heterocycles	Heteroatom (s)	Chemical Structure	MW (g/mol)	HBA	HBD
Pyrrolidine	N	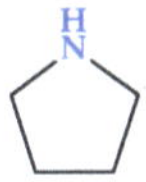	71.12	1	1
Imidazole	N(2)	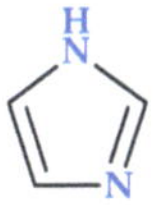	68.08	1	1
1,2,3-Triazole	N(3)	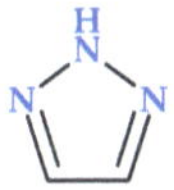	69.07	2	1
Tetrazole	N(4)	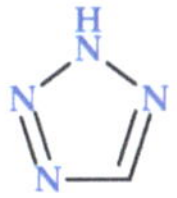	70.05	3	1
Furan	O(1)	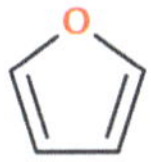	68.07	1	0
1,3-Oxazolidine	N(1),O(1)	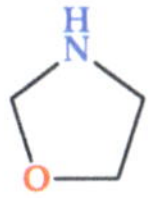	73.09	2	1
1,3-Oxazole	N(1),O(1)	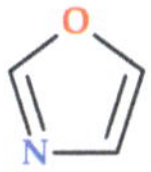	69.06	2	0
1,2-Oxazole (Isoxazole)	N(1),O(1)	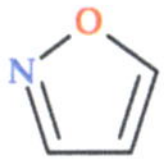	69.06	2	0
Thiophene	S(1)	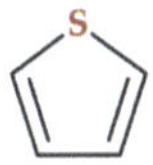	84.14	1	0
1,3-Thiazolidine	N(1),S(1)	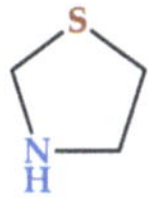	89.6	2	1
1,3-Thiazole	N(1),S(1)	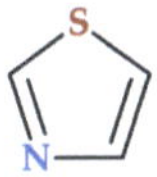	89.16	2	1
1,2,4-Thiadiazole	N(2),S(1)	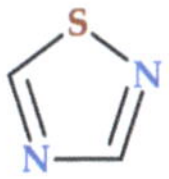	86.12	3	0
1,3,4-Thiadiazole	N(2),S(1)	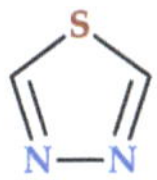	86.12	3	0

4. Five-Membered Heterocycles Containing Nitrogen Atoms

Five-membered heterocycles are believed to originate from the cyclopentadienyl compound. They possess properties such as conjugated dienes or acyclic amines, but with a nitrogen atom replacing the "-CH=" group. The characteristics of these compounds are closely linked to the non-participatory electron pair of the heteroatom. They have a planar pentagonal structure, with the six π electrons distributed over the five sp2 hybridized atoms. Each carbon atom contributes one electron, and the heteroatom donates two electrons to the aromatic sextet, which confers the aromaticity of the heterocyclic system. The two non-participating electrons of the nitrogen will contribute to the aromatic sextet and are delocalized throughout the heterocycle [1]. These heterocycles are less susceptible to being deprotonated at the nitrogen or carbon atom through the action of nucleophiles. Weak nucleophiles will react with the cation produced by electrophiles, leading to addition or ring-opening reactions. The most reactive compound in this class in terms of compound reactivity is pyrrole. The resonance structures' unevenly distributed energy causes greater reactivity [1].

According to an analysis conducted by Vitaku E. et al. (2014) on FDA-approved small compounds, N-heterocycles form the majority of the structural skeletons of pharmaceutical drugs on the market, accounting for about 84% of all molecules, and 59% of them contain at least one nitrogen heterocycle [23].

4.1. Pyrrolidine

Pyrrolidine is the first saturated family member of five-membered heterocycles with one nitrogen atom (Table 2). The heterocycle, commonly known as tetrahydropyrrole, is categorized as an aza cycloalkane (aza cyclopentane), a type of cyclic amine. The unsubstituted ones can participate in alkylation processes, while the substituted ones can be acylated or nitrosated. Pyrrolidine and N-substituted pyrrolidines go through reactions typical of secondary or tertiary alkylamines. Because they are cyclic amines, they can take part in these processes [22].

The compound is non-polar, flexible, and planar in structure. Its basicity is higher (pKa of 11.3) than that of the acyclic compound diethylamine (pKa of 10.49) [22,24]. Because the two alkyls "substituents" in the heterocycles, i.e., the ring carbons, are constrained back and away from the nitrogen lone pair, approach by an electrophile is made more accessible than in the case of diethylamine, where rotations of the C-N and C-C bonds interfere, pyrrolidine is a better nucleophile than diethylamine [25]. Both in natural and synthetic compounds, we can identify different modifications of pyrrolidines. The structure of several natural alkaloids, such as amathaspiramide A, B, and C, atropine, bgugaine and irniine, cocaine, codonopsinine and codonopsine, ficushispimine A and B, hygrine, nicotine, radicamine A and B, scalusamide A, and many more, have a pyrrolidine ring in their structure [24,26,27].

Five-membered heterocycles with nitrogen are employed more frequently as pharmacophores for various medicinal uses, free-standing rings, and spiro and polycyclic systems. Because of their capacity to interact with multiple essential enzymes, they have found particular use in pharmacotherapy for antibacterial or antiviral, antifungal, anticancer, and antidiabetic drugs [28]. As a pharmacophore group, pyrrolidine is found in the molecular structure of different classes of medicines, among them being an extensive series of antibiotics (Table 3) [29].

Pyrrolidine, as a structural element, is found in the molecule of some cephalosporins mentioned in Table 3, and its addition to their structure leads to numerous benefits.

Table 3. Groups of antibiotics with a pyrrolidine moiety in the chemical structures (Ref. = References).

No.	Therapeutic Class	Subclass	Reprezentatives	Ref.
1	Beta-lactam antibiotics	Carbapenemes	Doripenem	[30]
			Ertapenem	[30]
			Meropenem	[30]
		Cephalosporins	Cefepime	[31]
			Cefiderocol	[32]
			Ceftobiprole	[33]
2	Fluoroquinolones	-	Clinafloxacin	[34]
			Finafloxacin	[34]
			Gemifloxacin	[34]
			Lascufloxacin	[34]
			Premafloxacin	[35]
			Sitafloxacin	[34]
			Trovafloxacin	[34]
3	Lincosamides	-	Lincomycin	[31]
			Clindamycin	[31]
4	Streptogramins	-	Quinupristin/Dalfopristin	[36]
5	Tetracyclines	-	Rolitetracycline	[29]
		Glycylcyclines	Eravacycline	[37]

4.1.1. Beta-Lactam Antibiotics

Carbapenems

Thienamycin, ((5*R*,6*S*)-3-(2-aminoethylsulfanyl)-6-[(1*R*)-1-hydroxyethyl]-7-oxo-1-azabicyclo [3.2.0]hept-2-ene-2-carboxylic acid), was the first carbapenem isolated from *Streptomyces cattleya*, which became the model substance for all carbapenems. Thienamycin's chemical instability led to the development of similar compounds with improved stability. The first synthesized, more stable N-formimidoyl derivative was imipenem; several other optimized carbapenems have been developed lately [30,38]. Among the carbapenems that contain a pyrrolidine heterocycle in the molecular structure are doripenem, ertapenem, and meropenem (Figure 1). The pyrrolidine ring expanded the spectrum of activity and improved the potency and stability of these newly optimized compounds [30,39].

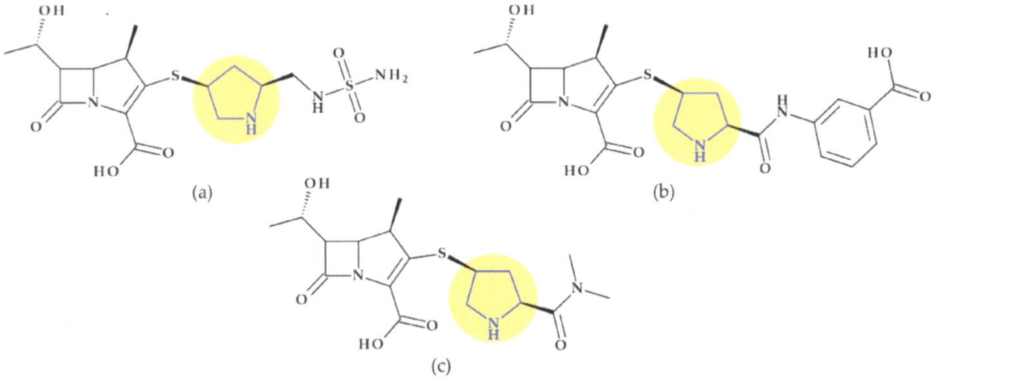

Figure 1. Chemical structure of carbapenems with the highlighted pyrrolidine nucleus: (**a**) doripenem, (**b**) ertapenem, and (**c**) meropenem.

Some details related to the spectrum of antibacterial activity of the three compounds are presented below. Compared to currently available penicillins, cephalosporins, and beta-lactam/beta-lactamase inhibitor combinations, carbapenems exhibit an overall larger antibacterial spectrum in vitro. Doripenem is effective against Gram-positive bacteria. Thus, doripenem, ertapenem, and meropenem are slightly more effective against Gram-negative bacteria. When used against *Pseudomonas aeruginosa* and *Acinetobacter baumannii*, doripenem is more efficient than meropenem and is least susceptible to hydrolysis by carbapenemases. Meropenem is more efficient than ertapenem against *Pseudomonas aeruginosa*. Also, meropenem is efficient against multidrug-resistant *Mycobacterium tuberculosis* if combined with clavulanic acid (a beta-lactamase inhibitor) [30]. Targeting severe hospital-acquired infections with uncertain etiologies is a common usage of meropenem. However, carbapenems are commonly used as the last choice of antibiotics [39].

Cephalosporins

Cefepime. The first approved cephalosporin that has a pyrrolidine fragment in its structure is cefepime, ((6*R*,7*R*,*Z*)-7-(2-(2-aminothiazol-4-yl)-2-(methoxyimino)acetamido)- 3-((1-methylpyrrolidinium-1-yl)methyl)-8-oxo-5-thia-1-aza-bicyclo [4.2.0]oct-2-ene-2-carboxylate) (Figure 2a), a fourth-generation cephalosporin for parenteral use [31,40]. The activity spectrum of cefepime includes Gram-positive and Gram-negative bacteria. Cefepime is a parenteral cephalosporin used to treat infections with susceptible pathogens such as infections of the skin and soft tissues, complex intra-abdominal infections (associated with metronidazole), complicated and uncomplicated urinary tract infections (UTIs), pneumonia, and empirically neutropenic fever. The molecule has an amphoteric character and passes through the porins found in the cell walls of Gram-negative bacteria due to the methyl-pyrrolidine residue, where the nitrogen atom is quaternary. At the same time, their ability to penetrate cell wall porins can be explained based on the low lipophilicity conferred by the pyrrolidine moiety (log P of 0.46) [31,40,41].

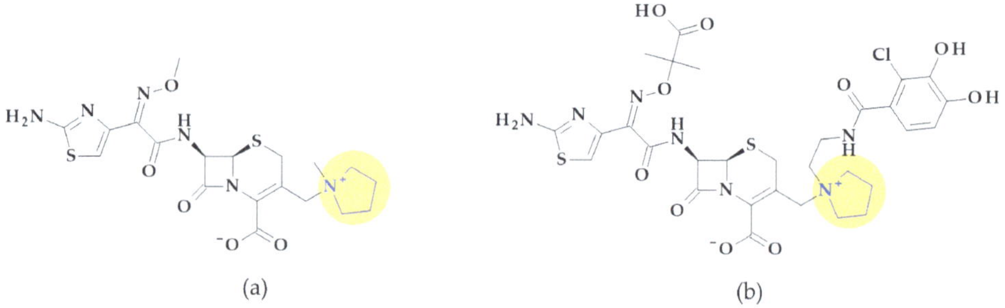

Figure 2. Chemical structure of cephalosporins with the highlighted pyrrolidine nucleus: (**a**) cefepime and (**b**) cefiderocol [31,42].

Cefiderocol. Another cephalosporin that contains a pyrrolidine ring is cefiderocol, ((6*R*,7*R*)-7-[[(2Z)-2-(2-amino-1,3-thiazol-4-yl)-2-(2-carboxypropan-2-yloxyimino)acetyl]amino]-3-[[1-[2-[(2-chloro-3,4-dihydroxybenzoyl)amino]ethyl]pyrrolidin-1-ium-1-yl]methyl]-8-oxo-5-thia-1-azabicyclo [4.2.0]oct-2-ene-2-carboxylate) (Figure 2b). This fifth-generation cephalosporin is particularly effective against Gram-negative bacteria, including carbapenem-resistant bacteria. Cefiderocol is a mixture of catechol-type siderophores and cephalosporins from a structural standpoint. This compound is carried over the bacterial cell's outer membrane and into the periplasm using specific iron transporter channels. Furthermore, cefiderocol has shown proven structural stability against hydrolysis by serine- and metallo-lactamases, including clinically significant carbapenemases [42,43]. The pyrrolidine nucleus confers increased antibacterial activity, increased stability of the nucleus against β-lactamases and an amphoteric character due to the quaternary nitrogen atom that increases the water solubility of the molecule [44].

With a minimum inhibitory concentration (MIC) of less than 4 mg/L for the majority of Enterobacteriaceae, *Pseudomonas aeruginosa*, and *Acinetobacter baumannii* isolates, cefiderocol exhibits high in vitro potency against pathogenic carbapenem-resistant Gram-negative bacteria [45] as a result of the high binding affinities for penicillin-binding proteins (PBP), especially PBP3 from *Escherichia coli, Klebsiella pneumoniae, Pseudomonas aeruginosa*, and *Acinetobacter baumannii* [46]. Cefiderocol's practical application in the treatment of Gram-negative infections as part of the early access program (PERSEUS Study) has just undergone a retrospective analysis [47].

Ceftobiprole. Pyrrolidine is also found in the molecular structure of ceftobiprole, ((6*R*,7*R*)-7-[[(2*Z*)-2-(5-amino-1,2,4-thiadiazol-3-ylidene)-2-nitroso-1-oxoethyl]amino]-8-oxo-3-[(E)-[2-oxo-1-[(3R)-3-pyrrolidinyl]-3-pyrrolidinylidene]methyl]-5-thia-1-azabicyclo [4.2.0] oct-2-ene-2-carboxylic acid), another fifth-generation cephalosporin (Figure 3). Because of its low solubility in water, ceftobiprole is administered as its water-soluble prodrug, ceftobiprole medocaril, which rapidly transforms into the active drug, diacetyl, and carbon dioxide; medocaril is the name of the fragment 5-methyl-2-oxo-1,3-dioxol-4-yl)methoxycarbonyl substituted at the nitrogen atom of the pyrrolidine heterocycle [48]. Due to its ability to inhibit abnormal PBP2a in methicillin-resistant *Staphylococcus aureus* (MRSA) and PBP2b and PBP2x in beta-lactam-resistant pneumococci, ceftobiprole is a unique parenteral extended-spectrum cephalosporin that is effective against both Gram-negative and Gram-positive bacteria that are resistant to antibiotics. Additionally, ceftobiprole is effective against *Pseudomonas aeruginosa* susceptible strains, AmpC overproducers, and Enterobacteriaceae that are not producing extended-spectrum beta-lactamases or carbapenemases [48–50].

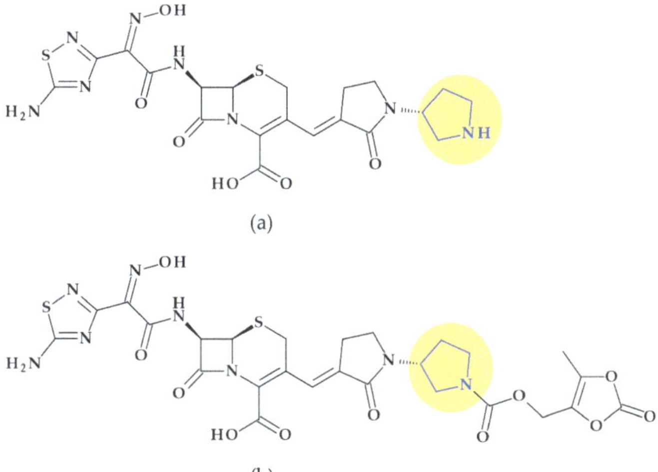

(a)

(b)

Figure 3. Chemical structure of (**a**) ceftobiprole and (**b**) ceftobiprole medocaril (prodrug), with the highlighted pyrrolidine nucleus [48].

The ceftobiprole molecule resembles the pentaglycine fragment due to the planarity of the pyrrolidine residue [50]. The MRSA's high resistance to beta-lactam antibiotics is known to be facilitated by the expression of PBP2a, a penicillin-binding protein (PBP) [51]. Ceftobiprole interacts with the PBP2a and PBP2x to attach to their active sites, forming an antibiotic-acyl PBP2a complex. Between the residues of tyrosine Tyr446, methionine Met641, and threonine Thr600, respectively, is the pyrrolidine residue, which participates in a hydrogen bond with the sulfur atom of Met641. Pyrrolidine forms a π-π interaction with the tyrosine residue Tyr446 and hydrophobic interactions with the Thr600 threonine residue. The molecule's planarity and hydrophobicity are crucial to access the active site of PBP2a enzymes. These types of interactions have been highlighted by molecular docking studies [50].

4.1.2. Fluoroquinolones

Fluoroquinolones constitute a different class of antibacterial significant for antibacterial therapy. The pyrrolidine moiety in position C7 is an essential structural component for some representatives such as clinafloxacin, finafloxacin, gemifloxacin, lascufloxacin, moxifloxacin, sitafloxacin, and zabofloxacin (Figure 4).

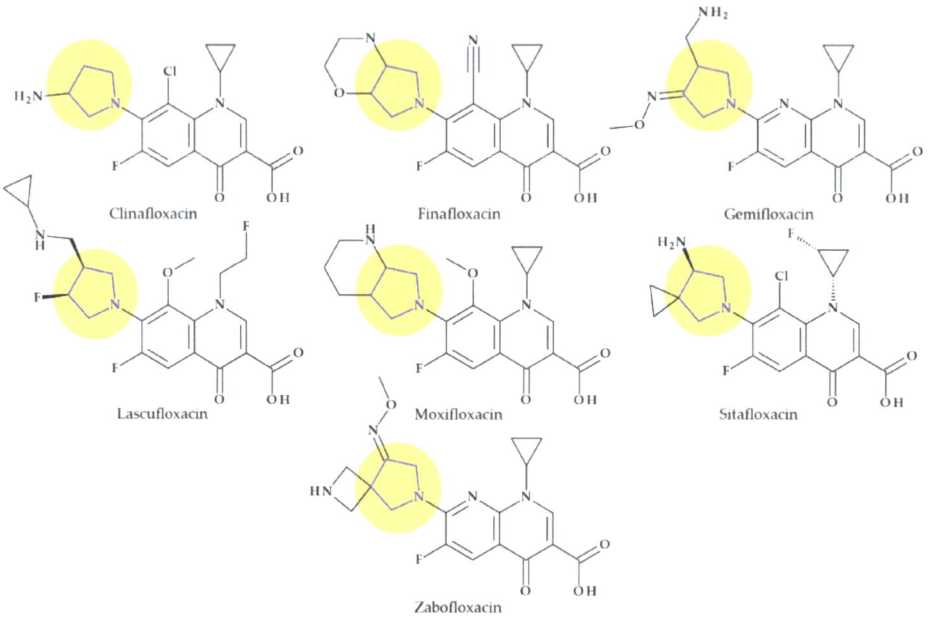

Figure 4. Chemical structures of fluoroquinolones with the highlighted pyrrolidine nucleus.

Among the benefits of pyrrolidine moiety is an increased spectrum of activity against Gram-positive bacteria, including MRSA, improved pharmacokinetic profile (increased half-life) and bioavailability [34,52,53]. However, the pyrrolidine substituent in the C7 position of fluoroquinolones has been associated by several authors with some of the side effects comprised in Table 4 [54].

Table 4. Associated side-effects of pyrrolidine moiety in comparison with other possible substituents in the C7 position of fluoroquinolones [54].

Associated Side-Effects	Comparison with Other Substituents in the C7 Position
Genotoxicity	Pyrrolidine > Piperazine > Alkyl Pyrrolidine (unsubstituted) > Piperazine (unsubstituted) > Pyrrolidine (substituted) > Piperazine (substituted)
Neuropsychiatric toxicity, seizures (GABA receptor binding)	Alkyl > Piperazine (unsubstituted) > Pyrrolidine (unsubstituted) > Piperazine (substituted) or Pyrrolidine (substituted)
Some NSAIDs interactions	Piperazine (unsubstituted) > Pyrrolidine (unsubstituted) > Piperazine (substituted) or Pyrrolidine (substituted)
Theophylline interactions	Pyrrolidine (unsubstituted) > Piperazine (unsubstituted) > Piperazine (substituted) or Pyrrolidine (substituted)

The antibacterial fluoroquinolones that contain a pyrrolidine nucleus in their chemical structure are briefly presented below.

Clinafloxacin. Clinafloxacin (7-(3-aminopyrrolidin-1-yl)-8-chloro-1-cyclopropyl-6-fluoro-4-oxoquinoline-3-carboxy-lic acid) is a fourth-generation fluoroquinolone antibacterial agent. In the C7 position, clinafloxacin presents a 3-amino pyrrolidine substituent (Figure 4) [55]. Clinafloxacin proved efficient against most Gram-positive, Gram-negative, and anaerobic bacteria. Numerous studies have shown that clinafloxacin has a wide range of antibacterial activity, good tissue penetration and bioavailability, a prolonged serum half-life, enhanced safety and tolerability, and acceptable pharmacokinetics. However, clinafloxacin has several drawbacks, including poor solubility in its original form and insufficient stability in aqueous solution. Also, clinafloxacin was associated with severe side effects such as phototoxicity and the prevalence of hypoglycemia and, consequently, it was withdrawn from the market in 1999 [55–57].

Finafloxacin. Finafloxacin, 7-[(4a*S*,7a*S*)-3,4,4a,5,7,7a-hexahydro-2*H*-pyrrolo [3,4-b][1,4] oxazin-6-yl]-8-cyano-1-cyclopropyl-6-fluoro-4-oxoquinoline-3-carboxylic acid, has a chiral cyano-substituent, pyrrole-oxazine component, with a zwitterionic chemical structure (Figure 4) [58,59]. Under acidic environments, finafloxacin exhibits higher antibacterial activity. This property differentiates finafloxacin from other fluoroquinolones and is appropriate for specific infection sites, including the skin, soft tissues, vagina, and urinary tract. The highest level of bactericidal activity was found at pH 5–6. The approved indication as otic suspension of finafloxacin is acute otitis externa produced by *Pseudomonas aeruginosa* and *Staphylococcus aureus* [59].

Gemifloxacin. Gemifloxacin, 7-[(4Z)-3-(aminomethyl)-4-methoxyiminopyrrolidin-1-yl]-1-cyclopropyl-6-fluoro-4-oxo-1,8-naphthyridine-3-carboxylic acid, is a fourth-generation fluoroquinolone antibiotic [60], a 1,4-dihydro-1,8-naphthyridine derivative. The spectrum of activity is improved by heterocyclic substitution at C7, especially against Gram-negative bacteria. At the C7 position, gemifloxacin presents an unusual substituent: a methoxyiminopyrrolidine substituted with an aminomethyl fragment (at the pyrrolidine C3 position) (Figure 4) [31,61]. This fluoroquinolone was used orally to treat mild to moderate respiratory tract infections from susceptible microorganisms. However, gemifloxacin has been connected to a few cases of acute liver damage [60]. Though gemifloxacin had improved antibacterial action compared to moxifloxacin, it was withdrawn in 2009 by the producer due to adverse effects, primarily rash [61–63].

Lascufloxacin. The oral version of this lascufloxacin, 7-[(3*S*,4*S*)-3-[(cyclopropylamino) methyl]-4-fluoropyrrolidin-1-yl]-6-fluoro-1-(2-fluoroethyl)-8-methoxy-4-oxoquinoline-3-carboxylic acid, was licensed in Japan in 2019 to treat respiratory diseases, including community-acquired bacterial pneumonia (CABP) and ear, nose, and throat infections. An uncommon structural fragment can be found in the lascufloxacin chemical structure at position C7. It is about a primary pyrrolidine heterocycle 3-substituted with a (cyclopropyl amino)methyl moiety and 4-substituted with a fluorine atom (Figure 4). The interaction with DNA gyrase or topoisomerase IV requires this position. Previously, the representative of clinafloxacin also demonstrated that an amino pyrrolidine fragment enhances activity against Gram-positive pathogens. Lascufloxacin showed a strong affinity for phosphatidylserine, the primary surfactant in alveolar epithelial fluid and a component of human cell membranes. Compared to levofloxacin, garenoxacin, and moxifloxacin, lascufloxacin has better tissue penetration (head and neck infections). Also, lascufloxacin is shown to be quite effective when used against Gram-positive bacteria, including resistant strains [34,64].

Moxifloxacin. Moxifloxacin is a fourth-generation fluoroquinolone antibiotic [65]. Structurally, moxifloxacin, 7-[(4a*S*,7a*S*)-1,2,3,4,4a,5,7,7a-octahydropyrrolo [3,4-b]pyridin-6-yl]-1-cyclopropyl-6-fluoro-8-methoxy-4-oxoquinoline-3-carboxylic acid, is an 8-methoxy fluoroquinolone with a bulky moiety at the C7 position (Figure 4) [61,65]. This fragment is a fused bicycle of pyrrolidine and piperidine. Because of this C7-azabicyclo side chain, it is more challenging to efflux the moxifloxacin out of the bacterial cell [66], [67]. Moxifloxacin is characterized by a broad-spectrum activity against Gram-positive and Gram-negative bacteria and anaerobes. Compared to other fluoroquinolones from older generations, moxifloxacin has increased efficacy against Gram-positive organisms such as pneumococci and is very potent against anaerobes [65].

Sitafloxacin. Sitafloxacin, (7-[(7*S*)-7-amino-5-azaspiro [2.4]heptan-5-yl]-8-chloro-6-fluoro-1-[(1R,2S)-2-fluorocyclopropyl]-4-oxoquinoline-3-carboxylic acid, is a fourth-generation derivative, a chloro-fluoroquinolone that has received approval in Japan (2008) and Thailand (2012). It includes the [(*7S*)-7-amino-5-azaspiro [2.4]heptanyl fragment, a pyrrolidinyl fragment enclosed in a spiro substituent at the C7 position (Figure 4) [34]. Sitafloxacin could be considered a clinafloxacin analog, which underwent optimization at N1 and C7 positions. In vitro, sitafloxacin proved efficacy against Gram-positive, Gram-negative, anaerobic bacteria and atypical pathogens. Furthermore, it is effective against strains that are resistant to other fluoroquinolones and multi-drug-resistant bacteria [68–70].

Zabofloxacin. A brand-new broad-spectrum fluoroquinolone that can be orally administered is zabofloxacin, 1-cyclopropyl-6-fluoro-7-[(8*Z*)-8-methoxyimino-2,6-diazaspiro [3.4]octan-6-yl]-4-oxo-1,8-naphthyridine-3-carboxylic acid (Figure 4) [59]. This novel fluoroquinolone has similarities to the fourth-generation antibiotic gemifloxacin. Zabofloxacin contains an unusual heterocycle at the C7 position, a spiro substituent (2,6-diazaspiro [3.4]octan) substituted with an imino methoxy group; a pyrrolidinyl fragment is present in the structure of the spiro substituent of zabofloxacin [34]. Zabofloxacin has two different forms in development: hydrochloride and aspartate. The principal bacterial strains that zabofloxacin acts against include Gram-negative and Gram-positive respiratory pathogens (a broad spectrum against respiratory pathogens), particularly drug-resistant *Neisseria gonorrhoeae* and *Streptococcus pneumoniae*. According to its approved indications, zabofloxacin can be orally taken to treat acute bacterial chronic obstructive pulmonary disease exacerbations [34,59].

4.1.3. Lincosamides (Lincomycin and Clindamycin)

Pyrrolidine is an essential pharmacophore group in the molecular structure of antibacterial lincosamides, lincomycin and clindamycin (Figure 5) [29]. Structurally, lincosamides consist of a thio-methylated carbohydrate unit joined by an amide bond to an N-methyl-pyrrolidine-carboxylic acid (proline) residue [31,71]. A fundamental function of pyrrolidine nitrogen is the formation of water-soluble salts with an apparent pKa of 7.6. Lincomycin, ((2*S*,4*R*)-N-[(1*R*,2*R*)-2-hydroxy-1-[(2*R*,3*R*,4*S*,5*R*,6*R*)-3,4,5-trihydroxy-6-(methylsulfanyl)oxan-2-yl]propyl]-1-methyl-4-propylpyrrolidine-2-carboxamide), is transformed into methyl α-thiolincosamide (the sugar moiety) and *trans*-L-4-n-propylhygric acid (the pyrrolidine moiety) when it is subjected to hydrazinolysis [29].

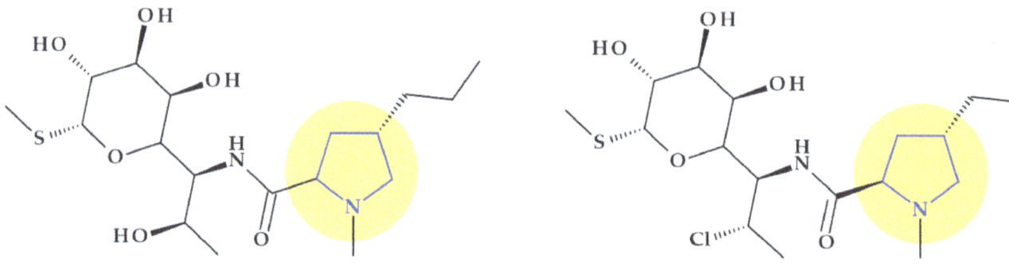

(a) (b)

Figure 5. Chemical structure of lincosamides with the highlighted pyrrolidine nucleus: (**a**) lincomycin and (**b**) clindamycin.

However, reports of severe diarrhea and the emergence of pseudomembranous colitis in patients receiving lincomycin (or clindamycin) have forced a reevaluation of the therapeutic use of these antibiotics [29]. Today, lincomycin is rarely used, replaced by its semisynthetic analog, clindamycin. Clindamycin, (2*S*,4*R*)-N-[(1*S*,2*S*)-2-chloro-1-[(2*R*,3*R*,4*S*,5*R*,6*R*)-3,4,5-trihydroxy-6-methylsulfanyloxan-2-yl]propyl]-1-methyl-4-propylpyrrolidine-2-carboxamide, is the only medication successfully used in clinical practice, although hundreds of lincomycin derivatives, including those created through total chemical synthesis, were obtained [71]. Also, pyrrolidine appears in the structure of clindamycin, a lincosamide with a broader spectrum of antibacterial activity and favorable pharmacokinetic profile versus lincomycin [29].

The timing and specificity of microbial protein synthesis stages are disrupted by lincosamides, which slow the growth or are fatal to the bacterium. Clindamycin's three-dimensional structure closely resembles *L*-Pro-Met and the *D*-ribosyl ring of adenosine, which are found nearby at the 3′-ends of *L*-Pro-Met-tRNA and deacylated-tRNA for a brief period after the formation of a peptide bond between. This similarity could be explained by *L*-Pro-tRNA and *L*-Met-tRNA, which are involved in the molecular process through which clindamycin suppresses the synthesis of ribosomal proteins. The 3′ ends of *L*-Pro-Met-tRNA and deacylated-tRNA may, therefore, function as structural analogs of clindamycin and other lincosamides at the first stage of pre-translocation in the peptide elongation cycle [71].

4.1.4. Streptogramins

Quinupristin/Dalfopristin. Antibiotics known as streptogramins are naturally produced by several species of the Streptomyces genus. The same bacterial species simultaneously produces the two subgroups of this class of antibiotics, type A and type B, at a ratio of roughly 70:30 [72,73]. Semi-synthetic water-soluble derivatives of pristinamycin IA (type B) and pristinamycin IIA (type A) were developed. Therefore, the formulation quinupristin-dalfopristin, marketed as Synercid® (Pfizer, New York, NY, USA), exhibits activity against Gram-positive bacteria that are typically resistant to other medications, including MRSA and vancomycin-resistant *Enterococcus faecium*. The bacterial 50S ribosome is the primary target, and the formulation works by preventing the synthesis of bacterial proteins. In the bacterial ribosome, quinupristin and dalfopristin inhibit protein synthesis's early and late stages. Both antibiotics contain a pyrrolidine heterocycle in their molecular structure (into a proline amino acid fragment) [36,74].

4.1.5. Tetracyclines

Tetracyclines are recognized antibacterial agents with excellent broad-spectrum activity. They are effective against Gram-positive and Gram-negative bacteria and various spirochetes, *Mycoplasma*, *Rickettsiae*, and *Chlamydiae* [29,37].

Rolitetracycline. N-(pyrrolidinomethyl)tetracycline or rolitetracycline, (4*S*,4a*S*,5a*S*,6*S*,12a*R*)-4-(dimethylamino)-1,6,10,11,12a-pentahydroxy-6-methyl-3,12-dioxo-N-(pyrrolidin-1-yl-methyl)-4,4a,5,5a-tetrahydrotetracene-2-carboxamide (Figure 6a) is a member of the first generation of tetracyclines characterized by high solubility in water. It was designed to be intravenously or intramuscularly injected. Tetracycline was combined with pyrrolidine, formaldehyde, and *tert*-butyl alcohol to obtain this derivative. Although it has been recommended when oral dosage forms are inappropriate, it is currently only used in exceptional cases [29].

Eravacycline. Eravacycline, (4*S*,4a*S*,5a*R*,12a*R*)-4-(dimethylamino)-7-fluoro-1,10,11,12a-tetrahydroxy-3,12-dioxo-9-[(2-pyrrolidin-1-ylacetyl)amino]-4a,5,5a,6-tetrahydro-4*H*-tetracene-2-carboxamide, is a synthetic fluorocycline created using a complete synthesis. Specific alterations were added to the naphtacen nucleus' D ring. The D ring of eravacycline (the analog of tigecycline) has two essential modifications: the insertion of a fluorine atom in the C7 position, an electron-withdrawing substituent, and a pyrrolidin-acetamido group in the C9 position (Figure 6b). Eravacycline is very efficient against Gram-positive and Gram-negative bacteria, including resistant strains to tetracyclines. It was approved in 2018 to treat adults with complex intra-abdominal infections [37,75–77].

Eravacycline demonstrated an 8 to 16 times higher potency against *Klebsiella pneumoniae* and a 4 to 8 times higher potency against *Escherichia coli* when compared to tertiary alkylamine, dimethyl, azetidine, and piperidine counterparts. Eravacycline is also 4 to 64 times more effective than piperidine and azetidine homologs against tested bacterial isolates with known tetracycline-resistant genes *Enterococcus faecalis* [tet(M)], *Streptococcus pneumoniae* [tet(M)], *Escherichia coli* [tet(A)], and *Klebsiella pneumoniae* [tet(A)]), except (*Staphylococcus aureus* [tet(M) and tet(K)]. Compared to unsubstituted pyrrolidine analogs, adding polar substituents, fluorine atoms, or pyrrolidine bicycles did not result in any enhancements and had no adverse effects on the effectiveness against pneumococcal bacteria. The fluoro and pyrrolidine substitutions at C7 and C9 positions, respectively, had a beneficial impact on the antibacterial range and efficacy [78–80].

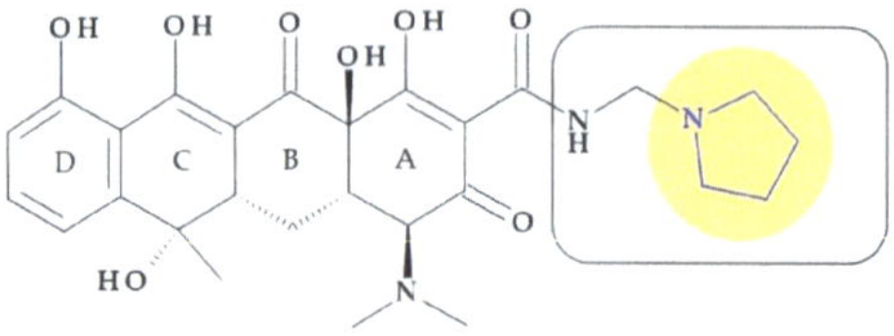

(a)

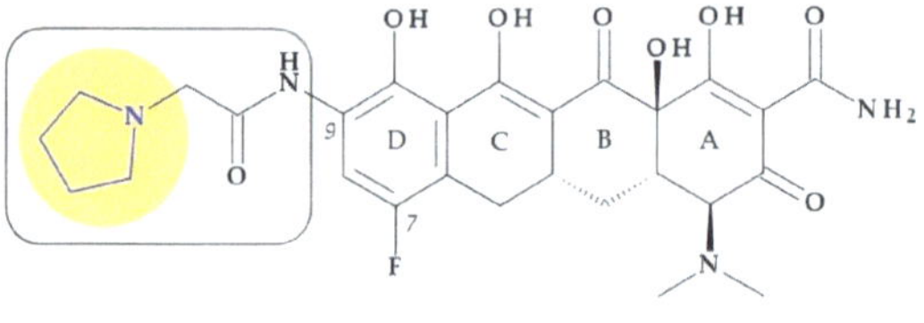

(b)

Figure 6. Chemical structure of tetracyclines with the highlighted pyrrolidine nucleus: (**a**) rolitetracycline and (**b**) eravacycline.

4.1.6. Other Antibacterials

A new antibacterial compound is very close to receiving approval to treat infections. Therefore, we thought it appropriate for it to be mentioned here.

Rifaquizinone (TNP-2092). A rifamycin-quinolone hybrid compound with dual action (TNP-2092, formerly CBR-2092) was identified as a drug candidate currently in clinical development. The hybrid is 3-[(*E*)-[[4-[[1-[(3*R*)-1-(3-carboxy-1-cyclopropyl-7-fluoro-9-methyl-4-oxo-4*H*-quinolizin-8-yl)-3-pyrrolidinyl]cyclopropyl]methylamino]-1-piperidinyl]imino] methyl]rifamycin (Figure 7) [81–83]. Pyrrolidine compounds were used as starting materials for synthesizing the quinolizinone core (the lead ABT-714 compound) [81]. ABT-719 was previously synthesized at Abbott Laboratories [84]. TenNor Therapeutics (Suzhou, China) conducts clinical testing on TNP-2092, which completed Phase 2 for Acute Bacterial Skin and Skin Structure Infection (ABSSSI) (https://www.clinicaltrials.gov/show/NCT03964493, accessed on 24 October 2023). Both oral and intravenous routes are used to deliver the hybrid candidate [85–87].

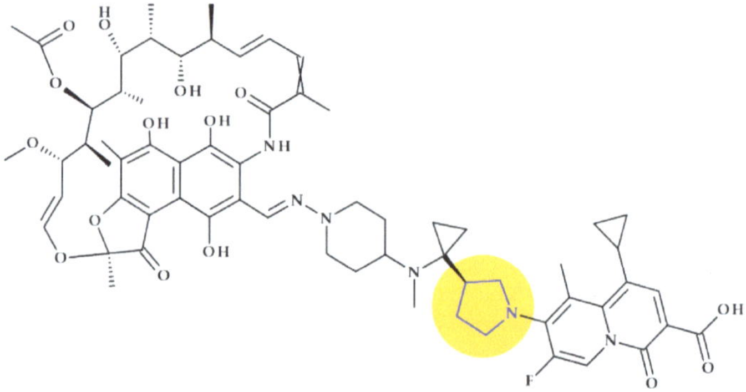

Figure 7. The molecular structure of Rifaquizinone (TNP-20292) with highlighted pyrrolidine heterocycle [82,83].

4.2. Imidazole

Imidazole is a five-membered heterocyclic moiety with two double bonds, three carbon, and two nitrogen atoms, also known as 1, 3-diazole (Table 2). It has two nitrogen atoms, one of which has a hydrogen atom and the other is referred to as pyrrole-type nitrogen. The compound has in position 1 a pyrrolic-type nitrogen atom with acidic properties and in position 3 a pyridinic-type nitrogen atom with basic properties. Imidazole has acidic and basic properties due to its amphoteric nature [88]. There are two equivalent tautomeric forms of imidazole, and one of them allows the hydrogen atom to be located on one of the two nitrogen atoms [89].

The six extra electrons in this cycle are dispersed among the five other atoms but are mainly concentrated on the nitrogen atoms. This heterocycle has an excess of electrons. Positions 4 and 5 experience electrophilic replacements as a result of the electron excess, while position 2, where the electron density is lower, is susceptible to nucleophilic substitutions [22,24,25]. Despite electron density being concentrated on nitrogen atoms and classified as π-excessive heterocycle, the ring system's electrons are delocalized. Easy protonation in strong acid, a sign of a strong base, is caused by a lone pair of electrons on N3. Also, a strong acid is indicated by the production of imidazolide in a strong base. As a result, imidazole has an amphoteric character [24]. The imidazole ring unsubstituted at the N1 position can be considered a weak acid. Considering these aspects, imidazole is amphoteric; it can function both as a base (iminic N3 atom) and as an acid (it can donate the proton from the secondary amino group (position N1)). Due to the abovementioned properties, imidazole can function as a hydrogen bond donor and acceptor, with the pyridinic N3 atom functioning as an electron pair donor and the N1 atom functioning as an acceptor. Thus, numerous mechanisms of action of some enzymes and drugs can be explained [22,89,90].

The imidazole can interact with numerous organic molecules via hydrogen bonds, van der Waals forces, ion-dipole, coordination, cation–π, π–π stacking, or hydrophobic effects [89]. Imidazole may create hydrogen bonds with its two nitrogen atoms, which increases its water solubility. The imidazole core's strong polarity and capacity to complex various metal ions are two additional significant characteristics [22,25]. It serves as the fundamental building block of many natural products, including DNA-based structures, histidine, purines, and histamine [88].

Imidazole is a significant five-membered heterocycle in drug design. According to reports in the literature, the 1,3-diazole derivatives present a variety of biological activities [88,89]. Notably, a large number of imidazole-based compounds have been extensively used as clinical drugs, including anticancer, antifungal, antiparasitic, antihistaminic, antineuropathic, and antihypertensive medications, due to their high therapeutic potency and significant potential for future development [29,89].

4.2.1. Macrolides (Ketolides Subclass)

Telithromycin. The macrolide class of antibiotics comprises the novel chemical class of ketolides, which includes the semisynthetic erythromycin derivative telithromycin (the first ketolide) [91]. Telithromycin, (1*S*,2*R*,5*R*,7*R*,8*R*,9*R*,11*R*,13*R*,14*R*)-8-[(2*S*,3*R*,4*S*,6*R*)-4-(dimethylamino)-3-hydroxy-6-methyloxan-2-yl]oxy-2-ethyl-9-methoxy-1,5,7,9,11,13-hexamethyl-15-[4-(4-pyridin-3-ylimidazol-1-yl)butyl]-3,17-dioxa-15-azabicyclo [12.3.0] heptadecane-4,6,12,16-tetrone, chemically differs from the macrolide group of antibacterials by the lack of α-*L*-cladinose at position 3 of the erythronolide A ring, resulting in a 3-keto function. This new ketolide lacks *L*-cladinose at position 3 of the erythronolide A ring and has a 3-keto action (differences from the macrolides group) [92]. Telithromycin has an additional pyridyl-imidazole-butyl side chain versus erythromycin. In telithromycin, the carbamate is linked to an alkyl-aryl extension, which gives the drug more potency than macrolides (Figure 8). As a result, telithromycin proved to be efficient against erythromycin-susceptible and resistant organisms, pneumococcus, as well against respiratory bacteria (*Haemophilus influenzae* and *Moraxella catarrhalis*) [91,93,94].

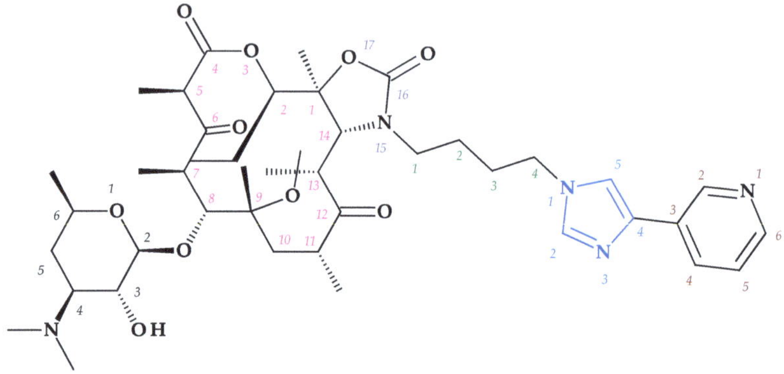

Figure 8. Telithromycin, chemical structure and atoms numbering by the IUPAC name.

The mechanism of action of telithromycin is based on stopping bacterial growth by preventing their ability to synthesize proteins. Older macrolides only firmly bind to one domain of the 50S ribosomal subunit's 23S RNA and weakly to the second domain, while telithromycin simultaneously strongly binds to both domains. Unfortunately, the presence of the pyridine-imidazole group of the telithromycin side chain was associated with uncommon but severe side effects (e.g., hepatotoxic effects) [94,95]. Consequently, to increase patient safety, the FDA (2007) announced a change to the telithromycin (Ketek®, Munich, Germany) use, the only indications being the treatment of CABP. In the European Union (EU), telithromycin was withdrawn from therapy [94–96].

4.2.2. Nitroimidazoles

After azomycin (2-nitroimidazole) was isolated from streptomycetes (1953) and its anti-trichomonas action was demonstrated (1956), multiple chemical synthesis methods and biological experiments for other nitroimidazole compounds were carried out. Thus, 1-(β-hydroxyethyl)-2-methyl-5-nitroimidazole compound, also known as metronidazole, was discovered. Metronidazole proved activity in vitro and in vivo against the anaerobic protozoa *Trichomonas vaginalis* and *Entamoeba histolytica*. Later tests found that metronidazole was particularly effective in treating various anaerobic infections, including Gram-positive and Gram-negative bacteria and the protozoa *Giardia lamblia* [97].

Metronidazole, ornidazole, secnidazole, nimorazole, and tinidazole are examples of imidazole derivative drugs. These 5-nitroimidazole compounds (Figure 9) are frequently used in clinical settings to treat protozoa and anaerobic bacteria infections [29,89]. According to a theory, the fatal impact of pathogens is caused when a reactive intermediate created during the microbial reduction of the 5-nitro group of imidazole derivatives covalently attaches to the microorganism's DNA. The nitroxide, nitroso, hydroxylamine, and amine are examples of potential reactive intermediates [29].

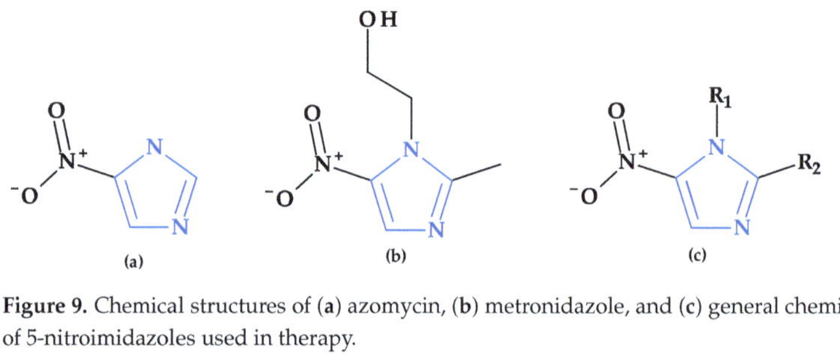

Figure 9. Chemical structures of (**a**) azomycin, (**b**) metronidazole, and (**c**) general chemical structure of 5-nitroimidazoles used in therapy.

4.3. 2-Imidazolidinone

Found in antibacterial drugs, such as some beta-lactamase inhibitors, 2-Imidazolidinone is another five-membered heterocycle (Table 2).

Beta-Lactamase Inhibitors

Relebactam. Relebactam, [(2*S*,5*R*)-7-oxo-2-(piperidin-4-ylcarbamoyl)-1,6-diazabicyclo [3.2.1]octan-6-yl] hydrogen sulfate, is a beta-lactamase inhibitor that does not contain a beta-lactam ring. It is structurally similar to avibactam, with the only difference being the presence of a piperidine ring attached to the carbonyl group at the 2-position (Figure 10a) [98]. This new beta-lactamase inhibitor has been demonstrated to covalently bind and with high affinity to the active site of Ambler classes A and C serine beta-lactamases and specific class D enzymes [38]. Relebactam is a compound belonging to the diazabicyclooctane class of beta-lactamase inhibitors, similar to avibactam. The central diazabicyclooctane core comprises piperidine and a 2-imidazolidinone heterocycle, with two carbon and one nitrogen atom in common. The high reactivity of the diazabicyclooctane pharmacophore, which is influenced by the electron-withdrawing properties of an aminoxy-sulfate group and the strained nature of the bridged bicyclic urea core structure, contributes to its ability to greatly enhance the potency of beta-lactamase inhibition [38].

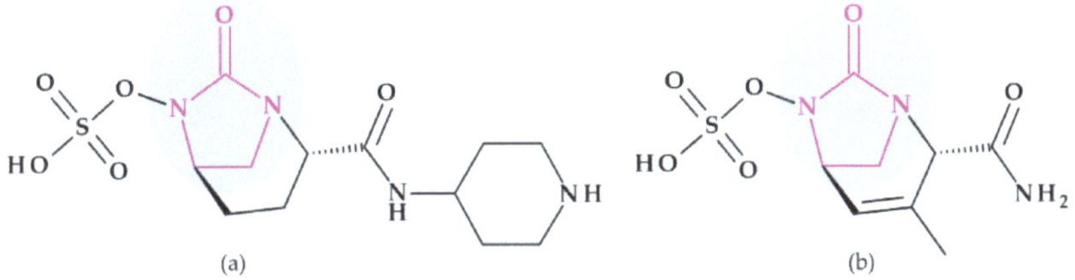

Figure 10. Chemical structure of beta-lactamase inhibitors with the highlighted 2-imidazolidinone heterocycle: (**a**) Relebactam and (**b**) Durlobactam.

Recarbrio® is a combination of imipenem (a carbapenem antibiotic), cilastatin (a renal dehydropeptidase inhibitor), and relebactam (a beta-lactamase inhibitor) approved by the FDA in 2019. This combination is prescribed to treat certain infections caused by susceptible Gram-negative bacteria, such as complicated UTIs (including pyelonephritis) and complicated intra-abdominal infections (cIAI), mainly when other treatment options are limited or unavailable. Moreover, it was also approved (in 2020) for the treatment of hospital-acquired bacterial pneumonia and ventilator-associated bacterial pneumonia (HABP/VABP) [99].

Durlobactam. Durlobactam, [(2*S*,5*R*)-2-carbamoyl-3-methyl-7-oxo-1,6-diazabicyclo [3.2.1]oct-3-en-6-yl] hydrogen sulfate, belongs to the diazabicyclooctane class of beta-lactamase inhibitors and exhibits wide-ranging effectiveness against Ambler class A, C, and D serine beta-lactamases. In contrast to the relebactam, the central diazabicyclooctane core comprises 1,2,3,6-tetrahydropyridine and a 2-imidazolidinone heterocycle, with two carbon and one nitrogen atom in common (Figure 10b) [100]. Unlike other beta-lactamase inhibitors, durlobactam's molecular structure is characterized by endocyclic double bonds and methyl substituent. Durlobactam, a polar compound, can enter Gram-negative cells through outer membrane porins [101].

On 23 May 2023, the FDA approved a new drug called Xacduro® for hospital-acquired bacterial pneumonia (HABP) and ventilator-associated bacterial pneumonia (VABP) cases. Specific strains of *Acinetobacter baumannii*-calcoaceticus complex produce these infections. Xacduro® is composed of two components: sulbactam and durlobactam. Sulbactam, a beta-lactam antibiotic and a beta-lactamase inhibitor, is responsible for activity against *Acinetobacter baumannii* bacteria. At the same time, durlobactam protects sulbactam from being hydrolyzed by enzymes that the same bacteria may produce. It is administered through intravenous infusion [100].

4.4. 1,2,3-Triazole

The 1,2,3-triazole heterocycle is a planar, cyclic structure containing two carbon atoms and three nitrogen atoms (two are pyridinic and one is pyrrole type) (Table 2). There are three tautomeric forms of triazole—*1H*- and *2H*- and 4-forms, the *2H* form being the most stable. The *4H*-1,2,3-triazole is a nonaromatic form. The *1H*- and *2H*-1,2,3-triazoles are in equilibrium in the gas phase and the solution. Electrophilic replacements at the level of the three nitrogen or carbon atoms are preferred in this heterocycle. Although 1,2,3-triazole is a weak base, it also has the strength of phenol when acting as a weak acid (Figure 11) [1,24].

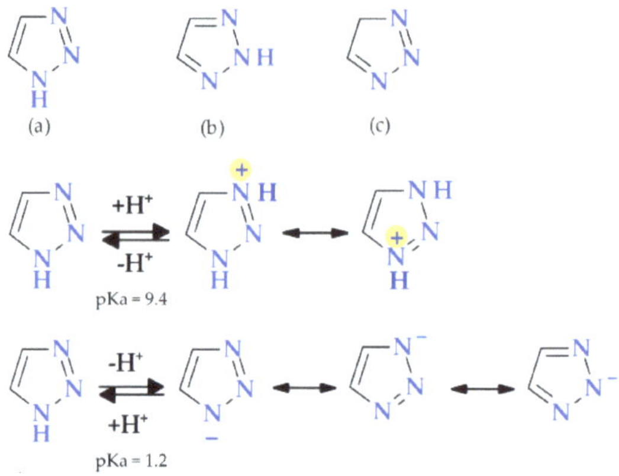

Figure 11. Tautomeric forms: (**a**) *1H*-1,2,3-Triazole, (**b**) *2H*-1,2,3-Triazole, (**c**) *4H*-1,2,3-Triazole, and amphoteric behavior of 1,2,3-triazole [1,24].

The 1,2,3-triazole is aromatic because all of its atoms are sp2 hybridized, and its available six electrons are delocalized around the ring. The ionization energy of 1,2,3-triazole (10.06 eV) is greater than imidazole (8.78 eV) and pyrazole (9.15 eV). Although reductive cleavages are possible, the 1,2,3-triazole ring is exceedingly stable and can resist reductive, oxidative, and acidic/basic hydrolysis processes. Also, due to their aromatic nature, triazoles resist enzymatic degradation and participate in hydrogen bond formations, and dipole-dipole and π-stacking interactions. Due to the two nitrogen atoms in the ring that are of the pyridine type, quaternization is more complex and demands aggressive conditions [24,102,103]. Many standard and non-traditional methods have been used to synthesize 1,2,3-triazole derivatives [104]. Triazole can enhance a compound's solubility and pharmacokinetic and pharmacodynamic features by creating hydrogen bonds, also known as dipole-dipole interactions. The result is the design of molecules with improved biological activity and selectivity [105,106].

4.4.1. Beta-Lactamase Inhibitors

Tazobactam. Clavulanic acid was the first reported beta-lactamase inhibitor isolated in 1977 from *Streptomyces clavuligerus*. This was followed by the discovery of sulbactam and tazobactam in the 1980s. Sulbactam and tazobactam are penicillanic acid sulfones, whereas clavulanic acid is a clavam. Tazobactam, (2*S*,3*S*,5*R*)-3-methyl-4,4,7-trioxo-3-(triazol-1-ylmethyl)-4λ^6-thia-1-azabicyclo [3.2.0]heptane-2-carboxylic acid, is considered the analog of sulbactam [107]. The heterocycle 1,2,3,-triazole is found in the structure of tazobactam (a beta-lactamase inhibitor) in the C3 position as 3-(triazol-1-ylmethyl) (Figure 12).

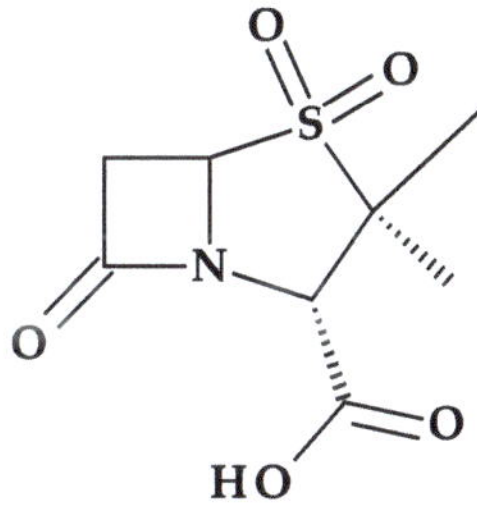

Figure 12. The chemical structure of tazobactam.

In addition, tazobactam has a broader spectrum of activity than clavulanic acid (an oxapenam beta-lactamase inhibitor with (2-hydroxy ethylidene) moiety at C3). It is more effective than sulbactam (a beta-lactamase inhibitor with dimethyl substituents at C3) and other usual beta-lactamase inhibitors. Thus, its antibacterial activity is minimal [29,107].

4.5. Tetrazole

Tetrazole is a type of five-membered nitrogen heterocycle in which four nitrogen atoms are present next to each other and are connected by a single carbon bond and two double bonds (Table 2) [24]. Tetrazole presents two tautomeric forms, 1*H*-tetrazole and 2*H*-tetrazole, and is an aromatic aza pyrrolic system with six π delocalized electrons, and three pyridinic and one pyrrolic nitrogen atoms [1,24,108]. While the 2*H*-form is more stable in the gas phase, the 1*H*-form is more stable and appears more frequently in solution (Figure 13) [24].

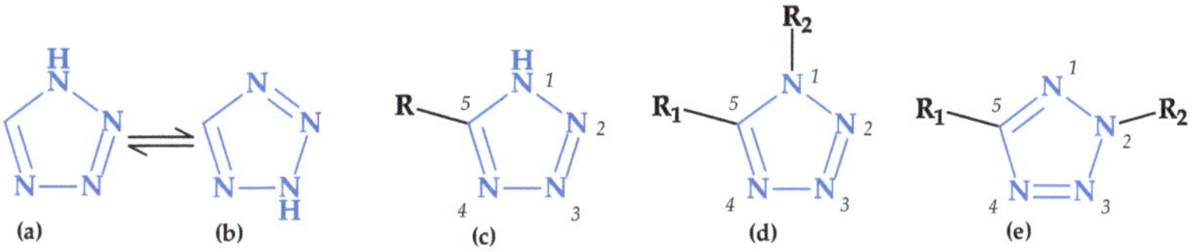

Figure 13. Tetrazole forms: (**a**) 1*H*-tautomer, (**b**) 2*H*-tautomer, (**c**) 5-monosubstituted, (**d**) 1,5-disubstituted, and (**e**) 2,5-disubstituted [24,109].

A substantial electron-withdrawing inductive action is more significant than the mesomeric effect in the tetrazole heterocycle. The planar tetrazole anion has a strong aromatic property. As a result, it can contribute to the development of ion-dipole, ion-ion interactions with various electron-deficient compounds [1,109]. The unsubstituted tetrazole rings can establish intermolecular hydrogen bonds because the nitrogen atoms of the pyridinic type -N= act as proton acceptors. Some molecules' structures allow the hydrogen atom, which comes from the pyrrolic type of nitrogen, to create intermolecular hydrogen bonds with specific electro-negative atoms. Despite having a weak basic nature, tetrazole can establish hydrogen bonds comparable to those formed by purine and pyrimidine bases [109].

Tetrazole is an acidic substance with a pKa of 4.89, similar to acetic acid's pKa of 4.76 [24]. Tetrazolate anion has a planar structure and high aromaticity. This form can actively interact with partner molecules' electron-deficient centers through ion-ion and ion-dipole interactions. Tetrazole rings that are NH-unsubstituted and 1,5-disubstituted are structural analogs of the carboxy and cisamide moieties that are metabolically stable [109].

Tetrazole is often used as a proline substitute due to increased solubility compared to proline [1]. Thereby, it is widely used as an isosteric replacement for carboxyl groups in the structure of several drugs due to the similarity to carboxylic acids and metabolic stability [1,25,109–111]. Also, tetrazole can interact with amidines at two points, like carboxylic acid. However, the tetrazole-amidine combination is less stable than the comparable carboxylate-amidine salt [111]. Tetrazole, as a bioisoster of natural amino acids and carboxylic acids, can enhance the pharmacokinetic profile of drugs with therapeutic efficacy by lowering their polarity and raising their lipophilicity for improved membrane permeability [109,111,112]. Tetrazole's lack of involvement in phase II reactions during the metabolic process can be associated with the improvement of the pharmacokinetic profile of the new compound; it is advantageous for using it as a substitute for the carboxyl group to extend the compounds' half-lives [113].

There are some tetrazole-based synthetic drugs from the classes of analeptics, antihypertensives, antifungals, antidiabetics, anti-inflammatories, anti-ulcers, metalloprotease inhibitors, growth hormone stimulators, opioid agonists, and chloride channel blockers used in clinical settings [24,29,114]. Also, a series of antibiotics containing the tetrazole heterocycle in their molecular structure are used in therapy [29].

4.5.1. Beta-Lactam Antibiotics

Cephalosporins

Cephalosporins with this moiety at the C3 position (such as cefamandole, cefmetazole, cefoperazone, cefotetan, and moxalactam) have been linked to a higher prevalence of hypoprothrombinemia in comparison to cephalosporins without the N-methyl-5-thiotetrazole group, by subsequently inhibiting glutamic acid's gamma-carboxylation [29,115]. Another cephalosporin, cefazolin, presents a tetrazolyl acetylamino fragment at the C7 position (Figure 14), also associated with a higher prevalence of hypoprothrombinemia [29,115].

Additionally, this group has been linked to the alcohol intolerance produced by several injectable cephalosporins, including cefamandole, cefotetan, cefmetazole, and cefoperazone. As a result, patients who have consumed alcohol before, during, or after the beginning of therapy may experience disulfiram-like reactions that are attributed to acetaldehyde and brought on by the inhibition of the aldehyde dehydrogenase-catalyzed oxidation of ethanol by N-methyl-5-thiotetrazole-containing cephalosporins [29,31]. Cephalosporin-induced coagulation deficiencies or bleeding can be produced by several mechanisms such as: (a) the induction of vitamin K-responsive hypoprothrombinemia, (b) the production of an acquired platelet defect, and (c) thrombocytopenia secondary to bone marrow suppression, and others [116].

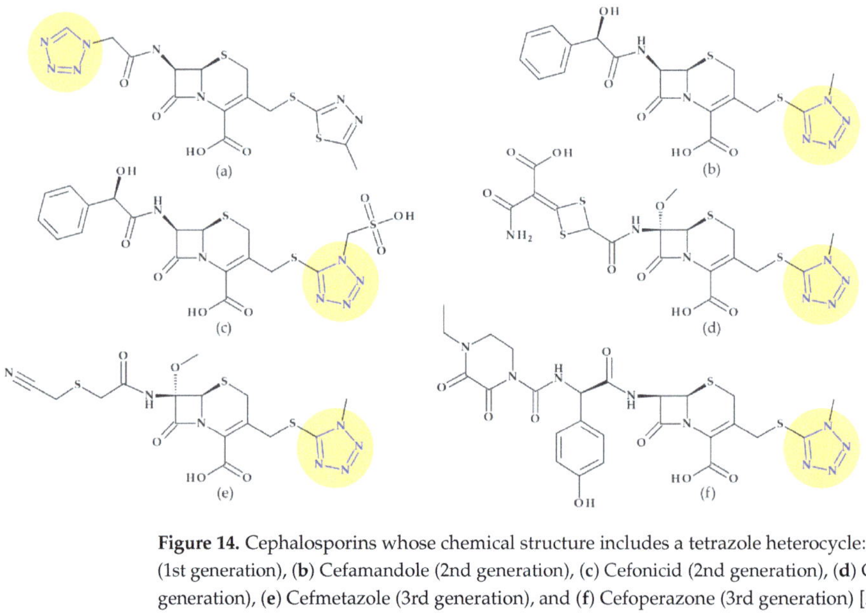

Figure 14. Cephalosporins whose chemical structure includes a tetrazole heterocycle: (**a**) Cefazolin (1st generation), (**b**) Cefamandole (2nd generation), (**c**) Cefonicid (2nd generation), (**d**) Cefotetan (3rd generation), (**e**) Cefmetazole (3rd generation), and (**f**) Cefoperazone (3rd generation) [29,31,117].

Cefazolin (1st generation). Cefazolin, (6*R*,7*R*)-3-[(5-methyl-1,3,4-thiadiazol-2-yl) sulfanylmethyl]-8-oxo-7-[[2-(tetrazol-1-yl)acetyl]amino]-5-thia-1-azabicyclo [4.2.0]oct-2-ene-2-carboxylic acid, is a semisynthetic cephalosporin approved in 1973 as a water-soluble sodium salt for parenteral administration. In addition to the 1,3,4-thiadiazole heterocycle at the C3 substituent, cefazolin contains an unusual tetrazolyl acetyl acylating moiety in the C7 position (Figure 14a) associated with a higher prevalence of hypoprothrombinemia [29,31,115]. Like first-generation cephalosporins, which demonstrated good action against Gram-positive bacteria and limited activity against Gram-negative bacteria, cephazolin's activity spectrum and therapeutic uses are the same [117,118]. Cefazolin was often selected among the first-generation cephalosporins because its prolonged half-live (2.2 h) allows a more advantageous administration schedule [118].

Cefamandole (2nd generation). Cefamandole, (6*R*,7*R*)-7-[[(2*R*)-2-hydroxy-2-phenylacetyl] amino]-3-[(1-methyltetrazol-5-yl)sulfanylmethyl]-8-oxo-5-thia-1-azabicyclo [4.2.0]oct-2-ene-2-carboxylic acid, is a second-generation cephalosporin used as a nafate ester. Cefamandole nafate spontaneously hydrolyses to cefamandole at neutral to alkaline pH. Esterification of the α-hydroxyl group of the *D*-mandeloyl function overcomes the instability of cefamandole in solid-state dosage forms. It gives adequate concentrations of the parent antibiotic in vivo. The characteristic groups of cefamandole are a *D*-mandelic acid fragment and a (1-methyltetrazol-5-yl) sulfanyl methyl at the C3 position (Figure 14b). Also, cefamandole has a tetrazole-thiomethyl side chain associated with side effects. When combined with alcohol, cefamandole may (rarely) lengthen the prothrombin time and produces a disulfiram-like reaction [29,119]. Compared to the first-generation cephalosporins, cefamandole exhibits higher activity against Gram-negative bacteria [118].

Cefonicid (2nd generation). Cefonicid, (6*R*,7*R*)-7-[[(2*R*)-2-hydroxy-2-phenylacetyl] amino]-8-oxo-3-[[1-(sulfomethyl)tetrazol-5-yl]sulfanylmethyl]-5-thia-1-azabicyclo [4.2.0]oct-2-ene-2-carboxylic acid, is a second-generation cephalosporin with an almost similar structure to cefamandole. Compared to cefamandole, cefonicid has a methane sulfonic acid group linked to the N-1 position of the tetrazole ring (Figure 14c). Cefonicid and cefamandole have nearly equal antibacterial activity and limited lactamase stability. Thus, cefonicid has superior pharmacokinetic characteristics versus cefamandole. In comparison to other second-generation cephalosporins, cefonicid differentiates due to its relatively extended serum half-life of around 4.5 h [29,120,121]. The pharmacological action and indications for use are analogous to those of cefamandole [117].

Cefotetan (3nd generation). Third-generation cephalosporin cefotetan, (6*R*,7*S*)-7-[[4-(2-amino-1-carboxy-2-oxoethylidene)-1,3-dithietane-2-carbonyl]amino]-7-methoxy-3-[(1-methyltetrazol-5-yl)sulfanylmethyl]-8-oxo-5-thia-1-azabicyclo [4.2.0]oct-2-ene-2-carboxylic acid, is unaffected by beta-lactamases due to a methoxy moiety at the C7 position of the cephalosporanic system (a cephamycin antibiotic). Also, the 1-methyltetrazol-5-yl group in cefotetan (Figure 14d) has been linked to hypoprothrombinemia and alcohol intolerance [29,31,119]. Third-generation cephalosporins are usually less effective than first-generation representatives against Gram-positive cocci. However, they are substantially more effective against Enterobacteriaceae despite beta-lactamase-producing strains, causing a significant increase in resistance [118].

Cefmetazole (3rd generation). Another third-generation cephalosporin for parenteral use is cefmetazole, (6*R*,7*S*)-7-[[2-(cyanomethylsulfanyl)acetyl]amino]-7-methoxy-3-[(1-methyltetrazol-5-yl)sulfanylmethyl]-8-oxo-5-thia-1-azabicyclo [4.2.0]oct-2-ene-2-carboxylic acid. This cephalosporin belongs to the cephamycin family. Like other cephamycins, the C7-methoxy group offers resistance to various beta-lactamases. However, the methyl tetrazole moiety (Figure 14e) has been linked to increased bleeding in some high-risk patients, similar to other cephalosporins [29,122].

Cefoperazone (3rd generation). Cefoperazone, (6*R*,7*R*)-7-[[(2*R*)-2-[(4-ethyl-2,3-dioxopiperazine-1-carbonyl)amino]-2-(4-hydroxyphenyl)acetyl]amino]-3-[(1-methyltetrazol-5-yl)sulfanylmethyl]-8-oxo-5-thia-1-azabicyclo [4.2.0]oct-2-ene-2-carboxylic acid, exhibits chemical and biological properties with piperacillin (a broad-spectrum beta-lactam antibiotic of the ureidopenicillin class) [29]. Additionally, cefoperazone contains a side chain of methyl thiotetrazole (Figure 14f) and can lead to bleeding, especially when taken in quantities larger than 4 g daily [115,116]. Cefoperazone is efficient against *Pseudomonas aeruginosa* but less efficient against Gram-positive cocci than other third-generation representatives [118].

Oxacephalosporins

Latamoxef/Moxalactam (1st generation). Latamoxef, (6*R*,7*R*)-7-[[2-carboxy-2-(4-hydroxyphenyl)acetyl]amino]-7-methoxy-3-[(1-methyltetrazol-5-yl)sulfanylmethyl]-8-oxo-5-oxa-1-azabicyclo [4.2.0]oct-2-ene-2-carboxylic acid, is an oxacephalosporin from the first generation, a cephamycin antibiotic (with a C7-methoxy moiety). The oxygen atom in the 7-aminocephalosporanic acid nucleus of latamoxef replaced the sulfur atom in the nucleus of the genuine cephalosporins (Figure 15a) [123]. Latamoxef more frequently induces coagulopathy and bleeding than other cephalosporins [116]. Like cefamandole, it has an N-methylthiotetrazole side-chain and may cause hypoprothrombinaemia [115,123].

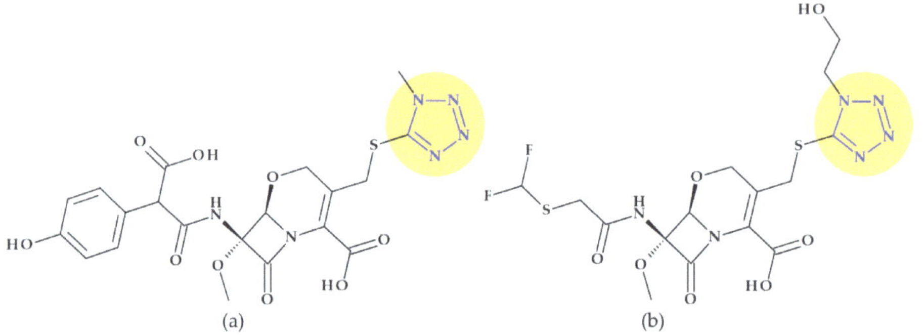

Figure 15. Oxacephalosporins the chemical structure of which includes a tetrazole heterocycle: (**a**) Latamoxef (1st generation), and (**b**) Flomoxef (2nd generation) [29,123,124].

Thereby, latamoxef has been linked to severe bleeding episodes. Therefore, prophylaxis with vitamin K and monitoring of bleeding time has been indicated throughout therapy. Inhibition of platelet function and, less frequently, immune-mediated thrombocytopenia may also interfere with hemostasis and hypoprothrombinemia. Also, a disulfiram-like reaction to alcohol is possible, similar to cephalosporins that include the methylthiotetrazole heterocycle [123]. These potentially fatal side effects ultimately led to Latamoxef medication being discontinued [125]. Identical to the third-generation cephalosporin cefotaxime, latamoxef exhibits antibacterial activity, albeit it tends to be less effective against Gram-positive bacteria and more effective against *Bacteroides fragilis* [123].

Flomoxef (2nd generation). Flomoxef, ((6*R*,7*R*)-7-[[2-(difluoromethylsulfanyl) acetyl]amino]-3-[[1-(2-hydroxyethyl)tetrazol-5-yl]sulfanylmethyl]-7-methoxy-8-oxo-5-oxa-1-azabicyclo [4.2.0]oct-2-ene-2-carboxylic acid) [126], is also an oxacephalosporin from the second generation, similar to latamoxef [29,123]. This antibiotic includes an extra C7-β-difluoromethyl-thioacetamido side chain substitution (Figure 15b), resulting in significant activity levels against Gram-positive and Gram-negative bacteria (including anaerobes) and a lower toxicity profile. In addition, the N-methyl tetrazole thiol group linked to the C3 position of the oxacephem nucleus is replaced with a methyl thiadiazole-thiol group, which is presumed to be the cause of the disulfiram- and coumarin-like adverse effects associated with latamoxef therapy [124].

4.5.2. Oxazolidinones

Tedizolid (2nd generation). In 2014, the FDA approved tedizolid, (5*R*)-3-{3-fluoro-4-[6-(2-methyl-2*H*-1,2,3,4-tetrazol-5-yl)pyridin-3-yl]phenyl}-5-(hydroxymethyl)-1,3-oxazolidin-2-one [127], a second-generation oxazolidinone synthesized as the phosphate prodrug, for treating acute bacterial skin and skin structure infections (ABSSSIs) produced by susceptible Gram-positive organisms, such as MRSA. Compared to linezolid, tedizolid is 4- to 16-fold more effective against MRSA [110,128]. The optimizations of linezolid (the first approved oxazolidinone) by replacing the morpholine ring with a pyridine one and an additional methyl tetrazole ring were responsible for the enhanced potency of tedizolid (Figure 16) [128,129].

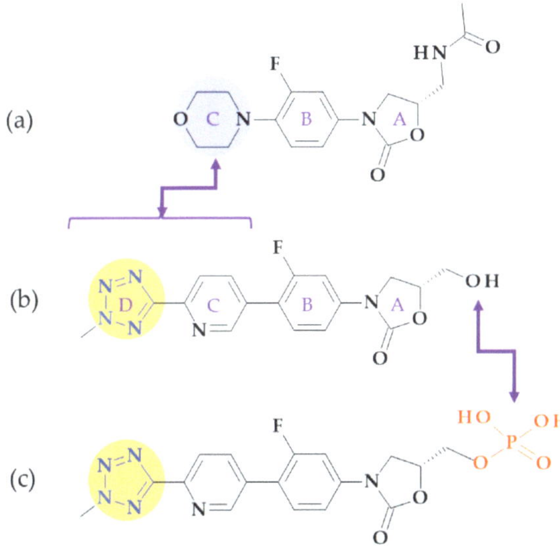

Figure 16. Structural differences between (**a**) linezolid, (**b**) tedizolid, and (**c**) tedizolid phosphate; the morpholine ring in linezolid was replaced with a pyridine and a methyl tetrazole ring in tedizolid [31,128,130].

Due to these structural optimizations, tedizolid can engage in additional binding interactions with the upper region of the peptidyltransferase center of the 50S ribosomal subunit, inhibiting protein synthesis. Tedizolid's pyridine and methyl tetrazole rings add two hydrogen bonds to the residues A2451 and U2584 of the sugar backbone. The antimicrobial potency of tedizolid has been linked to the formation of more target site interactions at the peptidyltransferase center [128,129].

It is well known that several prodrugs containing tetrazole heterocycle as a bioisoster of carboxylic acid have received enhanced oral bioavailability, lipophilicity, and bioavailability while lowering its adverse effects [110]. Given that tedizolid has a mean half-life of 12 h, which is twice as long as linezolid's (5.4 h), it can be used once daily, which is more convenient. Tedizolid has an excellent pharmacokinetic profile, a half-life for once-daily treatment, and absent steady-state nonlinearities. The administration of tedizolid phosphate can be undertaken regardless of food [130–132]. In addition to more favorable pharmacokinetics and enhanced antimicrobial potency, tedizolid phosphate proves a lower incidence of side effects, including thrombocytopenia [130].

Although it is in development (two phase 2 clinical trials), we consider it appropriate to discuss the following compound that has the potential to be shortly approved.

Radezolid. Melinta scientists developed the second-generation oxazolidinone antibacterial drug radezolid, N-[[(5S)-3-[3-fluoro-4-[4-[(2*H*-triazol-4-ylmethylamino)methyl]phenyl] phenyl]-2-oxo-1,3-oxazolidin-5-yl]methyl]acetamide, to increase ribosomal binding affinity and lower off-target activity [21,133]. In Figure 17, it is shown that the molecular building blocks of radezolid are the triazole ring, methylamino methyl link, biaryl ring system, oxazolidinone ring, and acetamide fragment. Radezolid is entirely synthesized and has one stereocenter in the oxazolidinone ring (position C5) [134]. Abscesses, bacterial skin illnesses, streptococcal infections, infectious skin disorders, and staphylococcal skin infections have all been studied in clinical trials with radezolid [21,133]. Two phase 2 clinical trials were completed to treat pneumonia and uncomplicated skin infections [135], [136]. This new oxazolidinone derivative possesses enhanced antibacterial potency against antibiotic-resistant Gram-positive bacteria compared with linezolid. Its action mechanism consists of forming π-π stacking interactions with the 50S subunit of the bacteria [137].

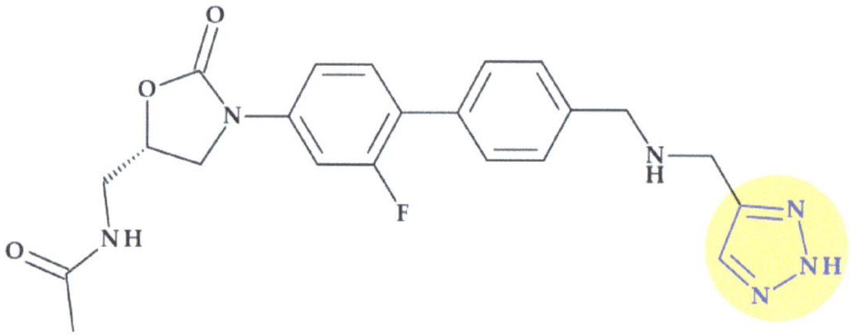

Figure 17. Chemical structure of radezolid with highlighted triazole heterocycle.

5. Five-Membered Heterocycles Containing Oxygen Atoms

5.1. Furan

The word furan, which indicates bran, is derived from the Latin *furfur* [24]. Furan is an aromatic five-membered heterocycle with a centrally positioned sp2 hybridized oxygen atom that is planar and pentagonal (Table 2). Furan's ring atoms all lay in a plane, forming a pentagon with minor distortion. The bond length between C-3 and C-4 is more extended than between C-2 and C-3 and between C-4 and C-5. Therefore, the C-C bond length averages the single and double bond lengths, while the C-O bond is shorter by 0.05 Å. The C-C bond length is approximately the same (1.33 Å). The places next to the heteroatom were previously denoted as α and α'. Furyl is the name attributed to the monovalent residue [1,22,24].

One of the two pairs of non-participating electrons is in an sp2 hybridized orbital, while the other pair is in a π orbital. These two pairings are in separate orbitals. The ring's bonds are comparable to those in the pyrrolic ring, and the heterocycle displays six delocalized electrons [1]. Furan reacts with electrophilic reagents similarly to benzene, frequently with substitution. However, depending on the reagent and reaction circumstances, it can also react via addition and/or ring-opening [22]. Furan is faster than benzene to participate in electrophilic substitution reactions because it is a heterocycle with excess electrons. Therefore, furan is more reactive than thiophene but less reactive than pyrrole in reactivity [1,22]. Thus, furan is less stable than thiophene due to its lower resonance energy [24].

Primarily, furan serves as a precursor in synthesizing and manufacturing numerous chemical components necessary for the synthesis of drugs [24]. Several drugs from different therapeutic classes contain the furan heterocycle in their chemical structure: 5-nitrofuran derivatives and cefuroxime (antibacterials), darunavir (HIV protease inhibitor), furosemide (diuretic), lapatinib (antineoplastic agent and tyrosine kinase inhibitor), prazosin (alpha-blocker used to treat hypertension), and ranitidine (histamine H2 antagonist) [24,29,31,138].

Drug discovery frequently uses structural alerts to detect compounds likely to produce harmful metabolites. Le Dang N. et al. (2017) showed that mathematical models of P450 metabolism can forecast the context-specific possibility that a structural alarm will be biologically activated in a particular molecule. Furan heterocycles were found in 17 approved or withdrawn drugs. Among these, thirteen were in the literature-derived Accelrys Metabolite Database, and three were bioactivated through epoxidation. In this study, three 5-nitrofuran derivatives (furazolidone, nitrofural, and nitrofurantoin) and a cephalosporin (cefuroxime) were targeted from the class of antibiotics. None of these compounds showed metabolism by epoxidation [139].

5.1.1. Beta-Lactam Antibiotics

Cephalosporins

Cefuroxime/Cefuroxime axetil (2nd generation). Cefuroxime, (6*R*,7*R*)-3-(carbamoyloxym ethyl)-7-[[(2Z)-2-(furan-2-yl)-2-methoxyiminoacetyl]amino]-8-oxo-5-thia-1-azabicyclo [4.2.0] oct-2-ene-2-carboxylic acid, is a second-generation cephalosporin with a similar antibacterial activity spectrum to cefamandole [29]. The C-7 position of cefuroxime has a *Z*-oriented methoxy imino moiety into a (2*Z*)-2-(furan-2-yl)-2-methoxyiminoacetyl]amino fragment, which confers significant resistance from attack by many but not all beta-lactamases [31,140]. The 1-acetyoxyethyl ester of cefuroxime is known as cefuroxime axetil (Figure 18). This lipophilic, acid-stable oral prodrug derivative of cefuroxime is hydrolyzed to cefuroxime during intestinal and/or plasma enzyme absorption [29]. *Escherichia coli*, *Klebsiella pneumoniae*, *Neisseria gonorrhoea*, and *Haemophilus influenzae* are beta-lactamase-producing bacteria resistant to cefamandole and susceptible to cefuroxime. Thus, Serratia and Proteus species (indole-positive), *Pseudomonas aeruginosa*, and *Bacteroides fragilis* are Gram-negative pathogens resistant to cefuroxime [31].

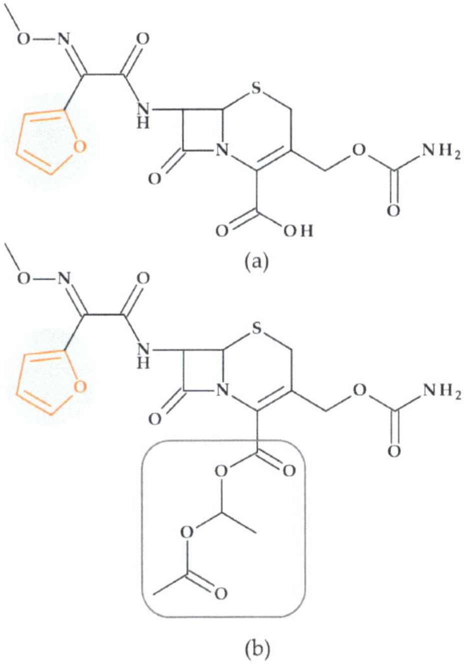

Figure 18. Cephalosporins: (**a**) Cefuroxime and (**b**) Cefuroxime axetyl (acetyoxyethyl ester of cefuroxime), whose chemical structure include a furan heterocycle.

5.1.2. Nitrofurans

According to chemical structure–biological activity relationship studies, the 5-nitrofural element and the azomethine group are essential for nitrofurans' antibacterial, antifungal, and antiprotozoal activity. In addition, the rest of the heterocyclic amine determines its activity spectrum and pharmacokinetic properties (Figure 19) [29]. Nitrofurans exhibit activity against Gram-positive and Gram-negative bacteria, particularly the Enterobacter, Citrobacter, Escherichia, and Klebsiella species. Additionally, it shows antiprotozoal and antimycotic effects against *Giardia lamblia* and *Trichomonas vaginalis*, respectively. Nitrofurans' mode of action is based on the production of superoxide ions, nitroso derivatives, and highly reactive free radical species that result from the activity of certain reductases in bacterial cells. The bacterial ribosomal proteins will attach to the compound produced by reductases. As a result, bacterial nucleic acid structure and function, or bacterial metabolism, are affected [29,118].

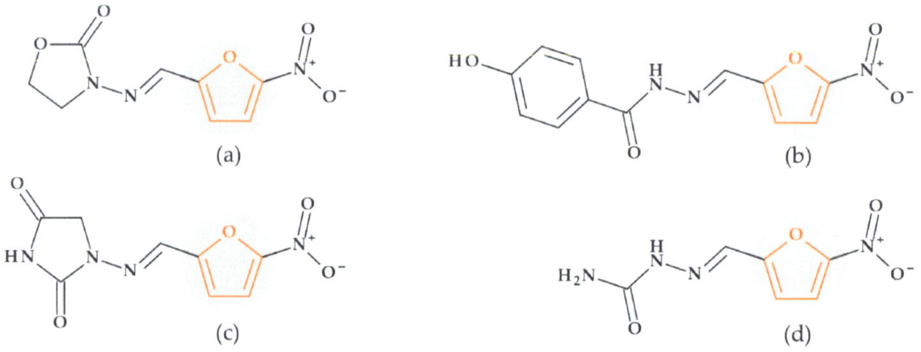

Figure 19. Nitrofurans, the chemical structure of which includes a furan heterocycle: (**a**) Furazolidone, (**b**) Nifuroxazide, (**c**) Nitrofurantoin, and (**d**) Nitrofurazone.

5.1.3. Oxazolidinones

Although the following compound is an investigational drug, this may be a "lead" compound for other oxazolidinones.

Ranbezolid. The 'piperazinyl-phenyl-oxazolidinone' core of eperezolid was used to synthesize new oxazolidinones that had a variety of substituted five-membered heterocycles connected to it. These optimizations resulted from several compounds with strong action against various resistant and sensitive Gram-positive pathogens [141]. Thus, a 2-substituted-5-nitro-furyl derivative was identified as ranbezolid (RBx 7644) with the IUPAC name N-[[(5S)-3-[3-fluoro-4-[4-[(5-nitrofuran-2-yl)methyl]piperazin-1-yl]phenyl]-2-oxo-1,3-oxazolidin-5-yl]methyl]acetamide (Figure 20) [141]. The compound in this group with the highest in vivo activity was ranbezolid, which also had in vitro activity comparable with or slightly better than linezolid. Additionally, ranbezolid is active against Gram-positive and Gram-negative anaerobes [141,142].

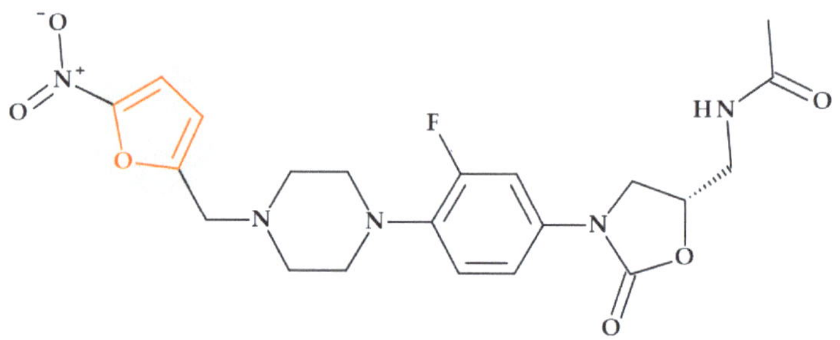

Figure 20. Ranbezolid, the chemical structure of which includes a furan heterocycle.

6. Five-Membered Heterocycles Containing Oxygen and Nitrogen Atoms

6.1. 1,3-Oxazolidine

Oxazolidine is a five-membered heterocycle with two heteroatoms, one represented by oxygen in position 1 and the other by nitrogen in position 3 (Table 2). There are two isomers of this heterocycle: 1,3-oxazolidine and 1,2-isoxazolidine. Tetrahydro-oxazole, or oxazole, is represented by the heterocycle in its fully reduced state [24]. 1,3-Oxazolidine-2-one derivatives were created and developed to cure infections produced by Gram-positive bacteria resistant to different antibiotics. First, the antibacterial properties of linezolid and other oxazolidinone compounds that prevented bacterial protein synthesis were discovered [143].

Oxazolidinones

In 1987, oxazolidinones (DuP 721 and DuP 105) were introduced as a new class of antibiotics [144]. Currently, they are used in therapy with two representatives: linezolid (1st generation) and tedizolid (2nd generation). The five-membered heterocycle oxazolidine, which has a 2-oxazolidinone carbonyl group attached (A cycle), is the pharmacophore for this class of drugs (Figure 16) [145]. The 1,3-oxazolidin-2-onic nucleus represents oxazolidinone's basic structure, essential to antibacterial activity [146]. Thus, the C5 acyl aminomethyl group, the 5*S* configuration, and the N-aryl substituent were all necessary for antibacterial properties. Although it was not necessary, the meta-fluoro substitution of the phenyl ring typically increased antibacterial activity, and the para substitution might be modified to broaden the antibacterial spectrum [147].

Oxazolidinone antibiotics act by inhibiting the formation of the initiation complex, which inhibits the start of bacterial protein synthesis. The 30S and 50S ribosomal subunits, rRNA, and mRNA are part of the initiation complex. The 50S ribosomal subunit's peptidyl-transferase enzyme center can interact with the 1,3-oxazolidin-2-onic ring. The peptidyl transferase enzyme is the catalytic center and plays a fundamental role in bacterial protein synthesis [145,146,148].

Oxazolidinones are a relatively recent class of antibiotics developed to mainly treat Gram-positive bacterial infections [149]. They are active on a broad spectrum of aerobic and anaerobic Gram-positive bacteria, including bacteria resistant to other antibiotics - methicillin- and vancomycin-resistant staphylococci, vancomycin-resistant enterococci, penicillin-resistant pneumococci, and *Mycobacterium tuberculosis* [118,146].

Linezolid is the "first-in-class" representative of oxazolidinones approved by the FDA in 1999 [145] for treating skin infections, nosocomial pneumonia, and drug-resistant tuberculosis [149]. Therefore, infections caused by *Enterococcus faecalis*, pneumonia caused by *Staphylococcus aureus* and *Streptococcus pneumoniae*, and complicated skin infections caused by methicillin-resistant *Staphylococcus aureus* and *Staphylococcus pyogenes* are all treated with linezolid [150]. Tedizolid phosphate is the inactive prodrug of tedizolid [147] approved by the FDA in 2014 for treating skin and skin structure infections [128,130,147]. Both oxazolidinones were previously discussed in Section 4.5.2. regarding structural features correlated with pharmacological and toxicological aspects.

Notably, other oxazolidinones such as posizolid, sutezolid, radezolid, eperezolid, delpazolid, torezolid, and TBI-223 are in different phases of clinical trials [146].

6.2. Oxazoles and Isoxazoles

With five atoms, including the heteroatoms oxygen and nitrogen, oxazole is an unsaturated molecule belonging to the 1,3 azole class (Table 2) [1]. Because a -CH= group was substituted for an azomethine group, which has a nitrogen atom of the pyridinic type, it is regarded as a furan derivative; this is considered a heterocycle since it has an excess of electrons and an aromatic π sextet [1,24]. However, the existence of an electronegative oxygen atom limits the total delocalization of electrons. Since the oxazole's nitrogen atom exhibits pyridine-type behavior and its oxygen atom exhibits furan-type behavior, it is regarded as a hybrid heteroaromatic system [24]. It has been noticed that the aromaticity order is comparable to that of the five-membered heterocycles with a single heteroatom (thiophene > pyrrole > furan). Among the 1,3-azoles, oxazole has the least aromatic content and has diene-like characteristics. Following the bond lengths in oxazole (with a noticeable difference in the C2-N and C4-N bonds), the oxazole ring is planar and has significant bond fixation [1].

Isoxazoles are an essential type of five-membered aromatic heterocycles that include three conventional sp2 carbon atoms and two electronegative heteroatoms, nitrogen and oxygen, in a 1,2 relationship (Table 2) [24]. Isoxazole is a monocyclic heteroarene (1-oxa-2-azacyclopentadiene). It is a heterocycle with excess electrons and an oxygen atom of the furan type in position 1 and a nitrogen atom of the pyridinic type in position 2. As a result, it will develop features unique to those two types of atoms [1].

Isoxazole is a π-excessive heterocycle with characteristics similar to pyridine and furans. The electrophilic substitution of isoxazole develops more frequently than pyridine due to the electron-attracting quality of the pyridine type of nitrogen and the electron-donating characteristic of oxygen. Isoxazoles can be modified to produce a variety of complex structures. As oxazole, it is an aromatic system, and the oxygen and nitrogen heteroatoms in the five-membered ring significantly impact the aromatic feature. Various reactions, including electrophilic substitution, nucleophilic substitution, oxidation, reduction, etc., are carried out in this heteroaromatic system [24].

Oxazole is regarded as a hybrid of both heterocyclic systems. It demonstrates characteristics of both (i) pyridine-type nitrogen, which includes protonation, N-alkylation, and the reactivity of the halogen atom at position 2, and (ii) furan-type oxygen, which includes diene-type characteristics as a result of bond localization [1]. Similar to imidazoles, oxazoles are weakly basic compounds that can be either partially reduced (2,5-dihydro oxazole or 4,5-dihydro oxazole) or totally reduced (oxazolidine) [24].

Because it is capable of producing weak non-covalent bonds, including hydrogen bonds, ion-dipole interactions, and van der Waals interactions, the oxazole nucleus has the potential to be biologically active. Oxazole is used to structure several compounds with pharmacological effects because it binds to receptors and interacts with various enzymes [24]. Also, the isosteres of oxazole are thiazole, imidazole, benzimidazole, triazole, and tetrazole. The pharmacokinetic profile of multiple drugs is enhanced, their range of activity is expanded, and their toxicity is decreased due to oxazole heterocycle in the molecular structure [151].

Oxazole has been identified as a critical molecular building block for developing new drugs. Numerous structurally complex natural compounds have this ring system. Oxazole-containing drugs have been obtained from marine and plant sources [24]. Oxazoles, in particular, can bind with a wide range of enzymes and biological receptors and exhibit a wide range of pharmacological activities, being included in antibacterial, antifungal, antiviral, antitubercular, anticancer, and anti-inflammatory medicines [24,151]. Isoxazoles have also been discovered to be essential components in many synthetic items used daily and as a pharmacophore present in many medications and bioactive natural products. Additionally, isoxazoles have shown they can interact with several enzymes and receptors in hydrogen bond donor/acceptor interactions. Isoxazoles are helpful building blocks for many different compounds, including many natural compounds, when synthetically created [24].

6.2.1. Beta-Lactam Antibiotics

Isoxazolyl penicillins (Antistaphylococcal penicillins)

The beta-lactam cycle is hydrolyzed by bacteria into inactive molecules by hydrolytic enzymes known as beta-lactamases (penicillinases). Researchers made structural modifications at the level of the radical linked to the carbonyl bond to avoid this phenomenon. The carbonyl group is shielded and given steric hindrance by adding a sizeable heterocyclic residue (e.g., isoxazole) [29]. The bioisosteric substitution of the benzene ring (isoxazolyl) in benzylpenicillin has resulted in the biosynthesis of isoxazolyl penicillins. Chemical differences between isoxazolyl penicillins include fluorine or chlorine substituents on the benzene ring [31]. Including the isoxazole heterocycle in their molecular structure improves beta-lactamase resistance and resistance in the acidic stomach environment [29,118].

Oxacillin and its derivatives, cloxacillin, dicloxacillin, and flucloxacillin (Figure 21), are rarely used in therapy. Pulcini et al. (2012) named these antibiotics "forgotten antibiotics".

Unfortunately, economic motives are the primary cause for the discontinuation of the marketing of these antibiotics [13].

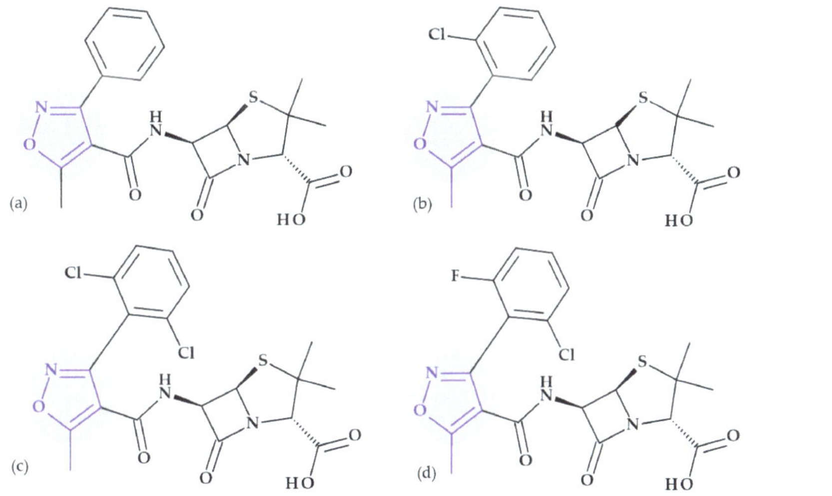

Figure 21. Isoxazolyl penicillins including 1,2-oxazole heterocycle in their molecular structures: (**a**) Oxacillin, (**b**) Cloxacillin, (**c**) Dicloxacillin, and (**d**) Flucloxacillin.

Isoxazolyl penicillins are typically less effective than benzylpenicillin against Gram-positive pathogens (staphylococci and streptococci) that do not develop a beta-lactamase. Still, they retain their effectiveness against those that do. Since isoxazolyl penicillins are more acid-stable than natural penicillins, they can be orally administered and have a higher potency. However, they are poor options for treating septicemia due to their high serum protein binding. The isoxazolyl group of penicillins are highly lipophilic compounds active against bacteria resistant to methicillin and methicillin-sensitive *Staphylococcus aureus* (MSSA). Due to their inability to pass through Gram-negative bacteria's cell walls, these antibiotics have a limited spectrum of activity. Penicillins from the isoxazolyl group are mainly utilized to treat infections with *Staphylococcus aureus*, which produces beta-lactamase [29,31,118,152]. Although their spectrum of activity is comparable to benzylpenicillin, isoxazolyl penicillins should be restricted to treating infections induced by Staphylococci resistant to benzylpenicillin [153].

6.2.2. Izoxazolidinones

Cycloserine. Cycloserine, *D*-(+)-4-amino-3-isoxazolidinone, is an antibiotic from the isoxazolidinones class and second-line therapy for tuberculosis [31,154]. The antibiotic has been isolated from three different Streptomyces species' fermenting beer (Figure 22). Later, it was synthesized, being a relatively simple structure. The stereochemistry of cycloserine and *D*-serine is similar. However, the *L*-form exhibits comparable antibiotic action [29].

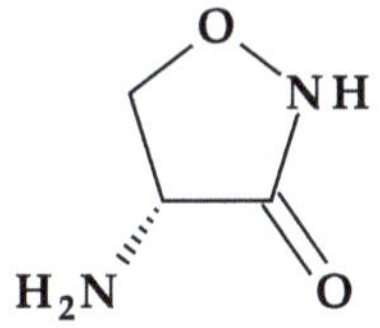

Figure 22. Chemical structure depiction of Cycloserine.

As a mechanism of action, cycloserine inhibits the synthesis of the bacterial wall. The inhibition occurs in the early phase of peptidoglycan synthesis, a cell wall constituent [31,154]. The peptidoglycan of the mycobacterial cell wall contains a significant amount of *D*-alanine. *D*-alanine racemase is an enzyme that converts naturally available *L*-alanine to D-alanine in Mycobacteria [31]. The enzymes alanine racemase and *D*-alanyl-*D*-alanyl synthetase are involved in the production of the dipeptide *D*-alanyl-*D*-alanine, a precursor of the pentapeptide chain in the development of mycobacterial cell walls. Both enzymes are inhibited by cycloserine. It has been suggested that cycloserine has a better probability of binding to the enzyme because the isoxazole ring has a more rigid structure than *D*-alanine (a more flexible structure) [154]. So, the rigid analog *D*-cycloserine competitively inhibits *D*-alanine binding to both of these enzymes and, consequently, its inclusion into the peptidoglycan [31].

Despite antibiotic efficacy in vitro against various Gram-positive and Gram-negative pathogens, cycloserine is limited to treating tuberculosis due to its relatively low potency and frequent side effects due to the excellent penetration of cerebrospinal fluid [29,155,156]. A series of central nervous system (CNS) side effects are due to the binding of *D*-cycloserine to neuronal N-methylasparate (NMDA) receptors and affecting the synthesis and metabolism of γ-aminobutyric acid (GABA) [31,155].

Some antibacterials in development, such as posizolid and zoliflodacin, include in their molecular structure an isoxazole heterocycle.

Posizolid. Posizolid, (5*R*)-3-[4-[1-[(2S)-2,3-dihydroxypropanoyl]-3,6-dihydro-2*H*-pyridin-4-yl]-3,5-difluorophenyl]-5-(1,2-oxazol-3-yloxymethyl)-1,3-oxazolidin-2-one, includes an extra 1,2-oxazole heterocycle in its molecular structure in addition to the oxazolidinone nucleus (Figure 23); it is in phase I of clinical trials [149].

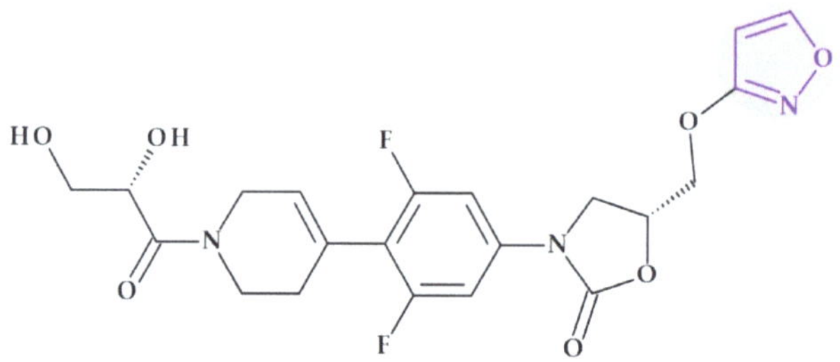

Figure 23. Chemical structure depiction of Posizolid.

Zoliflodacin. The novel antibacterial class spiro-pyrimidinetrione includes zoliflodacin, 4′*R*,6′*S*,7′*S*)-17′-fluoro-4′,6′-dimethyl-13′-[(4*S*)-4-methyl-2-oxo-1,3-oxazolidin-3-yl]spiro [1,3-diazinane-5,8′-5,15-dioxa-2,14-diazatetracyclo [8.7.0.02,7.012,16]heptadeca-1(17),10,12(16),13-tetraene]-2,4,6-trione, as its first representative. Zoliflodacin contains the spirocyclic pyrimidinetrione pharmacophore. Izoxazole is present in the molecular structure of this promising novel antibiotic currently undergoing a global phase 3 randomized controlled trial to treat gonorrhea (Figure 24) [157,158].

6.2.3. Sulfonamides

Antibacterial sulfonamides are bacteriostatic agents that work as antimetabolites of para-aminobenzoic acid (PABA), which competitively inhibit dihydropteroate synthetase, an enzyme involved in the synthesis of bacterial folic acid [31]. Microorganisms considered sensitive must produce folic acid; bacteria that can utilize preformed folate are unaffected. Sulfonamides are bacteriostatic when used alone; nevertheless, complete infection eradication requires the host's cellular and humoral defensive mechanisms [118]. Some sulfonamides contain 1,2-oxazole heterocycle in their chemical structure, such as sulfisoxazole and sulphamethoxazole.

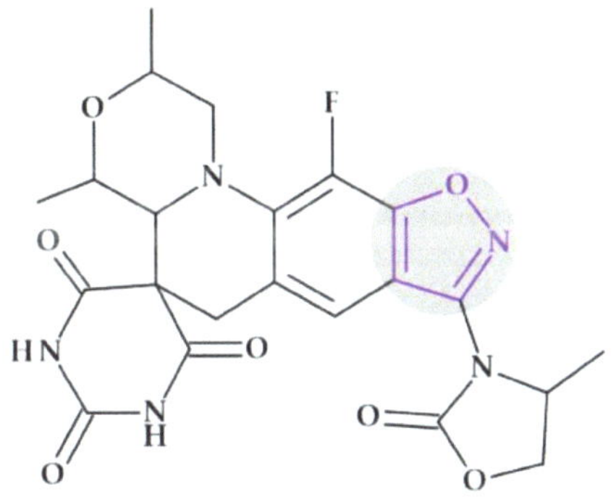

Figure 24. Chemical structure depiction of Zoliflodacin.

Sulfisoxazole (Sulfafurazole). Sulfisoxazole, 4-amino-N-(3,4-dimethyl-1,2-oxazol-5-yl) benzenesulfonamide, or sulfafurazole contains a 1,2-oxazole heterocycle in its chemical structure (Figure 25a). In the studies of the structure-activity relationship (SAR), replacing one of the amino function hydrogens with an electron-withdrawing heteroaromatic ring (1,2-isoxazole) enhanced the remaining hydrogen's acidity and potency. Sulfisoxazole has a pKa of approximately 5.0. It is a short-acting sulfonamide, the half-life of sulfisoxazole being about 5 to 8 h. It enters the fetal circulation through the placenta and is released into the breast milk. Sulfisoxazole treats infections caused by sulfonamide-sensitive bacteria since it has the same effects and applications as other sulfonamides. Gram-negative urine infections have responded well to this sulphonamide therapy [29,31,123].

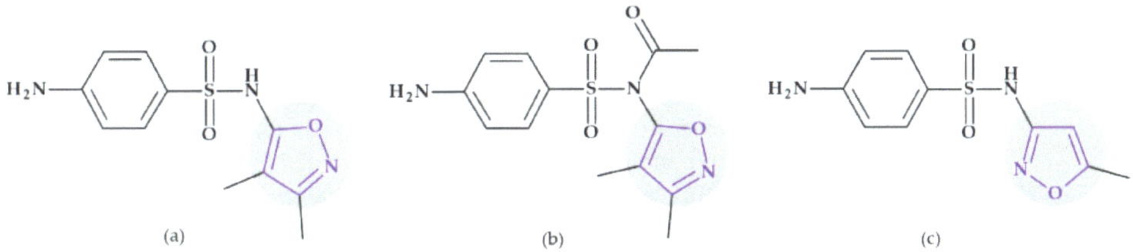

Figure 25. Sulfonamides including 1,2-oxazole heterocycle in their molecular structures: (**a**) Sulfisoxazole, (**b**) Sulfisoxazole acetyl, and (**c**) Sulfamethoxazole.

Sulfisoxazole diolamine. The 2,2′-iminodiethanol (diolamine) salt of sulfisoxazole is prepared (1:1 ratio) to make the sulfonamide more soluble in the physiological pH. When it cannot be maintained by oral treatment, the diolamine salt is used in solution for systemic delivery by slow intravenous, intramuscular, or subcutaneous injection. Additionally, it is utilized for applying drops or ointments to the eye to treat localized infections that are susceptible to sulfisoxazole [29].

Sulfisoxazole acetyl. Like its parent chemical, sulfisoxazole, sulfisoxazole acetyl (Figure 25b) exhibits the same properties and applications. Since the acetyl derivative has no taste, it can be orally administered, especially in liquid solutions. The acetyl molecule functions as a prodrug for sulfisoxazole, splits in the intestinal system, and is absorbed as sulfisoxazole. It is essential to distinguish between acetyl sulfafurazole and the N4-acetyl derivative of sulfafurazole produced through conjugation in the body [29,123].

Sulfamethoxazole. In terms of chemical structure and antibacterial activity, sulfamethoxazole, 4-amino-N-(5-methyl-1,2-oxazol-3-yl)benzenesulfonamide, is a sulfonamide medication that is related to sulfisoxazole. The difference is given by the methyl substituent on the oxazole ring and the 3-position of the heterocycle linked to the sulfonamide amino (N1) group (Figure 25c). The plasma half-life of sulfamethoxazole is 6 to 12 h, longer than that of sulfisoxazole (about 6 h) [29,123].

The sulfamethoxazole and trimethoprim combination (cotrimoxazole) represented a significant step forward in the design of antimicrobial drugs that were both clinically efficacious and synergistic. Trimethoprim inhibits the bacterial enzyme dihydrofolate reductase from converting dihydrofolate to tetrahydrofolate [118,159]. The sulfamethoxazole and trimethoprim combination can be bactericidal because it inhibits two processes in the bacterial biosynthesis of vital proteins and nucleic acids. Gram-positive and Gram-negative bacteria, Nocardia, *Chlamydia trachomatis,* and certain protozoa are all inhibited by sulfonamides. Also, some enteric bacteria are inhibited, including *Escherichia coli*, Klebsiella, Salmonella, Shigella, and Enterobacter species. Unfortunately, many previously susceptible species' strains have developed resistance. Among the FDA-approved indications are acute infective exacerbation of chronic bronchitis, otitis media (only in children), prevention and treatment of travelers' diarrhea, UTIs, Shigellosis, prophylaxis, and therapy of *Pneumocystis pneumonia* and Toxoplasmosis [29,159].

7. Five-Membered Heterocycles Containing One Sulfur Atom

Tiophene

Thiophene is a five-membered unsaturated aromatic heterocycle often referred to as furan's sulfur analog (Table 2) [1]. The sulfur atom's presence has a specific impact on the aromatic nature of the compound as well as its characteristics and reactions. In the π electron system, sulfur's "electron pairs" are strongly delocalized and behave as highly reactive, similar to a benzene derivative [160].

Thiophene exhibits an electron cloud, making it similarly reactive to benzene. Due to the weakly electronegative sulfur atom, it is the least reactive to the action of electrophilic agents when compared to furan and pyrrole. However, compared to benzene, its electrophilic substitutions occur significantly more quickly [1,161]. The bioisosterism link between thiophene and benzene is explained by the discovery of thiophene as an impurity in benzene and the remarkable similarity between the two chemicals' physicochemical features. Therefore, thiophene can be effectively used to replace the benzene nucleus in the structure of molecules of medicinal interest as a bioequivalent [160].

Chemical structures known as structural alerts or toxicophores can be bioactivated to produce reactive metabolites. Le Dang N. et al. (2017) indicated that the thiophene structural alert is unclear. Currently, it is known that thiophenes can be bioactivated by epoxidation. Different oxidative metabolic processes can convert thiophenes into electrophilic, unstable intermediates such as S-oxides, epoxides, and sulfenic acids. Toxicity can result from the oxidative metabolism of thiophenes, which produces reactive, electrophilic intermediates [139].

Thiophene is found in various natural compounds, such as biotin (vitamin H) [1]. The biological activity of thiophene and its derivatives include antiviral, antifungal, antibacterial, antileishmanial, antimicrotubule, anti-inflammatory, antioxidant, anticancer, and anti-HIV effects. Because of these effects, thiophene is a critical structural component in several therapeutically relevant drugs [161,162].

Beta-Lactam Antibiotics

Carboxypenicillins

The presence of an extra carboxyl group at the acylamino group (at the C6 position) of these semisynthetic penicillins led to the generic name of carboxypenicillins. Compared to other penicillins, the carboxyl moiety enhances the molecule's ability to penetrate through Gram-negative bacilli's cell wall barriers. Carboxypenicillins are typically used to treat infections produced by Gram-negative, ampicillin-resistant bacilli [29]. Two carboxypenicillins containing thiophene in the molecular structure are ticarcillin and their analog, temocillin.

Ticarcillin. Ticarcillin, (2*S*,5*R*,6*R*)-6-[[(2*R*)-2-carboxy-2-thiophen-3-ylacetyl]amino]-3,3-dimethyl-7-oxo-4-thia-1-azabicyclo [3.2.0]heptane-2-carboxylic acid, is an isostere of carbenicillin in which a thiophene heterocycle substitutes the phenyl. It is also known as α-carboxy-3-thienylpenicillin (Figure 26a) and is formulated as a disodium salt. Because this semisynthetic penicillin derivative is unstable in acid, parenteral administration is required [29]. Ticarcillin is a fourth-generation extended-spectrum penicillin previously used to treat mild to severe infections caused by sensitive Gram-positive and Gram-negative organisms. Ticarcillin's broad spectrum made it a suitable antibiotic against *Pseudomonas aeruginosa*. Additionally, ticarcillin exhibits efficacy against a few Enterobacter and Proteus species. Ticarcillin is active against most bacteria susceptible to natural penicillins but is frequently less effective [163].

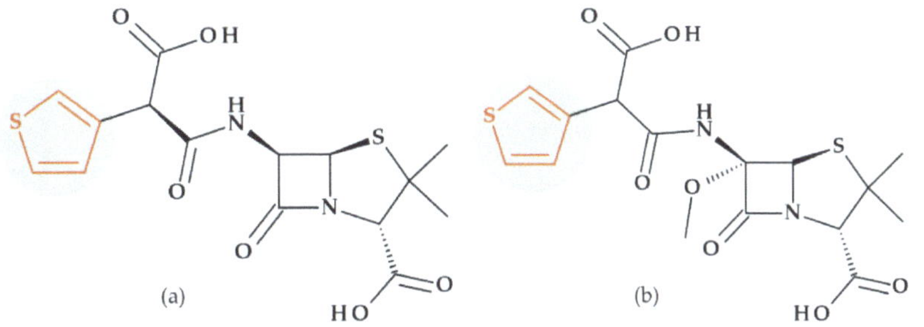

Figure 26. Carboxypenicillins including thiophene heterocycle in their molecular structures: (**a**) Ticarcillin and (**b**) Temocillin.

This semisynthetic penicillin is less effective than piperacillin (a ureidopenicillin) but more effective than carbenicillin against *Pseudomonas aeruginosa*. A combination of ticarcillin and clavulanate has been used to treat intra-abdominal UTIs and has activity against Gram-negative aerobic and anaerobic pathogens. Currently, ticarcillin and its combination with clavulanate are no longer manufactured [118]. In 2004, ticarcillin was withdrawn from the United States (US) market [163].

Temocillin. In the 1980s, the semisynthetic 6-methoxy derivative of ticarcillin, known as temocillin, (2*S*,5*R*,6*S*)-6-[(2-carboxy-2-thiophen-3-ylacetyl)amino]-6-methoxy-3,3-dimethyl-7-oxo-4-thia-1-azabicyclo [3.2.0]heptane-2-carboxylic acid (Figure 26b), was commercialized in Belgium and the United Kingdom [164]. Temocillin was immediately discontinued because of what was considered to be significant limitations, including a lack of action against anaerobes, *Pseudomonas aeruginosa*, and Gram-positive pathogens [12]. Although temocillin is an old antibiotic, given its unique properties, it may be an efficient substitute for carbapenems when treating infections caused by Enterobacteriaceae that produce extended-spectrum beta-lactamase (ESBL) and uncomplicated UTIs caused by carbapenemase-producing *Klebsiella pneumoniae* (KPC) producers [164].

Cephalosporins

Cephaloridine (Cefaloridine) (1st generation). Cephaloridine, (6R,7R)-8-oxo-3-(pyridin-1-ium-1-ylmethyl)-7-[(2-thiophen-2-ylacetyl)amino]-5-thia-1-azabicyclo [4.2.0]oct-2-ene-2-carboxylate (Figure 27a) was the first successful semisynthetic cephalosporin [165]. Cephaloridine has properties comparable to cephalotin, briefly discussed below [123]. Thus, cefaloridine was the first cephalosporin with noticeable dose-related nephrotoxicity. Cephaloridine builds up in the proximal renal tubular cell, most likely through active anionic transport [166]. It is not available for therapeutic purposes due to the availability of newer cephalosporins and concerns about potential side effects and bacterial resistance [123].

Cephalothin (*Cefalotin*) (1st generation). The first-generation cephalosporins have moderate effectiveness against Gram-negative bacteria but considerable efficacy against Gram-positive bacteria [118]. Structurally, cephalothin is 7-(thiophene-2-acetamido) cephalosporanic acid, respectively (6*R*,7*R*)-3-[(acetyloxy)methyl]-8-oxo-7-[2-(thiophen-2-yl)acetamido]-5-thia-1-azabicyclo [4.2.0]oct-2-ene-2-carboxylic acid (Figure 27b) [167]. In the presence of sodium bicarbonate, cephalothin was produced through the direct reaction of the 2-

thienylacetic acid chloride with 7-aminocephalosporanic acid [117]. The spectrum of activity of cephalothin is more comparable to ampicillin than benzylpenicillin. Cephalothin, in contrast to ampicillin, is resistant to the penicillinase produced by *Staphylococcus aureus*, offering an option for the use of penicillins that are penicillinase-resistant for the treatment of infections produced by such strains [29]. Cephalothin has been used to treat various blood, bone or joints, respiratory tract, skin, and UTI infections and to avoid infection during surgery [117,168]. In therapy, it has currently been replaced by new generations of cephalosporins.

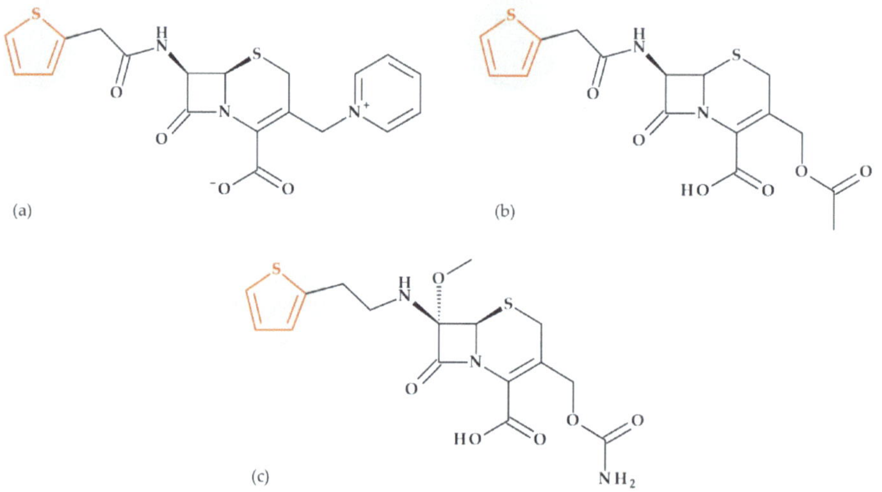

Figure 27. Cephalosporins including thiophene heterocycle in their molecular structures: (**a**) Cephaloridine, (**b**) Cephalotine, and (**c**) Cefoxitin.

Cefoxitin (2nd generation). Among beta-lactamase–resistant 7-α-methoxy cephalosporins (cephamycins) is cefoxitin, (6*R*,7*S*)-3-(carbamoyloxymethyl)-7-methoxy-8-oxo-7-[(2-thiophen-2-ylacetyl)amino]-5-thia-1-azabicyclo [4.2.0]oct-2-ene-2-carboxylic acid [29], a compound that contains a thiophene heterocycle in the side chain from the C6 position (Figure 27c). One of the first cephamycins available was cefoxitin (as sodium salt) [123]. The ability of cefoxitin (and cephamycins in general) to kill resistant bacterial strains is due to the 7-α-methoxyl substituent's protection against hydrolysis by beta-lactamases. Even though cefoxitin is less effective than cephalothin against Gram-positive bacteria and cefamandole against the majority of Enterobacteriaceae, it is nevertheless effective against some strains of Gram-negative bacteria that are resistant to these cephalosporins. *Neisseria gonorrhoeae* and penicillin-resistant *Staphylococcus aureus* are also resistant to it. A disadvantage of cefoxitin is its short half-live (about one hour), and therefore, cefoxitin needs to be parenterally given three to four times daily [29,123].

8. Five-Membered Heterocycles Containing Sulfur and Nitrogen Atoms

8.1. 1,3-Thiazolidine

1,3-Thiazolidine is a saturated five-membered heterocycle with sulfur and nitrogen in positions 1 and 3, respectively (Table 2); it is considered an analog of oxazolidine [161]. When thiazolidines are present in an acidic or basic aqueous solution, they hydrolyze to form aldehyde and amino thiol. The production of an iminium thiolate zwitterion intermediate has led researchers to conclude that the reaction involves breaking the C-S bond. Thiazolidines can be hydrolyzed to aldehydes under neutral conditions with metal ions such as Hg(II) or Cu(II). The existence of this moiety in penicillin derivatives was the main motive for the mechanistic research of thiazolidine ring opening [169].

Beta-Lactam Antibiotics: Natural and Semisynthetic Penicillins

The penicillin antibiotics contain a fused ring system, a substituted five-membered thiazolidine ring fused to the beta-lactam ring (cyclic amide with four atoms) [29,31], essential for antibacterial activity. This heterocycle proved to be the main component of the pharmacophore [31]. Penicillin's unsubstituted bicyclic ring structure is named "penam" because it makes it simpler to comprehend (Figure 28a). The penicillins are referred to as 4-thia-1-azabicyclo (3.2.0) heptanes (Figure 28b) [153].

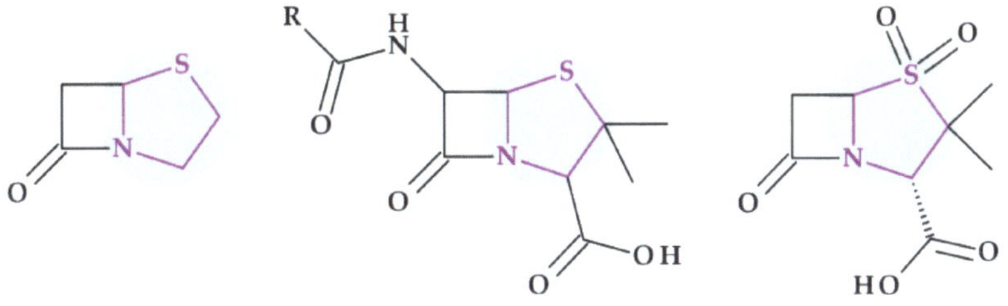

Figure 28. The thiazolidine heterocycle (purple) depiction in (**a**) Penam bicycle, (**b**) Penicillins molecular structure, and (**c**) Sulbactam.

Sulbactam, (2*S*,5R)-3,3-dimethyl-4,4,7-trioxo-4λ^6-thia-1-azabicyclo [3.2.0]heptane-2-carboxylic acid, is penicillanic acid sulfone. The 1,3-thiazolidine 1,1-dioxide is a fragment of the central core of sulbactam, which replaced thiazolidine in the "penam" heterocycle of penicillins (Figure 28c) [104].

Sulbactam is a potent inhibitor of beta-lactamases produced by *Staphylococcus aureus* and Gram-negative bacilli. While it has limited antibacterial activity, it enhances the effectiveness of ampicillin and carbenicillin against beta-lactamase-producing *Staphylococcus aureus* and certain species in the Enterobacteriaceae family. However, it does not synergize with carbenicillin or ticarcillin on *Pseudomonas aeruginosa* strains resistant to these drugs [29].

Xacduro® (sulbactam for injection and durlobactam for injection), a recent drug approved by the FDA in 2023, was previously discussed in Section 4.4.1. Sulbactam is responsible for activity against *Acinetobacter baumannii*, whereas durlobactam protects sulbactam from being degraded by beta-lactamases that may be produced by *Acinetobacter baumannii* [100].

8.2. 1,3-Thiazole

With one sulfur atom and one nitrogen atom of the pyridine type at position 3 of the cyclic ring system, thiazole is a five-membered, unsaturated, planar, and excessive heteroaromatic (Table 2) [1,22]. Thiazole is believed to be generated from thiophene by substituting a pyridine-type nitrogen (azomethine) at position 3 for the -CH= group. The structure of thiazole is quite comparable to the average of the structures of thiophene and 1,3,4-thiadiazole, although it is predicted to be structurally related to thiophene and pyridine. Therefore, it is anticipated that the chemical reactions of thiazole will be comparable to those of pyridine and thiophene [1] due to the presence of thiophene-type sulfur at position 1 and pyridine-type nitrogen at position 3 of the thiazole ring. Electrophilic reactions have three possible sites: sulfur, nitrogen, and the C5 position. Though, the electronically weak site C2 is vulnerable to nucleophilic assault [22].

Thiazole is considered a planar, aromatic ring due to the delocalization of a pair of nonparticipating electrons from the sulfur atom (position 1). It has an excess of π electrons concentrated on the heteroatoms. Given this, electrophilic attacks will occur at the 1, 3, 4, and 5 positions, and nucleophilic attacks will appear at the C2 position [22,170,171].

According to molecular orbital calculations, the thiazole molecule is aromatic with some dienic characteristics. Thiazole's ring current corresponds to its aromatic nature [1].

Considering acid-base properties, thiazole (pKa of 2.5) is a weak base compared to pyridine (pKa of 5.2) but is more basic than oxazole (pKa of 0.8) [1]. The compound is miscible with water. It can form stable salts with strong acids by protonating the imine nitrogen (position 3) [25,161]. Thiazole is a substance that is highly stable and does not autoxidize. By protonating the imine nitrogen, thiazole forms stable crystalline salts with strong acids known as thiazolium salts [25].

There are many natural substances having thiazole rings exhibiting diverse biological properties. For example, vitamin B1 (thiamine) has a thiazole ring connected to 2-methylpyrimidine-4-amine [22]. Additionally, many thiazole synthetic derivatives have pharmacological activity. Numerous thiazole-containing drugs are successfully utilized in therapy [172]. Other compounds are in various stages of development [172–175]. Among antibacterials, several beta-lactam antibiotics and sulphonamides include thiazole in their molecular structure [1,172].

8.2.1. Beta-Lactam Antibiotics

Cephalosporins

Cephalosporins' aminoacyl moiety appears to become more stable against some beta-lactamases' action when polar substituents are added [29]. Various heterocycles associated with better pharmacokinetics and antibacterial activity can take place in the side chain of cephalosporins; amino-thiazoles are among these (Table 5) [153,172]. Unusual, cefditoren, a third-generation cephalosporin, contains an extra thiazole heterocycle at the C3 position as a 4-methyl-1,3-thiazol moiety. The antibacterial activity of cefditoren is similar to cefixime. In addition, cefditoren is efficient against *Staphylococcus aureus* [123].

Monobactams

Unlike penicillins and cephalosporins, which fuse the four-membered antibacterial beta-lactam structure to another heterocyclic ring, monobactams contain unfused beta-lactam heterocycle. It represents the most basic beta-lactam with antibacterial properties [165]. Including an aminothiazole oxime side chain as the 3-acyl substituent, typical to several third-generation cephalosporins, they have resulted in the most notable increase in Gram-negative antibacterial activity. This fragment is responsible for the drugs' remarkable activity against Gram-negative bacteria through increased affinity for their PBPs. Aztreonam was the first monobactam generated through side-chain modifications [177]. Further, several antibacterial drugs with the (*S*)-3-[2-(2-aminothiazol-4-yl)-2-(oxyimino) acetamido]-2-oxoazetidine-1-sulfonate structure were developed. To further widen the antibacterial activity and improve the stability of beta-lactamase hydrolysis, several modifications have been added at the 3- or 4-position of the beta-lactam ring or the oxime side chain [177].

Aztreonam. The FDA and European regulatory agencies approved the monobactam antibiotic aztreonam in 1986 [178]. Aztreonam, 2-[(*Z*)-[1-(2-amino-1,3-thiazol-4-yl)-2-[[(2S,3S)-2-methyl-4-oxo-1-sulfoazetidin-3-yl]amino]-2-oxoethylidene]amino]oxy-2-methylpropanoic acid, has been created using a total synthesis [29]. Antibacterial spectrum and resistance to beta-lactamases are determined by the 3-side chain amino thiazolyl oxime moiety and the 4-methyl group (Figure 29a) [29]. Aztreonam only presents a strong affinity for PBP 3 in Gram-negative bacteria but has no activity against Gram-positive bacteria and anaerobes. Beta-lactamase resistance is similar to ceftazidime's, which possesses the same isobutyric acid oximinoacyl moiety [29]. Thus, the beta-lactamases with a broad spectrum hydrolyze aztreonam [165]. In the past, aztreonam was mainly used to treat infections of the lower respiratory tract, the urinary tract, and intra-abdominal infections, as well as septicemia, endometritis, pelvic cellulitis, and infections of the skin and skin structures caused by aerobic Gram-negative bacteria [178]. Although it is considered an old antibiotic, aztreonam has become a particular area of interest when combined with beta-lactamase inhibitors and other antimicrobials [179].

Table 5. Cephalosporins containing a 2-amin-1,3 thiazole heterocycle in the 7-acyl side chain [21,29,123,176].

No.	Cephalosporin	Generation	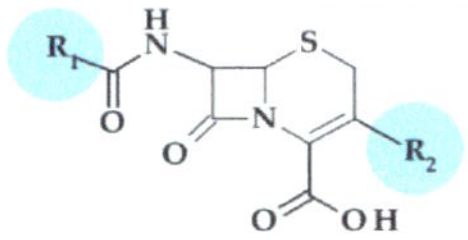 R1	R2	Administration	$t_{1/2}$ (Hours)	Acid Resistant	Resistance to β-lactamases	Antibacterial Spectrum	Activity against *Pseudomonas* sp.
1	Cefpodoxime (proxetil)	3rd	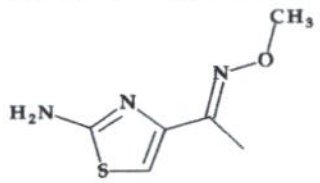	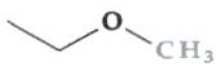	Oral	2.2	Yes	Good	Extended	No
2	Cefotaxime	3rd	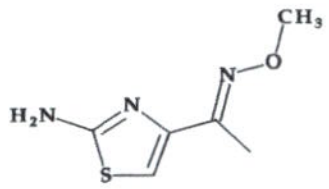	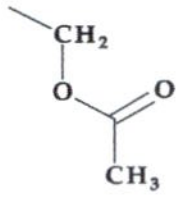	Parenteral	1	No	Good	Extended	Yes
3	Ceftazidime	3rd	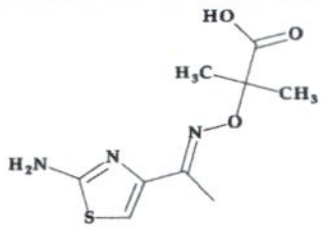	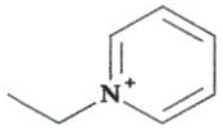	Parenteral	2	No	Good	Extended	Yes
4	Ceftriaxone	3rd	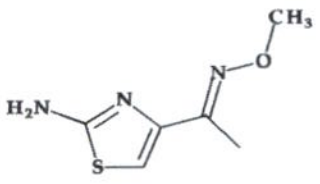	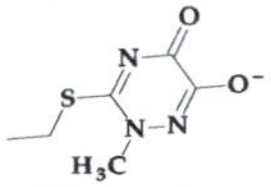	Parenteral	6–9	No	Good	Extended	Yes
5	Cefixime	3rd	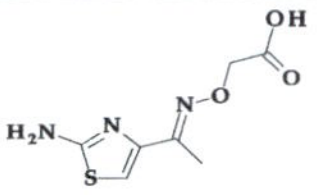	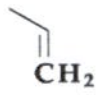	Oral	3–4	Yes	Good	Extended	No
6	Cefdinir	3rd	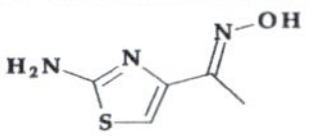	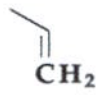	Oral	1.7	Yes	Good	Extended	No

Table 5. *Cont.*

7	Cefditoren (pivoxil)	3rd	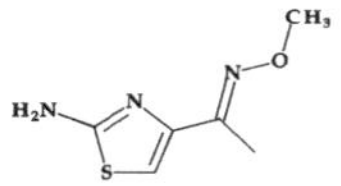	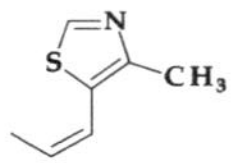	Oral	1.6	Yes	Good	Extended	No
8	Ceftibuten	3rd	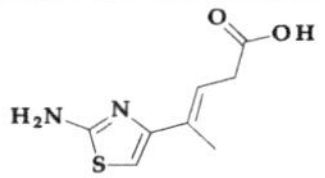	-H	Oral	2–2.3	Yes	Good	Extended	No
9	Ceftizoxime	3rd	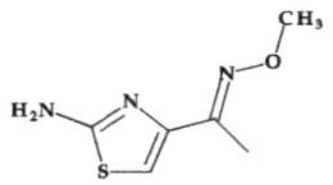	-H	Parenteral	1.7	No	Good	Extended	Yes
10	Cefepime	4th	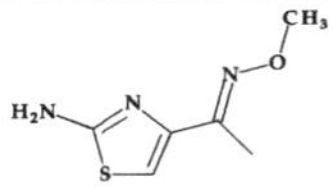	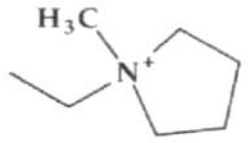	Parenteral	2	No	Good	Extended	Yes
11	Cefpirome	4th	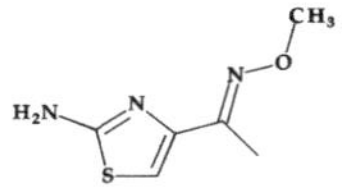	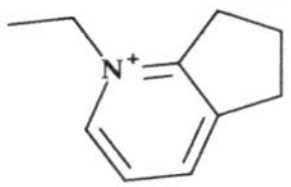	Parenteral	2	No	Good	Extended	Yes

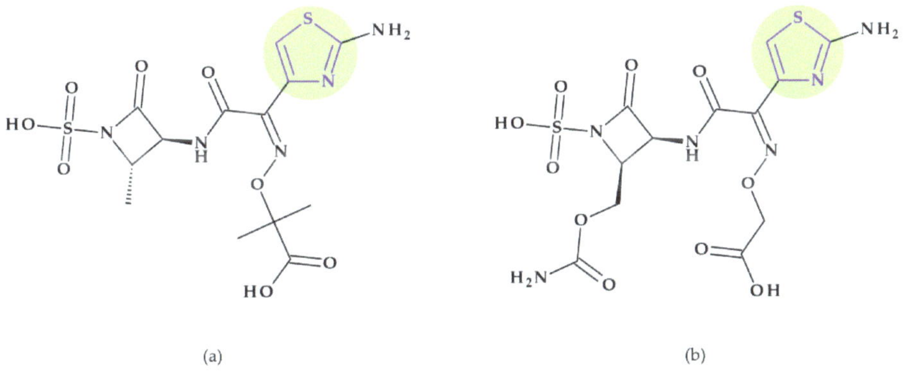

Figure 29. The thiazole heterocycle (purple) depiction in (**a**) Aztreonam and (**b**) Carumonam molecular structure.

Carumonam. Carumonam, 2-[(Z)-[1-(2-amino-1,3-thiazol-4-yl)-2-[[(2S,3S)-2-(carbamoyl oxymethyl)-4-oxo-1-sulfoazetidin-3-yl]amino]-2-oxoethylidene]amino]oxyacetic acid, is an N-sulfonated monobactam (Figure 29b) that is relatively stable against beta-lactamases. When a carbamoyloxymethyl group was added in a 3,4-cis configuration at the 4-position, the antibacterial activity against Gram-negative bacteria, including strains that produce beta-lactamases, was greatly improved. It has a similar broad antibacterial spectrum to aztreonam against common bacteria like Enterobacteriaceae, *Pseudomonas aeruginosa*, and *Haemophilus influenzae* [177,180]. When those pathogen agents produce respiratory or urinary tract infections, carumonam is a therapy option [180].

Some monobactams containing 1,3-thiazole, such as pirazmonam and tigemonam, are under development.

Pirazmonam. The first monocyclic β-lactam-siderophore conjugate prepared from the monobactams was pirazmonam, 2-[(Z)-[1-(2-amino-1,3-thiazol-4-yl)-2-[[1-[[3-[(5-hydroxy -4-oxo-1H-pyridine-2-carbonyl)amino]-2-oxoimidazolidin-1-yl]sulfonylcarbamoyl]-2-oxoazetidin-3-yl]amino]-2-oxoethylidene]amino]oxy-2-methylpropanoic acid (Figure 30a). The new compound had a 3-hydroxy-4-pyridone iron-chelating fragment included in the N1-activating group. Thus, it retained many beneficial properties characteristic of aztreonam but had significantly improved activity against *Pseudomonas aeruginosa* [177].

Tigemonam. Tigemonam, 2-[(Z)-[1-(2-amino-1,3-thiazol-4-yl)-2-[[(3S)-2,2-dimethyl-4-oxo-1-sulfooxyazetidin-3-yl]amino]-2-oxoethylidene]amino]oxyacetic acid (Figure 30b), is an oral monobactam; its oral absorption is excellent in comparison to the poor oral bioavailability of aztreonam. Moreover, it exhibits a strong resistance against beta-lactamases. Tigemonam demonstrates a similar antibacterial effectiveness as aztreonam. However, it is not highly effective against Gram-positive or anaerobic bacteria and has no activity against *Pseudomonas aeruginosa* [29].

8.2.2. Sulphonamides

Sulfathiazole. Sulphathiazole, 4-amino-N-(1,3-thiazol-2-yl)benzenesulfonamide, includs a 1,3-thiazole heterocycle (Figure 31a). Further, its derivatives, including succinylsulphathiazole monohydrate and phthalylsulphathiazole, have been developed [181]. Sulfathiazole is a sulfonamide with a short half-life (8 h) and characteristics comparable to sulfamethoxazole (Section 6.2.3). Due to its toxicity, it is rarely systemically utilized [29,123]. Later, sulfadiazine replaced sulfathiazole due to its broad antibacterial range, potent in vivo activity, low toxicity, and relatively long duration of action [182]. Thus, sulfathiazole is used with other medications to treat skin infections. It is used in formulations for the topical treatment of vaginal infections. For treating ocular infections, sulfathiazole sodium has been topically administered with other medications [123].

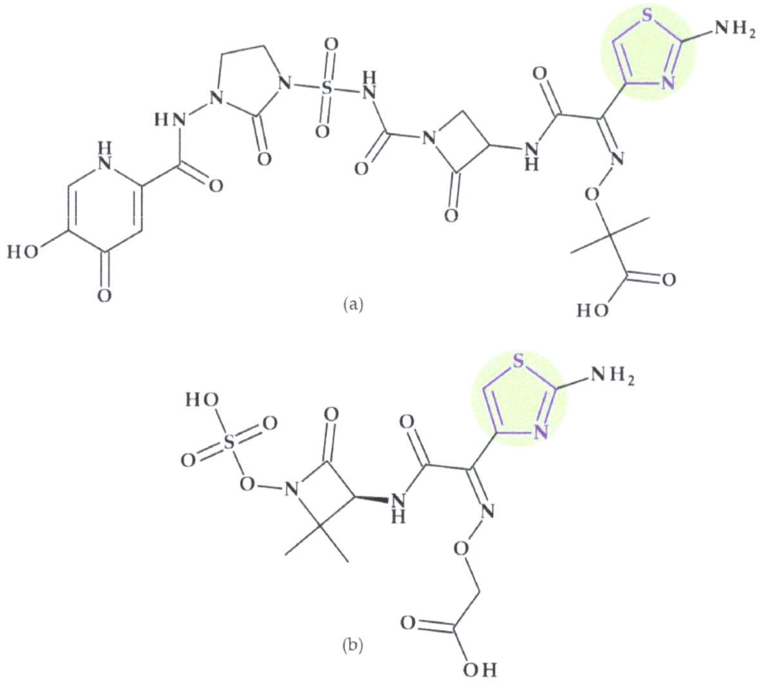

Figure 30. The thiazole heterocycle (purple) depiction in (**a**) Pirazmonam and (**b**) Tigemonam molecular structure.

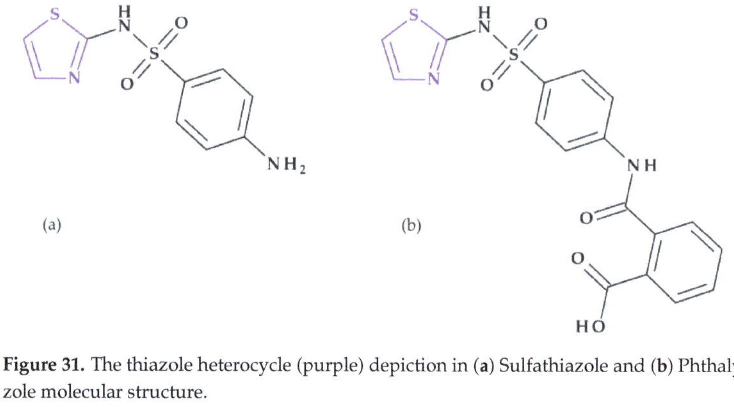

Figure 31. The thiazole heterocycle (purple) depiction in (**a**) Sulfathiazole and (**b**) Phthalylsulfathiazole molecular structure.

Phthalylsulfathiazole. Phthalylsulfathiazole, 2-[[4-(1,3-thiazol-2-ylsulfamoyl)phenyl] carbamoyl] benzoic acid, is an N4-acylated sulfonamide (Figure 31b). It is considered a prodrug of sulfathiazole containing a phthalic acid residue at the N4 position [183]. Sulfathiazole is released from phthalylsulfathiazole by bacterial enzymes in the colon through amide hydrolysis [31]. Only around 5% of phthalylsulfathiazole is slowly hydrolyzed to sulfathiazole and is absorbed, leaving about 95% in the colon. It is administered with other antibacterials to treat gastrointestinal tract infections and clean the bowels before surgery [123,183].

8.3. Thiadiazoles

Thiadiazoles are five-membered, aromatic, weakly basic, planar, electron-deficient heterocyclic ring systems composed of two carbon atoms, one sulfur atom, and two nitrogen atoms (Table 2). Four non-interconvertible regioisomeric configurations of thiadiazole are achievable: 1,2,3-, 1,2,4-, 1,2,5-, and 1,3,4-thiadiazole [24,184,185]. Among them, 1,2,4-thiadiazoles and 1,3,4-thiadiazoles are found in the structure of some antibacterial compounds.

- *1,2,4-Thiadiazoles.* A five-membered, unsaturated, conjugated heteroaromatic with one sulfur atom and two nitrogen atoms, one of which is next to the sulfur and the other of which is one carbon distinct from it, is known as 1,2,4-thiadiazole. It is a π-excessive ring though relatively π deficient at the two carbon atoms. The nucleophilic substitution is easy at the C5 position due to the lowest π-electron density [24]. In nucleophilic substitution reactions, the C5 position of 1,2,4-thiadiazoles is the most reactive. The 1,2,4-thiadiazoles exhibit extremely few electrophilic reactions. Considering acid-base properties, 1,2,4-thiadiazoles are weak bases. They produce salts with mineral acids, and with heavy metal salts generate additional compounds [186]. Derivatives of 1,2,4-thiadiazoles are useful as antibiotics, cysteine protease inhibitors (cysteine protease cathepsin K), melanocortin-4-receptor agonists, and modulators of adenosine A3 receptors. Also, agrochemicals such as pesticides, soil fungicides, lubricating greases and vulcanization agents are found as derivatives of 1,2,4-thiadiazoles [24,186,187].
- *1,3,4-Thiadiazoles.* 1,3,4-Thiadiazoles are a five-membered, aromatic, weakly basic, planar, electron-deficient heterocyclic ring system composed of two carbon atoms, one sulfur atom, and two nitrogen atoms that resemble pyridine in the N3- and N4-positions of the ring. The 1,3,4-thiadiazole's dipole moment indicates that it is a polar, symmetric molecule with pseudo-aromatic properties. Due to the inductive influence of nitrogen and sulfur, the carbon atoms at the C2- and C5-positions are electron deficient, so they're inert to electrophilic substitution but reactive to nucleophilic attack. The high aromaticity of the ring and the inductive action of sulfur are responsible for the 1,3,4-thiadiazole's weak basicity. In aqueous acidic media, it is relatively stable. However, in an aqueous base, it does not undergo ring cleavage [24]. Numerous medications, including antibiotic, anti-inflammatory, anti-hypertensive, anti-HIV, anti-depressant, local anesthetic, and anti-convulsant drugs, have been discovered based on the 1,3,4-thiadiazole ring [24,29,184].

8.3.1. Beta-Lactam Antibiotics

Cefalosporins

A 1,2,4-thiadiazole ring is included in the chemical structure of three fourth-generation cephalosporins: cefozopran, ceftaroline fosamil, and ceftobiprole. The 1,2,4-thiadiazole moiety has been added to modulate the pharmacokinetic characteristics of these antibiotics [186]. In addition, the 1,2,4-thiadiazole enables these cephalosporins to penetrate Gram-negative bacteria and promote transpeptidase action [188,189].

Cefozopran (4th generation). Cefozopran, (6*R*,7*R*)-7-[[(2Z)-2-(5-amino-1,2,4-thiadiazol-3-yl)-2-methoxyiminoacetyl]amino]-3-(imidazo [1,2-b]pyridazin-1-ium-1-ylmethyl)-8-oxo-5-thia-1-azabicyclo [4.2.0]oct-2-ene-2-carboxylate, is a parenteral fourth-generation cephalosporin used as the hydrochloride salt in Japan since the late (Figure 32a) 1990s [123,190,191]. Cefozopran is characterized by a broad spectrum activity against Gram-positive and Gram-negative bacteria. Also, cefozopran exhibits potent activity against Enterococci and *Pseudomonas aeruginosa*, two bacteria resistant to other cephalosporins. Clinically, cefozopran has been approved for the parenteral treatment of various adult patients, including pneumonia, sepsis, urinary tract infections, and intra-abdominal infections [191].

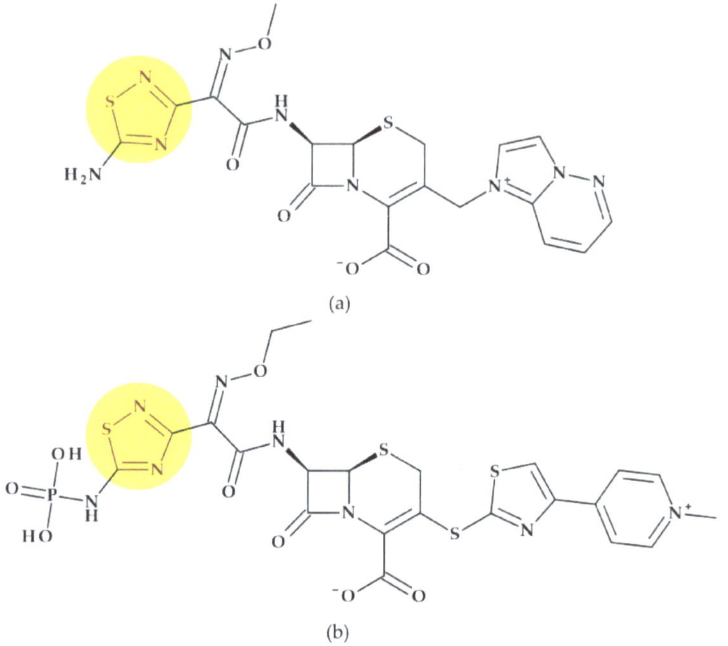

Figure 32. Cephalosporins including thiadiazole heterocycle in their molecular structures: (**a**) Cefozopran, and (**b**) Ceftaroline fosamil.

Ceftaroline fosamil (5th generation). Ceftaroline fosamil, (6*R*,7*R*)-7-[[(2*Z*)-2-ethoxyimino-2-[5-(phosphonoamino)-1,2,4-thiadiazol-3-yl]acetyl]amino]-3-[[4-(1-methylpyridin-1-ium-4-yl)-1,3-thiazol-2-yl]sulfanyl]-8-oxo-5-thia-1-azabicyclo [4.2.0]oct-2-ene-2-carboxylate, is a cephalosporin antibiotic from the fifth-generation (Figure 32b) [192,193]. The prodrug ceftaroline fosamil is transformed in vivo into ceftaroline, the active metabolite. An additional phosphonic group in the chemical structure of ceftaroline fosamil is the component that confers its name. The advantage of the resulting prodrug is the increased water solubility [188]. Based on the structure of fourth-generation cefozopran, ceftaroline is an oxyimino compound [188,193]. The enhanced action against MRSA is achieved by the existence of the oxime group in the C7 acyl moiety and a 1,3-thiazole ring linked to the central ore (C3 position) [188]. Both common Gram-negative (G(-)) and Gram-positive (G(+)) pathogens, such as MRSA and *Streptococcus pneumoniae*, are susceptible to ceftaroline fosamil [188,193]. Ceftaroline fosamil has received approval to treat ABSSSI and CABP [194].

Ceftobiprole (4th generation). Ceftobiprole was briefly discussed in Section 4.1.1 regarding beta-lactam antibiotics, including pyrrole in their molecular structure (Figure 3a). Its C7-side chain contains a 5-amino-1,2,4-thiadiazole heterocycle.

A representative from the class of cephalosporins includes in its chemical structure a 1,3,4-thiadiazole ring.

Cefazolin (1st generation). This first-generation cephalosporin was previously briefly discussed in Section 4.5.1. In addition to the tetrazole heterocycle from the C7-side-chain, cefazolin contains a [(5-methyl-1,3,4-thiadiazol-2-yl)sulfanylmethyl] fragment at C3 position (Figure 14a) that resembles vitamin-K antagonists in certain respects [195]. To obtain this cephalosporin, this structural fragment has replaced the C3 acetoxy function, including a 1,3,4-thiadiazole heterocycle [29]. Among the adverse reactions of cefazolin that have been reported are coagulation issues linked to hypovitaminosis K. These effects would be exacerbated in impaired renal function when high doses are administered, resulting in the accumulation of its active metabolite. According to some researchers, certain cefazolin-treated patients may benefit from systematic vitamin-K therapy [195].

8.3.2. Sulfonamides

Furthermore, one member of the sulphonamide class has a 1,3,4-thiadiazole ring in its chemical structure.

Sulfamethizole. Sulfamethizole is known as 4-amino-N-(5-methyl-1,3,4-thiadiazol-2-yl)benzenesulfonamide (Figure 33) [29]. Approximately 90% of sulfamethizole has been bound to plasma proteins and is easily absorbed from the gastrointestinal system. The half-life of this sulfonamide is between 1.5 and 3 h (a short-acting sulfonamide). Sulfamethizole was orally used to treat urinary tract infections, often combined with other antibacterials. However, because the drug only reaches relatively low concentrations in the blood and tissues, it is ineffective in treating systemic infections [123].

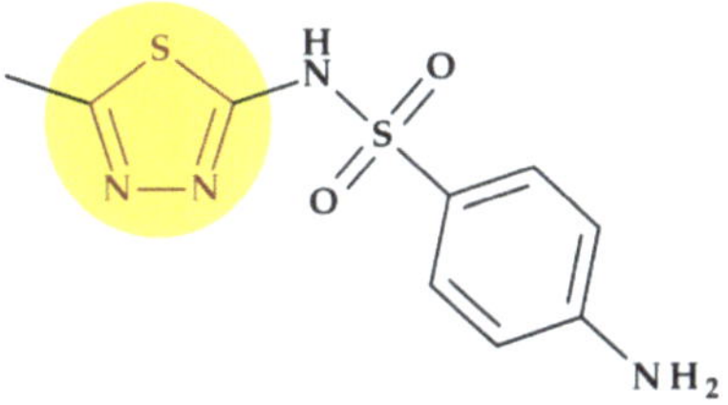

Figure 33. Sulfamethizole molecular structure highlighting 1,3,4-thiadiazole ring.

9. Conclusions

The role of five-membered heterocycles in the molecular structure of antibacterial drugs used in therapy is a highly relevant and promising area of research in medicinal chemistry and pharmaceutical sciences. Designing antibacterial compounds heavily relies on heterocycles. Incorporating five-membered heterocycles into drug molecules holds promise for improving the antibacterial activity of these drugs. These heterocyclic rings introduce critical structural elements that enable interactions with specific bacterial targets, potentially increasing the efficacy of antibacterial therapies. We have identified the classes of antibacterials of which some representatives include in their molecular structure one or more five-membered heterocycles such as beta-lactam antibiotics, beta-lactamase inhibitors, antibacterial fluoroquinolones, lincosamides, macrolides, nitroimidazoles, oxazolidinones, streptogramins, sulfonamides, and tetracyclines.

The five-membered heterocycles used in antibacterial design contain one to four heteroatoms such as nitrogen, oxygen, or sulfur atoms. We identified in the structure of antibacterials five-membered heterocycles containing:

- One or more nitrogen atoms: pyrrolidine, imidazole, 2-imidazolidinone, 1,2,3-triazole, and tetrazole;
- One oxygen atom: furan;
- Oxygen and nitrogen atoms: 1,3-oxazolidine, oxazole, and isoxazole;
- One sulfur atom: thiophene;
- One sulfur and nitrogen atoms: 1,3-thiazolidine, 1,3-thiazole, and thiadiazoles.

The physicochemical properties of a five-membered heterocycle can play an essential role in determining the biological activity of an antibacterial drug. These properties can affect the antibacterials' spectrum of activity and potency and their pharmacokinetic, pharmacologic, and toxicological properties. The size and shape of the heterocycle can influence its interaction with target bacterial enzymes, leading to different potency levels against specific bacteria. The presence of certain functional groups on the heterocycle can also impact its ability to penetrate through bacterial cell membranes, affecting its spectrum of activity.

Additionally, the physicochemical properties of the heterocycle can affect the antibacterials' pharmacokinetic characteristics. For example, pyrrolidine moiety increased the spectrum of activity against Gram-positive bacteria, including MRSA, and improved pharmacokinetic profile with increased half-life and bioavailability of fluoroquinolones. Triazole enhanced a compound's solubility and pharmacokinetic and pharmacodynamic features by creating hydrogen bonds (dipole-dipole interactions). Tetrazole acted as a bioisoster of natural amino acids and carboxylic acids, enhancing the pharmacokinetic profile of drugs with therapeutic efficacy. It lowered polarity and raised lipophilicity for improved membrane permeability. An oxazole heterocycle decreases the toxicity of a compound. The 1,2,4-thiadiazole addition to some cephalosporins, such as cefozopran and ceftaroline fosamil, modulates their pharmacokinetic characteristics. Furthermore, the physicochemical properties of the heterocycle can also influence the drug's pharmacologic and toxicological properties. Certain chemical features may contribute to specific biological effects, such as the inhibition of bacterial enzymes or disruption of essential cellular processes in bacteria.

Particular heterocycles can affect the drug's potential toxicity. Several examples are the pyrrolidine substituent in the C7 position of several fluoroquinolones associated with multiple side effects, tetrazolyl acetylamino moiety at the C7 position in some cephalosporins associated with a higher prevalence of hypoprothrombinemia, and pyridine-imidazole group in the telithromycin side chain associated with severe side effects (e.g. hepatotoxic effects).

In summary, an antibacterial with enhanced biological activity, pharmacokinetic profiles, and safety can be designed by comprehending and improving the physicochemical characteristics of the five-membered heterocycles. Incorporating five-membered heterocycles into the molecular structure of antibacterial drugs represents a promising avenue for advancing antibacterial drug development. It offers opportunities to enhance drug efficacy, safety, and diversity, which is crucial in the ongoing battle against bacterial infections and antibiotic resistance. Continued research in this area is essential to translating these promising findings into effective treatments that can benefit global public health.

Author Contributions: Conceptualization, A.R. and I.-M.M.; methodology, A.R. and I.-M.M.; software, A.R. and I.-M.M.; writing—original draft preparation, A.R., I.-M.M., L.U. and G.H.; writing—review and editing, A.R., L.U. and G.H.; visualization, L.U. and G.H.; supervision, A.R. and G.H. All authors have read and agreed to the published version of the manuscript.

Funding: This research received no external funding.

Conflicts of Interest: The authors declare no conflict of interest.

References

1. Gupta, R.R.; Kumar, M.; Gupta, V. *Heterocyclic Chemistry: Volume II: Five-Membered Heterocycles*; Springer Science & Business Media: Berlin/Heidelberg, Germany, 2013; ISBN 978-3-662-07757-3.
2. Gomtsyan, A. Heterocycles in Drugs and Drug Discovery. *Chem. Heterocycl. Comp.* **2012**, *48*, 7–10. [CrossRef]
3. Barreca, M.; Spanò, V.; Rocca, R.; Bivacqua, R.; Gualtieri, G.; Raimondi, M.V.; Gaudio, E.; Bortolozzi, R.; Manfreda, L.; Bai, R.; et al. Identification of Pyrrolo [3′,4′:3,4]Cyclohepta[1,2-d][1,2]Oxazoles as Promising New Candidates for the Treatment of Lymphomas. *Eur. J. Med. Chem.* **2023**, *254*, 115372. [CrossRef]
4. Grillone, K.; Riillo, C.; Rocca, R.; Ascrizzi, S.; Spanò, V.; Scionti, F.; Polerà, N.; Maruca, A.; Barreca, M.; Juli, G.; et al. The New Microtubule-Targeting Agent SIX2G Induces Immunogenic Cell Death in Multiple Myeloma. *Int. J. Mol. Sci.* **2022**, *23*, 10222. [CrossRef]
5. Lee, B.; Kim, D.G.; Lee, A.; Kim, Y.M.; Cui, L.; Kim, S.; Choi, I. Synthesis and Discovery of the First Potent Proteolysis Targeting Chimaera (PROTAC) Degrader of AIMP2-DX2 as a Lung Cancer Drug. *J. Enzym. Inhib. Med. Chem.* **2023**, *38*, 51–66. [CrossRef]
6. Bivacqua, R.; Barreca, M.; Spanò, V.; Raimondi, M.V.; Romeo, I.; Alcaro, S.; Andrei, G.; Barraja, P.; Montalbano, A. Insight into Non-Nucleoside Triazole-Based Systems as Viral Polymerases Inhibitors. *Eur. J. Med. Chem.* **2023**, *249*, 115136. [CrossRef]
7. Fesatidou, M.; Petrou, A.; Athina, G. Heterocycle Compounds with Antimicrobial Activity. *Curr. Pharm. Des.* **2020**, *26*, 867–904. [CrossRef] [PubMed]

8. Chinemerem Nwobodo, D.; Ugwu, M.C.; Oliseloke Anie, C.; Al-Ouqaili, M.T.S.; Chinedu Ikem, J.; Victor Chigozie, U.; Saki, M. Antibiotic Resistance: The Challenges and Some Emerging Strategies for Tackling a Global Menace. *J. Clin. Lab. Anal.* **2022**, *36*, e24655. [CrossRef]
9. Chin, K.W.; Michelle Tiong, H.L.; Luang-In, V.; Ma, N.L. An Overview of Antibiotic and Antibiotic Resistance. *Environ. Adv.* **2023**, *11*, 100331. [CrossRef]
10. Tacconelli, E.; Carrara, E.; Savoldi, A.; Harbarth, S.; Mendelson, M.; Monnet, D.L.; Pulcini, C.; Kahlmeter, G.; Kluytmans, J.; Carmeli, Y.; et al. Discovery, Research, and Development of New Antibiotics: The WHO Priority List of Antibiotic-Resistant Bacteria and Tuberculosis. *Lancet Infect. Dis.* **2018**, *18*, 318–327. [CrossRef] [PubMed]
11. Dutescu, I.A.; Hillier, S.A. Encouraging the Development of New Antibiotics: Are Financial Incentives the Right Way Forward? A Systematic Review and Case Study. *Infect. Drug Resist.* **2021**, *14*, 415–434. [CrossRef]
12. Livermore, D.M.; Tulkens, P.M. Temocillin Revived. *J. Antimicrob. Chemother.* **2008**, *63*, 243–245. [CrossRef] [PubMed]
13. Pulcini, C.; Bush, K.; Craig, W.A.; Frimodt-Møller, N.; Grayson, M.L.; Mouton, J.W.; Turnidge, J.; Harbarth, S.; Gyssens, I.C.; the ESCMID Study Group for Antibiotic Policies. Forgotten Antibiotics: An Inventory in Europe, the United States, Canada, and Australia. *Clin. Infect. Dis.* **2012**, *54*, 268–274. [CrossRef]
14. Miljković, N.; Polidori, P.; Kohl, S. Managing Antibiotic Shortages: Lessons from EAHP and ECDC Surveys. *Eur. J. Hosp. Pharm.* **2022**, *29*, 90–94. [CrossRef] [PubMed]
15. Urban-Chmiel, R.; Marek, A.; Stępień-Pyśniak, D.; Wieczorek, K.; Dec, M.; Nowaczek, A.; Osek, J. Antibiotic Resistance in Bacteria—A Review. *Antibiotics* **2022**, *11*, 1079. [CrossRef]
16. WHO Antibiotic Resistance. Available online: https://www.who.int/news-room/fact-sheets/detail/antibiotic-resistance (accessed on 20 July 2023).
17. Sun, G.; Zhang, Q.; Dong, Z.; Dong, D.; Fang, H.; Wang, C.; Dong, Y.; Wu, J.; Tan, X.; Zhu, P.; et al. Antibiotic Resistant Bacteria: A Bibliometric Review of Literature. *Front. Public Health* **2022**, *10*, 1002015. [CrossRef]
18. Research Center for Drug Evaluation and Drug Approvals and Databases. Available online: https://www.fda.gov/drugs/development-approval-process-drugs/drug-approvals-and-databases (accessed on 22 August 2023).
19. Research Center for Drug Evaluation and New Drugs at FDA: CDER's New Molecular Entities and New Therapeutic Biological Products. Available online: https://www.fda.gov/drugs/development-approval-process-drugs/new-drugs-fda-cders-new-molecular-entities-and-new-therapeutic-biological-products (accessed on 22 August 2023).
20. BIOVIA Draw for Academics. Available online: https://discover.3ds.com/biovia-draw-academic (accessed on 9 August 2023).
21. NIH PubChem. Available online: https://pubchem.ncbi.nlm.nih.gov/ (accessed on 12 July 2023).
22. Eicher, T.; Hauptmann, S. *The Chemistry of Heterocycles: Structure, Reactions, Syntheses and Applications*; Wiley: Hoboken, NJ, USA, 2002; ISBN 978-3-527-30887-3.
23. Vitaku, E.; Smith, D.T.; Njardarson, J.T. Analysis of the Structural Diversity, Substitution Patterns, and Frequency of Nitrogen Heterocycles among U.S. FDA Approved Pharmaceuticals. *S. FDA Approved Pharmaceuticals. J. Med. Chem.* **2014**, *57*, 10257–10274. [CrossRef] [PubMed]
24. Ji Ram, V.; Sethi, A.; Nath, M.; Pratap, R. Chapter 5—Five-Membered Heterocycles. In *The Chemistry of Heterocycles*; Ji Ram, V., Sethi, A., Nath, M., Pratap, R., Eds.; Elsevier: Amsterdam, The Netherlands, 2019; pp. 149–478. ISBN 978-0-08-101033-4.
25. Joule, J.A.; Mills, K. *Heterocyclic Chemistry*; Wiley: Hoboken, NJ, USA, 2010; ISBN 978-1-4051-3300-5.
26. Islam, M.T.; Mubarak, M.S. Pyrrolidine Alkaloids and Their Promises in Pharmacotherapy. *Adv. Tradit. Med.* **2020**, *20*, 13–22. [CrossRef]
27. Johari, S.A.; Mohtar, M.; Syed Mohammad, S.A.; Sahdan, R.; Shaameri, Z.; Hamzah, A.S.; Mohammat, M.F. In Vitro Inhibitory and Cytotoxic Activity of MFM 501, a Novel Codonopsinine Derivative, against Methicillin-Resistant Staphylococcus Aureus Clinical Isolates. *Biomed. Res. Int.* **2015**, *2015*, 823829. [CrossRef]
28. Łowicki, D.; Przybylski, P. Tandem Construction of Biological Relevant Aliphatic 5-Membered N-Heterocycles. *Eur. J. Med. Chem.* **2022**, *235*, 114303. [CrossRef]
29. *Wilson and Gisvold's Textbook of Organic Medicinal and Pharmaceutical Chemistry*, 12th ed.; Beale, J.M., Jr.; Block, J.H. (Eds.) Wolters Kluwer Health: Baltimore, MD, USA, 2010; ISBN 978-0-7817-7929-6.
30. Papp-Wallace, K.M.; Endimiani, A.; Taracila, M.A.; Bonomo, R.A. Carbapenems: Past, Present, and Future. *Antimicrob. Agents Chemother.* **2011**, *55*, 4943–4960. [CrossRef]
31. Foye, W.O. *Foye's Principles of Medicinal Chemistry*; Lippincott Williams & Wilkins: Philadelphia, PA, USA, 2013; ISBN 978-1-4511-7572-1.
32. El-Lababidi, R.M.; Rizk, J.G. Cefiderocol: A Siderophore Cephalosporin. *Ann. Pharmacother.* **2020**, *54*, 1215–1231. [CrossRef] [PubMed]
33. Rusu, A.; Lungu, I.-A. The New Fifth-Generation Cephalosporins—A Balance between Safety and Efficacy. *Rom. J. Pharm. Pract.* **2020**, *13*, 121–126. [CrossRef]
34. Rusu, A.; Lungu, I.-A.; Moldovan, O.-L.; Tanase, C.; Hancu, G. Structural Characterization of the Millennial Antibacterial (Fluoro)Quinolones—Shaping the Fifth Generation. *Pharmaceutics* **2021**, *13*, 1289. [CrossRef] [PubMed]
35. Schinzer, W.C.; Bergren, M.S.; Aldrich, D.S.; Chao, R.S.; Dunn, M.J.; Jeganathan, A.; Madden, L.M. Characterization and Interconversion of Polymorphs of Premafloxacin, a New Quinolone Antibiotic. *J. Pharm. Sci.* **1997**, *86*, 1426–1431. [CrossRef] [PubMed]

36. Quinupristin-Dalfopristin. In *LiverTox: Clinical and Research Information on Drug-Induced Liver Injury*; National Institute of Diabetes and Digestive and Kidney Diseases: Bethesda, MD, USA, 2012.
37. Rusu, A.; Buta, E.L. The Development of Third-Generation Tetracycline Antibiotics and New Perspectives. *Pharmaceutics* **2021**, *13*, 2085. [CrossRef]
38. Smith, J.R.; Rybak, J.M.; Claeys, K.C. Imipenem-Cilastatin-Relebactam: A Novel β-Lactam–β-Lactamase Inhibitor Combination for the Treatment of Multidrug-Resistant Gram-Negative Infections. *Pharmacother. J. Hum. Pharmacol. Drug Ther.* **2020**, *40*, 343–356. [CrossRef]
39. Armstrong, T.; Fenn, S.J.; Hardie, K.R. JMM Profile: Carbapenems: A Broad-Spectrum Antibiotic. *J. Med. Microbiol.* **2021**, *70*, 001462. [CrossRef]
40. O'Connor, A.; Lopez, M.J.; Eranki, A.P. Cefepime. In *StatPearls*; StatPearls Publishing: Treasure Island, FL, USA, 2023.
41. Chapman, T.M.; Perry, C.M. Cefepime: A Review of Its Use in the Management of Hospitalized Patients with Pneumonia. *Am. J. Respir. Med.* **2003**, *2*, 75–107. [CrossRef]
42. Sato, T.; Yamawaki, K. Cefiderocol: Discovery, Chemistry, and In Vivo Profiles of a Novel Siderophore Cephalosporin. *Clin. Infect. Dis.* **2019**, *69*, S538–S543. [CrossRef]
43. FDA FETROJA (Cefiderocol) for Injection, for Intravenous Use. Available online: https://www.accessdata.fda.gov/drugsatfda_docs/label/2019/209445s000lbl.pdf (accessed on 23 June 2023).
44. Wu, J.Y.; Srinivas, P.; Pogue, J.M. Cefiderocol: A Novel Agent for the Management of Multidrug-Resistant Gram-Negative Organisms. *Infect. Dis. Ther.* **2020**, *9*, 17–40. [CrossRef]
45. Yamano, Y. In Vitro Activity of Cefiderocol Against a Broad Range of Clinically Important Gram-Negative Bacteria. *Clin. Infect. Dis.* **2019**, *69*, S544–S551. [CrossRef] [PubMed]
46. Ito, A.; Sato, T.; Ota, M.; Takemura, M.; Nishikawa, T.; Toba, S.; Kohira, N.; Miyagawa, S.; Ishibashi, N.; Matsumoto, S.; et al. In Vitro Antibacterial Properties of Cefiderocol, a Novel Siderophore Cephalosporin, against Gram-Negative Bacteria. *Antimicrob. Agents Chemother.* **2017**, *62*, e01454-17. [CrossRef] [PubMed]
47. Shionogi Use of Cefiderocol in the Management of Gram-Negative Infections (PERSEUS). Available online: https://www.clinicaltrials.gov/study/NCT05789199?term=cefiderocol&rank=2 (accessed on 27 June 2023).
48. El Solh, A. Ceftobiprole: A New Broad Spectrum Cephalosporin. *Expert. Opin. Pharmacother.* **2009**, *10*, 1675–1686. [CrossRef] [PubMed]
49. Giacobbe, D.R.; Rosa, F.G.D.; Bono, V.D.; Grossi, P.A.; Pea, F.; Petrosillo, N.; Rossolini, G.M.; Tascini, C.; Tumbarello, M.; Viale, P.; et al. Ceftobiprole: Drug Evaluation and Place in Therapy. *Expert Rev. Anti-Infect. Ther.* **2019**, *17*, 689–698. [CrossRef] [PubMed]
50. Morosini, M.-I.; Díez-Aguilar, M.; Cantón, R. Mechanisms of Action and Antimicrobial Activity of Ceftobiprole. *Rev. Esp. Quim.* **2019**, *32*, 3–10.
51. Shalaby, M.-A.W.; Dokla, E.M.E.; Serya, R.A.T.; Abouzid, K.A.M. Penicillin Binding Protein 2a: An Overview and a Medicinal Chemistry Perspective. *Eur. J. Med. Chem.* **2020**, *199*, 112312. [CrossRef]
52. Pham, T.D.M.; Ziora, Z.M.; Blaskovich, M.A.T. Quinolone Antibiotics. *Medchemcomm* **2019**, *10*, 1719–1739. [CrossRef]
53. Zhang, G.-F.; Zhang, S.; Pan, B.; Liu, X.; Feng, L.-S. 4-Quinolone Derivatives and Their Activities against Gram Positive Pathogens. *Eur. J. Med. Chem.* **2018**, *143*, 710–723. [CrossRef]
54. Rusu, A.; Munteanu, A.-C.; Arbănași, E.-M.; Uivarosi, V. Overview of Side-Effects of Antibacterial Fluoroquinolones: New Drugs versus Old Drugs, a Step Forward in the Safety Profile? *Pharmaceutics* **2023**, *15*, 804. [CrossRef]
55. Liu, J.; Ren, Z.; Fan, L.; Wei, J.; Tang, X.; Xu, X.; Yang, D. Design, Synthesis, Biological Evaluation, Structure-Activity Relationship, and Toxicity of Clinafloxacin-Azole Conjugates as Novel Antitubercular Agents. *Bioorganic Med. Chem.* **2019**, *27*, 175–187. [CrossRef]
56. Zhanel, G.G.; Ennis, K.; Vercaigne, L.; Walkty, A.; Gin, A.S.; Embil, J.; Smith, H.; Hoban, D.J. A Critical Review of the Fluoroquinolones. *Drugs* **2002**, *62*, 13–59. [CrossRef]
57. W-L Withdraws Clinafloxacin NDA—Pharmaceutical Industry News. Available online: https://www.thepharmaletter.com/article/w-l-withdraws-clinafloxacin-nda (accessed on 4 July 2023).
58. Kocsis, B.; Domokos, J.; Szabo, D. Chemical Structure and Pharmacokinetics of Novel Quinolone Agents Represented by Avarofloxacin, Delafloxacin, Finafloxacin, Zabofloxacin and Nemonoxacin. *Ann. Clin. Microbiol. Antimicrob.* **2016**, *15*, 34. [CrossRef] [PubMed]
59. Kocsis, B.; Gulyás, D.; Szabó, D. Delafloxacin, Finafloxacin, and Zabofloxacin: Novel Fluoroquinolones in the Antibiotic Pipeline. *Antibiotics* **2021**, *10*, 1506. [CrossRef] [PubMed]
60. Gemifloxacin. In *LiverTox: Clinical and Research Information on Drug-Induced Liver Injury*; National Institute of Diabetes and Digestive and Kidney Diseases: Bethesda, MD, USA, 2012.
61. Saravolatz, L.D.; Leggett, J. Gatifloxacin, Gemifloxacin, and Moxifloxacin: The Role of 3 Newer Fluoroquinolones. *Clin. Infect. Dis.* **2003**, *37*, 1210–1215. [CrossRef] [PubMed]
62. EMA Factive: Withdrawn Application. Available online: https://www.ema.europa.eu/en/medicines/human/withdrawn-applications/factive (accessed on 9 August 2023).
63. WHO Gemifloxacin: Withdrawal of Marketing Authorization Application. Available online: https://apps.who.int/iris/handle/10665/74447 (accessed on 9 August 2023).

64. Tanaka, K.; Vu, H.; Hayashi, M. In Vitro Activities and Spectrum of lascufloxacin (KRP-AM1977) against Anaerobes. *J. Infect. Chemother.* **2021**, *27*, 1265–1269. [CrossRef]
65. Limberakis, C. Quinolone Antibiotics: Levofloxacin (Levaquin®), Moxifloxacin (Avelox®), Gemifloxacin (Factive®), and Garenoxacin (T-3811). In *The Art of Drug Synthesis*; John Wiley & Sons, Ltd.: Hoboken, NJ, USA, 2007; pp. 39–69. ISBN 978-0-470-13497-9.
66. Wise, R. A Review of the Clinical Pharmacology of Moxifloxacin, a New 8-Methoxyquinolone, and Its Potential Relation to Therapeutic Efficacy. *Clin. Drug Investig.* **1999**, *17*, 365–387. [CrossRef]
67. Miravitlles, M. Moxifloxacin in the Management of Exacerbations of Chronic Bronchitis and COPD. *Int. J. Chron. Obs. Pulmon. Dis.* **2007**, *2*, 191–204.
68. Keating, G.M. Sitafloxacin: In Bacterial Infections. *Drugs* **2011**, *71*, 731–744. [CrossRef]
69. Chen, C.-K.; Cheng, I.-L.; Chen, Y.-H.; Lai, C.-C. Efficacy and Safety of Sitafloxacin in the Treatment of Acute Bacterial Infection: A Meta-Analysis of Randomized Controlled Trials. *Antibiotics* **2020**, *9*, 106. [CrossRef]
70. Guo, S.; Li, X.; Li, Y.; Tong, H.; Wei, M.; Yan, B.; Tian, M.; Xu, B.; Shao, J. Sitafloxacin Pharmacokinetics/Pharmacodynamics against Multidrug-Resistant Bacteria in a Dynamic Urinary Tract Infection in Vitro Model. *J. Antimicrob. Chemother.* **2023**, *78*, 141–149. [CrossRef]
71. Spížek, J.; Řezanka, T. Lincosamides: Chemical Structure, Biosynthesis, Mechanism of Action, Resistance, and Applications. *Biochem. Pharmacol.* **2017**, *133*, 20–28. [CrossRef] [PubMed]
72. Mukhtar, T.A.; Wright, G.D. Streptogramins, Oxazolidinones, and Other Inhibitors of Bacterial Protein Synthesis. *Chem. Rev.* **2005**, *105*, 529–542. [CrossRef] [PubMed]
73. Johnston, N.J.; Mukhtar, T.A.; Wright, G.D. Streptogramin Antibiotics: Mode of Action and Resistance. *Curr. Drug Targets* **2002**, *3*, 335–344. [CrossRef] [PubMed]
74. Manzella, J.P. Quinupristin-Dalfopristin: A New Antibiotic for Severe Gram-Positive Infections. *Am. Fam. Physician* **2001**, *64*, 1863–1867.
75. Scott, L.J. Eravacycline: A Review in Complicated Intra-Abdominal Infections. *Drugs* **2019**, *79*, 315–324. [CrossRef]
76. FDA XERAVA (Eravacycline) for Injection. Available online: https://www.accessdata.fda.gov/drugsatfda_docs/label/2018/211109lbl.pdf (accessed on 1 August 2023).
77. European Medicines Agency Xerava. Available online: https://www.ema.europa.eu/en/medicines/human/EPAR/xerava (accessed on 3 August 2021).
78. Clark, R.B.; Hunt, D.K.; He, M.; Achorn, C.; Chen, C.-L.; Deng, Y.; Fyfe, C.; Grossman, T.H.; Hogan, P.C.; O'Brien, W.J.; et al. Fluorocyclines. 2. Optimization of the C-9 Side-Chain for Antibacterial Activity and Oral Efficacy. *J. Med. Chem.* **2012**, *55*, 606–622. [CrossRef]
79. Zhanel, G.G.; Cheung, D.; Adam, H.; Zelenitsky, S.; Golden, A.; Schweizer, F.; Gorityala, B.; Lagacé-Wiens, P.R.S.; Walkty, A.; Gin, A.S.; et al. Review of Eravacycline, a Novel Fluorocycline Antibacterial Agent. *Drugs* **2016**, *76*, 567–588. [CrossRef]
80. Lee, Y.R.; Burton, C.E. Eravacycline, a Newly Approved Fluorocycline. *Eur. J. Clin. Microbiol. Infect. Dis.* **2019**, *38*, 1787–1794. [CrossRef]
81. Ma, Z.; Lynch, A.S. Development of a Dual-Acting Antibacterial Agent (TNP-2092) for the Treatment of Persistent Bacterial Infections. *J. Med. Chem.* **2016**, *59*, 6645–6657. [CrossRef]
82. NCATS Inxight Drugs Rifaquizinone. Available online: https://drugs.ncats.io/drug/W2P7EF7O6O (accessed on 29 August 2023).
83. DrugBank TNP-2092. Available online: https://go.drugbank.com/drugs/DB16312 (accessed on 29 August 2023).
84. Meulbroek, J.A.; Oleksijew, A.; Tanaka, S.K.; Alder, J.D. Efficacy of ABT-719, a 2-Pyridone Antimicrobial, against Enterococci, *Escherichia Coli*, and *Pseudomonas Aeruginosa* in Experimental Murine Pyelonephritis. *J. Antimicrob. Chemother.* **1996**, *38*, 641–653. [CrossRef]
85. Butler, M.S.; Henderson, I.R.; Capon, R.J.; Blaskovich, M.A.T. Antibiotics in the Clinical Pipeline as of December 2022. *J. Antibiot.* **2023**, *76*, 431–473. [CrossRef]
86. GlobalData TNP-2092 by TenNor Therapeutics for Bacterial Infections: Likelihood of Approval. *Pharmaceutical Technology* 2023. Available online: https://www.pharmaceutical-technology.com/data-insights/tnp-2092-tennor-therapeutics-bacterial-infections-likelihood-of-approval/ (accessed on 8 August 2023).
87. TenNor Therapeutics Limited Phase 2, Double-Blind, Randomized, Multicenter, Parallel, Controlled Study to Evaluate the Safety, Tolerability, Pharmacokinetics, and Efficacy of TNP-2092 to Treat Acute Bacterial Skin and Skin Structure Infection in Adults; clinicaltrials.gov. 2020. Available online: https://clinicaltrials.gov/study/NCT03964493 (accessed on 24 October 2023).
88. Siwach, A.; Verma, P.K. Synthesis and Therapeutic Potential of Imidazole Containing Compounds. *BMC Chem.* **2021**, *15*, 12. [CrossRef] [PubMed]
89. Zhang, L.; Peng, X.-M.; Damu, G.L.V.; Geng, R.-X.; Zhou, C.-H. Comprehensive Review in Current Developments of Imidazole-Based Medicinal Chemistry. *Med. Res. Rev.* **2014**, *34*, 340–437. [CrossRef] [PubMed]
90. Molina, P.; Tárraga, A.; Otón, F. Imidazole Derivatives: A Comprehensive Survey of Their Recognition Properties. *Org. Biomol. Chem.* **2012**, *10*, 1711–1724. [CrossRef]
91. Tran, M.P. Telithromycin: A Novel Agent for the Treatment of Community-Acquired Upper Respiratory Infections. *Bayl. Univ. Med. Cent. Proc.* **2004**, *17*, 475–479. [CrossRef] [PubMed]

92. FDA Ketek (Telithromycin) Label NDA 21-144/S-012. Available online: https://www.accessdata.fda.gov/drugsatfda_docs/label/2007/021144s012lbl.pdf (accessed on 15 July 2023).
93. Douthwaite, S.; Champney, W.S. Structures of Ketolides and Macrolides Determine Their Mode of Interaction with the Ribosomal Target Site. *J. Antimicrob. Chemother.* **2001**, *48*, 1–8. [CrossRef]
94. Wu, Y.-J. Chapter 1—Heterocycles and Medicine: A Survey of the Heterocyclic Drugs Approved by the U.S. FDA from 2000 to Present. In *Progress in Heterocyclic Chemistry*; Gribble, G.W., Joule, J.A., Eds.; Elsevier: Amsterdam, The Netherlands, 2012; Volume 24, pp. 1–53.
95. Ross, D.B. The FDA and the Case of Ketek. *N. Engl. J. Med.* **2007**, *356*, 1601–1604. [CrossRef]
96. European Medicines Agency Ketek. Available online: https://www.ema.europa.eu/en/medicines/human/EPAR/ketek (accessed on 15 July 2023).
97. Wetzel, D.M.; Phillips, M.A. Chemotherapy of Protozoal Infections: Amebiasis, Giardiasis, Trichomoniasis, Trypanosomiasis, Leishmaniasis, and Other Protozoal Infections. In *Goodman & Gilman's: The Pharmacological Basis of Therapeutics*; Brunton, L.L., Hilal-Dandan, R., Knollmann, B.C., Eds.; McGraw-Hill Education: New York, NY, USA, 2017.
98. Zhanel, G.G.; Lawrence, C.K.; Adam, H.; Schweizer, F.; Zelenitsky, S.; Zhanel, M.; Lagacé-Wiens, P.R.S.; Walkty, A.; Denisuik, A.; Golden, A.; et al. Imipenem–Relebactam and Meropenem–Vaborbactam: Two Novel Carbapenem-β-Lactamase Inhibitor Combinations. *Drugs* **2018**, *78*, 65–98. [CrossRef]
99. FDA Drugs@FDA: FDA-Approved Drugs, New Drug Application (NDA): 212819, RECARBRIO. Available online: https://www.accessdata.fda.gov/scripts/cder/daf/index.cfm?event=overview.process&varApplNo=212819 (accessed on 22 August 2023).
100. Research Center for Drug Evaluation and FDA Approves New Treatment for Pneumonia Caused by Certain Difficult-to-Treat Bacteria. Available online: https://www.fda.gov/news-events/press-announcements/fda-approves-new-treatment-pneumonia-caused-certain-difficult-treat-bacteria (accessed on 22 August 2023).
101. Granata, G.; Taglietti, F.; Schiavone, F.; Petrosillo, N. Durlobactam in the Treatment of Multidrug-Resistant Acinetobacter Baumannii Infections: A Systematic Review. *J. Clin. Med.* **2022**, *11*, 3258. [CrossRef]
102. Kolb, H.C.; Sharpless, K.B. The Growing Impact of Click Chemistry on Drug Discovery. *Drug Discov. Today* **2003**, *8*, 1128–1137. [CrossRef]
103. Whiting, M.; Muldoon, J.; Lin, Y.-C.; Silverman, S.M.; Lindstrom, W.; Olson, A.J.; Kolb, H.C.; Finn, M.G.; Sharpless, K.B.; Elder, J.H.; et al. Inhibitors of HIV-1 Protease by Using In Situ Click Chemistry. *Angew. Chem.* **2006**, *118*, 1463–1467. [CrossRef]
104. Masood, M.M. Progress in Synthetic Trends Followed for the Development of 1,2,3-Triazole Derivatives: A Review. *Polycycl. Aromat. Compd.* 2023. [CrossRef]
105. Phetsang, W.; Blaskovich, M.A.T.; Butler, M.S.; Huang, J.X.; Zuegg, J.; Mamidyala, S.K.; Ramu, S.; Kavanagh, A.M.; Cooper, M.A. An Azido-Oxazolidinone Antibiotic for Live Bacterial Cell Imaging and Generation of Antibiotic Variants. *Bioorganic Med. Chem.* **2014**, *22*, 4490–4498. [CrossRef] [PubMed]
106. Zhou, C.-H.; Wang, Y. Recent Researches in Triazole Compounds as Medicinal Drugs. *Curr. Med. Chem.* **2012**, *19*, 239–280. [CrossRef] [PubMed]
107. Eiamphungporn, W.; Schaduangrat, N.; Malik, A.A.; Nantasenamat, C. Tackling the Antibiotic Resistance Caused by Class A β-Lactamases through the Use of β-Lactamase Inhibitory Protein. *Int. J. Mol. Sci.* **2018**, *19*, 2222. [CrossRef] [PubMed]
108. Patowary, P.; Deka, B.; Bharali, D. Tetrazole Moiety as a Pharmacophore in Medicinal Chemistry: A Review. *Malar. Contr. Elimination* **2021**, *10*, 1–11.
109. Ostrovskii, V.A.; Trifonov, R.E.; Popova, E.A. Medicinal Chemistry of Tetrazoles. *Russ. Chem. Bull.* **2012**, *61*, 768–780. [CrossRef]
110. Zou, Y.; Liu, L.; Liu, J.; Liu, G. Bioisosteres in Drug Discovery: Focus on Tetrazole. *Future Med. Chem.* **2020**, *12*, 91–93. [CrossRef]
111. Ballatore, C.; Huryn, D.M.; Smith, A.B. Carboxylic Acid (Bio)Isosteres in Drug Design. *ChemMedChem* **2013**, *8*, 385–395. [CrossRef]
112. Brown, N. *Bioisosteres in Medicinal Chemistry*; John Wiley & Sons: Hoboken, NJ, USA, 2012; ISBN 978-3-527-65432-1.
113. Stevens, E. *Medicinal Chemistry: The Modern Drug Discovery Process*; Pearson: London, UK, 2014; ISBN 978-0-321-71048-2.
114. Kaushik, N.; Kumar, N.; Kumar, A.; Singh, U.K. Tetrazoles: Synthesis and Biological Activity. *Immunol. Endocr. Metab. Agents Med. Chem.* **2018**, *18*, 3–21. [CrossRef]
115. Lipsky, J.J. N-Methyl-Thio-Tetrazole Inhibition of the Gamma Carboxylation of Glutamic Acid: Possible Mechanism for Antibiotic-Associated Hypoprothrombinaemia. *Lancet* **1983**, *2*, 192–193. [CrossRef]
116. Fekety, F.R. Safety of Parenteral Third-Generation Cephalosporins. *Am. J. Med.* **1990**, *88*, S38–S44. [CrossRef] [PubMed]
117. Vardanyan, R.S.; Hruby, V.J. 32—Antibiotics. In *Synthesis of Essential Drugs*; Vardanyan, R.S., Hruby, V.J., Eds.; Elsevier: Amsterdam, The Netherlands, 2006; pp. 425–498. ISBN 978-0-444-52166-8.
118. *Goodman and Gilman's The Pharmacological Basis of Therapeutics*, 13th ed.; McGraw-Hill Education: New York, NY, USA, 2018; ISBN 978-1-259-58474-9.
119. Castle, S.S. Cefamandole. In *xPharm: The Comprehensive Pharmacology Reference*; Enna, S.J., Bylund, D.B., Eds.; Elsevier: New York, NY, USA, 2007; pp. 1–4. ISBN 978-0-08-055232-3.
120. Saltiel, E.; Brogden, R.N. Cefonicid. *Drugs* **1986**, *32*, 222–259. [CrossRef] [PubMed]
121. McLeod, D.C.; Tartaglione, T.A.; Polk, R.E. Review of the New Second-Generation Cephalosporins: Cefonicid, Ceforanide, and Cefuroxime. *Drug Intell. Clin. Pharm.* **1985**, *19*, 188–198. [CrossRef]
122. Jones, R.N. Cefmetazole (CS-1170), a "New" Cephamycin with a Decade of Clinical Experience. *Diagn. Microbiol. Infect. Dis.* **1989**, *12*, 367–379. [CrossRef] [PubMed]

123. *Martindale: The Complete Drug Reference*, 36th ed.; Pharmaceutical Press: London, UK; Chicago, IL, USA, 2009; ISBN 978-0-85369-840-1.
124. Darlow, C.A.; da Costa, R.M.A.; Ellis, S.; Franceschi, F.; Sharland, M.; Piddock, L.; Das, S.; Hope, W. Potential Antibiotics for the Treatment of Neonatal Sepsis Caused by Multidrug-Resistant Bacteria. *Paediatr. Drugs* **2021**, *23*, 465–484. [CrossRef]
125. DrugBank Latamoxef. Available online: https://go.drugbank.com/drugs/DB04570 (accessed on 31 July 2023).
126. DrugBank Flomoxef. Available online: https://go.drugbank.com/drugs/DB11935 (accessed on 16 September 2023).
127. DrugBank Tedizolid. Available online: https://go.drugbank.com/drugs/DB14569 (accessed on 16 September 2023).
128. Zhanel, G.G.; Love, R.; Adam, H.; Golden, A.; Zelenitsky, S.; Schweizer, F.; Gorityala, B.; Lagacé-Wiens, P.R.S.; Rubinstein, E.; Walkty, A.; et al. Tedizolid: A Novel Oxazolidinone with Potent Activity Against Multidrug-Resistant Gram-Positive Pathogens. *Drugs* **2015**, *75*, 253–270. [CrossRef]
129. Michalska, K.; Karpiuk, I.; Król, M.; Tyski, S. Recent Development of Potent Analogues of Oxazolidinone Antibacterial Agents. *Bioorganic Med. Chem.* **2013**, *21*, 577–591. [CrossRef] [PubMed]
130. Rybak, J.M.; Roberts, K. Tedizolid Phosphate: A Next-Generation Oxazolidinone. *Infect. Dis. Ther.* **2015**, *4*, 1–14. [CrossRef]
131. Flanagan, S.D.; Bien, P.A.; Muñoz, K.A.; Minassian, S.L.; Prokocimer, P.G. Pharmacokinetics of Tedizolid Following Oral Administration: Single and Multiple Dose, Effect of Food, and Comparison of Two Solid Forms of the Prodrug. *Pharmacotherapy* **2013**, *34*, 240–250. [CrossRef] [PubMed]
132. Brier, M.E.; Stalker, D.J.; Aronoff, G.R.; Batts, D.H.; Ryan, K.K.; O'Grady, M.; Hopkins, N.K.; Jungbluth, G.L. Pharmacokinetics of Linezolid in Subjects with Renal Dysfunction. *Antimicrob. Agents Chemother.* **2003**, *47*, 2775–2780. [CrossRef] [PubMed]
133. DrugBank Radezolid. Available online: https://go.drugbank.com/drugs/DB12339 (accessed on 19 July 2023).
134. Michalska, K.; Bednarek, E.; Gruba, E.; Lewandowska, K.; Mizera, M.; Cielecka-Piontek, J. Comprehensive Spectral Identification of Key Intermediates to the Final Product of the Chiral Pool Synthesis of Radezolid. *Chem. Cent. J.* **2017**, *11*, 82. [CrossRef]
135. Melinta Therapeutics, Inc. *A Phase 2, Multicenter, Randomized, Open-Label, Comparative Study to Evaluate the Safety and Efficacy of RX-1741 Versus Linezolid in the Outpatient Treatment of Adult Patients With Uncomplicated Skin and Skin Structure Infection*; Melinta Therapeutics, Inc.: Troy Hills, NJ, USA, 2014.
136. Melinta Therapeutics, Inc. *A Phase 2, Multicenter, Randomized, Double-Blind Study to Evaluate the Safety and Efficacy of RX-1741 in the Treatment of Adult Patients With Mild to Moderate Severity of Community-Acquired Pneumonia (CAP)*; Melinta Therapeutics, Inc.: Troy Hills, NJ, USA, 2016.
137. Wang, L.; Zhang, Y.; Liu, S.; Huang, N.; Zeng, W.; Xu, W.; Zhou, T.; Shen, M. Comparison of Anti-Microbic and Anti-Biofilm Activity Among Tedizolid and Radezolid Against Linezolid-Resistant Enterococcus Faecalis Isolates. *Infect. Drug Resist.* **2021**, *14*, 4619–4627. [CrossRef]
138. DrugBank Furans | DrugBank Online. Available online: https://go.drugbank.com/categories/DBCAT000766 (accessed on 1 August 2023).
139. Le Dang, N.; Hughes, T.B.; Miller, G.P.; Swamidass, S.J. Computational Approach to Structural Alerts: Furans, Phenols, Nitroaromatics, and Thiophenes. *Chem. Res. Toxicol.* **2017**, *30*, 1046–1059. [CrossRef] [PubMed]
140. PubChem Cefuroxime. Available online: https://pubchem.ncbi.nlm.nih.gov/compound/5479529 (accessed on 4 August 2023).
141. Das, B.; Rudra, S.; Yadav, A.; Ray, A.; Rao, A.V.S.R.; Srinivas, A.S.S.V.; Soni, A.; Saini, S.; Shukla, S.; Pandya, M.; et al. Synthesis and SAR of Novel Oxazolidinones: Discovery of Ranbezolid. *Bioorganic Med. Chem. Lett.* **2005**, *15*, 4261–4267. [CrossRef] [PubMed]
142. Mathur, T.; Kalia, V.; Barman, T.K.; Singhal, S.; Khan, S.; Upadhyay, D.J.; Rattan, A.; Raj, V.S. Anti-Anaerobic Potential of Ranbezolid: Insight into Its Mechanism of Action against Bacteroides Fragilis. *Int. J. Antimicrob. Agents* **2013**, *41*, 36–40. [CrossRef]
143. Karaman, N.; Adil Zainel, R.; Kapkaç, H.A.; Karaca Gençer, H.; Ilgın, S.; Karaduman, A.B.; Karaküçük-İyidoğan, A.; Oruç-Emre, E.E.; Koçyiğit-Kaymakçıoğlu, B. Design and Evaluation of Biological Activities of 1,3-Oxazolidinone Derivatives Bearing Amide, Sulfonamide, and Thiourea Moieties. *Arch. Pharm.* **2018**, *351*, e1800057. [CrossRef]
144. Neu, H.C.; Novelli, A.; Saha, G.; Chin, N.-X. In Vitro Activities of Two Oxazolidinone Antimicrobial Agents DuP 721 and DuP 105. *Antimicrob. Agents Chemother.* **1988**, *32*, 580–583. [CrossRef]
145. Matsingos, C.; Al-Adhami, T.; Jamshidi, S.; Hind, C.; Clifford, M.; Mark Sutton, J.; Rahman, K.M. Synthesis, Microbiological Evaluation and Structure Activity Relationship Analysis of Linezolid Analogues with Different C5-Acylamino Substituents. *Bioorganic Med. Chem.* **2021**, *49*, 116397. [CrossRef]
146. Foti, C.; Piperno, A.; Scala, A.; Giuffrè, O. Oxazolidinone Antibiotics: Chemical, Biological and Analytical Aspects. *Molecules* **2021**, *26*, 4280. [CrossRef]
147. Chellat, M.F.; Raguž, L.; Riedl, R. Targeting Antibiotic Resistance. *Angew. Chem. Int. Ed.* **2016**, *55*, 6600–6626. [CrossRef] [PubMed]
148. Polacek, N.; Mankin, A.S. The Ribosomal Peptidyl Transferase Center: Structure, Function, Evolution, Inhibition. *Crit. Rev. Biochem. Mol. Biol.* **2005**, *40*, 285–311. [CrossRef] [PubMed]
149. Pathania, S.; Petrova-Szczasiuk, K.; Pentikäinen, O.; Singh, P.K. Oxazolidinones: Are They Only Good for the Discovery of Antibiotics? A Worm's Eye View. *J. Mol. Struct.* **2023**, *1286*, 135630. [CrossRef]
150. Hashemian, S.M.R.; Farhadi, T.; Ganjparvar, M. Linezolid: A Review of Its Properties, Function, and Use in Critical Care. *Drug Des. Dev. Ther.* **2018**, *12*, 1759. [CrossRef] [PubMed]
151. Zhang, H.-Z.; Zhao, Z.-L.; Zhou, C.-H. Recent Advance in Oxazole-Based Medicinal Chemistry. *Eur. J. Med. Chem.* **2018**, *144*, 444–492. [CrossRef]
152. Bush, K. CHAPTER 14-β-Lactam Antibiotics: Penicillins. In *Antibiotic and Chemotherapy*, 9th ed.; Finch, R.G., Greenwood, D., Norrby, S.R., Whitley, R.J., Eds.; W.B. Saunders: London, UK, 2010; pp. 200–225. ISBN 978-0-7020-4064-1.

153. Alagarsamy, V. *Textbook of Medicinal Chemistry Vol II—E-Book*; Elsevier: Amsterdam, The Netherlands, 2012; ISBN 978-81-312-3259-0.
154. Thomas, G. *Fundamentals of Medicinal Chemistry*; John Wiley & Sons: Hoboken, NJ, USA, 2004; ISBN 978-0-470-87169-0.
155. Cotrina-Santome, A.; Ulloa-Esquivel, L.; Vásquez-Quispe, S.; Arevalo-Flores, M.; Pedraz-Petrozzi, B. Cycloserine-Induced Psychosis in Patients with Drug-Resistant Tuberculosis: A Systematic Review of Case Reports. *Egypt. J. Neurol. Psychiatry Neurosurg.* **2023**, *59*, 37. [CrossRef]
156. Deshpande, D.; Alffenaar, J.-W.C.; Köser, C.U.; Dheda, K.; Chapagain, M.L.; Simbar, N.; Schön, T.; Sturkenboom, M.G.G.; McIlleron, H.; Lee, P.S.; et al. D-Cycloserine Pharmacokinetics/Pharmacodynamics, Susceptibility, and Dosing Implications in Multidrug-Resistant Tuberculosis: A Faustian Deal. *Clin. Infect. Dis.* **2018**, *67*, S308–S316. [CrossRef]
157. Bradford, P.A.; Miller, A.A.; O'Donnell, J.; Mueller, J.P. Zoliflodacin: An Oral Spiropyrimidinetrione Antibiotic for the Treatment of Neisseria Gonorrheae, Including Multi-Drug-Resistant Isolates. *ACS Infect. Dis.* **2020**, *6*, 1332–1345. [CrossRef]
158. Golparian, D.; Jacobsson, S.; Ohnishi, M.; Unemo, M. Complete Reference Genome Sequence of the Clinical Neisseria Gonorrhoeae Strain H035, with Resistance to the Novel Antimicrobial Zoliflodacin, Identified in Japan in 2000. *Microbiol. Resour. Announc.* **2023**, *12*, e0113022. [CrossRef]
159. Kemnic, T.R.; Coleman, M. Trimethoprim Sulfamethoxazole. In *StatPearls*; StatPearls Publishing: Treasure Island, FL, USA, 2023.
160. Shah, R.; Verma, P.K. Therapeutic Importance of Synthetic Thiophene. *Chem. Cent. J.* **2018**, *12*, 137. [CrossRef]
161. Pathania, S.; Narang, R.K.; Rawal, R.K. Role of Sulphur-Heterocycles in Medicinal Chemistry: An Update. *Eur. J. Med. Chem.* **2019**, *180*, 486–508. [CrossRef] [PubMed]
162. Scott, K.A.; Njardarson, J.T. Analysis of US FDA-Approved Drugs Containing Sulfur Atoms. *Top. Curr. Chem.* **2018**, *376*, 5. [CrossRef] [PubMed]
163. Ticarcillin. In *LiverTox: Clinical and Research Information on Drug-Induced Liver Injury*; National Institute of Diabetes and Digestive and Kidney Diseases: Bethesda, MD, USA, 2012.
164. Lupia, T.; De Benedetto, I.; Stroffolini, G.; Di Bella, S.; Mornese Pinna, S.; Zerbato, V.; Rizzello, B.; Bosio, R.; Shbaklo, N.; Corcione, S.; et al. Temocillin: Applications in Antimicrobial Stewardship as a Potential Carbapenem-Sparing Antibiotic. *Antibiotics* **2022**, *11*, 493. [CrossRef]
165. Sköld, O. Penicillins and Other Betalactams. In *Antibiotics and Antibiotic Resistance*; John Wiley & Sons, Ltd.: Hoboken, NJ, USA, 2011; pp. 69–94. ISBN 978-1-118-07560-9.
166. Norrby, S.R. CHAPTER 5—Antimicrobial Agents and the Kidneys. In *Antibiotic and Chemotherapy*, 9th ed.; Finch, R.G., Greenwood, D., Norrby, S.R., Whitley, R.J., Eds.; W.B. Saunders: London, UK, 2010; pp. 60–67. ISBN 978-0-7020-4064-1.
167. Godzeski, C.W.; Brier, G.; Pavey, D.E. Cephalothin, a New Cephalosporin with a Broad Antibacterial Spectrum. I. In Vitro Studies Employing the Gradient Plate Technique. *I. In Vitro Studies Employing the Gradient Plate Technique. Appl. Microbiol.* **1963**, *11*, 122–127. [CrossRef]
168. DrugBank Cefalotin. Available online: https://go.drugbank.com/drugs/DB00456 (accessed on 16 August 2023).
169. Dondoni, A.; Merino, P. 3.06—Thiazoles. In *Comprehensive Heterocyclic Chemistry II*; Katritzky, A.R., Rees, C.W., Scriven, E.F.V., Eds.; Pergamon: Oxford, UK, 1996; pp. 373–474. ISBN 978-0-08-096518-5.
170. Li, J.J. *Heterocyclic Chemistry in Drug Discovery*; Wiley: Hoboken, NJ, USA, 2013; ISBN 978-1-118-35442-1.
171. Ayati, A.; Emami, S.; Asadipour, A.; Shafiee, A.; Foroumadi, A. Recent Applications of 1,3-Thiazole Core Structure in the Identification of New Lead Compounds and Drug Discovery. *Eur. J. Med. Chem.* **2015**, *97*, 699–718. [CrossRef]
172. Sharma, P.C.; Bansal, K.K.; Sharma, A.; Sharma, D.; Deep, A. Thiazole-Containing Compounds as Therapeutic Targets for Cancer Therapy. *Eur. J. Med. Chem.* **2020**, *188*, 112016. [CrossRef] [PubMed]
173. Borcea, A.-M.; Ionuț, I.; Crișan, O.; Oniga, O. An Overview of the Synthesis and Antimicrobial, Antiprotozoal, and Antitumor Activity of Thiazole and Bisthiazole Derivatives. *Molecules* **2021**, *26*, 624. [CrossRef]
174. Ayati, A.; Emami, S.; Moghimi, S.; Foroumadi, A. Thiazole in the Targeted Anticancer Drug Discovery. *Future Med. Chem.* **2019**, *11*, 1929–1952. [CrossRef] [PubMed]
175. Arshad, M.F.; Alam, A.; Alshammari, A.A.; Alhazza, M.B.; Alzimam, I.M.; Alam, M.A.; Mustafa, G.; Ansari, M.S.; Alotaibi, A.M.; Alotaibi, A.A.; et al. Thiazole: A Versatile Standalone Moiety Contributing to the Development of Various Drugs and Biologically Active Agents. *Molecules* **2022**, *27*, 3994. [CrossRef]
176. Singh, A.; Malhotra, D.; Singh, K.; Chadha, R.; Bedi, P.M.S. Thiazole Derivatives in Medicinal Chemistry: Recent Advancements in Synthetic Strategies, Structure Activity Relationship and Pharmacological Outcomes. *J. Mol. Struct.* **2022**, *1266*, 133479. [CrossRef]
177. Decuyper, L.; Jukič, M.; Sosič, I.; Žula, A.; D'hooghe, M.; Gobec, S. Antibacterial and β-Lactamase Inhibitory Activity of Monocyclic β-Lactams. *Med. Res. Rev.* **2018**, *38*, 426–503. [CrossRef]
178. Neu, H.C. Aztreonam Activity, Pharmacology, and Clinical Uses. *Am. J. Med.* **1990**, *88*, S2–S6. [CrossRef] [PubMed]
179. Ramsey, C.; MacGowan, A.P. A Review of the Pharmacokinetics and Pharmacodynamics of Aztreonam. *J. Antimicrob. Chemother.* **2016**, *71*, 2704–2712. [CrossRef] [PubMed]
180. Bulitta, J.B.; Duffull, S.B.; Landersdorfer, C.B.; Kinzig, M.; Holzgrabe, U.; Stephan, U.; Drusano, G.L.; Sörgel, F. Comparison of the Pharmacokinetics and Pharmacodynamic Profile of Carumonam in Cystic Fibrosis Patients and Healthy Volunteers. *Diagn. Microbiol. Infect. Dis.* **2009**, *65*, 130–141. [CrossRef] [PubMed]
181. Chatwal, G.R. *Medicinal Chemistry*; Himalaya Publishing House: Mumbai, India, 2010; ISBN 978-1-4416-6248-4.

182. Anand, N. Sulfonamides: Structure-Activity Relationships and Mechanism of Action. In *Inhibition of Folate Metabolism in Chemotherapy: The Origins and Uses of Co-trimoxazole*; Hitchings, G.H., Ed.; Handbook of Experimental Pharmacology; Springer: Berlin/Heidelberg, Germany, 1983; pp. 25–54. ISBN 978-3-642-81890-5.
183. Testa, B.; Mayer, J.M. *Hydrolysis in Drug and Prodrug Metabolism*; John Wiley & Sons: Hoboken, NJ, USA, 2003; ISBN 978-3-906390-25-3.
184. Ameta, K.L.; Kant, R.; Penoni, A.; Maspero, A.; Scapinello, L. *N-Heterocycles: Synthesis and Biological Evaluation*; Springer: Berlin/Heidelberg, Germany, 2022; ISBN 978-981-19083-2-3.
185. Hu, Y.; Li, C.-Y.; Wang, X.-M.; Yang, Y.-H.; Zhu, H.-L. 1,3,4-Thiadiazole: Synthesis, Reactions, and Applications in Medicinal, Agricultural, and Materials Chemistry. *Chem. Rev.* **2014**, *114*, 5572–5610. [CrossRef] [PubMed]
186. Wilkins, D.J. 5.08—1,2,4-Thiadiazoles. In *Comprehensive Heterocyclic Chemistry III*; Katritzky, A.R., Ramsden, C.A., Scriven, E.F.V., Taylor, R.J.K., Eds.; Elsevier: Oxford, UK, 2008; pp. 487–513. ISBN 978-0-08-044992-0.
187. Delgado, C.P.; Rocha, J.B.T.; Orian, L.; Bortoli, M.; Nogara, P.A. In Silico Studies of Mpro and PLpro from SARS-CoV-2 and a New Class of Cephalosporin Drugs Containing 1,2,4-Thiadiazole. *Struct. Chem.* **2022**, *33*, 2205–2220. [CrossRef]
188. Laudano, J.B. Ceftaroline Fosamil: A New Broad-Spectrum Cephalosporin. *J. Antimicrob. Chemother.* **2011**, *66*, iii11–iii18. [CrossRef] [PubMed]
189. Zhanel, G.G.; Sniezek, G.; Schweizer, F.; Zelenitsky, S.; Lagacé-Wiens, P.R.S.; Rubinstein, E.; Gin, A.S.; Hoban, D.J.; Karlowsky, J.A. Ceftaroline. *Drugs* **2009**, *69*, 809–831. [CrossRef]
190. Iizawa, Y.; Okonogi, K.; Hayashi, R.; Iwahi, T.; Yamazaki, T.; Imada, A. Therapeutic Effect of Cefozopran (SCE-2787), a New Parenteral Cephalosporin, against Experimental Infections in Mice. *Antimicrob. Agents Chemother.* **1993**, *37*, 100–105. [CrossRef]
191. Wu, G.L.; Shentu, J.Z.; Zhou, H.L.; Zhu, M.X.; Hu, X.J.; Liu, J.; Wu, L.H. Pharmacokinetics of Cefozopran by Single and Multiple Intravenous Infusions in Healthy Chinese Volunteers. *Drugs R&D* **2015**, *15*, 63–70. [CrossRef]
192. Bui, T.; Preuss, C.V. Cephalosporins. In *StatPearls*; StatPearls Publishing: Treasure Island, FL, USA, 2023.
193. Duplessis, C.; Crum-Cianflone, N.F. Ceftaroline: A New Cephalosporin with Activity against Methicillin-Resistant Staphylococcus Aureus (MRSA). *Clin. Med. Rev. Ther.* **2011**, *3*, a2466. [CrossRef] [PubMed]
194. FDA TEFLARO®(Ceftaroline Fosamil) for Injection, for Intravenous Use. Available online: https://www.accessdata.fda.gov/drugsatfda_docs/label/2015/200327s015lbl.pdf (accessed on 22 August 2023).
195. Kouki, I.; Montagner, C.; Mauhin, W.; London, J.; Lazard, T.; Grimbert, S.; Zeller, V.; Lidove, O. Coagulation Disorders during Treatment with Cefazolin and Rifampicin: Rare but Dangerous. *J. Bone Jt. Infect.* **2021**, *6*, 131–134. [CrossRef] [PubMed]

pharmaceutics

MDPI

Review

Synthetic Pathways to Non-Psychotropic Phytocannabinoids as Promising Molecules to Develop Novel Antibiotics: A Review

Silvana Alfei [1,*], Gian Carlo Schito [2] and Anna Maria Schito [2]

[1] Department of Pharmacy (DIFAR), University of Genoa, Viale Cembrano, 4, 16148 Genoa, Italy
[2] Department of Surgical Sciences and Integrated Diagnostics (DISC), University of Genoa, Viale Benedetto XV, 6, 16132 Genova, Italy; giancarlo.schito@unige.it (G.C.S.); amschito@unige.it (A.M.S.)
* Correspondence: alfei@difar.unige.it; Tel.: +39-010-355-2296

Abstract: Due to the rapid emergence of multi drug resistant (MDR) pathogens against which current antibiotics are no longer functioning, severe infections are becoming practically untreatable. Consequently, the discovery of new classes of effective antimicrobial agents with novel mechanism of action is becoming increasingly urgent. The bioactivity of *Cannabis sativa*, an herbaceous plant used for millennia for medicinal and recreational purposes, is mainly due to its content in phytocannabinoids (PCs). Among the 180 PCs detected, cannabidiol (CBD), Δ^8 and Δ^9-tetrahydrocannabinols (Δ^8-THC and Δ^9-THC), cannabichromene (CBC), cannabigerol (CBG), cannabinol (CBN) and some of their acidic precursors have demonstrated from moderate to potent antibacterial effects against Gram-positive bacteria (MICs 0.5–8 µg/mL), including methicillin-resistant *Staphylococcus aureus* (MRSA), epidemic MRSA (EMRSA), as well as fluoroquinolone and tetracycline-resistant strains. Particularly, the non-psychotropic CBG was also capable to inhibit MRSA biofilm formation, to eradicate even mature biofilms, and to rapidly eliminate MRSA persiter cells. In this scenario, CBG, as well as other minor non-psychotropic PCs, such as CBD, and CBC could represent promising compounds for developing novel antibiotics with high therapeutic potential. Anyway, further studies are necessary, needing abundant quantities of such PCs, scarcely provided naturally by *Cannabis* plants. Here, after an extensive overture on cannabinoids including their reported antimicrobial effects, aiming at easing the synthetic production of the necessary amounts of CBG, CBC and CBD for further studies, we have, for the first time, systematically reviewed the synthetic pathways utilized for their synthesis, reporting both reaction schemes and experimental details.

Keywords: bacterial resistance; methicillin-resistant *S. aureus* (MRSA); multi drug resistant (MDR) bacteria; *Cannabis sativa*; phytocannabinoids (PCs); endocannabinois (ECs); synthetic cannabinoids (SCs); synthetic procedures; cannabichromene (CBC); cannabigerol (CBG); cannabidiol (CBC)

Citation: Alfei, S.; Schito, G.C.; Schito, A.M. Synthetic Pathways to Non-Psychotropic Phytocannabinoids as Promising Molecules to Develop Novel Antibiotics: A Review. *Pharmaceutics* **2023**, *15*, 1889. https://doi.org/10.3390/pharmaceutics15071889

Academic Editors: Aura Rusu, Valentina Uivarosi and Thierry Vandamme

Received: 14 May 2023
Revised: 27 June 2023
Accepted: 1 July 2023
Published: 5 July 2023

1. Introduction

Given the rapid emergence of multi drug resistant (MDR), extensively drug-resistant (XDR) and pandrug-resistant (PDR) pathogens, against which current antibiotics are no longer functioning, we are rapidly moving into a post-antibiotic era where infections will be practically untreatable [1]. According to the definition of the World Health Organization (WHO), antimicrobial resistance is a natural event that occurs when microbes become tolerant to drugs originally active, thus rendering several infections more difficult or impossible to treat [2,3]. Particularly, WHO has identified twelve families of bacteria to be considered as the most dangerous to human health. These families have been assigned to three priority groups, comprising critical pathogens (*Acinetobacter*, *Pseudomonas*, and *Enterobacteriaceae*), high priority pathogens (*Enterococcus faecium*, *Staphylococcus aureus*, *Helicobacter pylori*, *Campylobacter*, *Salmonella* spp., and *Neisseria gonorrhoeae*), and medium priority pathogens (*Streptococcus pneumoniae*, and *Shigella* spp.) [3,4]. Resistance in bacteria can be acquired or natural, but several mechanisms exist by which pathogens can become resistant to antibiotics (Figure 1).

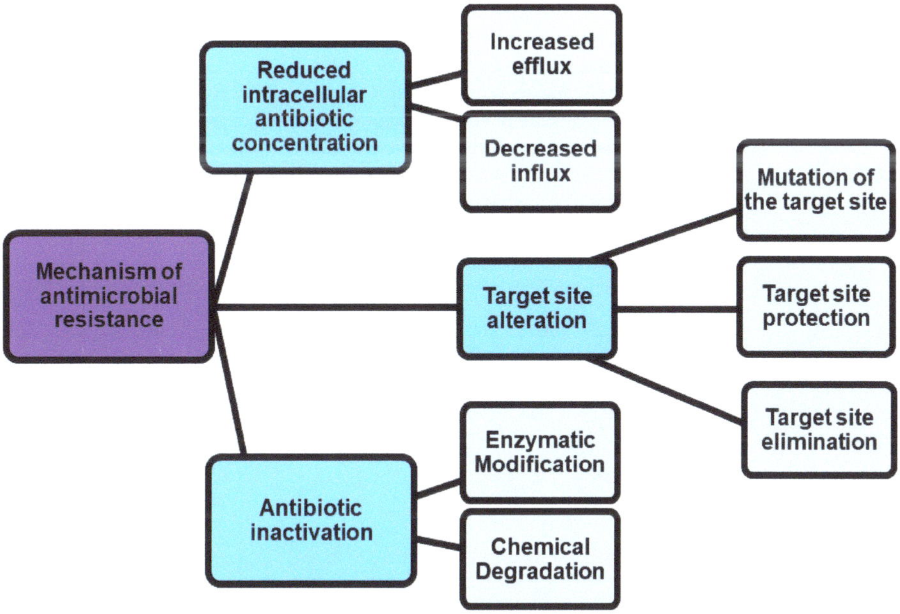

Figure 1. Mechanisms by which pathogens can become resistant.

As shown in Figure 1, antimicrobial resistance mechanisms include drug inactivation, decreased intracellular drug concentration, and altered drug targets [5].

1.1. Mechanism of Antimicrobial Resistance vs. Strategies to Develop Novel Antibiotics

Drug inactivation can occur either by enzymatic or chemical degradation, while decreased intracellular drug concentration can occur because of increasing drugs efflux and decreasing drugs influx [5]. In this regard, porin mutations in resistant strains alter the permeability of bacterial membranes, thus reducing the uptake of antibiotics into the bacterial cell. On the contrary, the hyperexpression of efflux pumps, which pump antibiotics out of the cell, dramatically reduces their concentration inside the cell [6]. Also, by the action of enzymes that chemically modify components of the bacterial outer membrane essential for antibiotic binding, some Gram-negative bacteria such as *P. aeruginosa*, *Acinetobacter baumannii* and others develop resistance to glycopeptide and polymyxin antibiotics. Furthermore, methyltransferases are a class of enzymes capable to modify the target thus promoting the resistance to antibiotics including aminoglycoside, lincosamide, macrolide, streptogramin, and oxazolidinone [7]. Another phenomenon known as "target protection" occurs when antibiotic target's resistance proteins, such as the tetracycline ribosomal protection proteins (TRPPs), protect bacteria from the antibiotic-induced inhibition [8]. Additionally, the antibiotic resistance could be caused by the use of antibiotics in feed diet for animal production. The overuse, abuse, and misuse of β-lactams, aminoglycosides, tetracyclines, macrolides, and other antibiotics, with the purpose of promoting the development of animals, can cause the presence of residual antibiotics in the products intended for human consumption obtained from those animals, and can determine antibiotics pollution into the environment [9–11]. It was reported that some bacterial infections in humans are sustained by animal pathogens, namely zoonotic pathogens, thus proving that antibiotic resistance can be directly or indirectly transmitted from animal to humans [9]. A few practices, including the improvement of animal feed, waste management, and animal natural immunity, as well as the use of antibiotic alternatives such as prebiotics, probiotic vaccines, and bacteriophages can regulate and limit the antibiotic resistance, thus maintaining the potency of the available drugs [12]. However, more strategies to counteract antibiotic resistance are necessary, and currently they include the use of nanotechnology, computational methods, the use of antibiotic alternatives, drug repurposing, the synthesis of novel antibacterial agents, prodrugs, the development of efficient diagnostic agents also named rapid diagnostic tests (RDTs), the use of combination therapy, as well as the awareness, and knowledge of antibiotic prescribing (Table 1).

Table 1. Strategies for combating antibiotic resistance.

Strategies for Combating Antibiotic Resistance		Ref.
Nanotechnology	Quality by design (QbD) approach	[13]
Computational methods	In silico modelling Fragment-based drug design (FBDD)	[14] [15]
Antibiotic alternatives	Antimicrobial peptides (AMPs) Essential oils Anti-Quorum Sensing (QS) Darobactins Vitamin B6 Bacteriophages Odilorhabdins 18-β-glycyrrhetinic acid Cannabinoids	[12]
Drug reproposing	Ticagrelor Mitomycin C (MMC) Auranofin Pentamidine Zidovudine (AZT)	[16]
Synthesis of novel antibacterial agents	Lactones Piperidinol Sugar-based bactericides Isoxazole derivatives Carbazole	[17] [18] [19] [20] [21]
Prodrugs	Siderophores Carbapenem-oxazolidinones Oral Gyrb/ParE dual binding inhibitor AMPs prodrugs	[22]
Development of efficient diagnostic agents (RDTs)	Point-of-care tests (POCTs) Molecular (genotyping) assays	[23]
Combination therapy	Penicillin with streptomycin * Rifampin–isoniazid–pyrazinamide ** Trimethoprim-sulfamethoxazole Quinupristin-dalfopristin Bacitracin-polymyxin B Bacitracin-polymyxin B-gramicidin Neomycin,-bacitracin-gramicidin	[24]
	β-Lactams antibiotics-β-Lactamase inhibitors ***	[25,26]
Awareness and knowledge of antibiotic prescribing		[27]

RDTs = rapid diagnostic tests; * For enterococcal infections; ** in the treatment of tuberculosis; *** ceftazidime/avibactam, meropenem/vaborbactam and imipenem/relebactam.

1.2. Cannabinoids as Strategic Compounds to Develop New Antibiotics

Omitting to comment on each strategy reported in Table 1, because it is out ofthe scope of this study, and instead focusing on the development of alternative antibiotics, we can observe that cannabinoids, better known for many other pharmacological and psychotropic effects are included in this category. Particularly, cannabinoids are prenylated polyketides produced in *Cannabis* plants and particularly in *Cannabis sativa*, which is an herbaceous plant that has been used for millennia for both medicinal and recreational purposes. *C. sativa* possesses a plethora of pharmacological properties and mind-altering effects, largely due to its content in cannabinoids, more precisely phytocannabinois (PCs), given their vegetable origin [28]. Collectively, more than 1600 chemical compounds have been isolated from *C. sativa*, of which over 500 are phytochemicals including cannabinoids, flavonoids terpenoids and sterols [28]. Among phytochemicals, more than 180 are cannabinoids, about 125 have been isolated, that can be classified into 11 structural families [28,29]. The most abundant representatives of these families are Δ^9-tetrahydrocannabinol (Δ^9-THC, also the main psychoactive cannabinoid), cannabidiol (CBD), and cannabichromene (CBC). Additionally, other classes whose prototypes are Δ^8-*E*-tetrahydrocannabinol (Δ^8-THC), cannabigerol (CBG), cannabinodiol (CBND), cannabielsoin (CBE), cannabicyclol (CBL), cannabinol (CBN), cannabitriol (CBT), and a miscellaneous group have been identified [28,29]. Currently, despite its psychotropic effects, Δ^9- THC is used as therapeutic agent in the treatment of chemotherapy-associated nausea and vomiting, AIDS related loss of appetite, as well as pain and muscle spasms in multiple sclerosis [30]. Also, its carboxylic acid precursor, THCA, not exerting psycho-active effects in humans, is currently examined for its immunomodulatory, anti-inflammatory, neuroprotective and anti-neoplastic effects as well for its effectiveness in reducing adiposity and preventing metabolic disease caused by diet-induced obesity [31]. CBD, non-psychotropic as well, is currently investigated for application in the treatment of Alzheimer's disease, Parkinson's disease, epilepsy, cancer and for its neuroprotective efficacy [32]. Although the most studied cannabinoids for medicinal purposes are CBD and Δ^9-THC, nowadays the research focus moves increasingly towards other PCs, such as the not psychoactive CBC, currently investigated for its anti-inflammatory, anti-fungal, antibiotic and analgesic effects [30], CBG and cannabigerolic acid (CBGA), which is the precursor of the decarboxylated CBG and could be considered as the "mother of all cannabinoids" (see later). Particularly, CBG has many putative benefits ranging from anti-inflammatory action to pain reliever [33]. Among other more investigated therapeutic properties, PCs including Δ^9-THC, Δ^8-THC, CBD, CBN, CBG, and CBC and some their correspondent carboxylic acids have shown from moderate to potent antimicrobial properties mainly against Gram-positive bacteria (MICs 0.5–8 µg/mL), and especially against strains of *S. aureus*, including MRSA, EMRSA, as well as fluoroquinolone and tetracycline-resistant strains, [34]. Particularly, even if the precise mechanisms used by PCs remains unknown so far, recent investigations have revealed that PCs inhibits bacteria by injuring their cytoplasmic membrane [35,36]. Recently, Luz-Veiga et al. have reported the antibacterial activity of both CBD and CBG, being CBG the most potent compound, and their capability to inhibit *Staphylococci* adherence to keratinocytes without compromising skin microbiota, thus being very promising as antibacterial agents to treat skin infection by topical administration [37]. Blaskovich et al., in addition to confirm the antibacterial activity of CBD on Gram-positive pathogens, including highly resistant *S. aureus*, *S. pneumoniae*, and *Clostridioides difficile*, demonstrated that CBD has excellent activity against biofilms, little propensity to induce resistance, and topical in vivo efficacy [38]. Moreover, the authors reported that CBD can selectively kill a subset of Gram-negative bacteria that includes the 'urgent threat' pathogen *Neisseria gonorrhoeae* [38]. Additionally, the interaction of CBD with broad-spectrum antibiotics such as ampicillin, kanamycin, and polymyxin B was studied by Gildea et al. [39]. By disrupting membrane integrity at extremely low dosages, CBD-antibiotic co-therapy showed synergistic activity against *Salmonella typhimurium*, offering an intriguing alternative in the treatment of this clinically relevant bacterium. The impressively strong antibacterial activity against MRSA of CBG has been reported by Farha et al. in the year 2020 [33]. Even in comparison with standard therapy with vancomycin, CBG outcompetes classical approaches against MRSA. Additionally, CBG demonstrated to inhibit the capability of MRSA to generate de novo biofilm, showed to succeed in disaggregating the pre-formed biofilm, to kill rapidly stationary phase cells (persisters), and to effectively inhibit MRSA also in vivo, in a murine model. The authors speculated that C.

sativa may produce PCs as a natural defense mechanism against pathogens and suggested PCs as a new compound class serving as novel antibiotic drug [33].

Unfortunately, since in *C. sativa*, CBGA is promptly and directly converted to CBDA and THCA, leaving no CBGA pool available to form CBG, the CBG levels in plants are exceptionally low. In this context, it has been suggested that a possible strategy to increase the CBG yield from hemp biomass could consist in harvesting much earlier in the ripening phase of the plants before the other cannabinoids are formed and detract the CBGA from the cannabinoid pool [40]. On the other hand, having available reliable synthetic procedures to prepare natural PCs would consent the accessibility to considerable quantities of CBG, as well as of other microbiologically promising minor cannabinoids, unlikely provided naturally by *Cannabis* plants, thus allowing further studies finalized to the development of novel PCs-based antibiotics.

Particularly, since deprived of psychoactive effects, the non-psychotropic CBG, CBD, and CBC could represent promising compounds or template molecules for developing novel antibiotics with high therapeutic potential. Here, to give the reader a comprehensive background on the topic, we have first reviewed cannabinoids, in terms of classification, chemical structures, mode of action, main pharmacological properties, current applications, clinical applicability, and antimicrobial properties. Doing this, CBC, CBG and CBD, known to exclusively possess beneficial non-mind-altering pharmacological effects and reported to have potent antibacterial effects, have emerged as the most promising compounds for the development of new efficient antibacterial agents. So, with the aim to ease the synthetic production of high amounts of CBC, CBG and CBD for favoring further studies and for promoting the development of new antimicrobial agents, we have systematically reviewed all the synthetic pathways utilized for their preparation, reporting both reaction schemes and experimental details.

2. Phytocannabinoids (PCs), Endocannabinoids (ECs) and Synthetic Cannabinoids (SCs)

2.1. *Phytocannabinoids (PCs) and Endocannabinoids (ECs)*

Generally, the term 'cannabinoids' refers to a heterogeneous family of compounds that exhibit activity upon particular human cannabinoid receptors, namely CB1 and CB2 [41,42]. They encompass the natural compounds present in the *Cannabis* plants, lipid mediators called ECs naturally produced by human cells, as well as by all vertebrates on planet Earth, and the synthetic analogs of both groups designed by scientist, called SCs [42]. Natural cannabinoids from *Cannabis* are more specifically called PCs referring to their original plant source, differently from ECs which are produced from human cells [43,44]. PCs and ECs could include compounds structurally very different both between the two families and inside the same class, as shown in Figures 2 and 3, which report the structure of the most relevant PCs and ECs, respectively.

Both PCs and ECs exert their effects by interacting with CB1 and CB2 receptors, found throughout the human body, and whose locations have been listed in Table 2. We have constructed Table 2 using the valuable information contained in the relevant work by Fraguas-Sánchez et al. [45].

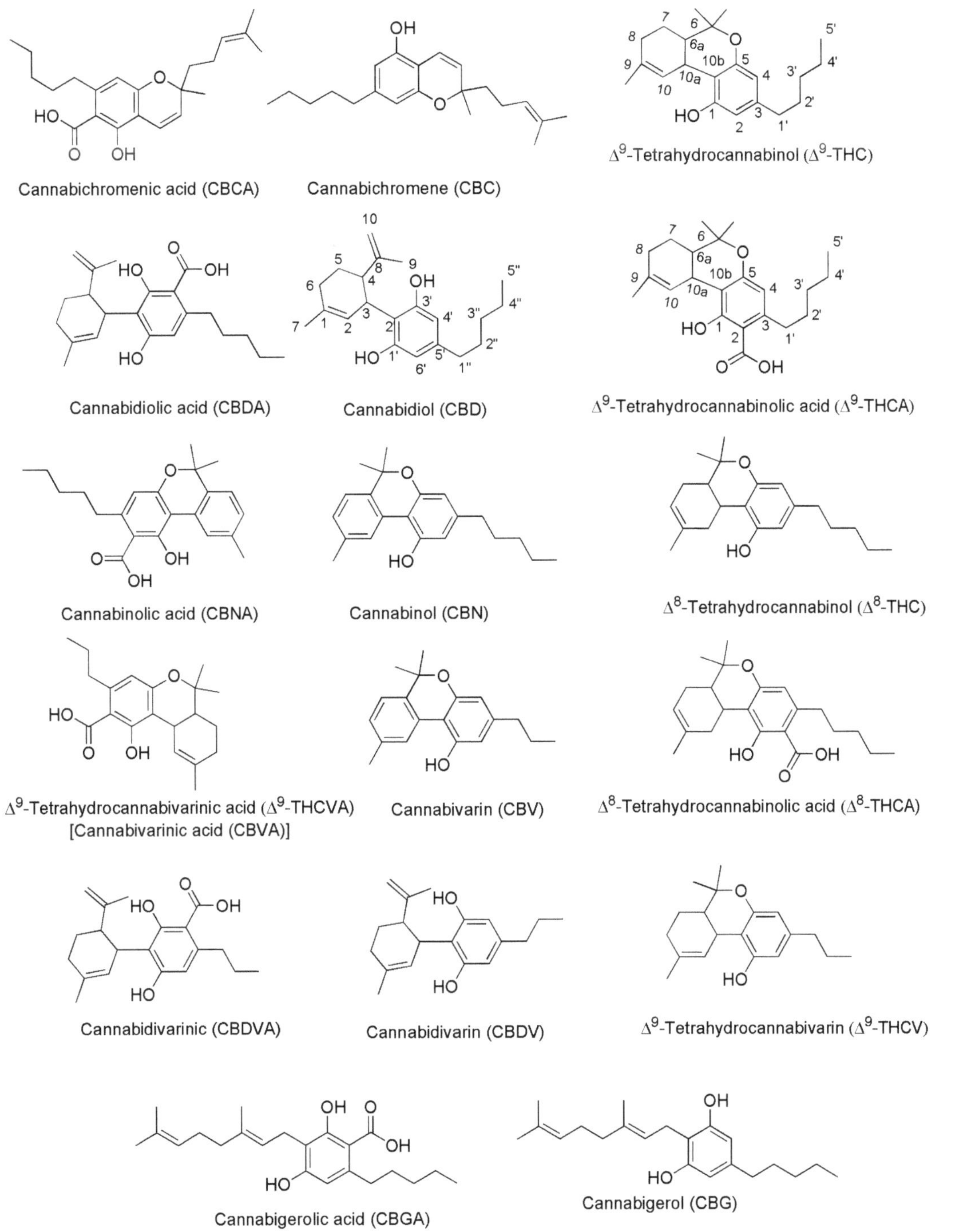

Figure 2. Chemical structure of the main PCs found in *C. sativa* acting on CB1 and/or CB2 receptors.

Table 2. Locations of CB1 and CB2 receptors in the human body.

Receptor Type	Location	Sublocation	Ref.
CB1	Central nervous system (CNS)	Hippocampus, cerebellum, basal ganglia, cortical regions Olfactory areas	[46]
	Peripheral nerve terminals Extra-neuronal sites	Eye, vascular endothelium, adipose tissue, lungs, liver Spleen, kidneys, uterus, prostate, testis, stomach, placenta Skeletal, muscles	
CB2	Peripheral immune system tissues	Spleen, tonsils, thymus, lymph nodes	[47]
	Peripheral immune system cells	B cells, natural killer cells, monocytes, macrophages Neutrophils, CD8+ T cells, CD4+ T cells	
	CNS *	Cerebellum, olfactory tubercle, striatum Thalamic nuclei (hippocampus and amygdala)	

* Under certain circumstances, most notably during inflammation.

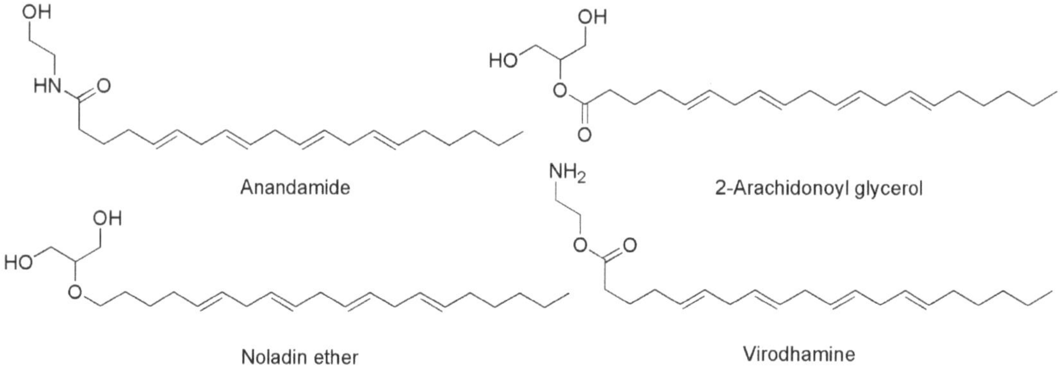

Figure 3. Chemical structure of the main ECs found in humans acting on CB1 and/or CB2 receptors.

The activation of CB1 receptor or the concurrent activation of both receptors by ECs or PCs leads to both psychotropic, undesired effects and therapeutic outcomes. Exactly, while mind alteration, psychotropic effects, cardiovascular adverse events can occur, analgesic, sedative, antidepressant, anti-inflammatory, anti-anorexic, anti-emetic, anticancer and antibacterial desirable effects can also arise. As an example, the FDA-approved drug formulations containing the synthetic versions of Δ^9-THC namely dronabinol (marketed as Marinol® or Syndros®) or nabilone (marketed as Cesamet™), as well as the extracted THC (marketed as Sativex®), possess affinity for both CB1 and CB2 [48]. Clinically, they are primarily used to treat the chemotherapy-induced nausea, to enhance appetite in cachexic AIDS-patients, and to alleviate the spasticity and pain associated with multiple sclerosis [30]. Unfortunately, evidence of undesired psychotropic and cardiovascular adverse effects strongly limits the therapeutic efficacy of such medicines [49]. Otherwise, the selective activation of CB2 receptors, occurring for example by CBG or CBD, could provide therapeutic effects, such as immuno-modulatory properties, anti-inflammatory, anti-emetic, and anti-anorexic effects without exerting the psychotropic actions deriving from the CB1 activation. In addition, the potent analgesic effects, associated with the activation of CB2, could be helpful in alleviating chronic widespread musculoskeletal pain (CWP) disorders, such as fibromyalgia syndrome [50]. Also, the selective activation of CB2 receptors could enhance severe human diseases as osteoporosis, atherosclerosis, cancer, chronic liver injuries and neurodegeneration [48]. Collectively, CB1 and CB2 receptors together with ECs make part of the so-called EC system (ECS), which was discovered in the 1990′s by scientists researching cannabinoids, which includes also several enzymes involved in producing and recycling ECs. In humans, ECs are naturally produced by cells within the body in response to external factors, like pain or temperature. As shown in Figure 3, among other molecules, ECs include the well-known compounds 2-arachidonoylglycerol (2-AG) and anandamide (ANA), as well as the less-known ECs like virodhamine, and 2-arachidonoyl glycerol ether [51]. Particularly 2-AG and ANA activate both CB1 and CB2 receptors with affinity for CB1 higher than that for CB2 [48]. Collectively, the interaction between ECs and their corresponding receptors is pivotal in maintaining the body's internal balance or homeostasis. ECs regulate some very important aspects of human health, as depicted in Figure 4.

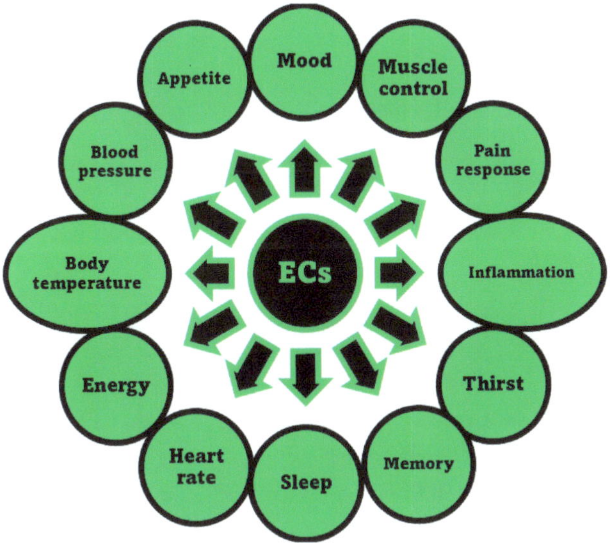

Figure 4. Aspects of humans' life regulated by the ECS, through the interaction of ECs with receptors CB1 and/or CB2, as reported in the relevant review by Sharma et al. [52].

Researchers suggest that ECs deficiencies could cause many refractory health conditions, such as depression, arthritis, fibromyalgia, and Crohn's disease that could ameliorate upon treatments with *Cannabis*, due to the activation by PCs of the same receptors activated in normal conditions by ECs. In fact, as reported above, PCs specifically produced by *Cannabis* plants and not by humans, when appropriately assumed can interact with CB1 and/or CB2 receptors triggering effects similar to those prompted by ECs, thus influencing the same aspects reported in Figure 4 and contributing to maintain or recover the body's internal balance or homeostasis [41]. Anyway, if abused, the psychotropic and undesired side effects of psychoactive PCs, such as THC and CBN may overwhelm the benefits. Figure 5 shows the chemical structure of two metabolites which form in the human body after *Cannabis* consumption, of cannabicyclolic acid (CBLA), a degradative byproduct of cannabichromenic acid (CBCA), and of cannabicyclol (CBL) which is the product of decarboxylation of CBLA [53]. Particularly, CBL is a non-psychoactive cannabinoid, which could also derive by degradation of CBC through natural irradiation or under acid conditions [54].

Particularly, CBLA, like CBCA and CBC, is a minor cannabinoid found in low concentrations in the *Cannabis* plant. It is not produced by *Cannabis* directly, but it forms when CBCA degrades after exposure to ultraviolet (UV) light or heat. CBLA is an acidic cannabinoid, like THCA, CBCA and CBDA, which produces CBL, upon decarboxylation and release of CO_2. CBLA is not considered intoxicating, is often deemed non-psychoactive or non-psychotropic, and curiously, it does not interact with receptors CB1 and CB2. There is little research into the effects and potential therapeutic uses of CBLA and CBL. Anyway, although more research is needed to confirm these attributes, some suggestions exist, that CBLA may have anti-inflammatory, antimicrobial, and antitumoral effects, due to its structural similarity to CBCA and CBN [53]. As for the metabolite 11-NCTHC, it is a no longer active secondary metabolite of THC, which forms in the body through the oxidation of the still psychoactive metabolite of THC, 11-HTHC, by liver enzymes [55].

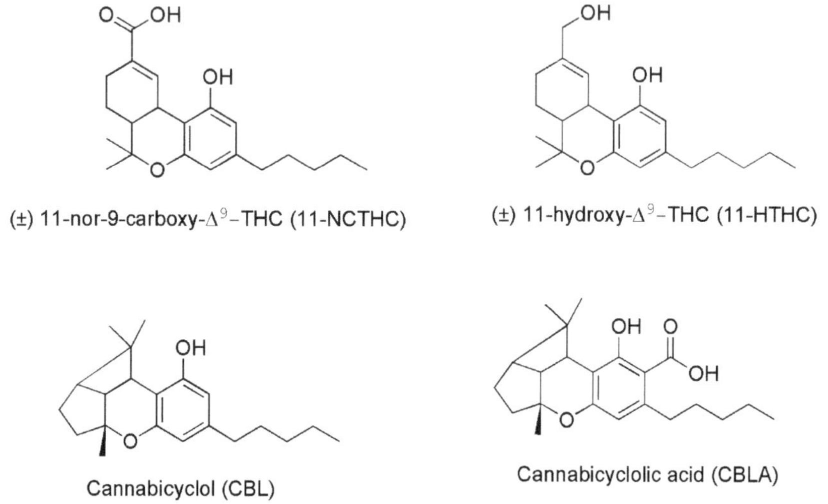

Figure 5. Chemical structure of two THC metabolites (11-NCTHC and 11-HTHC) and of two products deriving from CBCA degradation.

Structural Differences between Psychotropic and Not-Psychotropic PCs

It has been reported that the n-pentyl chain at the C-(3) position (Figure 2) works and essential role in the activity of psychotropic THC derivatives and that modification in this side chain leads to critical changes in the affinity, selectivity and pharmaco-potency of these ligands relating to the CB1 and CB2 cannabinoid receptors. Generally, while a shorter alkyl chain reduces the affinity of the compound for the cannabinoid receptor, an increase in the number of carbon atoms (hexyl, heptyl, or octyl) leads to an increase affinity for the same cannabinoid receptor [56,57]. Additionally, a number of other transformations in the tricyclic core of the THC cannabinoid structure have been carried out [58]. Particularly, the pyran ring-opening generally causes in the achieved compound a relative reduction in the affinity to the CB1/CB2 cannabinoid receptors, and in the psycho activity. In this regard, the absence of the tricyclic core in CBC, CBD and CBG for CB2 receptors, could be responsible for the for their higher affinity for CB2 receptors dealing with beneficial pharmacological properties, thus not exerting psychotropic effects [59].

2.2. Synthetic Cannabinoids (SCs)

The third group of cannabinoids consists of synthetic analogs of both ECs and PCs groups, appositely designed by scientists in the field, to enhance the benefits and therapeutic properties of ECs and PCs, while reducing the psychotropic and adverse effects. Among others, they include the compounds reported as examples in Figure 6 (chemical structures), and Table 3 (pharmacological properties and selectivity for receptors CB1 and CB2), which have demonstrated to be promising for treating severe humans' chronic diseases including breast and prostate tumors, the unpleasant side-effects of chemotherapy, and chronic pain [42].

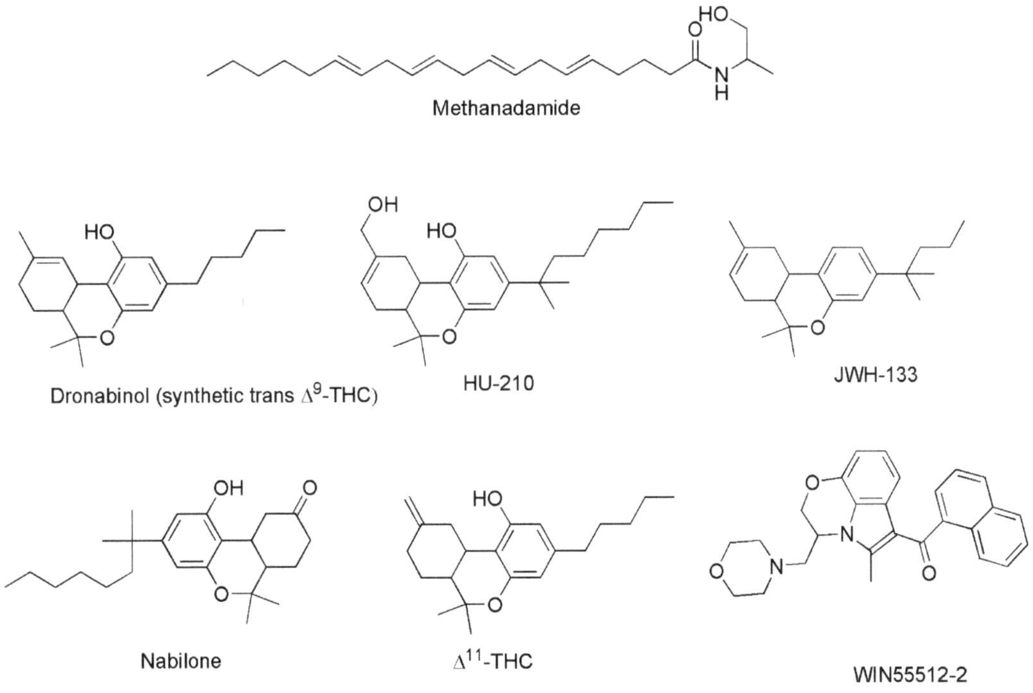

Figure 6. Structure of some SCs capable to act on CB1 and/or CB2 receptors.

Table 3. Selectivity of some SCs for CB1 and CB2 receptors, and their effects.

SCs	Binding Affinity		Effects	Refs.
	CB1 (Ki, nM)	CB2 (Ki, nM)		
Dronabinol *	15	51	Appetite stimulant Psychotropic effects Analgesic ↓ Nausea Antiemetic	[60]
Methanandamide (AM-356)	20	815		[61]
SR144528	280	0.1	Anti-inflammatory Analgesic ↓ Neuropathic pain	[48]
Cannabinor # (PRS-211,375)	5585	17.4		[62]
CP47,597	2.1 (Kd)	56	Analgesic	[48]
JTE907	490	2.2	Anti-inflammatory	[48]
JWH133	680	3.4	↓↓ Neurotoxicity Anti-inflammatory ↓ Alzheimer symptoms	[48]
AM1241	272	3.4	Analgesic effects ↓ Hyperalgesia ↓ Allodynia Amyotrophic lateral sclerosis	[48]
GW405,833	8640	7.2	↓ Hyperalgesia ↓ Allodynia	[48]

Table 3. *Cont.*

SCs	Binding Affinity		Effects	Refs.
	CB1 (Ki, nM)	CB2 (Ki, nM)		
L-759,633	1604	9.8	Analgesic Antianxiety Antidepressant Anti-inflammatory ↓ Alzheimer symptoms	[48]
JWH139	2290	14		
HU308	115,000	23		
AM630	3795	32		
HU-210	0.061	0.52		[63]
L-759,656	4888	↑11.8		[64]
WIN 55,212-2	1.9		Analgesic Anti-inflammatory ↓ Alzheimer symptoms	[65]
JWH015	383	13.8	Analgesic Anti-inflammatory	[66]
WIN 48,098 (Pravadoline)	4.9 (IC_{50})		Analgesic Anti-inflammatory	[67]

Ki = Defined kinetically as the ratio of rate constants koff/kon for the binding of a ligand to the receptor. This is the same as Kd; IC_{50} = the concentration of ligand required to saturate half of the receptor; * Approved by the FDA as safe and effective for HIV/AIDS-induced anorexia and chemotherapy-induced nausea and vomiting only; # failed in Phase IIb human clinical trials due to lack of efficacy; ↓ = reduction of; ↓↓ = strong reduction of.

On the base of their affinity and selectivity for receptors CB1 and CB2, they can exert both therapeutic and psychotropic effects, or mainly one of the two. Table 3 summarizes the selectivity of some SCs for CB1 and CB2, and their therapeutic effects.

The following Figure 7 shows the chemical structures of compounds in Table 3 not previously reported in Figure 6.

Methanandamide (AM-356) is a synthetically constructed stable chiral analog of anandamide. AM-356 acts on the cannabinoid receptors, and specifically on CB1-type receptors in the CNS found in mammals, fish, and certain invertebrates (e.g., Hydra), thus resulting also a psychoactive compound [68]. HU-210, as well as other SCs including L-759,656, HU-308, L-759,633, L-768,242 etc. are potent analgesic and anti-inflammatory compounds with many of the same effects as natural THC [44]. WIN 55,212-2 is an organic heterotricyclic SC. Particularly, it is the 5-methyl-3-(morpholin-4-ylmethyl)-2,3-dihydro [1,4]oxazine [2,3,4-hi]indole substituted at position 6 by a 1-naphthylcarbonyl group. It has a role as an analgesic, and neuroprotective agent, as well as an apoptosis inhibitor [69].

JWH-133 is a Δ^9-tetrahydrocannabinol lacking the hydroxy group and having a 1,1-dimethylbutyl group at position 3 in place of the pentyl group. It acts as potent and highly selective CB2 receptor agonist, thus exerting antineoplastic effects, and working as a vasodilator and an anti-inflammatory agent, as an apoptosis inhibitor, as well as an analgesic molecule [70].

Δ^{11}-THC, also known as exo-tetrahydrocannabinol, is a synthetic isomer of tetrahydrocannabinol, developed in the 1970s. It can be synthesized from Δ^8-THC by several different routes, and only the (6aR, 10aR) enantiomer is known. In animal studies in mice, it was found to exert the same effect of Δ^9-THC with around 1/4 its potency. It has been identified as a component of "vaping liquids" sold for use in humans [71].

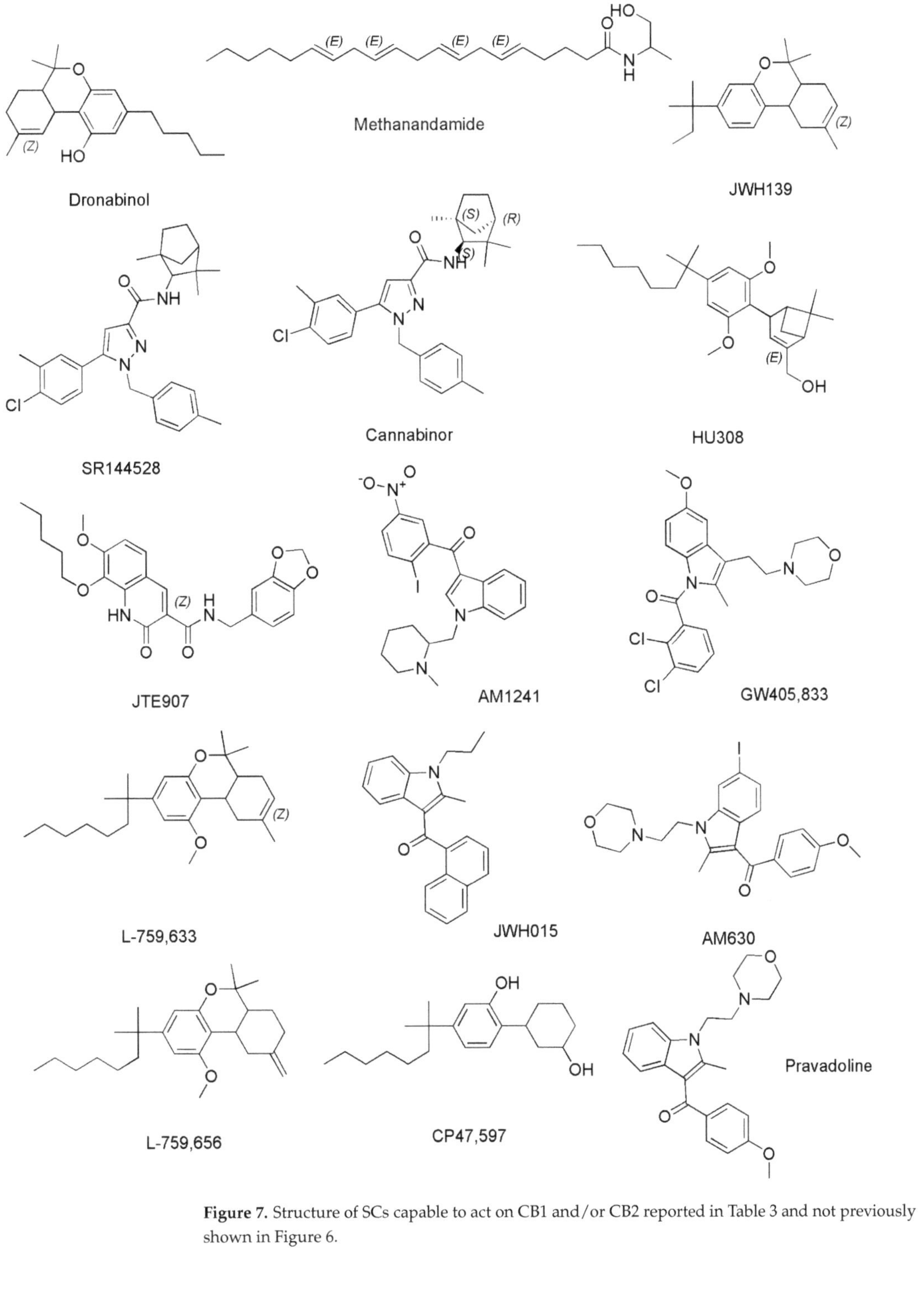

Figure 7. Structure of SCs capable to act on CB1 and/or CB2 reported in Table 3 and not previously shown in Figure 6.

2.3. Cannabinoids Clinically Approved

Collectively, PCs and the several developed SCs have proved to be useful in the treatment of chemotherapy side effects such as nausea, vomiting, pain, weight loss, and lack of appetite [30], but only few drugs based only on THC and CBD have been approved so far in some countries, as palliative agents in anticancer treatments. Dronabinol, the synthetic analogous of Δ^9-THC and nabilone, a SC similar to Δ^9-THC, are currently approved in Canada, United States, and several countries in Europe to treat nausea and vomiting associated with chemotherapeutic treatments [72]. An oromucosal spray containing a mixture 1:1 of Δ^9-THC and CBD marketed as Sativex® is approved in Europe and Canada for the treatment of spasticity associated with multiple sclerosis (MS), while in Canada Sativex is applied also as an adjunctive analgesic for the treatment of pain in patients with advanced cancer and MS [73,74]. An oral solution of CBD, marketed as Epidiolex® is an US FDA-approved prescription that is used in association with clobazam to treat refractory epilepsy due to Lennox–Gastaut or Dravet syndrome [75,76]. Finally, we signalize the case of Rimonabant (or SR141716), which was marketed as Acomplia®. It is an inverse agonist for the CB1 receptor, capable to reduce the appetite, and was clinically applied as an anorectic anti-obesity drug. It was withdrawn from the market in 2009, after a long dispute between the European Medicines Agency (EMA) and the Cochrane Collaboration, because it increased the risk of psychiatric problems and suicide [77].

3. Phytocannibinoids: Polyfunctional Molecules Promising to Develop Novel Antibiotics

3.1. Not Only THC and CBD

Wehave likely heard that *C. sativa* provides THC, having high medicinal value, but also mind-altering effects (psychotropic) and cannabidiol (CBD), which is praised for its medicinal benefits without being psychoactive [41]. Anyway, while these are the most well-known and abundant PCs, as mentioned above, there are a plethora of other cannabinoids produced by the *Cannabis* plants.

Particularly, *C. sativa* produces about 1600 chemical substances, 500 bioactive compounds, including approximately 180 cannabinoids (113–125 isolated), many terpenes, and flavonoids which could be promising as novel therapeutic agents [40,78].

More generally, the known different cannabinoids, are naturally present not only in *Cannabis*, but also in various other plants or in burned cannabis resin. Cannabinoids are found in certain species of flowering plants (Rhododendron), some species of liverworts, an ancient fern-like plant, as well as in certain types of fungi (myco-cannabinoids). Among PCs, cannabigerolic acid (CBGA) which is the direct precursor of the decarboxylated CBG, can be considered as the "mother of all major cannabinoids", according to the biosynthetic pathway in Figure 8 [40].

The most common misunderstanding about *Cannabis* consists in thinking that the plant produces THC, as well as the other major activated cannabinoids (red compounds in Figure 8), while it actually generates their acidic forms (raw cannabis), such as CBGA, THCA, CBDA, CBCA, which are converted in the decarboxylated forms (CBG, THC, CBD, CBC) only once the flower is heated. Actually, very little activated cannabinoids are found in fresh *Cannabis* flower, while most are in the acidic form and get decarboxylated into THC, CBD, CBC or CBG upon smoking or plant ageing [41]. Anyway, despite being most dismissed as inactive, because it is not absorbed in the brain, also acids cannabinoids may actually offer several therapeutic potentials, including antimicrobial activity.

3.2. Much More beyond the Psychotropic Effect of THC

Figure 9 shows the several pharmacologic activities of some relevant natural cannabinoids (PCs), including also some minor cannabinoids of the varin (V) family.

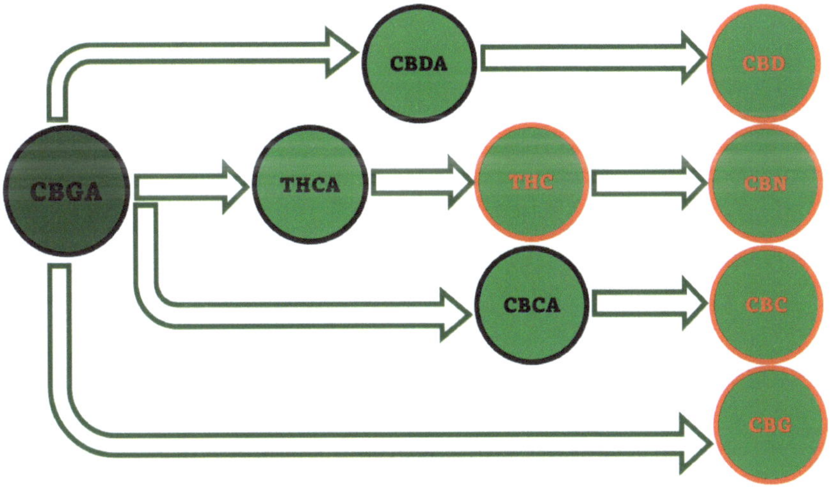

Figure 8. Biosynthetic pathway starting from CBGA and leading to the five major PCs. This image has been created by the authors exploiting information available online at https://www.openaccessgovernment.org/cbg-the-mother-of-all-cannabinoids-with-broad-antibacterial-activity/95824/ (accessed on 3 May 2023).

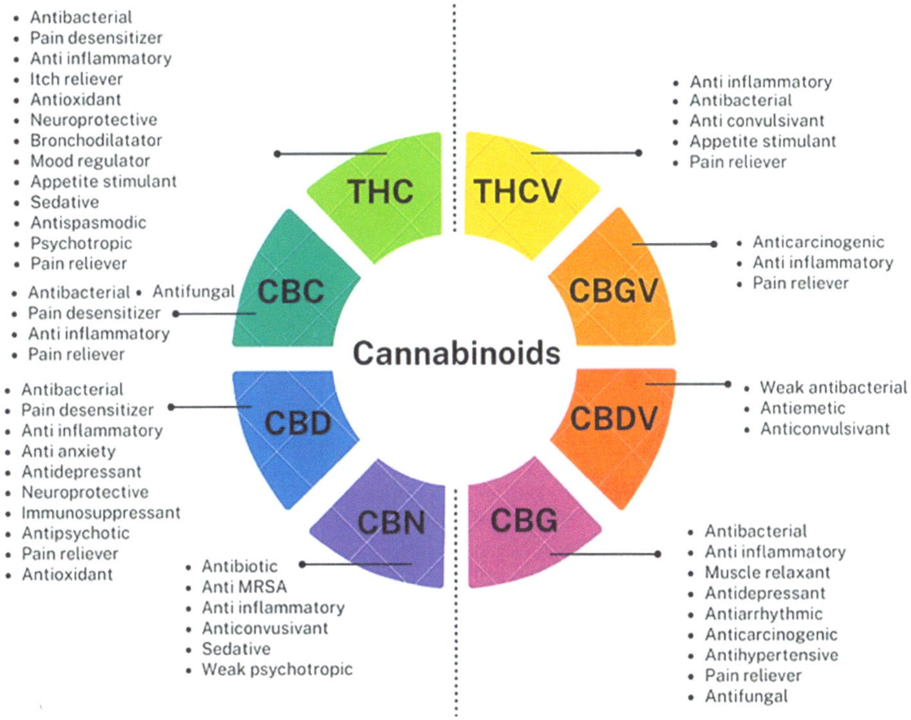

Figure 9. Pharmacological properties of some relevant major and minor PCs. Figure 9 has been originally created by the authors using information found online [41] and using Flipsnack, a free dowlodable application to produce PowerPoint professional designes, available online at https://app.flipsnack.com/editor/7uld8l9xu3 (accessed on 14 June 2023).

From a structural point of view, CBDV, THCV and CBGV reported in Figure 9 and CBCV (not reported), belonging to the varins (Vs), have two fewer carbon atoms in the alkyl chain with respect to the correspondent better-known cannabinoids CBD, THC, CBG and CBC. This shorter carbon chain strongly affects their pharmacologic activity, thus being promising compounds in managing weight loss, diabetes, cholesterol problems, autism, seizures, and more [79]. Particularly, THCV, although very structurally similar to THC has a totally different effects profile. The slight alteration in its chemical structure implies that, unlike THC, it acts as an antagonist to the receptor CB1 rather than an activator, thus not producing relaxing, euphoric, and energizing outcomes, but exerting antianxiety, anticonvulsant, appetite suppressant and anti-inflammatory effects [41]. THCV could be a weight-loss aid, by reducing appetite and boosting metabolism, and could be helpful in the treatment diabetes by controlling the blood sugar levels and the insulin production. Also, THCV may help promoting new bone cell growth, preventing weakening bones, and can even act as a neuroprotectant in conditions like Parkinson's disease [80].

Collectively, as observable both in Figure 9 and in the following Figure 10, all the reported cannabinoids, like many other phytochemicals, are multifunctional compounds owing several pharmacological activities, being THC, the cannabinoid possessing the highest number of effects on human body, followed by CBD and CBG.

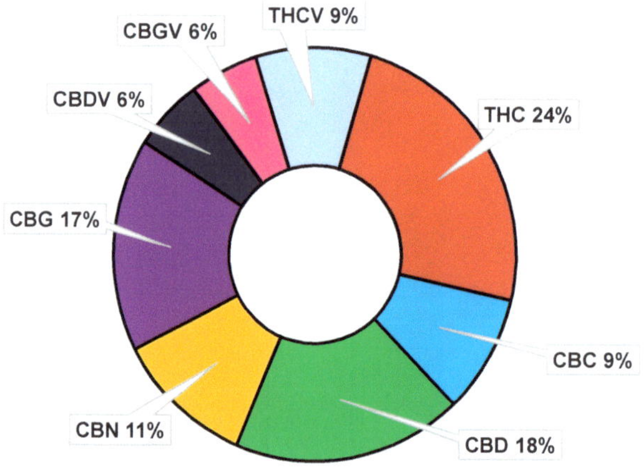

Figure 10. Percentages of pharmacological properties possessed by some major and minor cannabinoids.

Interestingly, only THC and CBN possess intoxicant effects (psychotropic actions), while all other PCs in Figures 9 and 10, except for CBGV, have demonstrated to possess antimicrobial properties, and especially antibacterial effects on MDR strains of Gram-positive species, thus being promising molecules or template compounds to develop novel antibiotics. The molecular mechanisms at the base of the antibacterial activity of PCs have yet to be fully unveiled. Anyway, the effects of structural modifications on the bactericidal effects of the more studied cannabinoids (CBD, CBC, CGB, THC, and CBN) have been recently investigated by Scott et al. [81]. All the considered cannabinoids demonstrated potent activity against a variety of MRSA strains, with MIC values in the range 0.5–2 μg/mL. Methylation and acetylation of the phenolic hydroxyls, esterification of the carboxylic group, as well as the introduction of a second prenyl group were detrimental to the cannabinoids' antibacterial activity. The antibacterial effects were maintained regardless the type of prenyl moiety, its relative position compared to the n-pentyl moiety (abnormal cannabinoids), and the carboxylation of the resorcinol moiety (pre-cannabinoids). Collectively, structural modification of the terpenoid moiety do not affect the antibacterial effects of PCs, suggesting that these residues serve mainly as modulators of lipid affinity, while the addition of further prenyl moiety may result in poorer aqueous solubility, leading to a loss of antibacterial activity [81].

3.3. Antimicrobial Cannabinoids

Table 4 reports the most relevant PCs, both in the acid forms and in the decarboxylated ones, ECs, and SCs (mainly prepared by scientist to study the structure-activity relationships (SARs), which were in the past or recently assayed as antimicrobial agents. Figure 11 shows the chemical structure of SCs present in Table 4 not showed previously, while the subsequent Table 5 reports the antimicrobial properties of compounds listed in Table 4, expressed as minimum inhibitory concentrations (MICs), as well as the target pathogens.

Table 4. The most relevant cannabinoids which were in the past or recently assayed to assess their antimicrobial properties.

Precannabinoids	Cannabinoids	Synthetic Compounds
Cannabichromenic acid (CBCA)	Cannabichromene (CBC) *	Δ^{11}-THC **S
Cannabidiolic acid (CBDA)	Cannabidiol (CBD) *	Me-CBD
Cannabigerolic acid (CBGA)	Cannabigerol (CBG) *	Me-CBG
		Ac-CBD
Δ^9-Tetrahydrocannabinolic acid A (THCAA)	Δ^9-Tetrahydrocannabinol (Δ^9-THC) *	Ac-CBG
Δ^9-Tetrahydrocannabinolic acid B (THCAB)		PhEO-CBD
		PhEO-CBG
Δ^9-tetrahydrocannabivarin acid (THCVA)	Δ^9-tetrahydrocannabivarin (THCV) *	MeO-CBD
Cannabidivarinic acid (CBDVA)	Cannabidivarin (CBDV) *	MeO-CBG
		Abn-CBD
	Δ^8-THC **N	Abn-CBG
	Cannabicyclol (CBL) #	Carmagerol °°
	(±)11-NCTHC °	BP-CBD
N.T.	(±)11-HTHC §	CBC isomer (ICBC)
		CBC-C_o
	Anantamide (ANA) ***,$	CBC-C_1
	Arachidonyl serine (AraS) $	ICBC-C_o

* From decarboxylation of acidic pre-cannabinoids; N.T. = not tested; **N natural isomer of Δ^9-THC; **S synthetic isomer of Δ^9-THC; Me-CBD = mono- di-methylated derivatives of CBD (Figure 11); Me-CBG = mono-di-methylated derivatives of CBG (Figure 11); Ac-CBD = acetylated derivative of CBD (Figure 11); Ac-CBG = acetylated derivative of CBG (Figure 11); PhEO-CBD = phenyl-ethyl ester of CBD (Figure 11); PhEO-CBG = phenyl-ethyl ester of CBG (Figure 11); MeO-CBD = methyl ester of CBD (Figure 11); MeO-CBG = methyl ester of CBG (Figure 11); Abn-CBD = abnormal (*orto*-isomer) CBD (Figure 11); Abn-CBG = abnormal (*orto*-isomer) CBG (Figure 11); °° polar analogue of CBG (Figure 11); BP-CBD = bis-prenylated analogue of CBD (Figure 11); ICBC, CBC-C_o, CBC-C_1, ICBC-C_o = isomers and analogous of CBC whose structures are available in Figure 11; # degradative product of CBC; ° not active secondary metabolite of THC which is formed in the body after cannabis is consumed; § main active metabolite of THC, which is formed in the body after Δ^9-THC is consumed; *** also known as N-arachidonoyl-ethanolamine (AEA); $ ECs.

Table 5. Antimicrobial effects against bacteria and fungi reported in the past and recently for several cannabinoids expressed as MICs (μg/mL) if not differently specified.

Compounds	Pathogens	MIC * (μg/mL)	Ref.	Comments
Δ^9-THC	*S. aureus*	1–5	[82]	Binding to plasma proteins ↓ Activity on Gram-negative Psychotropic
	Streptococcus pyogenes	5		
	S. milleri	2		
	Enterococcus faecalis	5		
	S. aureus	1	[83]	
	EMRSA	0.5–2		
	S. aureus SA-1199B	2		
	S. aureus RN-4220	1		
	S. aureus XU212	1		
	MRSA USA300	2	[33]	

Table 5. *Cont.*

Compounds	Pathogens	MIC * (μg/mL)	Ref.	Comments
Δ9-THC acid A (THCAA)	MRSA USA300	4	[33]	Binding to plasma proteins ↓ Activity on Gram-negative Non-psychotropic ↑ Therapeutic potential ↑ Effects without the carboxylate moiety
	S. aureus EMRSA *S. aureus* SA-1199B *S. aureus* RN-4220 *S. aureus* XU212	4 4–8 8 4 8	[83]	
Δ8-THC	MRSA USA300	2	[33]	Binding to plasma proteins ↓ Activity on Gram-negative Psychotropic Lack psychotropic effects ↑ Therapeutic potential ↓ Activity on Gram-negative ↑ Effects without the carboxylate moiety
Δ11-THC	MRSA USA300	2	[33]	
Δ9-THCV	MRSA USA300	4	[33]	
THCV acid (THCVA)	MRSA USA300	16	[33]	
CBD	*S. aureus*	1 1–5 0.5 1.25	[84] [82] [83] [85]	Binding to plasma proteins ↓ Activity on Gram-negative Antiepileptic Anti-inflammatory Non-psychotropic ↑ Therapeutic potential
	EMRSA *S. aureus* SA-1199B *S. aureus* RN-4220 *S. aureus* XU212	1	[83]	
	MRSA USA300	2 4	[33] [86]	
	S. epidermidis	2	[84]	
	S. pyogenes *S. milleri* *E. faecalis*	2 1 5	[82]	
	MRSE *Listeria monocytogenes* *E. faecalis*	4 4 8	[86]	
	E. coli	1.25	[85]	
CBN	MRSA USA300	2	[33]	Binding to plasma proteins ↓ Activity on Gram-negative Weakly psychotropic
	S. aureus EMRSA *S. aureus* SA-1199B *S. aureus* RN-4220 *S. aureus* XU212	1	[83]	
Abn-CBD	*S. aureus* EMRSA *S. aureus* SA-1199B *S. aureus* RN-4220 *S. aureus* XU212	1	[83]	Binding to plasma proteins ↓ Activity on Gram-negative Non-psychotropic ↑ Therapeutic potential
CBC	*B. subtilis* *S. aureus* *Mycobacterium smegmatis* *Candida albicans* *Saccharomyces cerevisiae* *Trichophyton mentagrophytes*	0.39 1.56 12.5 N.T. 25 25	[87]	↓ Activity on Gram-negative Non-psychotropic ↑ Therapeutic potential In case of acid compounds: ↑ Effects without the carboxylate moiety
	MRSA USA300	8	[33]	

Table 5. *Cont.*

Compounds	Pathogens	MIC * (μg/mL)	Ref.	Comments
CBC	EMRSA	2	[83]	↓ Activity on Gram-negative Non-psychotropic ↑ Therapeutic potential In case of acid compounds: ↑ Effects without the carboxylate moiety
	S. aureus	2		
	S. aureus SA-1199B	2		
	S. aureus RN-4220	2		
	S. aureus XU212	1		
CBCA	MRSA USA300	2	[33]	
CBC isomer (ICBC)	*B. subtilis*	0.78	[87]	
	S. aureus	N.T.		
	M. smegmatis	25		
	C. albicans	50		
	S. cerevisiae	N.T.		
	T. mentagrophytes	N.T.		
CBC-C_o	*B. subtilis*	6.25		
	S. aureus	12.5		
	M. smegmatis	12.5		
	C. albicans	50		
	S. cerevisiae	25		
	T. mentagrophytes	25		
CBC-C_1	*B. subtilis*	3.12		
	S. aureus	3.12		
	M. smegmatis	3.12		
	C. albicans	N.T.		
	S. cerevisiae	6.25		
	T. mentagrophytes	6.25		
ICBC-C_o	*B. subtilis*	6.25		
	S. aureus	12.5		
	M. smegmatis	12.5		
	C. albicans	12.5		
	S. cerevisiae	N.T.		
	T. mentagrophytes	6.25		
CBDA	*S. aureus* EMRSA *S. aureus* SA-1199B *S. aureus* RN-4220 *S. aureus* XU212	2	[83]	↑ Effects without the carboxylate moiety ↓ Activity on Gram-negative Non-psychotropic ↑ Therapeutic potential ↑ Effects without the carboxylate moiety
	S. epidermidis	4	[84]	
	S. aureus	2		
	MRSA USA300	16	[33]	
		4	[84]	
CBGA	MRSA USA300	4	[33]	Non-psychotropic ↑ Therapeutic potential ↑ Effects without the carboxylate moiety ↓ Activity on Gram-negative
	EMRSA	2–4	[83]	
	S. aureus	4		
	S. aureus SA-1199B	4		
	S. aureus RN-4220	2		
	S. aureus XU212	4		
CBG	*Streptococcus mutans*	2.5	[88]	Non-psychotropic ↑ Membrane permeability Cause membrane hyperpolarization ↓ Membrane fluidity Non-psychotropic ↑ Therapeutic potential ↓ Activity on Gram-negative
	S. sanguis	1		
	S. sobrinos	5		
	S. salivarius	5		

Table 5. *Cont.*

Compounds	Pathogens	MIC * (μg/mL)	Ref.	Comments
CBG	MRSA USA300	2	[33]	Non-psychotropic ↑ Membrane permeability Cause membrane hyperpolarization ↓ Membrane fluidity Non-psychotropic ↑ Therapeutic potential ↓ Activity on Gram-negative
	S. aureus EMRSA *S. aureus* SA-1199B *S. aureus* RN-4220 *S. aureus* XU212	1 1–2 1 1 1	[83]	
	C. albicans *S. cerevisiae* *T. mentagrophytes*	3 [a]; (4) [b] 6 [a]; (2) [b] 5 [a]; (4) [b]	[89]	
Abn-CBG	*S. aureus* EMRSA *S. aureus* SA-1199B *S. aureus* RN-4220 *S. aureus* XU212	1 2 2 1 0.5	[83]	
CBDV	MRSA USA300	8	[33]	Non-psychotropic ↑ Therapeutic potential ↓ Activity on Gram-negative
CBDVA	MRSA USA300	32	[33]	Non-psychotropic ↑ Therapeutic potential ↑ Effects without the carboxylate moiety ↓ Activity on Gram-negative
CBL (±) 11-NCTHC	MRSA USA300	>32	[33]	Non-psychotropic ↑ Therapeutic potential
(±) 11-HTHC	MRSA USA300	>32	[33]	Psychotropic
ANA	MRSA	>256 ** 64 *** (51–54) #	[90]	Psychotropic ↓ Membrane potential in bacteria ↓ Bacteria adhesion capacity ↓ Cells aggregation capacity Not bactericidal ↓ Activity on Gram-negative
AraS	MRSA	32->256 ** 64 *** (33–61) #	[90]	Psychotropic Neuroprotective ↓ Activity on Gram-negative Affect membrane potential in bacteria ↓ Bacteria adhesion capacity ↓ Cells aggregation capacity Not bactericidal

* After 24 h exposure on bacteria, after 48 h exposure on fungi; [a] activity was recorded as the width (in millimeters) of the inhibition zone measured from the edge of the agar well to the edge of the inhibition zone; [b] inhibition zone of Amphotericin B; ** on planktonic cells; *** on biofilm; # percentage of biofilm eradication; SA-1199B = fluoroquinolones-resistant; RN-4220 = macrolides-resistant; XU212 = tetracycline-resistant; MRSE = methicillin-resistant *S. epidermidis; S. aureus* = ATCC25923 strains; EMRSA = the major epidemic methicillin-resistant *S. aureus* occurring in U.K. hospitals; ↓ = low, lower, minor; ↑ = high, higher, strong.

Since except for compounds Δ^{11}-THC, Abn-CBD, Abn-CBG and CBC derivatives, the other SCs reported in Table 4 and Figure 11 demonstrated insignificant activity against the tested pathogens reported in Table 5 (MICs > 100 μg/mL), they were no longer reported in Table 5.

The first data we have found concerning the possible antibacterial activity of PCs were reported by Van Klingeren and Ham in the year 1976 [82]. The authors tested both THC and CBD on *S. aureus* and some isolates of *Streptococcus* genus, finding MICs in the range 1–5 μg/mL for both compounds against both species [82]. A weak antifungal activity was reported in the past (years 1981, 1982) only for CBC, some its synthetic derivatives [87] and for CBG [89], but no recent reports is present in the literature, thus demonstrating the poor interest of scientists, probably due to the scarce effects. On the contrary, in the year 1981, Turner found good antimicrobial activity for CBC against *Bacillus subtilis* (MIC = 0.4 μg/mL) and *S. aureus* (1.6 μg/mL), and for ICBC against *B. subtilis* (MIC = 0.8 μg/mL) [87]. Δ^9- THC, CBD, CBG, CBC, and CBN were assayed for their antimicrobial properties by Appendino et al. on the MDR *S. aureus* SA-1199B strain, which showed a high level of resistance to certain fluoroquinolones, on EMRSA isolates, which are the major epidemic methicillin-resistant *S. aureus* strains occurring in U.K. hospitals, on a macrolide-resistant strain (RN4220), on a tetracycline-resistant line (XU212), and on a standard laboratory *S. aureus* strain (ATCC25923) [83]. All compounds showed potent antibacterial activity, with MIC values in the 0.5–2 μg/mL range. Interestingly, also the acidic precursors of CBD, CBG, and THC (compounds CBDA, CBGA and THCA) maintained the activity substantially [83].

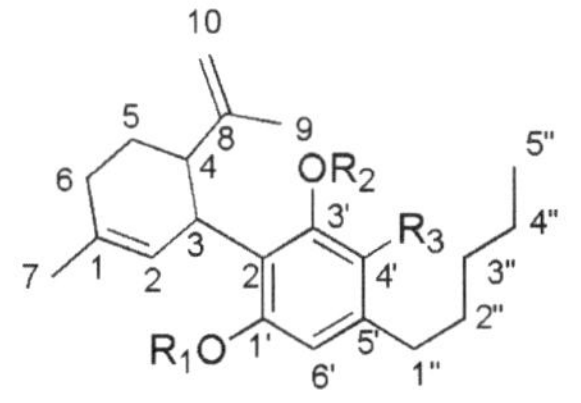

Me-CBD R_1 = Me; R_2 = H; R_3 = H
R_1 = Me; R_2 = Me; R_3 = H
Ac-CBD R_1 = Ac; R_2 = Ac; R_3 = H
PhEO-CBD R_1 = H; R_2 = H; R_3 = $PhCH_2CH_2COO$
MeO-CBD R_1 = H; R_2 = H; R_3 = MeCOO

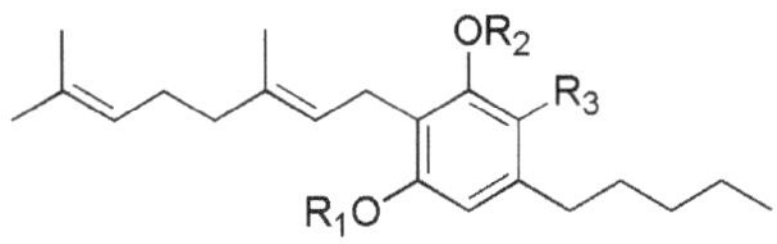

Me-CBG R_1 = Me; R_2 = H; R_3 = H
R_1 = Me; R_2 = Me; R_3 = H
Ac-CBG R_1 = Ac; R_2 = Ac; R_3 = H
PhEO-CBG R_1 = H; R_2 = H; R_3 = $PhCH_2CH_2COO$
MeO-CBG R_1 = H; R_2 = H; R_3 = MeCOO

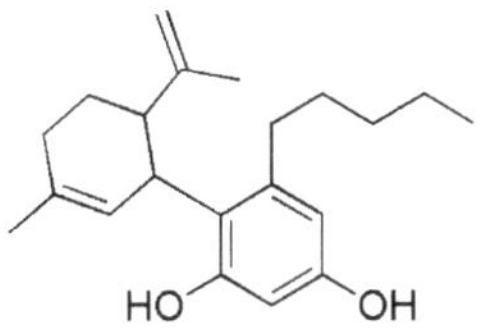

Abn-CBD

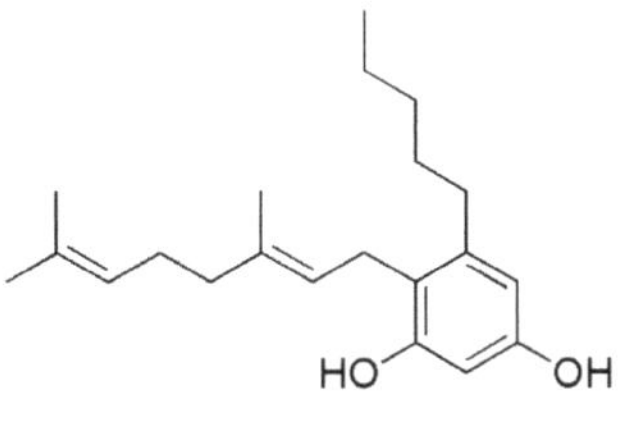

Abn-CBG

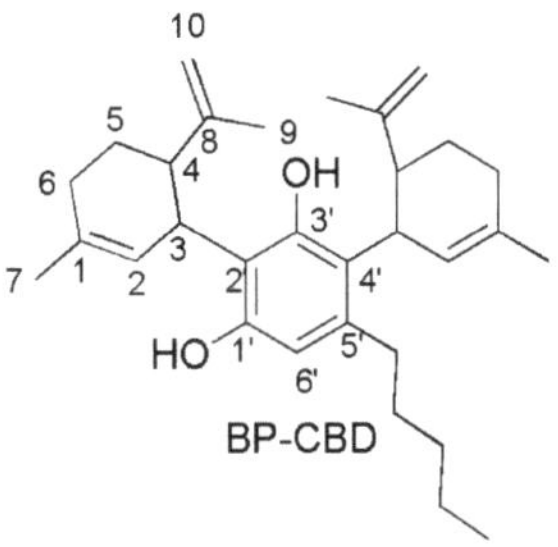

BP-CBD

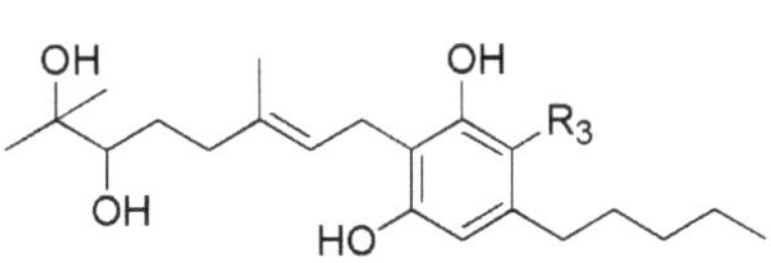

Carmagerol

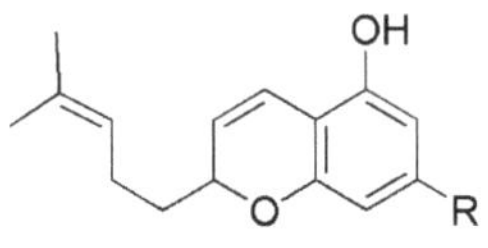

CBC-C_1 R = CH_3
CBC-Co R = H

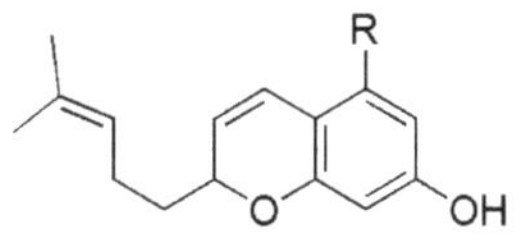

iso-CBC R = C_5H_{11}
iso-CBC-Co R = H

Figure 11. SCs reported in Table 4 whose chemical structure was not reported previously. Abn-CBD and Abn-CBG are defined as *orto*-isomers of *para*-derivatives CBD and CBG, being the *orto*- and *para*-positions those reciprocals to the pentyl chain.

Since given their non-psychotropic profiles, CBD and CBG can be considered especially promising, Appendino et al. performed structure-activity studies. Among the various synthetic derivatives, only the synthetic abnormal cannabinoids Abn-CBD and abn-CBG, although slightly less potent than CBD and CBG, showed antibacterial activity comparable to that of their corresponding natural products [83].

According to recent reports, 18 cannabinoids including CBC, CBD, CBG, CBN, Δ^9-THC and their carboxylic precursors (pre-cannabinoids CBCA, CBDA, CBGA, Δ^9-THCA), CBDV, THCV and their precursors (CBDVA, THCVA), Δ^8-THC, CBL, 11-NCTHC, 11-HTHC and Δ^{11}-THC were tested against MRSA USA300, a highly virulent and prevalent community-associated MRSA, by Farha et al. [33]. Susceptibility tests were conducted according to the Clinical and Laboratory Standards Institute (CLSI) protocol [91].

CBG, CBD, CBN, CBCA, Δ^9-THC, Δ^8-THC, and Δ^{11}-THC were potent antibiotics with MICs = 2 μg/mL. A moderate loss of potency was observed for their acidic precursors such as CBDA, CBGA and THCAA. THCV and CBDV were less active, displaying MICs = 4 and 8 μg/mL, respectively. It is well-known, that biofilm formation by MRSA, typically on necrotic tissues and medical devices, represents an important virulence factor influencing the persistence of MRSA and is typically associated with increased resistance to antimicrobial compounds. In this regard, Farha et al. investigated also the capability of the above-mentioned cannabinoids to inhibit the formation of biofilms by MRSA [33]. According to the results reported, the tested cannabinoids except for varins, clearly repressed MRSA biofilm formation, with CBG exhibiting the most potent antibiofilm activity. Indeed, at concentration of 0.5 μg/mL (1/4 MIC), CBG inhibited biofilm formation by ~50% [33].

When its effect was evaluated on preformed biofilms by determining its minimal biofilm eradication concentration (MBEC), CBG eradicated preformed biofilms of MRSA USA300 at concentration of 4 μg/mL. Additionally, on MRSA persister cells, which are a nongrowing, dormant cells subpopulations, which exhibit high levels of tolerance to antibiotics, and are responsible of chronic and relapsing *S. aureus* infections, such as osteomyelitis and endocarditis, the tested cannabinoids showed antipersisters activity which correlated with MIC values [33]. Again, CBG was the most potent cannabinoid against the persisters. In time-kill experiments, while the β-lactam oxacillin at 160 μg/mL (5 × MIC) did not show any activity, CBG killed persisters in a concentration-dependent manner starting at 5 μg/mL, and rapidly eradicated a population of $\sim 10^8$ CFU/mL MRSA persisters within 30 min of treatment.

As expected, the two most common human metabolites of THC, (±)11-NCTHC and (±) 11-HTHC, as well as CBL were inactive at the highest concentrations screened (MIC > 32 μg/mL). Unfortunately, in the study by Farha et al., none of these analogous displayed bactericidal effects against *E. coli* [33,78]. However, CBG was found to be effective also against Gram-negative bacteria when associated to polymyxin B or the less nephrotoxic polymyxin B nonapeptide [33,78] and acted as a sensitizing agent in combination with various antibiotics [92].

Concerning the association with polymyxin B, it was proposed that polymyxins permeabilize the outer membrane of Gram-negative pathogens, unassailable by CBG, thus enabling CBG to reach and damage the inner membrane [33,78]. Additionally, when *E. coli* VCS257 was treated with CBD in combination with erythromycin, vancomycin, rifampicin, kanamycin or colistin, an enhanced antimicrobial effect was observed [92]. In the year 2020, Martinenghi et al., tested CBDA and CBD against *S. aureus* and *S. epidermidis* finding very low MIC for CBD (MIC = 1 μg/mL and 2 μg/mL, respectively), and MICs twice as high for CBDA, while CBDA displayed MIC = 4 μg/mL against MRSA USA300 [80]. In the same year, Wassmann et. al. reported for CBD, MICs = 4, 4, 4, and 8 μg/mL against MRSA USA300, MRSE, *L. monocytogenes* and *E. faecalis* respectively [86]. One year later, MICs in the range 1–5 μg/mL were reported for CBG, against some species of *Streptococcus* genus [88].

Feldman and colleagues tested ANA and AraS, which are the main ECs found in humans against MRSA [90]. While they resulted completely inactive towards planktonic cells (MICs > 256 μg/mL), they demonstrated appreciable activity against MRSA biofilm, by reducing the biofilm formation by 51–54% (ANA) and 33–61% (AraS) at concentration 64 μg/mL [90]. Very recently, the antibacterial and antioxidant properties of CBD and its homologue, 8,9-dihydrocannabidiol (H2CBD), were also examined by Wu et al. against

S. aureus and *E. coli* with excellent results against both species with both compounds [85]. On these findings, *C. sativa* and its non-psychotropic cannabinoids, represent an interesting source of novel antibacterial agents which could help in addressing the problem of multidrug resistance in MRSA and other pathogenic bacteria.

4. Production of Phytocannabinoids: From Biosynthesis to Synthetic Procedures

4.1. Biosynthesis of Non-Psychotropic Cannabinoids (CBC, CBG and CBD)

The following Schemes 1 and 2 show the biosynthetic path to form geraniol pyrophosphate (GPP) and leading to CBG, CBC and CBD starting from CBGA, respectively [13]. As reported in the previous Figure 8, in *C. Sativa*, from CBGA, THCA is also produced, which provides THC upon decarboxylation, which in turn gives CBN, upon oxidation and aromatization. Although they have demonstrated interesting antibacterial effects, THCA, THC and CBN were not considered in this section because they possess from weak to strong psychotropic effects, which limit their possible therapeutic use [35]. On the contrary CBC, CBG and CBD, not exerting psychotropic actions have higher therapeutic potentials thus being more suitable to develop novel antibiotics [17].

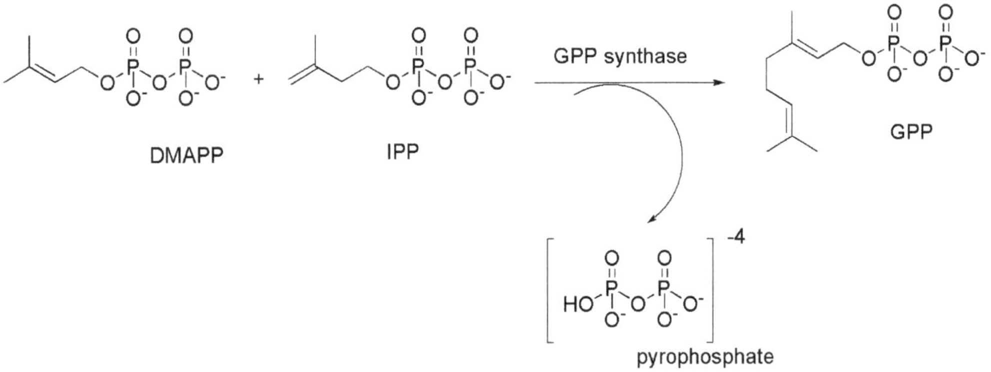

Scheme 1. Synthesis of geranyl pyrophosphate (GPP) from dimethylallyl pyrophosphate (DMAPP) and isopentenyl pyrophosphate (IPP) catalyzed by geranyl pyrophosphate synthase.

Briefly, the tetraketide synthase (TKS) catalyzed sequential condensation of hexanoyl-CoA with three molecules of malonyl-CoA yields 3,5,7-trioxododecaneoyl-CoA. By olivetolic acid cyclase (OAC), this compound cyclizes and aromatizes, through the loss of Coenzyme A, providing olivetolic acid (OLA) [13]. During these first steps, by hydrolytic processes and lactonization the side-products pentyl diacetic lactone (PDAL) (red square) and hexanoyl triacetic acid lactone (HTAL) (blue square) are also produced, while upon a decarboxylation TKS catalyzed, olivetol is formed (green square). Then, aromatic prenyltransferase inserts the prenyl group at the highly nucleophilic 2-resorcinol position to provide cannabigerolic acid (CBGA) [13]. Then, while CBGA provides CBG upon a non-enzymatic loss of CO_2, through reactions catalyzed by the opportune synthases, it provides the cannabinolic acids CBDA, and CBCA, which in turn provide the de-carboxylate (−)-CBD and CBC, by non-enzymatic decarboxylation [13].

4.2. Synthetic Procedures to Prepare Non-Psychotropic Cannabinoids CBC, CBG and (−)-CBD

The synthetic procedures for synthesizing CBC, CBD and CBG reported in the following sections have been found upon a survey carried out using SciFinder^{n} data base (Chemical Abstracts Service (CAS)), available online at https://scifinder-n.cas.org/ (accessed on 3 May 2023). The research was performed using the CAS registry number of the compounds, and all the synthesis reported so far have been described. Patents have been excluded.

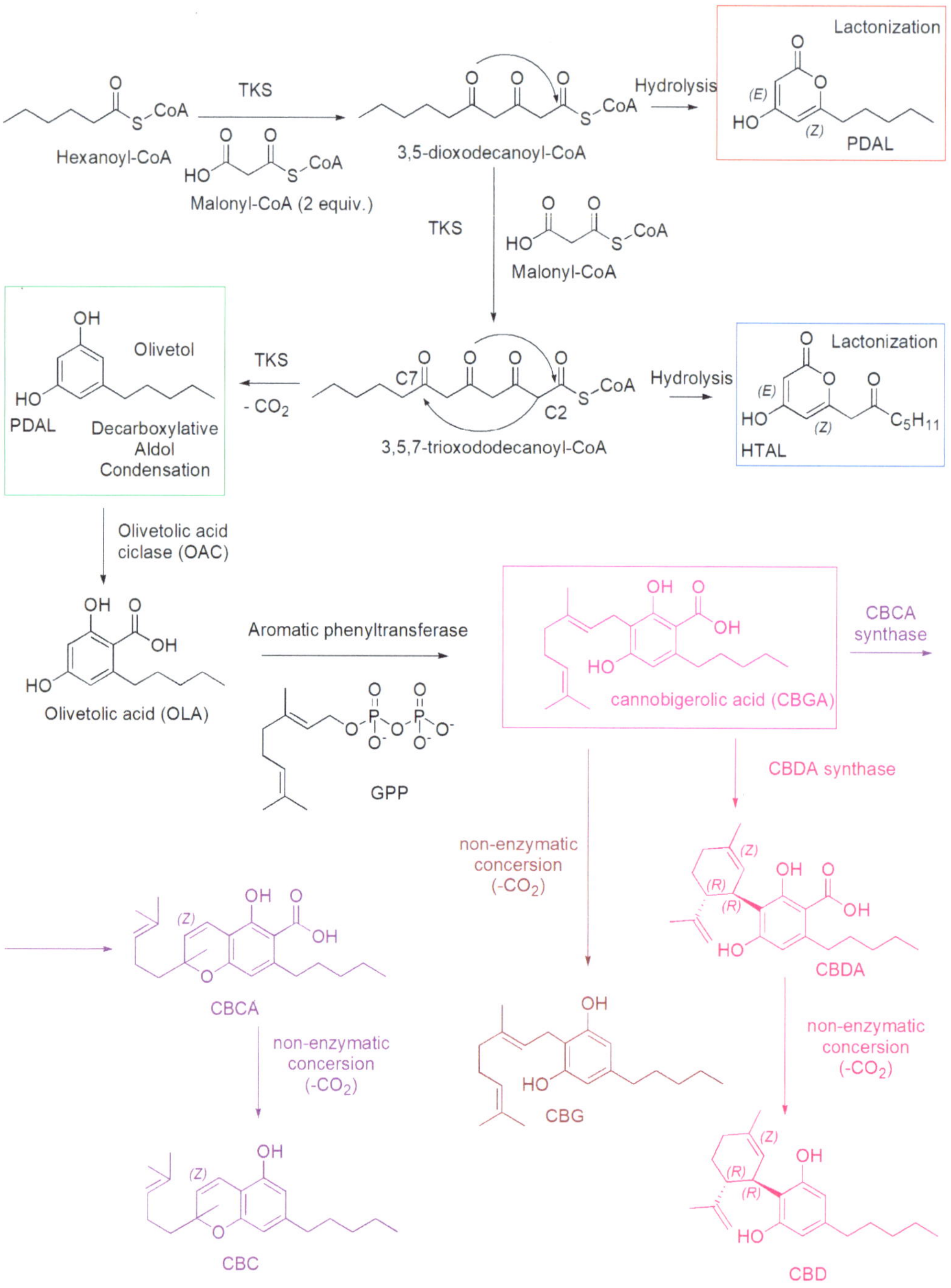

Scheme 2. Biosynthesis of non-psychotropic cannabinoids CBG (amaranth route), CBD (pink route) and CBC (light purple route), including the formation of the three by-products pentyl diacetic lactone (PDAL), hexanoyl triacetic acid lactone (HTAL), and olivetol.

4.2.1. Syntheses of CBC

The most recent synthetic procedures for preparing CBC were reported in the year 2021. Particularly, Seccamani et al. [93], who reproduced synthetic procedures previously reported [94–97], synthesized CBC starting from *E*-geraniol according to Scheme 3.

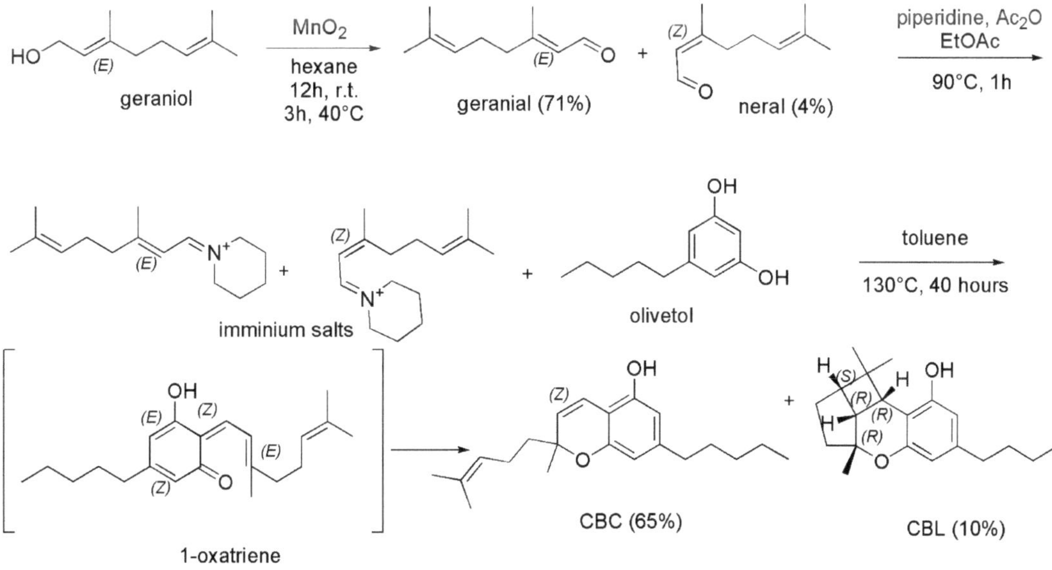

Scheme 3. Synthetic procedure to achieve CBC [93]. Ac_2O = acetic anhydride; EtOAc = ethyl acetate.

Briefly, *E*-geraniol dissolved in dry hexane was treated with manganese dioxide (MnO_2) under magnetic stirring at room temperature for about 12 h and then heated at 40 °C for further 3 h, to provide citral as crude product, which was purified by silica gel chromatographic column obtaining the purified aldehydes (with a yield of 75%) as an *E/Z* mixture (*E/Z* 95/5, GC-MS) of geranial (*E*-citral, 71%) and neral (*Z*-citral, 4%). Subsequently, the prepared mixture was treated with Ac_2O in EtOAc in the presence of piperidine and heated at 90 °C for 1 h, to give an iminium salt, which was added with a solution of olivetol in toluene and stirred at 130 °C for 40 h. Upon an oxa-annulation consisting of a Knoevenagel reaction providing the 1-oxatriene intermediate, followed by an oxa-electrocyclization, the crude CBC was obtained, which was then purified by chromatographic column. Pure CBC (yield 65%) and cannabicyclol (CBL, yield 10%) were finally isolated. Interestingly, Luo et al. [94], and Yeom et al. [96], who previously employed this procedure starting from a mixture of *E/Z*-citral, and from only geranial (*E*-citral) respectively, achieved CBC with a yield lower than Seccamani (50% vs. 65%). Similar procedures starting from *E/Z*-citral and olivetol were proposed in the same year (2021), by Schafroth, et al. [98] and by Anderson et al. [99], achieving CBC with yields of 50% and 35%, respectively. Particularly, the group of Schafroth evidenced that acidic or basic conditions were determinant to redirect the reaction towards the formation of CBC rather than towards that of Δ^9-THC (Scheme 4).

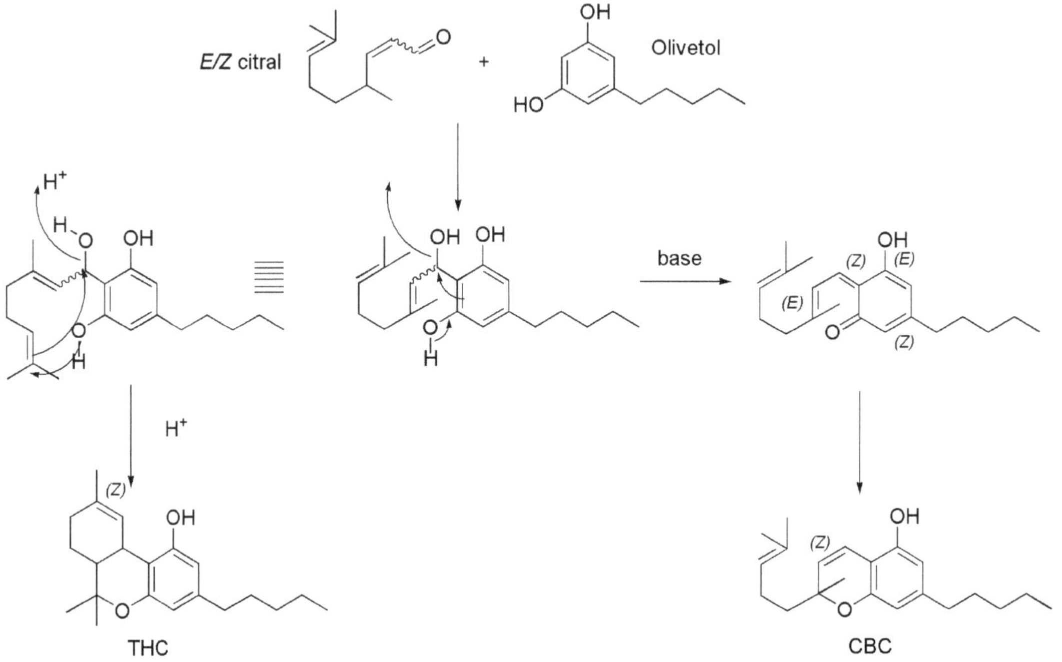

Scheme 4. Synthetic procedure to achieve either CBC in basic conditions or THC in acidic ones [98].

Differently and more specifically, Anderson et al. reacted olivetol and *E*/*Z*-citral in toluene using ethylenediamine diacetate as catalyst and heating the solution at reflux for 6 h (Scheme 5), as it was reported previously by Lee et al. [100], who prepared CBC with similar yield (40% vs. 35%).

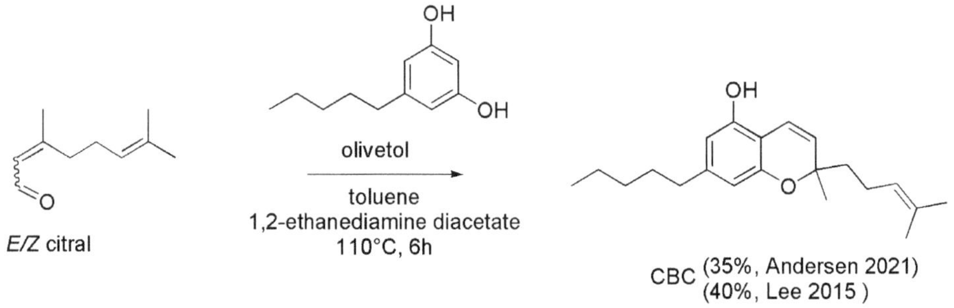

Scheme 5. Synthesis of CBC [99,100].

The use of ethylenediamine diacetate as catalyst had been reported in the past by Tietze et al. in the year 1982 [101], who achieved CBC in similar yield (37%) according to a different path (Scheme 6).

Briefly, geranial (**1**) was reacted with 5-pentyl-1,3-cyclohexandion (**2**) in methanol (CH_3OH) with catalytic amounts of ethylenediamine diacetate at 20 °C, achieving the intermediate **3**, which cyclized to the crude compound **4**. A chromatographic column was necessary to purify **4**, which was isolated in 62% yield. Compound **4** was treated with lithium di-isopropyl-amide (LDA) in tetrahydrofuran (THF) at −78 °C and phenylselenenyl chloride (C_6H_5SeCl), to afford the selenide intermediate **5**, which upon oxidation with 3-choloroperoxybenzoic acid in dichloromethane (DCM) followed by reaction with dimethoxy aniline, provided CBC in 37% yield.

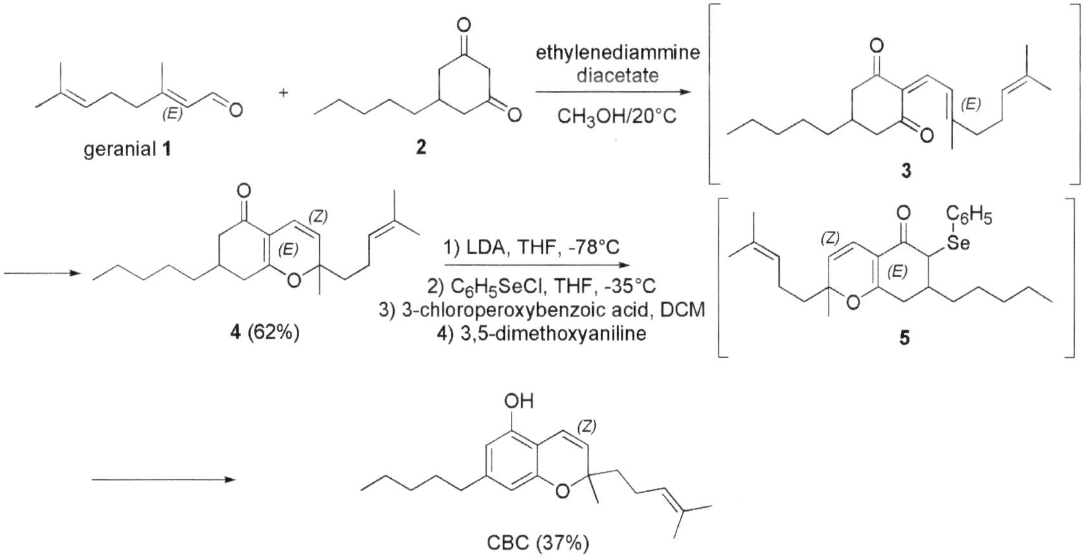

Scheme 6. Synthesis of CBC [101].

An analogous procedure, using *t*-butylamine in place of ethylenediamine diacetate, and at reflux time of 9 h in place of 6, had been reported in the years 1978 and 1982 by Elsohly et al. [89,102]. CBC was achieved in high yield (>60%), upon purification carried out reducing the unreacted citral with $NaBH_4$. In the 2008, the same reaction was exploited in their study by Appendino et al. [83]. Interestingly, CBC was prepared in very high yield (75%) by Quilez del Moral et al. [103], by a biomimetic green approach using water as solvent and ammonium chloride as catalyst, according to Scheme 7.

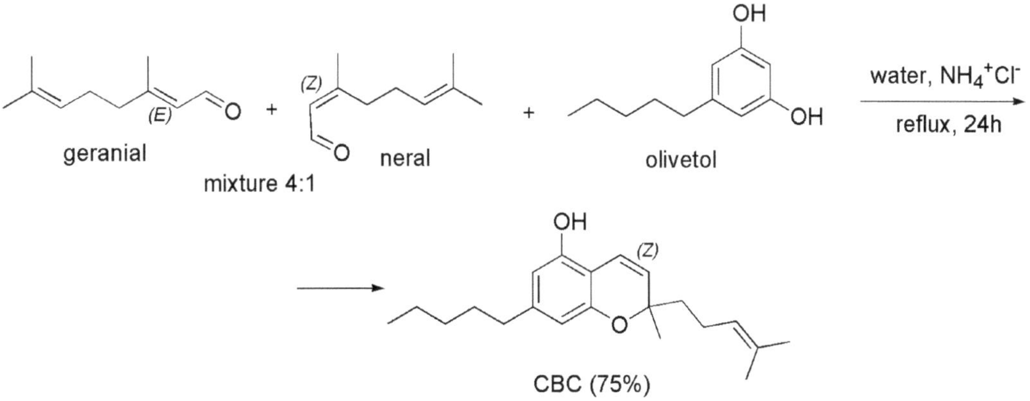

Scheme 7. Synthesis of CBC [103].

Particularly, working on a milligrams scale, the authors started from the commercial citral, as a mixture 4/1 of geranial (*E*-citral) and neral (*Z*-citral), which was reacted with olivetol in water using ammonium chloride ($NH_4^+Cl^-$) as catalyst for 24 h at reflux. The obtained crude product was purified by chromatographic column, thus isolating CBC in 75% yield. The procedure is interesting, because depending on the use of a surfactant as sodium dodecyl sulfate (SDS) or that of $NH_4^+Cl^-$ as catalyst, it was possible for the author to achieve an "in water" reaction thus obtaining ortho-THC as main product (CBC 45% yield), or an "on water" reaction achieving CBC as major compound (75% yield).

In the past (year 1995), a multi-step synthesis for CBC was reported by Yamaguchi et al. (Scheme 8) [104].

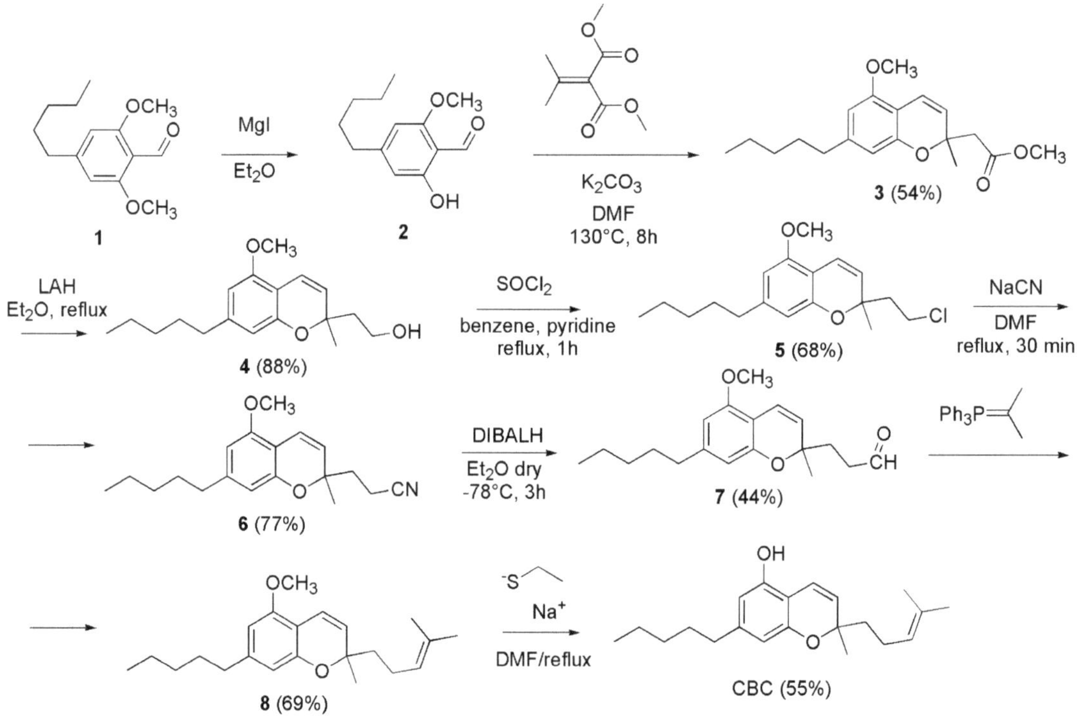

Scheme 8. Synthesis of CBC [104].

Briefly, the 2-hydroxy-6-methoxy-4-pentylbenzaldehyde (**2**) was prepared demethylating **1** with magnesium iodide etherate. Then, **2** was cyclized to **3** using dimethyl isopropylidenemalonate and K_2CO_3 in dimethylformamide (DMF) at 130 °C for 8 h, obtaining the chromene-2-acetate derivative **3** in 54% yield. Subsequently, **3** was converted to the aldehyde **7**, by reduction with lithium aluminum hydride (LAH), chlorination with $SOCl_2$, cyanation with NaCN and final reduction with diisobutylaluminium hydride (DIBALH). A Wittig reaction of **7** with isopropylidenetriphenylphosphorane provided *O*-methylcannabichromene (**8**) which was demethylated to CBC (yield 55%) by treatment with sodium ethanethiolate in refluxing DMF.

4.2.2. Synthesis of CBG

The oldest synthetic procedure to prepare CBG we found, not reporting the reaction yield, was described by Gaoni et al. in the year 1964 [105]. The authors synthesized CBG by boiling geraniol (**1**) with olivetol (**2**), in decalin for 36 h (Scheme 9).

Similarly, CBG was prepared by the condensation of geraniol and olivetol, using DCM in the presence of *p*-toluenesulfonic acid (PTSA) at 20° to achieve CBG as crystalline material in 52% yield, by Mechoulam et al. according to Scheme 10 [106].

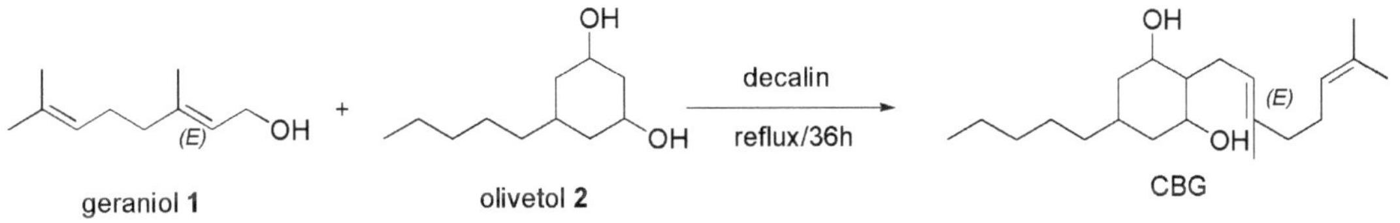

Scheme 9. Synthesis of CBG [105].

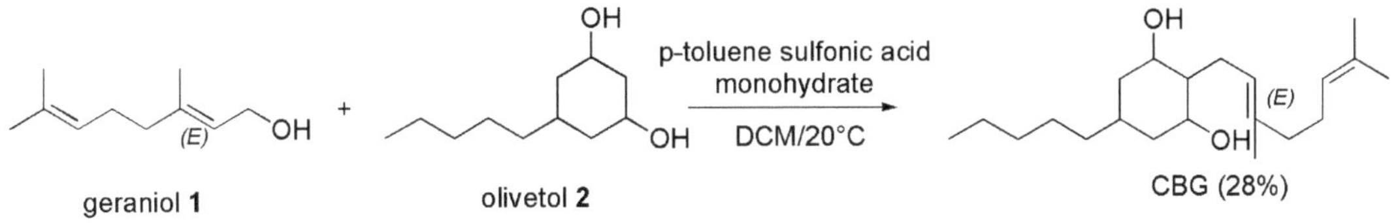

Scheme 10. Synthesis of CBG [102].

Starting from the same materials (geraniol and olivetol) and using DCM as solvent and PTSA monohydrate as catalyst, Farha et al. [33] prepared CBG like Mechoulam et al. [106] with the same yield, reproducing the procedure previously reported by Taura et al. [107].

The reaction was stirred at room temperature in the dark for 12 h, then added with aqueous saturated $NaHCO_3$. After evaporation of the separated organic phase, a crude residue was obtained, which was purified via flash column chromatography on silica gel, providing pure CBG as an off-white powder in 28% yield.

In 1985, it was reported that when BF_3-etherate on silica was used as condensing agent in the reaction of (+)-*p*-mentha-2,8-dien-l-ol (**1**) with olivetol (**2**), CBG could be obtained as the major product, in 29% yield (Scheme 11) [108].

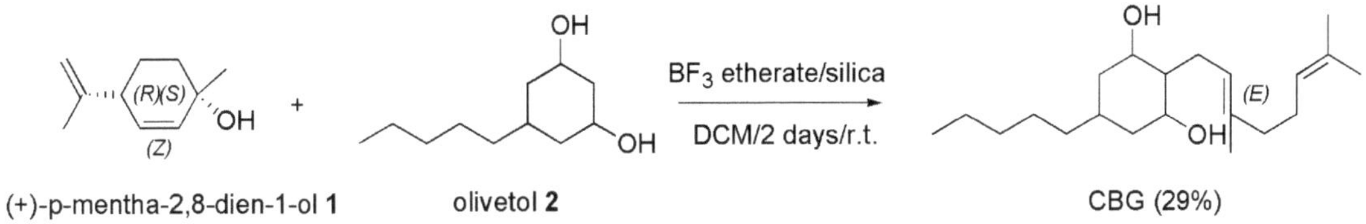

Scheme 11. Synthesis of CBG [108]. Silica = Si_2O_3.

Particularly, BF_3-etherate was added under nitrogen to a stirred suspension of silica in dry DCM, added with *Z*-(+)-*p*-mentha-2,8-dien-l-ol and olivetol dissolved in DCM and stirred at room temperature for 2 days. After having quenched the reaction with an aqueous solution of sodium bicarbonate followed by extraction with diethyl ether, CBG was achieved in 29% yield.

Later, the same authors used the above-reported procedure starting from geraniol and olivetol, as in Schemes 9 and 10, achieving CBG in 29% yield, as well [109,110].

A chemoenzymatic synthesis of CBG was reported by Kumano et al. in the year 2008 [111], which we did not discussed in the present work, because out of our scope aiming at describing only processes totally synthetic.

In the year 2020, Jentsch et al. reported the optimized synthesis of three phenolic natural products with unprecedented efficiency, using a new alumina-promoted regioselective aromatic allylation reaction [112]. As for CBG, it was prepared in one step from the inexpensive olivetol and geraniol, as in the reactions implemented previously by Farha et al. [33], Mechoulam et al. [106] and Taura et al. [107], but using different reagents and conditions, and achieving CBG in higher yield.

Briefly, to a solution of geraniol and olivetol in dichloroethane (DCE), acidic alumina (Al_2O_3) was added, and the heterogeneous mixture was stirred at reflux temperature for 6 h. After filtration of the alumina and the removal of the organic solvent, CBG was achieved as a yellow oil, that was purified via chromatography, thus obtaining pure CBG in 62% yield.

Like for CBC, the most recent synthetic procedures for preparing CBG have been reported in the year 2021. The group of Curtis et al. reported a multistep procedure based on a tandem Diels–Alder/retro-Diels–Alder cycloaddition which allowed to achieve CBG in very high yield (81%) (Scheme 12) [113].

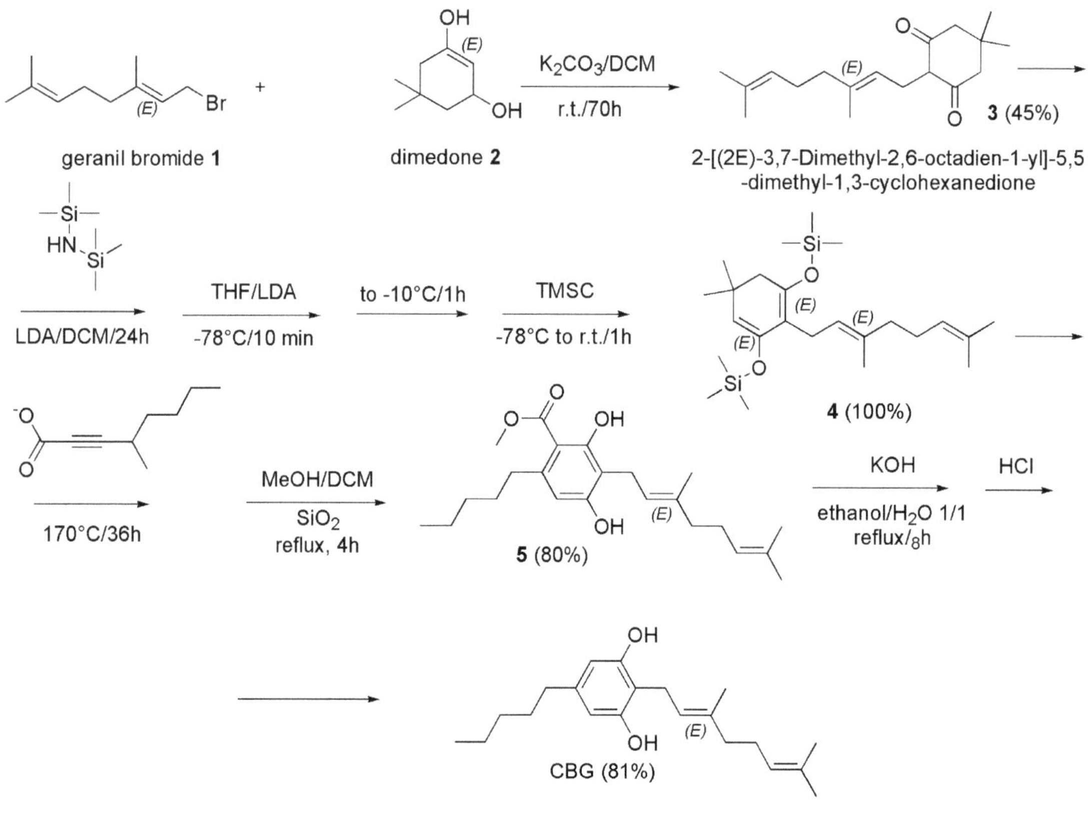

Scheme 12. Synthesis of CBG [113].

The group of Seccamani [93], reproposed the procedure previously described by Baek et al. in the year 1996 [110] (Scheme 13).

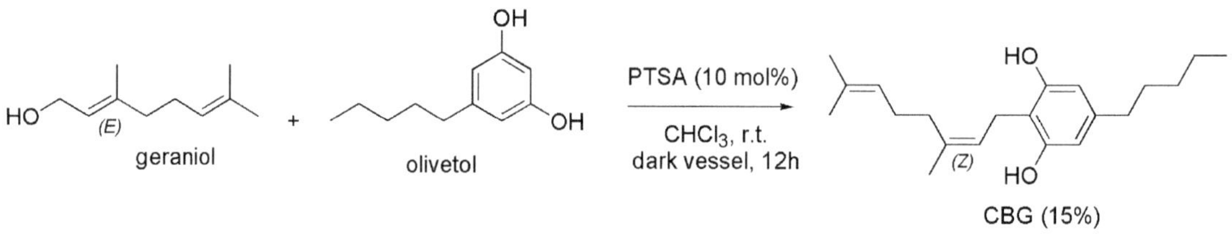

Scheme 13. Synthesis of CBG [93].

Briefly, CBG was prepared reacting olivetol dissolved in dry chloroform ($CHCl_3$) with geraniol, in the presence of PTSA for 12 h at room temperature. The crude CBG was achieved as an oil, which was purified by silica gel chromatographic column. CBG was isolated with a low 15% yield.

4.2.3. Synthesis of (−)-CBD

The first synthetic routes available to synthetize (−)-CBD [114–117] are of scarce practical value, as they lead to (−)-CBD in mediocre or even insignificant yields and the unnatural CBD isomer (Abn-CBD) (see Figure 11) was obtained in amounts considerably larger than those of (−)-CBD. Despite such poor results, the procedure proposed by Petrzilka et al. in the year 1969, but using *E*-(+)-*p*-mentha-2,8-dien-1-ol in place of *Z*-(+)-*p*-mentha-2,8-dien-1-ol and olivetol in benzene in the presence of catalytic amounts of PTSA was reproduced by Papahatjis et al. in the year 2002, achieving (−)-CBD in 31% yield [118]. The best route to (−)-CBD described is the condensation of (+)-*p*-mentha-diene-l-olo with olivetol in the presence of weak acids, reported by Razdan et al. in the year 1974 and Uliss et al. the next year [117,119]. In this case, the Abn-CBD obtained was converted to (−)-CBD with BF_3-etherate by a retro-Friedel-Crafts reaction, followed by recombination. However, with this reagent the reaction proceeded further causing cyclisation of (−)-CBD.

In the year 1985, it was reported that when BF_3-etherate on alumina is used as condensing agent in the reaction of *Z*-(+)-*p*-mentha-2, 8-dien-1-ol (**1**) with olivetol (**2**), (−)-CBD was obtained as the major product, in 55% yield as chromatographically pure oil, or in 41% yield as crystalline material (Scheme 14) [108].

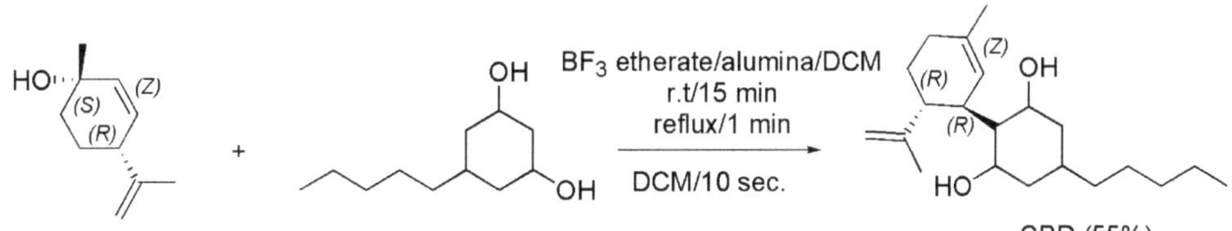

(+)-p-mentha-2,8-dien-1-ol **1** olivetol **2** CBD (55%)

Scheme 14. Synthesis of (−)-CBD [108]. Alumina = Al_2O_3.

No cyclization was observed, and side products were much more polar (14% yield) or much less polar (6% yield) than (−)-CBD.

Particularly, BF_3-etherate was added under nitrogen to a stirred suspension of basic aluminum oxide (Al_2O_3) in dry DCM, and after 15 min at room temperature and 1 min at 40–41 °C, (+)-*p*-mentha-2,8-dien-l-ol and olivetol dissolved in DCM were added. The reaction was quenched within 10 s with 10% aqueous solution of sodium bicarbonate (10 mL), and after evaporation of the organic extracts, (−)-CBD was obtained.

In 1988, Crombie et al. [120] reported the reaction of (1S,2S,3R,6R)-(+)-*E*-car-2-ene epoxide and that of *p*-menthadienol with olivetol in the presence of PTSA. Particularly, the starting material (1S,2S,3R,6R)-(+)-*E*-car-2-ene epoxide (**3**) was prepared starting from car-3-ene (**1**) by its treatment with potassium *tert*-butoxide to achieve the derivative **2**, which after epoxidation with *m*-chloroperoxybenzoic acid provided the desired compound **3** (Scheme 15). Otherwise, *p*-menthadienol was prepared by citral with HCl in water or with PTSA in water/DCM (reaction not reported). The authors observed that in both cases, among other minor compounds, (−)-CBD, Abn-CBD, 1-THC and 6-THC were obtained. In particular, when (1S,2S,3R,6R)-(+)-*E*-car-2-ene epoxide was reacted with olivetol in benzene in the presence of docosane as catalyst for 45 min at 40 °C, the main product which formed was *p*-menthadienol with traces of (−)-CBD, Abn-CBD and THC. The further reaction of the obtained *p*-menthadienol with olivetol for 1h at 50 °C in benzene with docosane as well, afforded (−)-CBD in 30% yield, together with THC (18%), Δ^8-THC (6%), and Abn-CBD (13%) (Scheme 15).

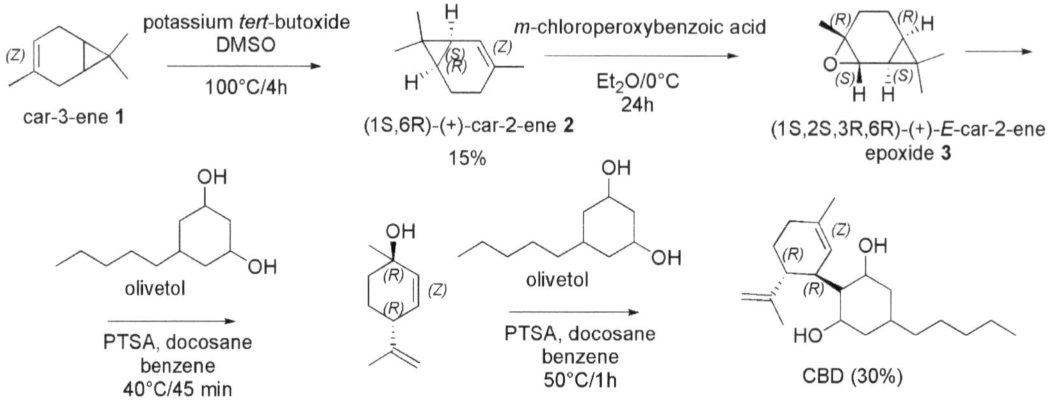

Scheme 15. Synthesis of (−)-CBD [120].

Rationally, the direct reaction of *p*-menthadienol (**1**) with olivetol in the conditions above reported afforded (−)-CBD in 30% yield (last part of Scheme 15).

Although in different conditions in terms of solvents, times, temperature, stereochemistry and catalysts, the reaction of *p*-menthadienol with olivetol was exploited by different research groups. Kinney et al. reacted *E*-(+)-*p*-mentha-2, 8-dien-1-ol with olivetol in toluene with PTSA for 1.5 h at 18–25 °C achieving (−)-CBD in 20% yield [121]. Also, Villano et al. in the year 2022 condensed olivetol with commercially available *Z*-(+)-*p*-mentha-2, 8-dien-1-ol in the presence of 33 mol% of wet PTSA in toluene at 0 °C for 3 h, affording a mixture of normal (−)-CBD and Abn-CBD, which were isolated in 26% and 38% yield respectively after a chromatographic column. Importantly, under these experimental conditions, no tricyclic structure was produced [122]. A different synthetic procedure was reported by Vaillancourt et al. in the year 1992 [123]. The authors described a new synthesis of (−)-CBD via the α-arylation of camphor, achieving both (−)-CBD and (−)-CBD mono methyl ether as shown in Scheme 16 [123].

Particularly, the authors prepared the endo-3-(2,5-dimethoxy-4-*n*-pentylphenyl)camphor (**2**), by reacting first olivetol dimethyl ether (**2**) dissolved in dry THF under nitrogen at −10 °C with *tert*-butyllithium (*tert*-BuLi) 1.7 M in hexanes for 3 h under stirring. Then the solution obtained was transferred to a solution of CuI in dry THF at 0 °C and the mixture was stirred for 20 min. Upon dilution with DMSO, the obtained solution was transferred dropwise to a solution of 3,9-dibromocamphor dissolved in dry THF/DMSO at 0 °C, and the reaction was then allowed to warm to room temperature and was stirred overnight. After the proper work-up and removal of the solvent in vacuo, the crude product was chromatographed and recrystallized from EtOH to achieve **2** in 71% yield. Compound **2** was transformed into the vinyl phosphate derivative **3**, by dissolving it in dry THF under nitrogen and titrating the obtained solution cooled to −78 °C with a freshly prepared 0.4 M Na-naphthalenide/0.4 M tetra-ethyleneglycol dimethyl ether solution (see later) in THF until a deep green color persisted. The green mixture was then added with diethyl chlorophosphate and hexamethylfosforamide (HMPA), was allowed to warm to −20 °C, and opportunely treated to provide the crude product which was subjected to a short silica column obtaining the desired enol phosphate **3** as a colorless oil (89%). (−)-CBD and (−)-CBD monomethyl ether (**4**), were finally obtained by adding the vinyl phosphate **3** dissolved in dry THF and *tert*-butanol (*t*-BuOH) to an excess of lithium foil in methylamine ($MeNH_2$) at −78 °C. When addition was complete, the reaction was allowed to stir at −10 °C for 1 h and treated by acidification with HCl 1M. After extraction and removal of organic solvent the crude reaction mixture was chromatographed on neutral alumina, achieving (−)-CBD monomethyl ether in 43% yield. Further elution afforded (−)-CBD in 35% yield. The 0.4 M Na-naphthalenide/0.4 M tetra-ethylene glycol dimethyl ether solution in THF was prepared adding naphthalene in dry THF with sodium metal. The mixture was allowed to stir for 2 h, and then 2.41 mL of tetra-ethylene glycol dimethyl ether was added. The mixture was allowed to stir an additional hour at room temperature before use (Scheme not reported).

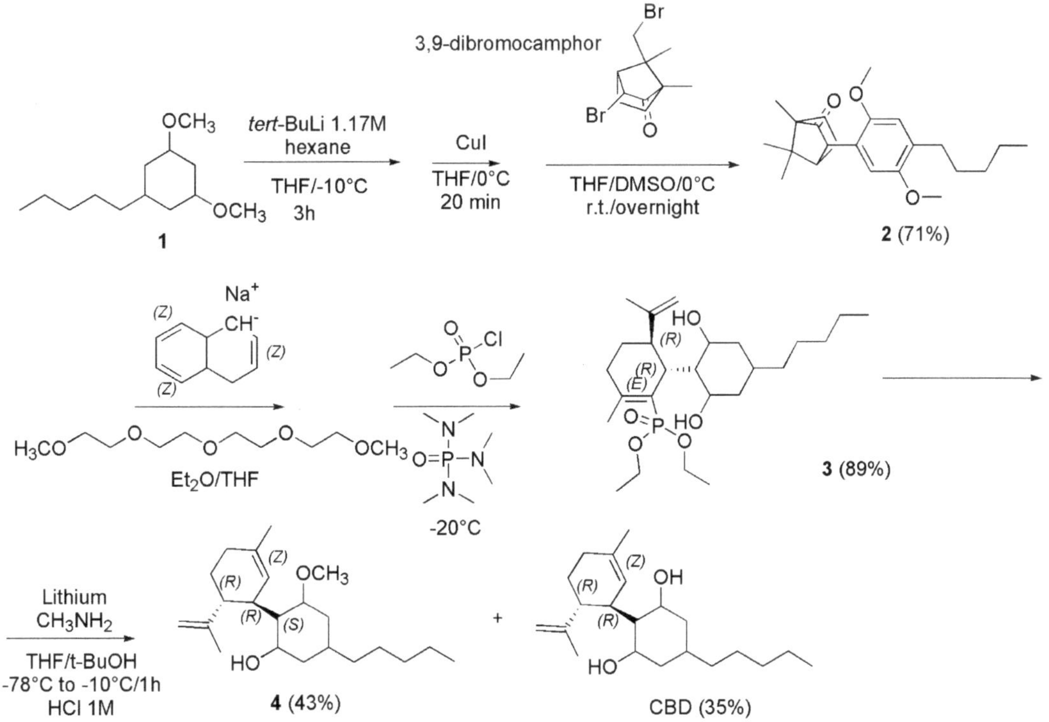

Scheme 16. Synthesis of (−)-CBD [123].

Later in the year 2002, Malkov et al. described the synthesis of (−)-CBD in 14–22% yield using *Z*-(+)-*p*-mentha-2, 8-dien-1-ol (**1**) or its acetate derivative **2** and olivetol in dichloromethane (DCM) and molybdenum catalysts (Scheme 17) [124].

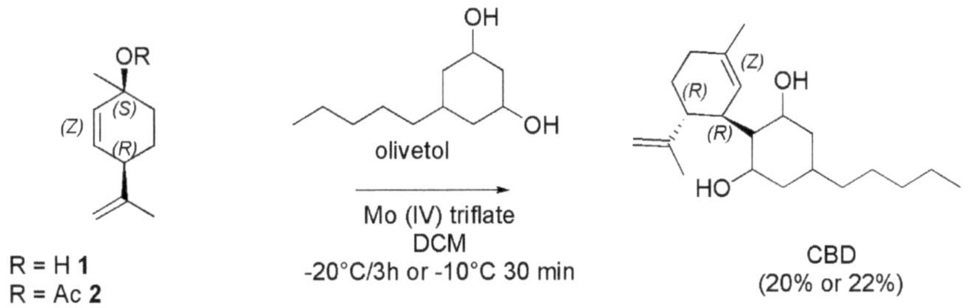

Scheme 17. Synthesis of (−)-CBD [124].

According to the reported results, starting from *Z*-(+)-*p*-mentha-2, 8-dien-1-ol **(1)** and olivetol dissolved in DCM and using the molybdenum Mo (IV) triflate complex as catalyst at −20 °C for 3 h (−)-CBD was obtained in 20% yield. Similar results (22% yield) were obtained starting from *Z*-(+)-*p*-mentha-2, 8-dien-1-ol acetate (**2**), olivetol and the same catalyst, and stirring the reaction mixture at −10 °C for 30 min. On the contrary, with the bimetallic Mo (II) catalyst V, and stirring **2** and olivetol at 20 °C for 4 h (−)-CBD was obtained in a lower yield (14%). Kobayashi et al. in the year 2001 reported the BF_3-promoted 1,4-addition of bulky aryl groups, including dimethoxy olivetol, to an α-iodo enone (**2**), prepared from the parent enone (**1**), thus affording a β-aryl-α-iodo ketone derivative (**3**). Its subsequent reaction with EtMgBr furnished the magnesium enolate (**4**), which upon reactions with $ClP(O)(OEt)_2$ gave an enol phosphate (**5**), which was applied successfully to the synthesis of (−)-CBD (Scheme 18) [125].

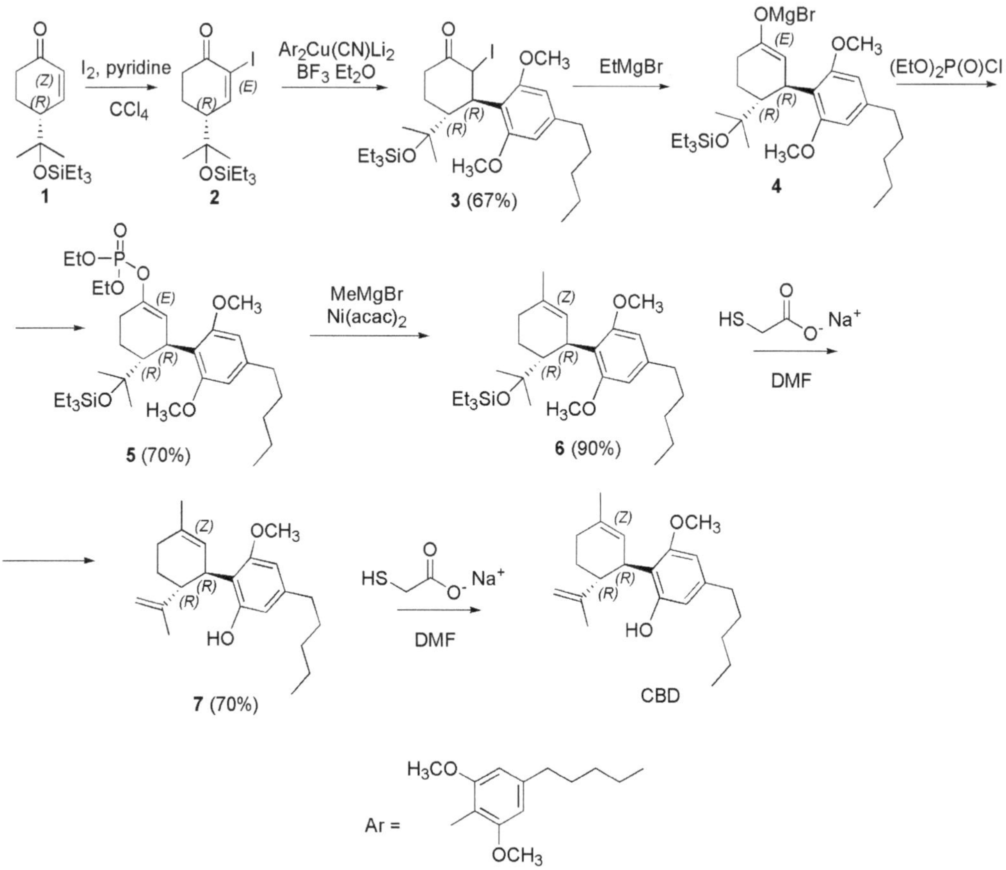

Scheme 18. Synthesis of (−)-CBD [125]. $Ni(acac)_2$ = nickel (II) acetylacetonate.

Particularly, the enone **1** was converted to the α-iodocyclohexenone (**2**) with I_2 and pyridine in CCl_4 with good yield. The 1,4-addition of $Ar_2Cu(CN)Li_2$ to **2** promoted by $BF_3{\cdot}OEt_2$ furnished ketone **3** in 67% yield, after aqueous workup and purification by chromatography. Then, EtMgBr was successful used to generate the corresponding enolate **4**, which provided the enol phosphate **5** by reaction with $(EtO)_2P(O)Cl$ in 70% yield (Scheme 18). Methylation of **5** with MeMgBr in the presence of nickel (II) acetylacetonate ($Ni(acac)_2$) afforded **6**, and its subsequent exposure to sodium ethyl thiolate (EtSNa) in DMF resulted in the deprotection of the triethylsilil (TES) group and of one of the MeO groups to furnish **7**. Attempted one-step deprotection of the two MeO groups under more vigorous conditions was unsuccessful, therefore **7** was converted in (−)-CBD by further exposure to EtSNa in DMF.

Later in 2006, the same group reported a new reagent system for synthesizing (−)-CBD and its analogues via alkenylation of cyclohexenyl diol monoacetate according to Scheme 19 [126].

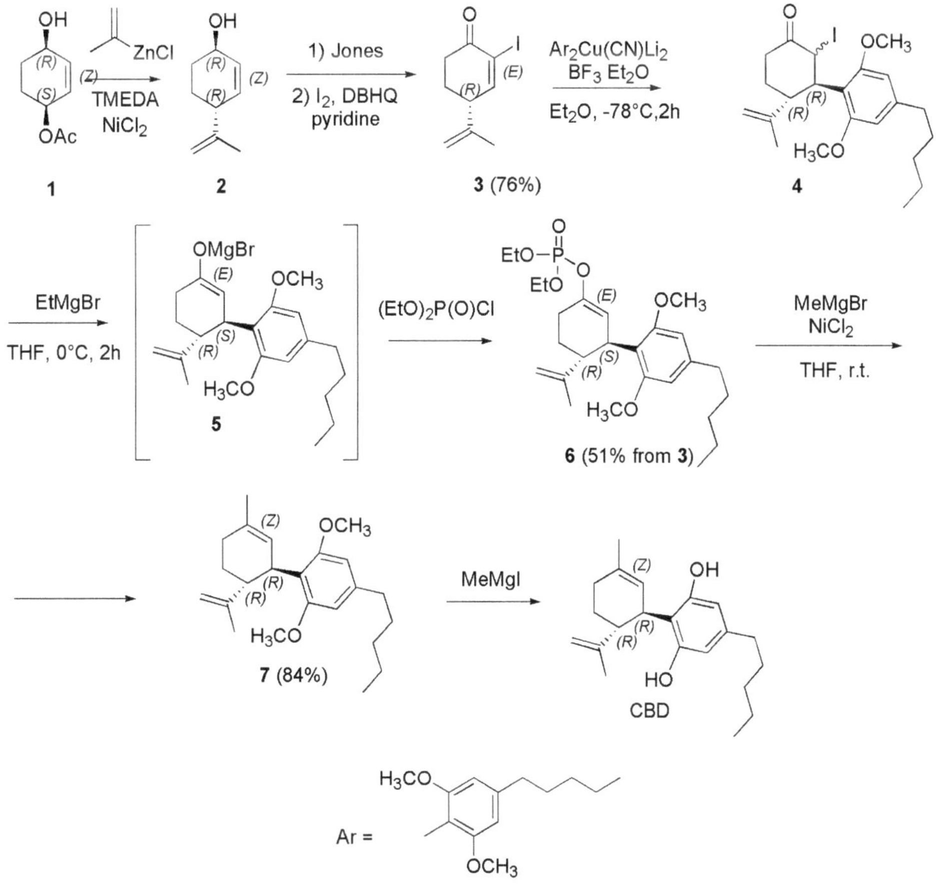

Scheme 19. Synthesis of (−)-CBD [126].

Briefly, by a nickel-catalyzed allylation of 2-cyclohexene-1,4-diol monoacetate (**1**) with a new reagent consisting of (alkenyl)ZnCl/TMEDA, the SN2-type product, namely *E*-(+)-*p*-mentha-2,8-dien-1-ol (**2**) was achieved with 94% regioselectivity in good yield. Oxidation of **2** afforded the intermediate enone, which underwent iodination at the α position by I_2 in the presence of 2,5-di-*tert*-butylhydroquinone (DBHQ) as a radical scavenger to produce the α-iodo enone (**3**) in 63% yield (two steps). Addition of the 2,6-dimethoxy-4-pentylphenyl group of olivetol (abbreviated as Ar in the first part of the Scheme) to **3** was performed with the higher-order cyanocuprate derivative ($Ar_2Cu(CN)Li_2$) in turn synthesized from the Aryl (Ar) lithium anion and CuCN (not reported), obtaining compound **4**, as a 1:1 stereoisomeric mixture at the α position. Compound **4** underwent reaction with EtMgBr to produce the reactive magnesium enolate **5**, which was quenched with $ClP(O)(OEt)_2$ to furnish enol phosphate **6** in 51% yield from **3**. Nickel-catalyzed coupling of **6** with MeMgCl afforded dimethyl ether **7** in good yield. Finally, (−)-CBD was obtained upon demethylation of **7** using MeMgI. Zachary et al. in the year 2018 reported a practical synthetic approach to synthetize Δ^9-THC, and (−)-CBD. Particularly, (−)-CBD was synthesized according to Scheme 20 [127].

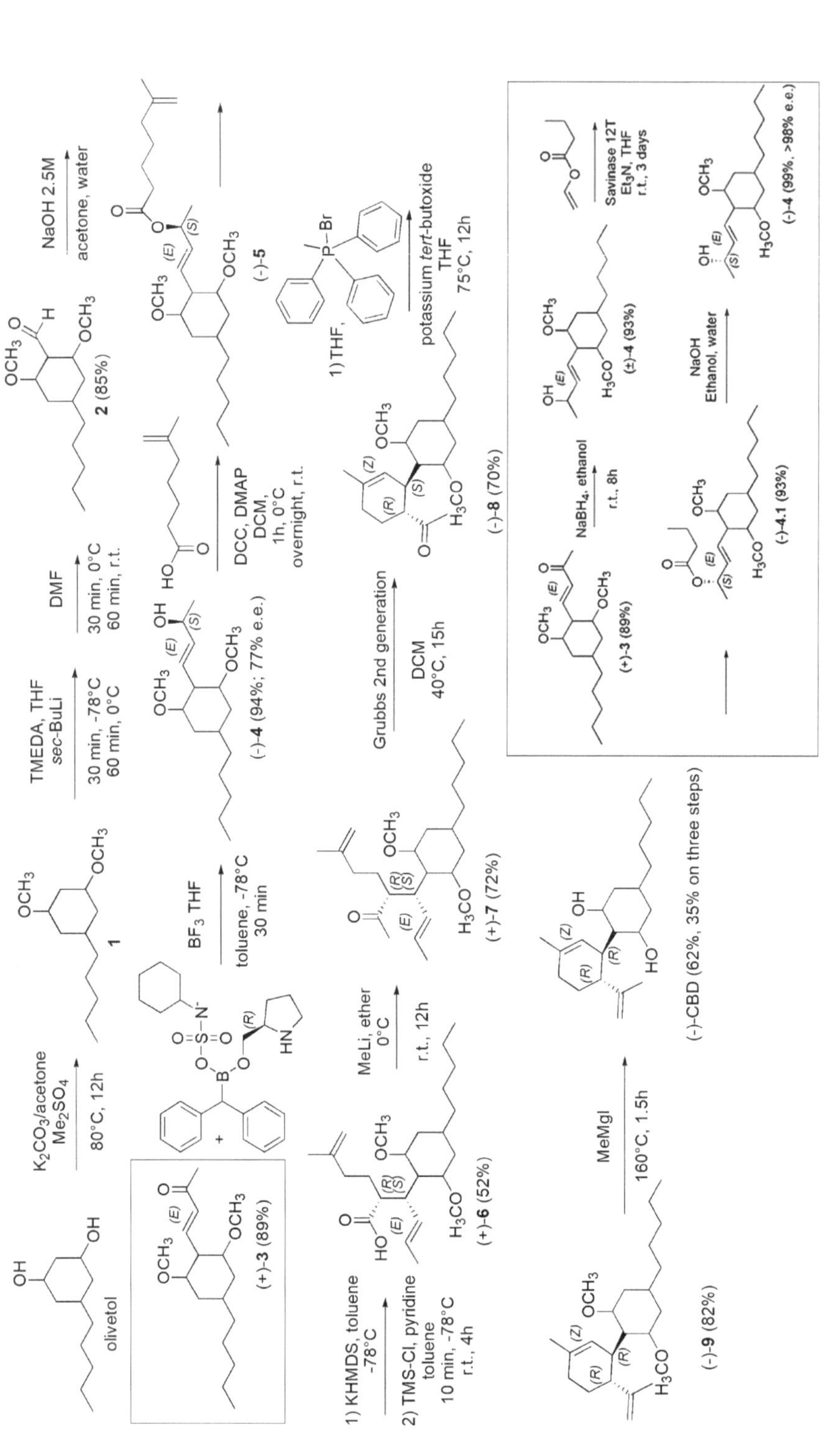

Scheme 20. Synthesis of (−)-CBD [127]. In the blue square the alternative route described in the main text starting from **3** has been reported.

Briefly, olivetol and K_2CO_3 in acetone were added with dimethyl sulphate (Me_2SO_4) in 5 min at room temperature and then the mixture was heated to 80 °C for 12 h under argon, achieving the crude olivetol dimethyl ether (**1**) as an oil which was purified by column chromatography (98% yield). A yellow solution of **1** and TMEDA in anhydrous THF at −78 °C under argon was added with *sec*-butyllithium (*sec*-BuLi) and was stirred for 30 min at −78 °C and for 60 min at 0 °C, before being added with anhydrous DMF. The mixture was stirred at 0 °C for 30 min and for additional 60 min at room temperature. Upon proper work up and silica gel column chromatography the pure aldehyde derivative **2** was obtained as a yellow oil in 85% yield. Aldehyde **2** was converted in the enone **3** via an aldolic condensation with acetone in water using a 2.5M NaOH solution and heating the reaction mixture to 60 °C for 12 h (89% yield). The carbonylic group of **3** was reduced in toluene at −78 °C under argon, using a solution of (R)-CBS oxazaborolidine ligand (see Scheme 20) and BH_3•THF complex. The reaction mixture continued to stir for 30 min at −78 °C obtaining the crude product (−)-**4** which was further purified by silica gel column chromatography achieving the pure compound (−)-**4** in 94% yield (77% enantiomeric excess (e.e.)) as a clear colorless oil that solidified upon standing. An alternative to generate a product with high enantiopurity consisted of an enzymatic approach using an inexpensive and readily available enzyme. In this regard, compound **3** in the blue square was reduced with sodium borohydride ($NaBH_4$) affording the racemic alcohol (±)-**4**, which was acylated with vinyl butyrate in the presence of Savinase 12T thus providing the ester (−)-**4.1** which was hydrolyzed with NaOH affording (−)-**4** with >98% e.e. in 38% overall yield for the three steps (blue square in Scheme 20).

Compound (−)-**4** was converted in the carboxylate (−)-**5** by its acylation with 5-methyl-5-hexencarboxylic acid in DCM in the presence of DCC and DMAP. After 1 h stirring at 0 °C and then overnight at room temperature, (−)-**5** was achieved as crude material which was purified by column chromatography. Compound (−)-**5** was treated with KHMDS in anhydrous toluene at −78 °C for 1 h, then a solution of anhydrous pyridine and tetramethylsilyl chloride (TMS-Cl) in anhydrous toluene was added and the mixture was stirred at −78 °C for 10 min and at room temperature for an additional 4 h. Upon the Ireland−Claisen rearrangement, compound (+)-**6** was achieved as a white crystalline solid that could be recrystallized using hexanes in a 52% overall yield. Treatment of (+)-**6** in ether at 0 °C with methyllithium (MeLi) and stirring overnight at room temperature led to the formation of ketone (+)-**7** as colorless oil in 71.8% yield, after chromatography column. Compound (+)-**7** could be cyclized and then converted into (−)-CBD, via Wittig methylenation and deprotection. Particularly, compound (+)-**7** and Grubbs 2nd generation catalyst in DCM were first stirred for a total of 15 h at 40 °C, thus achieving compound (−)-**8** in 69.6% yield. Then, by reaction at room temperature of (−)-**8** with bromo(methyl)triphenylphosphorane in THF, followed by the addition of potassium *tert*-butoxide and stirring at 75 °C for 12 h, compound (−)-**9** was isolated in 82% yield. After its demethylated in anhydrous ether under argon with MeMgI and heating to 160 °C for 1.5 h, (−)-CBD was obtained in 62% (35% on three steps) yield as a light-yellow oil.

In the year 2020, Gong et al. reported a novel synthetic procedure for making (−)-CBD on a 10 g scale, by a late-stage diversification method, starting from commercially available phloroglucinol. First, the key intermediate (−)-CBD-2OPiv-OTf was achieved which underwent Negishi cross-coupling with the pentyl chain to give (−)-CBD in 52% overall yield. By this approach using the symmetric phloroglucinol the generation of positional isomers (Abn-CBDs) was avoided (Scheme 21) [128].

Briefly, by a Friedel–Crafts alkylation of phloroglucinol with *Z*-(+)-*p*-mentha-2,8-dien-1-ol in a ratio of 1:10 in presence of BF_3 etherate gave the desired product **1** in an excellent 80% yield. By treatment of **1** with trifluoromethanesulfonic anhydride (Tf_2O) in the presence of 2,6-lutidine at −30 to −20 °C in DCM using 1.5 equivalent of **1**, to prevent double triflation, afforded the triflate derivative **2**, which was isolated by silica gel column chromatography in a 78.1% yield. Compound **2** was treated with a solution of pivaloyl chloride (Piv-Cl) in DCM and a solution of DMAP in pyridine at −10 to 0 °C. Subsequently, the mixture was stirred at 25 °C for 12 h, to obtain the O-protected derivative **3** in 95% yield after column chromatography as a yellow oil. Pentyl zinc chloride ($C_5H_{11}ZnCl$), was prepared in one step by the transmetalation of the correspondent Grignard $C_5H_{11}MgBr$. Particularly, anhydrous zinc chloride and anhydrous lithium chloride were dissolved in anhydrous THF and cooled to −10 °C, added with $C_5H_{11}MgBr$ and stirred first at −10 °C for 15 min and then at room temperature for 1.5 h. The obtained mixture was added with a solution of **3** in THF and then with [1,1′-Bis(diphenylphosphino)ferrocene]dichloropalladium(II) ($Pd(dppf)Cl_2$), as cross-coupling agent, to provide **4** in 90% yield after stirring at 55–60 °C for proper time and after column chromatography. (−)-CBD was finally obtained upon deprotection with MeMgBr (3 M in Et_2O) in toluene at 110 °C for 12 h in 99% yield after silica gel column chromatography.

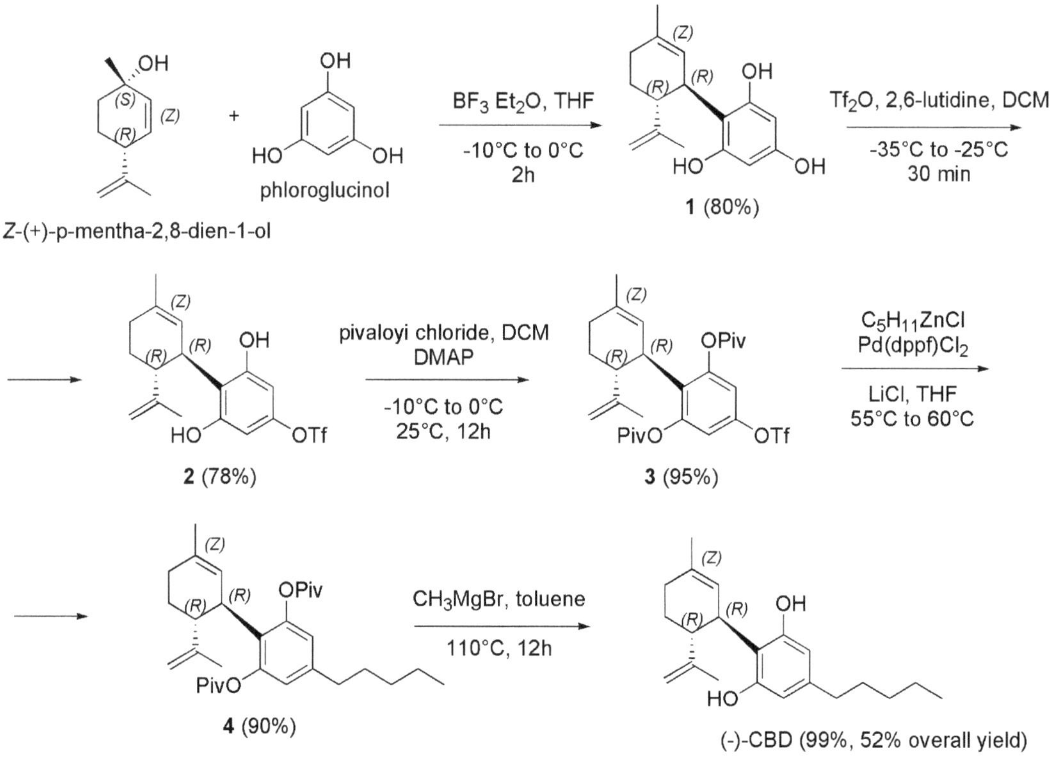

Scheme 21. Synthesis of (−)-CBD [128].

Chiurchiu et al. in the year 2021 reported an innovative and high yielding continuous approach for producing (−)-CBD, strongly reducing its cyclization into THC (traces), thus achieving (−)-CBD in 55% yield. Particularly, by means of flow chemistry, and following their studies concerning the use of this technology for synthesizing highly functionalized materials, the authors inserted acetyl isoperitenol and olivetol dissolved in DCM into a reservoir A, while $BF_3{\cdot}Et_2O$ dissolved in DCM into a reservoir B. Subsequently, they pumped the two solutions simultaneously into a T-connector before passing through a 3 mL PTFE coil reactor (7 min residence time). The outgoing solution was dropped into a flask containing a stirring saturated solution of $NaHCO_3$ from which (−)-CBD was extracted and purified by silica gel chromatography to provide pure (−)-CBD in 55% yield (Scheme 22) [129].

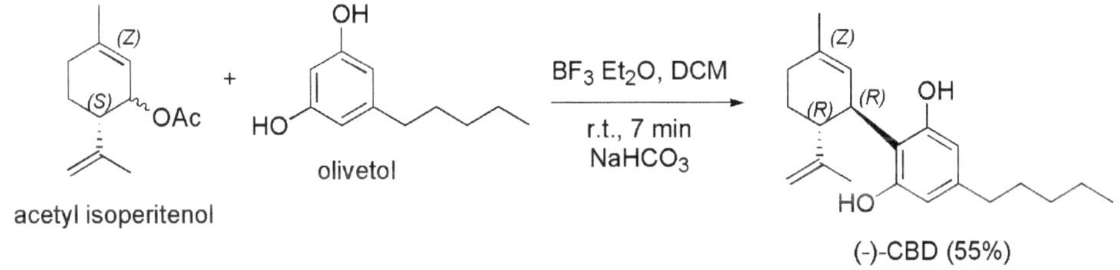

Scheme 22. Synthesis of (−)-CBD [129].

The main by-products were Abn-CBD and the dialkylated cannabidiol recovered in 19 % and 4 % of yield respectively, THC was observed in traces (GC < 0.4 %) and its isolation was unfeasible. In the same year, Navarro et al. followed a practical approach to prepare (−)-CBD that avoided the formation of the side abnormal regio-isomers by using protected 4,6-dihalo-olivetol in coupling reaction as shown in Scheme 23 [76].

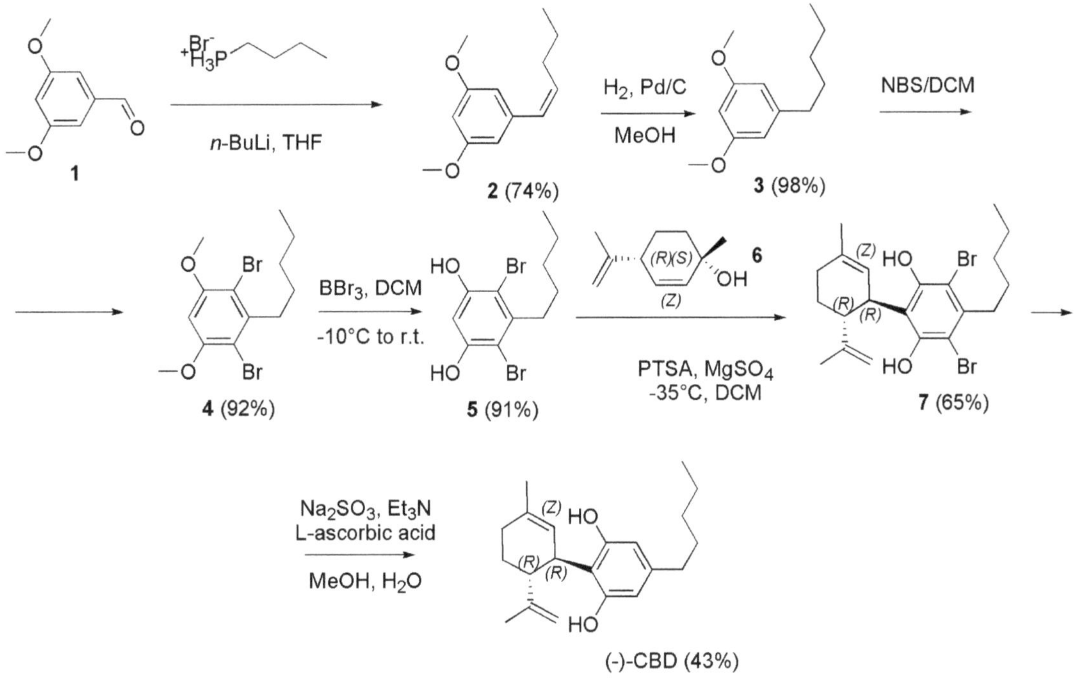

Scheme 23. Synthesis of (−)-CBD [76].

Briefly, the synthesis began by the Wittig reaction of butyl phosphonium bromide with commercially available 3,5-dimethoxybenzaldehyde (**1**), to deliver the olefin derivative **2** as mixture of Z and *E* isomers, which was conveniently reduced with hydrogen under pressure in presence of Pd/C as catalyst to the olivetol dimethyl ether (**3**). Regioselective electrophilic aromatic bromination of **3** using 2.3 equivalents of N-bromosuccinimide (NBS) in DCM at room temperature produced exclusively the 4,6-dibrominated product **4** in good yield. Then, the methyl ether-protecting groups were removed with boron tribromide to generate the key resorcinol intermediate **5** which was submitted to the Friedel–Craft alkylation with (1S,4R)-4-isopropenyl-1-methyl-2-cyclohexen-1-ol (**6**) in DCM, in the presence of PTSA as catalyst, thus affording the adduct **7** as single diastereomer. Finally, reductive dehalogenation using sodium sulfite in the presence of triethylamine (Et_3N) in a mixture of MeOH and H_2O at 75 °C delivered the targeted cannabinoid (−)-CBD in 43% yield. Anand et al. in the year 2022, developed a three-step concise and stereoselective synthesis route to (−)-CBD and (+)-CBD, using inexpensive and readily available starting material, such as R-(+)-limonene and S-(−)-limonene respectively. The synthesis involved the diastereoselective bi-functionalization of limonene, followed by effective elimination leading to the generation of the key chiral (+)- or (−)-*p*-mentha-2,8-dien-1-ols. Such dienols on coupling with olivetol under silver bis (trifluoromethanesulfonyl) imide ($AgN(SO_2CF_3)_2$) as catalysis provided regiospecific (−)-CBD or (+)-CBD in good yield (Scheme 24) [130].

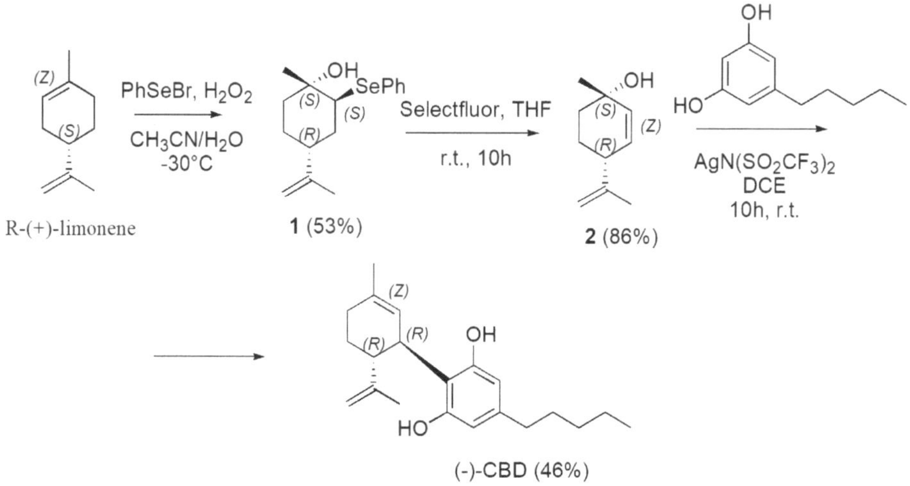

Scheme 24. Synthesis of (−)-CBD [130].

Briefly, the present approach started with the direct generation of diastereoselective bi-functionalized 2-phenylseleninyl-*p*-menth-8-en-1-ol (**1**) from readily available and inexpensive starting material R-(+)-limonene. Particularly, electrophilic phenyl selenium bromide and H_2O_2 in a mixture acetonitrile/water at −30 °C were used, thus achieving compound **1** in 53% yield. The removal of SePh to synthesize (+)-menthadienol **2** was carried out using Selectfluor in THF at room temperature for 10 h achieving optically pure (+)-*p*-mentha-2,8-dien-1-ol **2** in 86% yield. Compound **2** was then coupled with olivetol in DCM using $AgN(SO_2CF_3)_2$ at room temperature for 10 h achieving (−)-CBD in 46% yield. Similarly, starting from S-(−)-limonene, (+)-CBD was synthesized. Briefly, the synthesis began from commercially available S-(−)-limonene, which was subjected to stereoselective bifunctionalization and elimination cascade to afford (−)-*p*-mentha-2,8-dien-1-ol. Pleasingly, (−)-*p*-mentha-2,8-dien-1-ol on reaction with olivetol in the presence of $AgN(SO_2CF_3)_2$ afforded the single isomer of (+)-CBD. The last synthetic procedure we report here to obtain (−)-CBD was very recently described by Grimm et al. (Scheme 25) [131].

Briefly, neral (*Z*-citral) was cyclized to isopiperitrol using imino-imidodiphosphates (iIDP), featuring a bifunctional inner-core system with an acidic P=NHTf moiety and a basic P=O moiety, thus combining excellent reactivity and selectivity, and furnishing (1R,6S)-*E*-isopiperitenol (**1**) in good yield (77%) and excellent diastereo- and enantioselectivity. Interestingly, such cyclization can be performed easily on a multigram scale (>4 g) without any loss of selectivity or yield, and catalyst can be recovered in excellent yield (95%) and re-used in further cyclization reactions. Then, direct access to (−)-CBD from isopiperitenol (**1**) and olivetol was provided in 35% yield under mild conditions using PTSA as catalyst in DCM at room temperature for 5 days. It is noteworthy that no further reaction of (−)-CBD to the corresponding THC was observed.

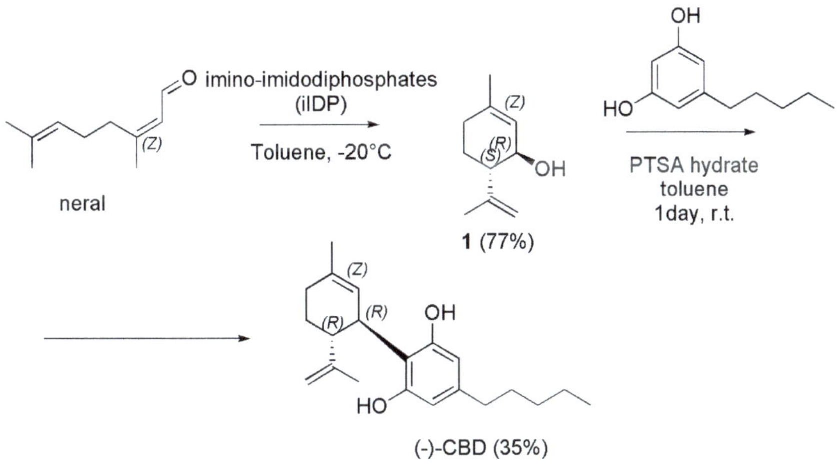

Scheme 25. Synthesis of (−)-CBD [131].

Following an overview scheme (Scheme 26) showing the synthetic procedures selected by us as the most convenient in terms of yields to obtain CBC (purple route) [103], CBD (pink route) [108] and CBG (amaranth route) [113]. Note that, while the synthetic paths leading to CBC and CBD are both one step processes shearing olivetol as reagent, that leading to CBG is a complicate multi-step process, using reagents completely different from those leading to CBC and CBD.

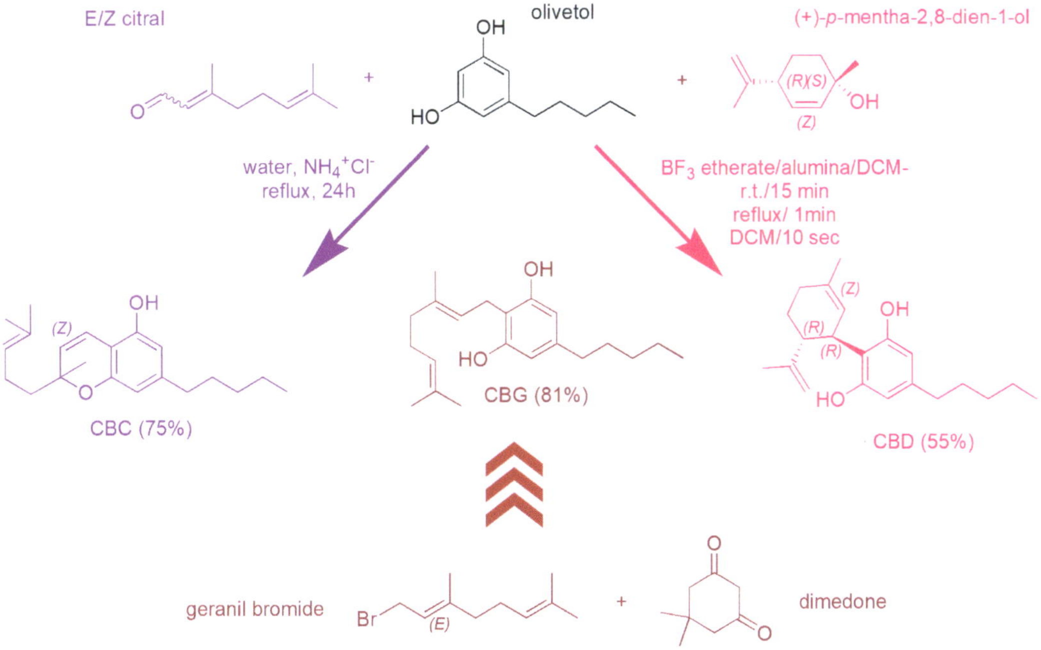

Scheme 26. Overview scheme showing the synthetic procedures selected by us as the most convenient in terms of yields to obtain CBC (purple route), CBD (pink route) and CBG (amaranth route). In the route to CBG, each arrow represents a reaction step.

5. Conclusions and Future Perspectives

Here, cannabinoids have been reviewed in terms of classification, chemical structures, mode of action, SARs, main pharmacological properties, current applications, clinical applicability, and antimicrobial properties, according to what has been reported so far. In doing so, we have detected the most promising compounds for the development of new efficient antibacterial agents to counteract MDR pathogens, promising as therapeutic agents because deprived of the psychotropic side effects, typical of the well-known THC. From the scenario that arose from this overture, it emerged that CBC, CBG and CBD, known to exclusively possess beneficial non-mind-altering pharmacological effects and reported to have potent antibacterial effects, may be the best candidates for the development of new antibiotics. So, we have systematically reviewed the synthetic pathways utilized for their preparation, thus providing a rich pool of different synthetic procedures, which can enable chemists to produce consistent amounts of these therapeutically promising PCs. Gathering in a single work the experience gained over the years by several scientists in the CBC, CBG and CBD synthesis, this review can represent a sort of manual where synthetic chemists can choose the most suitable procedure to prepare them, also according to their resources. An extensive synthetic work supported by this review will afford the material necessary for further studies and will encourage the development of new PCs-based antibiotics. Additionally, although already very potent as such, we think that additional SAR studies, specifically on CBC, CBG and CBD, are needed for detecting how these natural compounds could be modified, in order to focalize the plethora of their pharmacological properties only towards the antibacterial one, thus increasing their potency. Moreover, we think that, since these molecules have demonstrated only poor activity on bacteria of Gram-negative species, which are the ones that most endanger public health, proper structural modification could help to enhance their activity on frightening species such as resistant *E. coli*, *P. aeruginosa*, *Klebsiella* supp., *Salmonella* supp. Etc. Surely, starting from synthetic compounds obtainable in good amounts following the procedures reported here, the preparation of new and specialized cannabinoids might help to further elucidate the biological mode of action of cannabinoids on bacteria, which has not been clarified so far. In fact, although it is recognized that cannabinoids act by impairing the cytoplasmic membrane of bacteria, the mode exploited to achieve this damage remains unveiled. Note that, although a large collection of synthetically prepared cannabinoids has been reported, and the synthetic approaches employed for preparing THC have been analytically reviewed by Bloemendal and colleagues recently, those employed to prepare the non-psychotropic CBC, CBG and CBD have not yet been systematically reviewed.

Author Contributions: Conceptualization, investigation, resources, data curation, writing—original draft preparation, writing—review and editing, visualization, supervision, project administration, S.A.; writing—review and editing, A.M.S. and G.C.S. All authors have read and agreed to the published version of the manuscript.

Funding: This research received no external funding.

Data Availability Statement: All material and data related to this study is already available in the main text.

Conflicts of Interest: The authors declare no conflict of interest.

References

1. Vivas, R.; Barbosa, A.A.T.; Dolabela, S.S.; Jain, S. Multidrug-Resistant Bacteria and Alternative Methods to Control Them: An Overview. *Microb. Drug Resist.* **2019**, *25*, 890–908. [CrossRef]
2. Mancuso, G.; Midiri, A.; Gerace, E.; Biondo, C. Bacterial Antibiotic Resistance: The Most Critical Pathogens. *Pathogens* **2021**, *10*, 1310. [CrossRef]
3. WHO. Antimicrobial Resistance. Available online: https://www.who.int/news-room/fact-sheets/detail/antimicrobial-resistance (accessed on 3 May 2023).
4. Stojković, D.; Petrović, J.; Carević, T.; Soković, M.; Liaras, K. Synthetic and Semisynthetic Compounds as Antibacterials Targeting Virulence Traits in Resistant Strains: A Narrative Updated Review. *Antibiotics* **2023**, *12*, 963. [CrossRef]

5. Chancey, S.T.; Zahner, D.; Stephens, D.S. Acquired inducible antimicrobial resistance in Gram-positive bacteria. *Future Microbiol.* **2012**, *7*, 959–978. [CrossRef]
6. Spengler, G.; Kincses, A.; Gajdacs, M.; Amaral, L. New Roads Leading to Old Destinations: Efflux Pumps as Targets to Reverse Multidrug Resistance in Bacteria. *Molecules* **2017**, *22*, 468. [CrossRef]
7. Schaenzer, A.J.; Wright, G.D. Antibiotic Resistance by Enzymatic Modification of Antibiotic Targets. *Trends Mol. Med.* **2020**, *26*, 768–782. [CrossRef]
8. Wilson, D.N.; Hauryliuk, V.; Atkinson, G.C.; O'Neill, A.J. Target protection as a key antibiotic resistance mechanism. *Nat. Rev. Microbiol.* **2020**, *18*, 637–648. [CrossRef]
9. Larsson, D.G.J.; Flach, C.F. Antibiotic resistance in the environment. *Nat. Rev. Microbiol.* **2022**, *20*, 257–269. [CrossRef]
10. Guetiya Wadoum, R.E.; Zambou, N.F.; Anyangwe, F.F.; Njimou, J.R.; Coman, M.M.; Verdenelli, M.C.; Cecchini, C.; Silvi, S.; Orpianesi, C.; Cresci, A.; et al. Abusive use of antibiotics in poultry farming in Cameroon and the public health implications. *Br. Poult. Sci.* **2016**, *57*, 483–493. [CrossRef]
11. Baynes, R.E.; Dedonder, K.; Kissell, L.; Mzyk, D.; Marmulak, T.; Smith, G.; Tell, L.; Gehring, R.; Davis, J.; Riviere, J.E. Health concerns and management of select veterinary drug residues. *Food Chem. Toxicol. Int. J. Publ. Br. Ind. Biol. Res. Assoc.* **2016**, *88*, 112–122. [CrossRef]
12. Ghosh, C.; Sarkar, P.; Issa, R.; Haldar, J. Alternatives to Conventional Antibiotics in the Era of Antimicrobial Resistance. *Trend. Microbiol.* **2019**, *27*, 323–338. [CrossRef]
13. Gupta, A.; Mumtaz, S.; Li, C.H.; Hussain, I.; Rotello, V.M. Combatting antibiotic-resistant bacteria using nanomaterials. *Chem. Soc. Rev.* **2019**, *48*, 415–427. [CrossRef]
14. Sarkar, D.J.; Mohanty, D.; Raut, S.S.; Das, B.K. Antibacterial properties and in silico odelling perspective of nano ZnO transported oxytetracycline-Zn^{2+} complex $[ZnOTc]^+$ against oxytetracycline-resistant *Aeromonas hydrophila*. *J. Antibiot.* **2022**, *75*, 635–649. [CrossRef]
15. Li, Q. Application of Fragment-Based Drug Discovery to Versatile Targets. *Front. Mol. Biosci.* **2020**, *7*, 180. [CrossRef]
16. Boyd, N.K.; Teng, C.; Frei, C.R. Brief Overview of Approaches and Challenges in New Antibiotic Development: A Focus On Drug Repurposing. *Front. Cell. Infect. Microbiol.* **2021**, *11*, 684515. [CrossRef]
17. Mazur, M.; Masłowiec, D. Antimicrobial Activity of Lactones. *Antibiotics* **2022**, *11*, 1327. [CrossRef]
18. de Ruyck, J.; Dupont, C.; Lamy, E.; Le Moigne, V.; Biot, C.; Guérardel, Y.; Herrmann, J.L.; Blaise, M.; Grassin-Delyle, S.; Kremer, L.; et al. Structure-Based Design and Synthesis of Piperidinol-Containing Molecules as New *Mycobacterium abscessus* Inhibitors. *Chem. Open* **2020**, *9*, 351–365. [CrossRef]
19. Dias, C.; Pais, J.P.; Nunes, R.; Blázquez-Sánchez, M.-T.; Marquês, J.T.; Almeida, A.F.; Serra, P.; Xavier, N.M.; Vila-Viçosa, D.; Machuqueiro, M.; et al. Sugar-based bactericides targeting phosphatidylethanolamine-enriched membranes. *Nat. Commun.* **2018**, *9*, 4857. [CrossRef]
20. Thakur, A.; Verma, M.; Setia, P.; Bharti, R.; Sharma, R.; Sharma, A.; Negi, N.P.; Anand, V.; Bansal, R. DFT analysis and in vitro studies of isoxazole derivatives as potent antioxidant and antibacterial agents synthesized via one-pot methodology. *Res. Chem. Intermed.* **2023**, *49*, 859–883. [CrossRef]
21. Patil, S.A.; Patil, S.A.; Ble-González, E.A.; Isbel, S.R.; Hampton, S.M.; Bugarin, A. Carbazole Derivatives as Potential Antimicrobial Agents. *Molecules* **2022**, *27*, 6575. [CrossRef]
22. Jubeh, B.; Breijyeh, Z.; Karaman, R. Antibacterial Prodrugs to Overcome Bacterial Resistance. *Molecules* **2020**, *25*, 1543. [CrossRef] [PubMed]
23. Bassetti, M.; Kanj, S.S.; Kiratisin, P.; Rodrigues, C.; Van Duin, D.; Villegas, M.V.; Yu, Y. Early appropriate diagnostics and treatment of MDR Gram-negative infections. *JAC-Antimicrob. Resist.* **2022**, *4*, dlac089. [CrossRef]
24. Tyers, M.; Wright, G.D. Drug combinations: A strategy to extend the life of antibiotics in the 21st century. *Nat. Rev. Microbiol.* **2019**, *17*, 141–155. [CrossRef]
25. Alfei, S.; Schito, A.M. β-Lactam Antibiotics and β-Lactamase Enzymes Inhibitors, Part 2: Our Limited Resources. *Pharmaceuticals* **2022**, *15*, 476. [CrossRef]
26. Alfei, S.; Zuccari, G. Recommendations to Synthetize Old and New β-Lactamases Inhibitors: A Review to Encourage Further Production. *Pharmaceuticals* **2022**, *15*, 384. [CrossRef]
27. Karasneh, R.A.; Al-Azzam, S.I.; Ababneh, M.; Al-Azzeh, O.; Al-Batayneh, O.B.; Muflih, S.M.; Khasawneh, M.; Khassawneh, A.M.; Khader, Y.S.; Conway, B.R.; et al. Prescribers' Knowledge, Attitudes and Behaviors on Antibiotics, Antibiotic Use and Antibiotic Resistance in Jordan. *Antibiotics* **2021**, *10*, 858. [CrossRef]
28. Radwan, M.M.; Chandra, S.; Gul, S.; ElSohly, M.A. Cannabinoids, Phenolics, Terpenes and Alkaloids of *Cannabis*. *Molecules* **2021**, *26*, 2774. [CrossRef]
29. Tahir, M.N.; Shahbazi, F.; Rondeau-Gagné, S.; Trant, J.F. The biosynthesis of the cannabinoids. *J. Cannabis. Res.* **2021**, *3*, 7. [CrossRef]
30. Pagano, C.; Navarra, G.; Coppola, L.; Avilia, G.; Bifulco, M.; Laezza, C. Cannabinoids: Therapeutic Use in Clinical Practice. *Int. J. Mol. Sci.* **2022**, *23*, 3344. [CrossRef]
31. Palomares, B.; Ruiz-Pino, F.; Garrido-Rodriguez, M.; Eugenia Prados, M.; Sánchez-Garrido, M.A.; Velasco, I.; Vazquez, M.J.; Nadal, X.; Ferreiro-Vera, C.; Morrugares, R.; et al. Tetrahydrocannabinolic Acid A (THCA-A) Reduces Adiposity and Prevents Metabolic Disease Caused by Diet-Induced Obesity. *Biochem. Pharmacol.* **2020**, *171*, 113693. [CrossRef]

32. Pisanti, S.; Malfitano, A.M.; Ciaglia, E.; Lamberti, A.; Ranieri, R.; Cuomo, G.; Abate, M.; Faggiana, G.; Proto, M.C.; Fiore, D.; et al. Cannabidiol: State of the Art and New Challenges for Therapeutic Applications. *Pharmacol. Ther.* **2017**, *175*, 133–150. [CrossRef] [PubMed]
33. Farha, M.A.; El-Halfawy, O.M.; Gale, R.T.; MacNair, C.R.; Carfrae, L.A.; Zhang, X.; Jentsch, N.G.; Magolan, J.; Brown, E.D. Uncovering the Hidden Antibiotic Potential of Cannabis. *ACS Infect. Dis.* **2020**, *6*, 338–346. [CrossRef] [PubMed]
34. Breijyeh, Z.; Karaman, R. Design and Synthesis of Novel Antimicrobial Agents. *Antibiotics* **2023**, *12*, 628. [CrossRef] [PubMed]
35. Saleemi, M.A.; Yahaya, N.; Zain, N.N.M.; Raoov, M.; Yong, Y.K.; Noor, N.S.; Lim, V. Antimicrobial and Cytotoxic Effects of Cannabinoids: An Updated Review with Future Perspectives and Current Challenges. *Pharmaceuticals* **2022**, *15*, 1228. [CrossRef]
36. Chen, J.; Zhang, H.; Wang, S.; Du, Y.; Wei, B.; Wu, Q.; Wang, H. Inhibitors of Bacterial Extracellular Vesicles. *Front. Microbiol.* **2022**, *13*, 835058. [CrossRef]
37. Luz-Veiga, M.; Amorim, M.; Pinto-Ribeiro, I.; Oliveira, A.L.S.; Silva, S.; Pimentel, L.L.; Rodríguez-Alcalá, L.M.; Madureira, R.; Pintado, M.; Azevedo-Silva, J.; et al. Cannabidiol and Cannabigerol Exert Antimicrobial Activity without Compromising Skin Microbiota. *Int. J. Mol. Sci.* **2023**, *24*, 2389. [CrossRef]
38. Blaskovich, M.A.T.; Kavanagh, A.M.; Elliott, A.G.; Zhang, B.; Ramu, S.; Amado, M.; Lowe, G.J.; Hinton, A.O.; Pham, D.M.T.; Zuegg, J.; et al. The antimicrobial potential of cannabidiol. *Commun. Biol.* **2021**, *4*, 7. [CrossRef]
39. Gildea, L.; Ayariga, J.A.; Xu, J.; Villafane, R.; Robertson, B.K.; Samuel-Foo, M.; Ajayi, O.S. Cannabis sativa CBD Extract Exhibits Synergy with Broad-Spectrum Antibiotics against Salmonella enterica subsp. Enterica serovar typhimurium. *Microorganisms* **2022**, *10*, 2360. [CrossRef]
40. Calapai, F.; Cardia, L.; Esposito, E.; Ammendolia, I.; Mondello, C.; Lo Giudice, R.; Gangemi, S.; Calapai, G.; Mannucci, C. Pharmacological Aspects and Biological Effects of Cannabigerol and Its Synthetic Derivatives. *Evid.-Based Complement. Altern. Med.* **2022**, *2022*, 3336516. [CrossRef]
41. Whiting, P.F.; Wolff, R.F.; Deshpande, S.; Di Nisio, M.; Duffy, S.; Hernandez, A.V.; Keurentjes, J.C.; Lang, S.; Misso, K.; Ryder, S.; et al. Cannabinoids for Medical Use: A Systematic Review and Meta-analysis. *JAMA* **2015**, *313*, 2456–2473. [CrossRef]
42. Vučković, S.; Srebro, D.; Vujović, K.S.; Vučetić, Č.; Prostran, M. Cannabinoids and Pain: New Insights From Old Molecules. *Front. Pharmacol.* **2018**, *9*, 1259. [CrossRef] [PubMed]
43. Lafaye, G.; Karila, L.; Blecha, L.; Benyamina, A. Cannabis, Cannabinoids, and Health. *DCNS* **2017**, *19*, 309–316. [CrossRef]
44. Berman, P.; Futoran, K.; Lewitus, G.M.; Mukha, D.; Benami, M.; Shlomi, T.; Meiri, D. A New ESI-LC/MS Approach for Comprehensive Metabolic Profiling of Phytocannabinoids in Cannabis. *Sci. Rep.* **2018**, *8*, 14280. [CrossRef]
45. Fraguas-Sánchez, A.I.; Fernández-Carballido, A.; Torres-Suárez, A.I. Phyto-, Endo- and Synthetic Cannabinoids: Promising Chemotherapeutic Agents in the Treatment of Breast and Prostate Carcinomas. *Expert. Opin. Investig. Drugs.* **2016**, *25*, 1311–1323. [CrossRef]
46. Mackie, K. Cannabinoid Receptors: Where They are and What They do. *J. Neuroendocr.* **2008**, *20*, 10–14. [CrossRef]
47. Brennecke, B.; Gazzi, T.; Atz, K.; Fingerle, J.; Kuner, P.; Schindler, T.; Weck, G.; Nazaré, M.; Grether, U. Cannabinoid receptor type 2 ligands: An analysis of granted patents since 2010. *Pharm. Patent Anal.* **2021**, *10*, 111–163. [CrossRef]
48. Gertsch, J.; Raduner, S.; Altmann, K.-H. New Natural Noncannabinoid Ligands for Cannabinoid Type-2 (CB2) Receptors. *J. Recept. Signal Transduct.* **2006**, *26*, 709–730. [CrossRef]
49. Li, X.; Chang, H.; Bouma, J.; de Paus, L.V.; Mukhopadhyay, P.; Paloczi, J.; Mustafa, M.; van der Horst, C.; Kumar, S.S.; Wu, L.; et al. Structural Basis of Selective Cannabinoid CB2 Receptor Activation. *Nat. Commun.* **2023**, *14*, 1447. [CrossRef]
50. Lambert, D.M. Pharmacologic Targeting of the CB2 Cannabinoid Receptor for Application in Centrally-Mediated Chronic Pain. Ph.D. Thesis, University of British Columbia, Vancouver, BC, Canada, 2019. Available online: https://open.library.ubc.ca/collections/ubctheses/24/items/1.0376050 (accessed on 27 June 2023).
51. Fezza, F.; Bari, M.; Florio, R.; Talamonti, E.; Feole, M.; Maccarrone, M. Endocannabinoids, Related Compounds and Their Metabolic Routes. *Molecules* **2014**, *19*, 17078–17106. [CrossRef]
52. Sharma, D.S.; Paddibhatla, I.; Raghuwanshi, S.; Malleswarapu, M.; Sangeeth, A.; Kovuru, N.; Dahariya, S.; Gautam, D.K.; Pallepati, A.; Gutti, R.K. Endocannabinoid system: Role in blood cell development, neuroimmune interactions and associated disorders. *J. Neuroimmunol.* **2021**, *353*, 577501. [CrossRef]
53. Formato, M.; Crescente, G.; Scognamiglio, M.; Fiorentino, A.; Pecoraro, M.T.; Piccolella, S.; Catauro, M.; Pacifico, S. (−)-Cannabidiolic Acid, a Still Overlooked Bioactive Compound: An Introductory Review and Preliminary Research. *Molecules* **2020**, *25*, 2638. [CrossRef] [PubMed]
54. Nguyen, G.N.; Jordan, E.N.; Kayser, O. Synthetic Strategies for Rare Cannabinoids Derived from *Cannabis sativa*. *J. Nat. Prod.* **2022**, *85*, 1555–1568. [CrossRef] [PubMed]
55. Schwilke, E.W.; Schwope, D.M.; Karschner, E.L.; Lowe, R.H.; Darwin, W.D.; Kelly, D.L.; Goodwin, R.S.; Gorelick, D.A.; Huestis, M.A. Δ9-Tetrahydrocannabinol (THC), 11-Hydroxy-THC, and 11-Nor-9-Carboxy-THC Plasma Pharmacokinetics during and after Continuous High-Dose Oral THC. *Clin. Chem.* **2009**, *55*, 2180–2189. [CrossRef] [PubMed]
56. Martin, B.R.; Jefferson, R.; Winckler, R.; Wiley, J.L.; Huffman, J.W.; Crocker, P.J.; Saha, B.; Razdan, R.K. Manipulation of the tetrahydrocannabinol side chain delineates agonists, partial agonists, and antagonists. *J. Pharmacol. Exp. Ther.* **1999**, *290*, 1065–1079. [PubMed]

57. Andersson, D.A.; Gentry, C.; Alenmyr, L.; Killander, D.; Lewis, S.E.; Andersson, A.; Bucher, B.; Galzi, J.-L.; Sterner, O.; Bevan, S. TRPA1 mediates spinal antinociception induced by acetaminophen and the cannabinoid. δ 9-tetrahydrocannabiorcol. *Nat. Commun.* **2011**, *2*, 551. [CrossRef] [PubMed]
58. Bow, E.W.; Rimoldi, J.M. The structure–function relationships of classical cannabinoids: CB1/CB2 modulation. *Perspect. Med. Chem.* **2016**, *8*, 17–39. [CrossRef]
59. Thomas, A.; Ross, R.A.; Saha, B.; Mahadevan, A.; Razdan, R.K.; Pertwee, R.G. 6″-azidohex-2″-yne-cannabidiol: A potential neutral, competitive cannabinoid cb1 receptor antagonist. *Eur. J. Pharmacol.* **2004**, *487*, 213–221. [CrossRef]
60. O'Donnell, B.; Meissner, H.; Gupta, V. Dronabinol. In *StatPearls*; Updated 5 September 2022; StatPearls Publishing: Treasure Island, FL, USA, 2023. Available online: https://www.ncbi.nlm.nih.gov/books/NBK557531/ (accessed on 27 June 2023).
61. (R)-(+)-Methanandamide. Available online: https://www.tocris.com/products/r-methanandamide_1121 (accessed on 3 May 2023).
62. Gratzke, C.; Streng, T.; Stief, C.G.; Downs, T.R.; Alroy, I.; Rosenbaum, J.S.; Andersson, K.E.; Hedlund, P. Effects of cannabinor, a novel selective cannabinoid 2 receptor agonist, on bladder function in normal rats. *Eur. Urol.* **2010**, *57*, 1093–1100. [CrossRef]
63. D'Aquila, P.S. Microstructure analysis of the effects of the cannabinoid agents HU-210 and rimonabant in rats licking for sucrose. *Eur. J. Pharmacol.* **2020**, *887*, 173468. [CrossRef]
64. Ikeda, H.; Ikegami, M.; Kai, M.; Ohsawa, M.; Kamei, J. Activation of spinal cannabinoid CB2 receptors inhibits neuropathic pain in streptozotocin-induced diabetic mice. *Neuroscience* **2013**, *250*, 446–454. [CrossRef]
65. Du, J.J.; Liu, Z.Q.; Yan, Y.; Xiong, J.; Jia, X.T.; Di, Z.L.; Ren, J.J. The Cannabinoid WIN 55,212-2 Reduces Delayed Neurologic Sequelae After Carbon Monoxide Poisoning by Promoting Microglial M2 Polarization Through ST2 Signaling. *J. Mol. Neurosci. MN* **2020**, *70*, 422–432. [CrossRef]
66. Verty, A.N.; Stefanidis, A.; McAinch, A.J.; Hryciw, D.H.; Oldfield, B. Anti-Obesity Effect of the CB2 Receptor Agonist JWH-015 in Diet-Induced Obese Mice. *PLoS ONE* **2015**, *10*, e0140592. [CrossRef]
67. Howlett, A.C.; Thomas, B.F.; Huffman, J.W. The Spicy Story of Cannabimimetic Indoles. *Molecules* **2021**, *26*, 6190. [CrossRef] [PubMed]
68. Abadji, V.; Lin, S.; Taha, G.; Griffin, G.; Stevenson, L.A.; Pertwee, R.G.; Makriyannis, A. (R)-Methanandamide: A Chiral Novel Anandamide Possessing Higher Potency and Metabolic Stability. *J. Med. Chem.* **1994**, *37*, 1889–1893. [CrossRef]
69. WIN 55212-2. Available online: https://pubchem.ncbi.nlm.nih.gov/compound/5311501 (accessed on 3 May 2023).
70. JWH-133. Available online: https://pubchem.ncbi.nlm.nih.gov/compound/6918505 (accessed on 3 May 2023).
71. Hassenberg, C.; Clausen, F.; Hoffmann, G.; Studer, A.; Schürenkamp, J. Investigation of phase II metabolism of 11-hydroxy-Δ-9-tetrahydrocannabinol and metabolite verification by chemical synthesis of 11-hydroxy-Δ-9-tetrahydrocannabinol-glucuronide. *Int. J. Legal Med.* **2020**, *134*, 2105–2119. [CrossRef] [PubMed]
72. Engels, F.K.; de Jong, F.A.; Mathijssen, R.H.J.; Erkens, J.A.; Herings, R.M.; Verweij, J. Medicinal Cannabis in Oncology. *Eu. J. Cancer* **2007**, *43*, 2638–2644. [CrossRef]
73. Ward, S.J.; McAllister, S.D.; Kawamura, R.; Murase, R.; Neelakantan, H.; Walker, E.A. Cannabidiol Inhibits Paclitaxel-Induced Neuropathic Pain through 5-HT1A Receptors without Diminishing Nervous System Function or Chemotherapy Efficacy. *Br. J. Pharmacol.* **2014**, *171*, 636–645. [CrossRef] [PubMed]
74. Keating, G.M. Delta-9-Tetrahydrocannabinol/Cannabidiol Oromucosal Spray (Sativex®): A Review in Multiple Sclerosis-Related Spasticity. *Drugs* **2017**, *77*, 563–574. [CrossRef]
75. Reddy, D.S.; Golub, M.V. The Pharmacological Basis of Cannabis Therapy for Epilepsy. *J. Pharmacol. Exp. Ther.* **2016**, *357*, 45. [CrossRef]
76. Navarro, G.; Gonzalez, A.; Sánchez-Morales, A.; Casajuana-Martin, N.; Gómez-Ventura, M.; Cordomí, A.; Busqué, F.; Alibés, R.; Pardo, L.; Franco, R. Design of Negative and Positive Allosteric Modulators of the Cannabinoid CB2 Receptor Derived from the Natural Product Cannabidiol. *J. Med. Chem.* **2021**, *64*, 9354–9364. [CrossRef]
77. Luft, F.C. Rehabilitating rimonabant. *J. Mol. Med.* **2013**, *91*, 777–779. [CrossRef]
78. Karas, J.A.; Wong, L.J.M.; Paulin, O.K.A.; Mazeh, A.C.; Hussein, M.H.; Li, J.; Velkov, T. The Antimicrobial Activity of Cannabinoids. *Antibiotics* **2020**, *9*, 406. [CrossRef] [PubMed]
79. Stone, N.L.; Murphy, A.J.; England, T.J.; O'Sullivan, S.E. A Systematic Review of Minor Phytocannabinoids with Promising Neuroprotective Potential. *Br. J. Pharmacol.* **2020**, *177*, 4330–4352. [CrossRef] [PubMed]
80. Walsh, K.B.; McKinney, A.E.; Holmes, A.E. Minor Cannabinoids: Biosynthesis, Molecular Pharmacology and Potential Therapeutic Uses. *Front. Pharmacol.* **2021**, *12*, 777804. [CrossRef]
81. Scott, C.; Neira Agonh, D.; Lehmann, C. Antibacterial Effects of Phytocannabinoids. *Life* **2022**, *12*, 1394. [CrossRef]
82. van Klingeren, B.; ten Ham, M. Antibacterial Activity of Δ9-Tetrahydrocannabinol and Cannabidiol. *Antonie Leeuwenhoek* **1976**, *42*, 9–12. [CrossRef]
83. Appendino, G.; Gibbons, S.; Giana, A.; Pagani, A.; Grassi, G.; Stavri, M.; Smith, E.; Rahman, M.M. Antibacterial cannabinoids from Cannabis sativa: A structure-activity study. *J. Nat. Prod.* **2008**, *71*, 1427–1430. [CrossRef] [PubMed]
84. Martinenghi, L.D.; Jønsson, R.; Lund, T.; Jenssen, H. Isolation, purification, and antimicrobial characterization of cannabidiolic acid and cannabidiol from Cannabis sativa L. *Biomolecules* **2020**, *10*, 900. [CrossRef] [PubMed]
85. Wu, Q.; Guo, M.; Zou, L.; Wang, Q.; Xia, Y. 8,9-Dihydrocannabidiol, an Alternative of Cannabidiol, Its Preparation, Antibacterial and Antioxidant Ability. *Molecules* **2023**, *28*, 445. [CrossRef] [PubMed]

86. Wassmann, C.S.; Højrup, P.; Klitgaard, J.K. Cannabidiol Is an Effective Helper Compound in Combination with Bacitracin to Kill Gram-Positive Bacteria. *Sci. Rep.* **2020**, *10*, 4112. [CrossRef]
87. Turner, C.E.; Elsohly, M.A. Biological activity of cannabichromene, its homologs and isomers. *J. Clin. Pharmacol.* **1981**, *21*, 283s–291s. [CrossRef]
88. Aqawi, M.; Sionov, R.V.; Gallily, R.; Friedman, M.; Steinberg, D. Anti-Bacterial Properties of Cannabigerol Toward Streptococcus Mutans. *Front. Microbiol.* **2021**, *12*, 656471. [CrossRef]
89. Elsohly, H.N.; Turner, C.E.; Clark, A.M.; Elsohly, M.A. Synthesis and Antimicrobial Activities of Certain Cannabichromene and Cannabigerol Related Compounds. *J. Pharm. Sci.* **1982**, *71*, 1319–1323. [CrossRef] [PubMed]
90. Feldman, M.; Smoum, R.; Mechoulam, R.; Steinberg, D. Antimicrobial potential of endocannabinoid and endocannabinoid-like compounds against methicillin-resistant Staphylococcus aureus. *Sci. Rep.* **2018**, *8*, 17696. [CrossRef]
91. CLSI. Available online: https://clsi.org/ (accessed on 3 May 2023).
92. Kosgodage, U.S.; Matewele, P.; Awamaria, B.; Kraev, I.; Warde, P.; Mastroianni, G.; Nunn, A.V.; Guy, G.W.; Bell, J.D.; Inal, J.M.; et al. Cannabidiol Is a novel modulator of bacterial membrane vesicles. *Front. Cell. Infect. Microbiol.* **2019**, *9*, 324. [CrossRef]
93. Seccamani, P.; Franco, C.; Protti, S.; Porta, A.; Profumo, A.; Caprioglio, D.; Salamone, S.; Mannucci, B.; Merli, D. Photochemistry of Cannabidiol (CBD) Revised. A Combined Preparative and Spectrometric Investigation. *J. Nat. Prod.* **2021**, *84*, 2858–2865. [CrossRef] [PubMed]
94. Luo, G.-Y.; Wu, H.; Tang, Y.; Li, H.; Yeom, H.-S.; Yang, K.; Hsung, R.P. A Total Synthesis of (±)-Rhododaurichromanic Acid A via an Oxa-[3+3] Annulation of Resorcinols. *Synthesis* **2015**, *47*, 2713–2720. [CrossRef]
95. Lodewyk, M.W.; Lui, V.G.; Tantillo, D.J. Synthesis of (Sulfonyl)Methylphosphonate Analogs of Prenyl Diphosphates. *Tetrahedron Lett.* **2010**, *51*, 170–173. [CrossRef]
96. Yeom, H.-S.; Li, H.; Tang, Y.; Hsung, R.P. Total Syntheses of Cannabicyclol, Clusiacyclol A and B, Iso-Eriobrucinol A and B, and Eriobrucinol. *Org. Lett.* **2013**, *15*, 3130–3133. [CrossRef]
97. Crombie, L.; Ponsford, R.; Shani, A.; Yagnitinsky, B.; Mechoulam, R. Hashish Components. Photochemical Production of Cannabicyclol from Cannabichromene. *Tetrahedron Lett.* **1968**, *9*, 5771–5772. [CrossRef]
98. Schafroth, M.A.; Mazzoccanti, G.; Reynoso-Moreno, I.; Erni, R.; Pollastro, F.; Caprioglio, D.; Botta, B.; Allegrone, G.; Grassi, G.; Chicca, A.; et al. Δ9-Cis-Tetrahydrocannabinol: Natural Occurrence, Chirality, and Pharmacology. *J. Nat. Prod.* **2021**, *84*, 2502–2510. [CrossRef] [PubMed]
99. Andersen, L.L.; Ametovski, A.; Lin Luo, J.; Everett-Morgan, D.; McGregor, I.S.; Banister, S.D.; Arnold, J.C. Cannabichromene, Related Phytocannabinoids, and 5-Fluoro-Cannabichromene Have Anticonvulsant Properties in a Mouse Model of Dravet Syndrome. *ACS Chem. Neurosci.* **2021**, *12*, 330–339. [CrossRef]
100. Lee, Y.R.; Wang, X. Concise Synthesis of Biologically Interesting (′)-Cannabichromene, (′)-Cannabichromenic Acid, and (′)-Daurichromenic Acid. *Bull. Korean Chem. Soc.* **2005**, *26*, 1933–1936. [CrossRef]
101. Tietze, L.-F.; Kiedrowski, G.V.; Berger, B. A New Method of Aromatization of Cyclohexenone Derivatives; Synthesis of Cannabichromene. *Synthesis* **1982**, *8*, 683–684. [CrossRef]
102. Eisohly, M.A.; Boeren, E.G.; Turner, C.E. Constituents of Cannabis Sativa L. An Improved Method for the Synthesis of Dl-Cannabichromene. *J. Heterocycl. Chem.* **1978**, *15*, 699–700. [CrossRef]
103. Quílez del Moral, J.F.; Ruiz Martínez, C.; Pérez del Pulgar, H.; Martín González, J.E.; Fernández, I.; López-Pérez, J.L.; Fernández-Arteaga, A.; Barrero, A.F. Synthesis of Cannabinoids: "In Water" and "On Water" Approaches: Influence of SDS Micelles. *J. Org. Chem.* **2021**, *86*, 3344–3355. [CrossRef]
104. Yamaguchi, S.; Shouji, N.; Kuroda, K. A New Approach to Dl-Cannabichromene. *BCSJ* **1995**, *68*, 305–308. [CrossRef]
105. Gaoni, Y.; Mechoulam, R. The Structure and Synthesis of Cannabigerol, a New Hashish Constituent. *Proc. Chem. Soc.* **1964**, *82*.
106. Mechoulam, R.; Yagen, B. Stereoselective Cyclizations of Cannabinoid 1,5 Dienes. *Tetrahedron Lett.* **1969**, *10*, 5349–5352. [CrossRef] [PubMed]
107. Taura, F.; Morimoto, S.; Shoyama, Y. Purification and Characterization of Cannabidiolic-Acid Synthase from Cannabis Sativa L.: Biochemical analysis of a novel enzyme that catalyzes the oxidocyclization of cannabigerolic acid to cannabidiolic acid. *J. Biol. Chem.* **1996**, *271*, 17411–17416. [CrossRef]
108. Baek, S.H.; Srebnik, M.; Mechoulam, R. Boron Trifluoride Etherate on Alumina—A Modified Lewis Acid Reagent. An Improved Synthesis of Cannabidiol. *Tetrahedron Lett.* **1985**, *26*, 1083–1086. [CrossRef]
109. Baek, S.-H.; Yook, C.N.; Han, D.S. Boron trifluoride etherate on alumina—A modified Lewis acid reagent(V) a convenient single-step synthesis of cannabinoids. *Bull. Korean Chem. Soc.* **1995**, *16*, 293–296.
110. Baek, S.-H.; Du Han, S.; Yook, C.N.; Kim, Y.C.; Kwak, J.S. Synthesis and Antitumor Activity of Cannabigerol. *Arch. Pharm. Res.* **1996**, *19*, 228–230. [CrossRef]
111. Kumano, T.; Richard, S.B.; Noel, J.P.; Nishiyama, M.; Kuzuyama, T. Chemoenzymatic Syntheses of Prenylated Aromatic Small Molecules Using Streptomyces Prenyltransferases with Relaxed Substrate Specificities. *Bioorg. Med. Chem.* **2008**, *16*, 8117–8126. [CrossRef]
112. Jentsch, N.G.; Zhang, X.; Magolan, J. Efficient Synthesis of Cannabigerol, Grifolin, and Piperogalin via Alumina-Promoted Allylation. *J. Nat. Prod.* **2020**, *83*, 2587–2591. [CrossRef]
113. Curtis, B.J.; Micikas, R.J.; Burkhardt, R.N.; Smith, R.A.; Pan, J.Y.; Jander, K.; Schroeder, F.C. Syntheses of Amorfrutins and Derivatives via Tandem Diels–Alder and Anionic Cascade Approaches. *J. Org. Chem.* **2021**, *86*, 11269–11276. [CrossRef]

114. Mechoulam, R.; Gaoni, Y. A Total Synthesis of Dl-Δ1-Tetrahydrocannabinol, the Active Constituent of Hashish1. *J. Am. Chem. Soc.* **1965**, *87*, 3273–3275. [CrossRef]
115. Petrzilka, T.; Haefliger, W.; Sikemeier, C.; Ohloff, G.; Eschenmoser, A. Synthese Und Chiralität Des (−)-Cannabidiols Vorläufige Mitteilung. *Helvetica Chim. Acta* **1967**, *50*, 719–723. [CrossRef] [PubMed]
116. Petrzilka, T.; Haefliger, W.; Sikemeier, C. Synthese von Haschisch-Inhaltsstoffen. 4. Mitteilung. *Helvetica Chim. Acta* **1969**, *52*, 1102–1134. [CrossRef]
117. Razdan, R.K.; Dalzell, H.C.; Handrick, G.R. Hashish. X. Simple One-Step Synthesis of (−)-DELTA.1-Tetrahydrocannabinol (THC) from p-Mentha-2,8-Dien-1-Ol and Olivetol. *J. Am. Chem. Soc.* **1974**, *96*, 5860–5865. [CrossRef]
118. Papahatjis, D.P.; Nikas, S.P.; Andreou, T.; Makriyannis, A. Novel 1′,1′-Chain Substituted Δ8-Tetrahydrocannabinols. *Bioorg. Med. Chem. Lett.* **2002**, *12*, 3583–3586. [CrossRef]
119. Uliss, D.B.; Dalzell, H.C.; Handrick, G.R.; Howes, J.F.; Razdan, R.K. Hashish. Importance of the Phenolic Hydroxyl Group in Tetrahydrocannabinols. *J. Med. Chem.* **1975**, *18*, 213–215. [CrossRef]
120. Crombie, L.; Crombie, W.M.L.; Jamieson, S.V.; Palmer, C.J. Acid-Catalysed Terpenylations of Olivetol in the Synthesis of Cannabinoids. *J. Chem. Soc. Perkin Trans.* **1988**, *1*, 1243–1250. [CrossRef]
121. Kinney, W.A.; McDonnell, M.E.; Zhong, H.M.; Liu, C.; Yang, L.; Ling, W.; Qian, T.; Chen, Y.; Cai, Z.; Petkanas, D.; et al. Discovery of KLS-13019, a Cannabidiol-Derived Neuroprotective Agent, with Improved Potency, Safety, and Permeability. *ACS Med. Chem. Lett.* **2016**, *7*, 424–428. [CrossRef] [PubMed]
122. Villano, R.; Straker, H.; Di Marzo, V. Short and Efficient Synthesis of Alkylresorcinols: A Route for the Preparation of Cannabinoids. *New J. Chem.* **2022**, *46*, 20664–20668. [CrossRef]
123. Vaillancourt, V.; Albizati, K.F. A One-Step Method for the.Alpha.-Arylation of Camphor. Synthesis of (−)-Cannabidiol and (−)-Cannabidiol Dimethyl Ether. *J. Org. Chem.* **1992**, *57*, 3627–3631. [CrossRef]
124. Malkov, A.; Kocovsky, P. Tetrahydrocannabinol Revisited: Synthetic Approaches Utilizing Molybdenum Catalysts. *Collect. Czech. Chem. Commun.* **2001**, *66*, 1257–1268. [CrossRef]
125. William, A.D.; Kobayashi, Y. A Method To Accomplish a 1,4-Addition Reaction of Bulky Nucleophiles to Enones and Subsequent Formation of Reactive Enolates. *Org. Lett.* **2001**, *3*, 2017–2020. [CrossRef] [PubMed]
126. Kobayashi, Y.; Takeuchi, A.; Wang, Y.-G. Synthesis of Cannabidiols via Alkenylation of Cyclohexenyl Monoacetate. *Org. Lett.* **2006**, *8*, 2699–2702. [CrossRef] [PubMed]
127. Shultz, Z.P.; Lawrence, G.A.; Jacobson, J.M.; Cruz, E.J.; Leahy, J.W. Enantioselective Total Synthesis of Cannabinoids—A Route for Analogue Development. *Org. Lett.* **2018**, *20*, 381–384. [CrossRef] [PubMed]
128. Gong, X.; Sun, C.; Abame, M.A.; Shi, W.; Xie, Y.; Xu, W.; Zhu, F.; Zhang, Y.; Shen, J.; Aisa, H.A. Synthesis of CBD and Its Derivatives Bearing Various C4′-Side Chains with a Late-Stage Diversification Method. *J. Org. Chem.* **2020**, *85*, 2704–2715. [CrossRef] [PubMed]
129. Chiurchiù, E.; Sampaolesi, S.; Allegrini, P.; Ciceri, D.; Ballini, R.; Palmieri, A. A Novel and Practical Continuous Flow Chemical Synthesis of Cannabidiol (CBD) and Its CBDV and CBDB Analogues. *Eur. J. Org. Chem.* **2021**, *2021*, 1286–1289. [CrossRef]
130. Anand, R.; Cham, P.S.; Gannedi, V.; Sharma, S.; Kumar, M.; Singh, R.; Vishwakarma, R.A.; Singh, P.P. Stereoselective Synthesis of Nonpsychotic Natural Cannabidiol and Its Unnatural/Terpenyl/Tail-Modified Analogues. *J. Org. Chem.* **2022**, *87*, 4489–4498. [CrossRef] [PubMed]
131. Grimm, J.A.A.; Zhou, H.; Properzi, R.; Leutzsch, M.; Bistoni, G.; Nienhaus, J.; List, B. Catalytic Asymmetric Synthesis of Cannabinoids and Menthol from Neral. *Nature* **2023**, *615*, 634–639. [CrossRef] [PubMed]

pharmaceutics

Review

Bioactive ZnO Nanoparticles: Biosynthesis, Characterization and Potential Antimicrobial Applications

Md. Amdadul Huq [1,*], Md. Aminul Islam Apu [2], Md. Ashrafudoulla [3], Md. Mizanur Rahman [4], Md. Anowar Khasru Parvez [5], Sri Renukadevi Balusamy [6], Shahina Akter [7] and Md. Shahedur Rahman [8,*]

1 Department of Food and Nutrition, College of Biotechnology and Natural Resource, Chung-Ang University, Anseong 17546, Republic of Korea
2 Department of Nutrition and Hospitality Management, The University of Mississippi, Oxford, MS 38677, USA; aminul.btge@gmail.com
3 Department of Food Science and Technology, Chung-Ang University, Anseong 17546, Republic of Korea; ashrafmiu584@gmail.com
4 Department of Biotechnology and Genetic Engineering, Faculty of Biological Science, Islamic University, Kushtia 7003, Bangladesh; mmrahmanbtg79@hotmail.com
5 Department of Microbiology, Jahangirnagar University, Savar, Dhaka 1342, Bangladesh; khasru73@juniv.edu
6 Department of Food Science and Technology, Sejong University, Seoul 05006, Republic of Korea; renucoimbatore@gmail.com
7 Department of Food Science and Biotechnology, Gachon University, Seongnam 13120, Republic of Korea; shahinabristy16@gmail.com
8 Department of Genetic Engineering and Biotechnology, Jashore University of Science and Technology, Jashore 7408, Bangladesh
* Correspondence: amdadbge@gmail.com or amdadbge100@cau.ac.kr (M.A.H.); ms.rahman@just.edu.bd (M.S.R.)

Citation: Huq, M.A.; Apu, M.A.I.; Ashrafudoulla, M.; Rahman, M.M.; Parvez, M.A.K.; Balusamy, S.R.; Akter, S.; Rahman, M.S. Bioactive ZnO Nanoparticles: Biosynthesis, Characterization and Potential Antimicrobial Applications. *Pharmaceutics* **2023**, *15*, 2634. https://doi.org/10.3390/pharmaceutics15112634

Academic Editors: Patrick J. Sinko, Francisco Javier De La Mata and Dong Keun Han

Received: 7 June 2023
Revised: 22 July 2023
Accepted: 15 November 2023
Published: 16 November 2023

Abstract: In recent years, biosynthesized zinc oxide nanoparticles (ZnONPs) have gained tremendous attention because of their safe and non-toxic nature and distinctive biomedical applications. A diverse range of microbes (bacteria, fungi and yeast) and various parts (leaf, root, fruit, flower, peel, stem, etc.) of plants have been exploited for the facile, rapid, cost-effective and non-toxic synthesis of ZnONPs. Plant extracts, microbial biomass or culture supernatant contain various biomolecules including enzymes, amino acids, proteins, vitamins, alkaloids, flavonoids, etc., which serve as reducing, capping and stabilizing agents during the biosynthesis of ZnONPs. The biosynthesized ZnONPs are generally characterized using UV-VIS spectroscopy, TEM, SEM, EDX, XRD, FTIR, etc. Antibiotic resistance is a serious problem for global public health. Due to mutation, shifting environmental circumstances and excessive drug use, the number of multidrug-resistant pathogenic microbes is continuously rising. To solve this issue, novel, safe and effective antimicrobial agents are needed urgently. Biosynthesized ZnONPs could be novel and effective antimicrobial agents because of their safe and non-toxic nature and powerful antimicrobial characteristics. It is proven that biosynthesized ZnONPs have strong antimicrobial activity against various pathogenic microorganisms including multidrug-resistant bacteria. The possible antimicrobial mechanisms of ZnONPs are the generation of reactive oxygen species, physical interactions, disruption of the cell walls and cell membranes, damage to DNA, enzyme inactivation, protein denaturation, ribosomal destabilization and mitochondrial dysfunction. In this review, the biosynthesis of ZnONPs using microbes and plants and their characterization have been reviewed comprehensively. Also, the antimicrobial applications and mechanisms of biosynthesized ZnONPs against various pathogenic microorganisms have been highlighted.

Keywords: ZnONPs; biosynthesis; characterization; antimicrobial applications; antimicrobial mechanisms

1. Introduction

Nanoparticles (NPs) have been proposed as an intervention approach for suppressing microbial growth, as well as contamination, because of their high surface-to-volume ratio. They have distinctive chemical and physical properties that may interfere with bacterial adaptation [1]. Due to their numerous uses in disciplines of research like the health sector, agriculture, textiles, food technology, electronics, and so on, nanoparticles have attracted the attention of scientists [2–6]. However, due to their high propensity, NPs can survive in the environment, and this persistent attribute may be a viable tactic for preventing the bacterial growth used in the manufacturing of various food products including meat products, dairy or vegetables products, sausage products, etc. [7].

Numerous nanomaterials, such as zinc oxide nanoparticles (ZnONPs), silver nanoparticles (AgNPs), gold nanoparticles (AuNPs) and titanium dioxide nanoparticles (TiO_2NPs), have potent capacity to both fight bacteria and prevent microbial adhesion, as well as contamination [6–11]. Among them, ZnONPs have received a lot of attention due to their safe and non-toxic nature and powerful antibacterial characteristics, which are related to the release of reactive oxygen species (ROS) on their surface [12–15]. ZnONPs outperform their bulkier counterparts in terms of antibacterial activity because of quantum confinement and size effects [16]. Due to the multiple ways ZnONPs prevent bacterial development, they can succeed easily to protect bacterial-contamination-associated diseases in humans, whereas conventional antibiotics face difficulties to prevent the development of bacterial resistance [12]. Due to its benign properties, ZnO has "generally recognized as safe" (GRAS) classification, and the antimicrobial efficacy of ZnONPs indicates that they are a potent antimicrobial agent for preventing foodborne pathogen contamination in the food sector [17].

These nanoparticles are often created via physical and chemical processes like photochemistry, chemical reduction and microwave irradiation [18–20]. The main problems of these techniques are that they are costly, involve labor-intensive equipment and produce harmful consequences due to the use of poisonous substances [21,22]. Nowadays, scholars are focusing on biological strategies for affordable and simple production of nanoparticles due to the different limitations of physicochemical methods. Biological synthesis is a facile, rapid, cost effective, non-toxic and ecofriendly productive method because it is not very expensive, and it can also substitute toxic chemicals and decrease capping and stabilizing agents. A variety of biological resources such as plants and their various parts and different microbes (bacteria, algae, fungi, etc.) could be used for the facile and green synthesis of bioactive nanoparticles [23–27].

A serious problem for global public health is antibiotics resistance. Antibiotics resistance is mostly a result of the abuse of antibiotics. The overuse of antibiotics to treat bacterial infections in humans and aquatic animals has resulted in the spread of numerous antibiotic-resistant strains into the environment [28–30]. Since numerous infectious diseases that might be fatal are brought on by pathogenic bacteria, multidrug-resistant microorganisms pose a severe threat to public health globally [31–33]. Due to mutation, shifting environmental circumstances and high drug use, the number of multidrug-resistant bacterial strains is continuously rising. To solve this issue, researchers are working to create novel medications for the treatment of these microbial illnesses [9,34]. Biosynthesized ZnONPs could be novel and effective agents to control these multidrug-resistant pathogenic microorganisms because of their safe and non-toxic nature and powerful antibacterial characteristics. Many recent studies have shown that different pathogenic microorganisms can be successfully controlled using biosynthesized ZnONPs [15,35–38]. This review emphasizes the facile and rapid biological synthesis of ZnONPs using both microbes and plants and their characterizations, potential antimicrobial applications and antimicrobial mechanisms against pathogenic microorganisms.

2. Biosynthesis of ZnONPs

Biosynthesis of ZnONPs is a simple, facile, cost-effective and eco-friendly method compared to the physical and chemical methods that produce various toxic by-products that could be dangerous for our environment [39]. Moreover, biosynthesized nanoparticles are more biocompatible and show significantly higher antimicrobial activity than chemically or physically synthesized nanoparticles [40,41]. For these reasons, scientists are focusing more on utilizing different biological resources for the green, safe and effective synthesis of ZnONPs [3,8,23,36]. For the biosynthesis of ZnONPs, different microorganisms such as bacteria, fungi, yeast or various parts of plants such as leaf, root, fruit, flower, peel, stem, etc. could be used. Figure 1 shows the various steps of facile, cost-effective and eco-friendly biosynthesis of bioactive ZnONPs using the extracts of plants and microbes and their potential antimicrobial efficacy against pathogenic microorganisms.

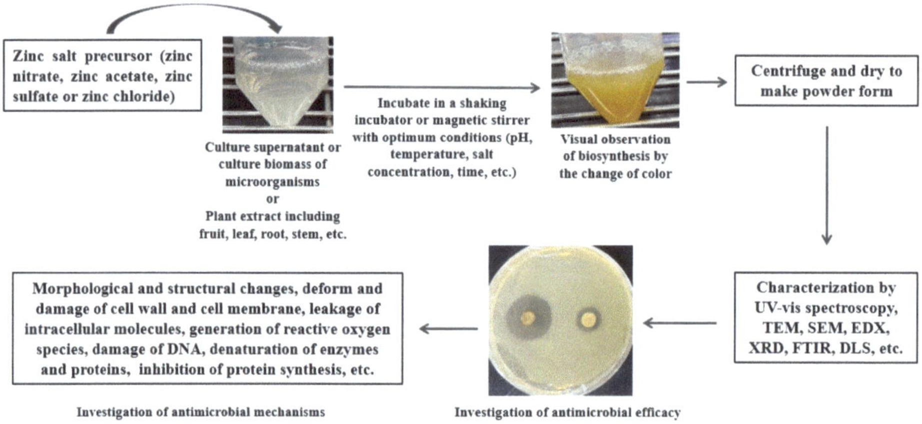

Figure 1. Schematic illustration of biosynthesis and potential antimicrobial applications of bioactive ZnONPs.

2.1. Microbe-Mediated Biosynthesis of ZnONPs

Microbe-mediated nanoparticles (NPs) have recently received a lot of attention because of the availability of microorganisms, their easy reproduction and their safe utilization for the biosynthesis of nanoparticles [27,39,42]. Chemical and physical methods can be used to produce NPs, but the microbial synthesis of ZnONPs is considerably more useful than other methods due to their environmental friendliness and low cost. Because of their prevalence in living microorganisms, ZnONPs have become quite popular among other nanoparticles. ZnONPs can be produced by microbial cells, proteins and a variety of enzymes in both prokaryotes and eukaryotes [43]. There are many recent studies on the cost-effective biosynthesis of ZnONPs using various microorganisms such as bacteria, fungi, yeast, algae, etc. (Table 1). Both intracellular and extracellular methods can be used for the facile and eco-friendly synthesis of ZnONPs using microbes [8,13,44]. The culture supernatant of microorganisms and the microbial biomass contain different bioactive compounds including enzymes, proteins, amino acids and many other biomolecules that serve as reducing, capping and stabilizing agents during the synthesis process [30,39]. Previous studies have reported that the bioreduction of Zn^{2+} was initiated by the electron transfer from NADH by an NADH dependent reductase enzyme that acts as an electron carrier. Consequently, the ZnONPs are formed. Subsequently, various biomolecules such as proteins, amino acids, flavonoids, etc. attached with ZnO and stabilized the ZnONPs [39]. It is also reported that the amino acids present in the proteins were found to interact with the Zn^{2+} ions to form ZnONPs [39].

Table 1. Microbe-mediated biosynthesis and potential antimicrobial applications of ZnONPs. NA, Not Available.

Microbes Used for Synthesis	Synthesis Method	Optimum Synthesis Conditions (Salt Concentration, Temperature, Incubation Time)	Size (nm, Nanoparticles/Crystallite)	Shape	Target Pathogens	Reference
Paraclostridium benzoelyticum	Extra cellular	0.1 M zinc nitrate, 80 °C for 24 h	50 (Average)	Spherical and rectangular	*Helicobacter suis*, *H. felis*, *H. bizzozeronii*, *H. salomonis*	[15]
Aspergillus sp.	Extra cellular	0.1 N zinc acetate, 40 °C for 6 h	80–100	Sphere shape	*Escherchia coli*, *Pseudomonas aeruginosa*, *Salmonella typhi*	[3]
Pseudomonas aeruginosa	Extra cellular	2 mM zinc acetate, 35 ± 2 °C for 24 h	14.9 ± 3.5	Spherical	*Staphylococcus aureus*, *Escherichia coli*, *Bacillus subtilis*, *Pseudomonas aeruginosa*, *Candida albicans*	[44]
Lactobacillus spp.	Intracellular	500 mM zinc salt, 37 °C for 24 h	32 (Average)	Spherical	*Clostridium difficile*, *E. coli*, *Clostridium perfringens*, *S. typhi*, *Aspergillus flavus*, *C. albicans*	[8]
Marinobacter sp. 2C8 and *Vibrio* sp. VLA	Extra cellular	0.1 M zinc sulfate, 30 °C for 24 h	10.2–20.3	Spherical	*E. coli*, *P. aeruginosa*, *Listeria innocua*, *S. aureus*, *Bacillus subtilis*	[35]
Bacillus cereus RNT6	Extra cellular	0.1 zinc sulfate, 80 °C for 15 min	21–35	Spherical	*Burkholderia glumae*, *B. gladioli*	[42]
Lactobacillus plantarum TA4	Extra and intracellular	500 mM zinc salt, 24 h at 37 °C	152.8–613.5	Flower pattern	*E. coli*, *Salmonella* sp., *S. aureus*, *S. epidermidis*	[13]
Endophytic fungus *Alternaria tenuissima*	Extra cellular	2 mM zinc sulphate, at room temperature for 20 min	10–30	Spherical	*P. aeruginosa*, *Klebsiella pneumoniae*, *E. coli*, *S. aureus*	[24]
Pseudomonas putida	Combine of intra and extracellular	100 mg zinc nitrate into 100 mL culture solution, 24 h at 37 °C	44.5 (Average)	Spherical	*Pseudomonas otitidis*, *Enterococcus faecalis*, *Acinetobacter baumannii*, *P. oleovorans*, *B. cereus*	[45]
Aeromonas hydrophila	Intracellular	Zinc salt, 37 °C, for 24 h	57.7 (Average)	Spherical	*P. aeruginosa*, *Aspergillus flavus*	[46]

Table 1. *Cont.*

Microbes Used for Synthesis	Synthesis Method	Optimum Synthesis Conditions (Salt Concentration, Temperature, Incubation Time)	Size (nm, Nanoparticles/Crystallite)	Shape	Target Pathogens	Reference
Bacillus megaterium	Intracellular	Zinc nitrate solution, 37 °C for 48 h	45–95	Rod and cubic	*Helicobacter pylori*	[47]
Halomonas elongate	Extracellular	Zinc chloride, 37 °C for one week	18.1 ± 8.9	Multiform	*E. coli, S. aureus*	[48]
Lactobacillus paracasei LB3	Intracellular	Zinc nitrate solution, 37 °C for 24 h	1179 ± 137	Spherical	*S. aureus, Acetinobacter baumannii*	[49]
Lactobacillus sporogens	Extracellular	0.1 M zinc sulfate, 37 °C for 24 h	145.7 (Average)	Hexagonal	*S. aureus*	[50]
Rhodococcus pyridinivorans NT2b	Extracellular	0.1 M zinc sulfate, 30 °C for 72 h	100–120	Roughly spherical	*S. epidermidis*	[51]
Sphingobacterium thalpophilum	Extracellular	Zinc nitrate solution, 37 °C for 24 h	40 (Average)	Triangle	*P. aeruginosa, Enterobacter aerogens*	[52]
Staphylococcus aureus	Extracellular	zinc acetate solution (1 mM), 37 °C.	10–50	Acicular	*S. aureus*	[53]
Streptomyces sp.	Extracellular	Zinc chloride solution, 28 °C for 7 days	20–50	Spherical	*E. coli, B. subtilis*	[54]
Pichia kudriavzevii	Extracellular	zinc acetate solution, 35 °C for 36 h	10–61	Hexagonal wurtzite	*B. subtilis, S. epidermidis, S. aurous, E. coli, Serratia marcescens*	[55]
Pichia fermentas JA2	Extracellular	1 mM zinc nitrate, 28 °C for 96 h	NA	Smooth and elongated	*P. aeruginosa*	[56]
Aspergillus fumigatus JCF	Extracellular	1.0 mM zinc sulfate, 32 °C for 96 h	60–80	Spherical	*K. pneumoniae, P. aeruginosa, E. coli, S. aureus, B. subtilis*	[57]
Aspergillus niger	Extracellular	5 mM Zinc nitrate, 32 °C for 48 h	61 ± 0.65	Spherical	*E. coli, S. aureus*	[58]
Aspergillus terreus	Extracellular	Zinc salt solution, 32 °C for 4 days	54.8–82.6	Spherical	*A. niger, A. fumigatus, A. aculeatus*	[59]

Yusof et al. [13] reported the *Lactobacillus plantarum* TA4 mediated the biosynthesis of ZnONPs using both intracellular and extracellular methods (Figure 2). They added the zinc nitrate solution to the cell-free supernatant (CFS) for the extracellular biosynthesis of ZnONPs; as well, the cell biomass (CB) was added to the zinc nitrate solution for the intracellular biosynthesis of the ZnONPs. The synthesis of NPs was confirmed by visual observation. The synthesized ZnONPs were collected by high-speed centrifugation and dried at 100 °C to obtain the powder form. Through the FTIR analysis, they found different biomolecules present both in the cell-free culture supernatant and in the cell biomass, as well as in the synthesized ZnONPs, and concluded that these biomolecules may be involved as reducing and capping agents during the biosynthesis process [13].

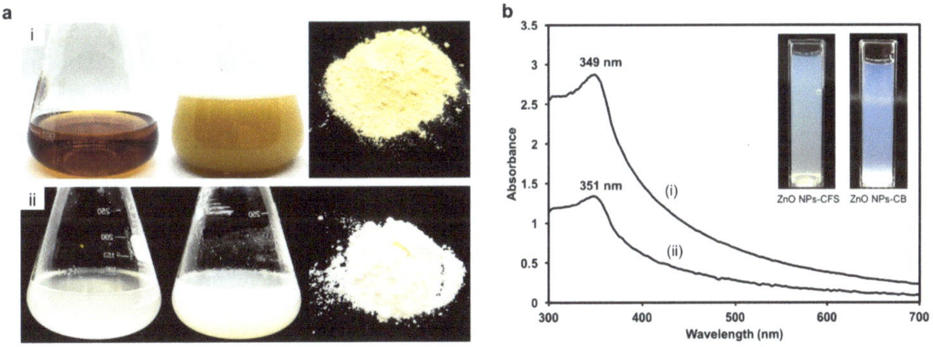

Figure 2. (**a**) Reduction of Zn^{2+} to ZnONPs by (i) cell-free supernatant and (ii) cell biomass of *L. plantarum* TA4. (**b**) UV-Vis spectrum of (i) ZnONPs-CFS and (ii) ZnONPs-CB. This figure has been reprinted with permission from Ref. [13], copyright 2020, Nature Portfolio.

Kumar et al., 2022 [3] reported the extracellular synthesis of bioactive ZnONPs using fungal isolate (*Aspergillus* sp.). The authors added the culture supernatant dropwise into the zinc acetate solution and confirmed the biosynthesis of ZnONPs by visual observation of color change [3]. Abdo et al. [44] successfully synthesized ZnONPs using cell-free filtrate of *P. aeruginosa*. They concluded that various metabolites present in the cell-free culture supernatant of *P. aeruginosa* are responsible for the formation and stabilization of the synthesized ZnONPs [44]. Suba et al. [8] demonstrated the intracellular biosynthesis of ZnONPs using the cell biomass of *Lactobacillus* spp. within 24 h of reaction and found spherical-shaped ZnONPs with a 32 nm average size. Abdelhakim et al. [24] used endophytic fungi *Alternaria tenuissima* for the extracellular production of spherical-shaped ZnONPs that possess significant antimicrobial activity against different pathogenic microbes. Table 1 summarizes the microbe-mediated biosynthesis of ZnONPs and their potential antimicrobial applications.

2.2. Plant-Mediated Biosynthesis of ZnONPs

Plant-extract-mediated biosynthesis of ZnONPs has been revealed as a viable option due to its convenience, stability and ease of synthesis compared to all other organisms. Mostly during the synthesis of ZnONPs, extracted phytochemicals function as reducing and capping agents. In the synthesis of ZnONPs as a natural green medium for metallic ion reduction, active bioorganic chemicals in plant extract were crucial [60]. Plant-based NP production has various advantages including minimal cost, ease of use, fast production time, reliability and the ability to scale up production volumes [61]. Furthermore, the availability of bioorganics with many active chemicals in plant components increases demand for ZnONPs, resulting in low-cost, secure and simple syntheses [60]. Various parts of plants such as the roots, shoots, fruits, seeds, leaves, etc. were utilized for the rapid, facile and eco-friendly synthesis of ZnONPs. There are many recent reports on the biosynthesis of ZnONPs and their potential antimicrobial applications using different parts of plants (Table 2). Abomuti et al. [62] reported the plant-mediated biosynthesis of bioactive ZnONPs using the leaf extract of *Salvia officinalis*. They added aqueous leaf extract to the zinc nitrate solution under constant stirring at a 50 °C temperature. In the second step, they added NaOH solution dropwise under continuous stirring at 50 °C to maintain the stable pH of the reaction mixture. Finally, the biosynthesized ZnONPs were collected by centrifugation and dried to obtain the powder form. Through the FTIR analysis, they found different biomolecules including phenolic and flavonoid compounds present in both the aqueous leaf extract of *Salvia officinalis* and the synthesized ZnONPs and concluded that these biomolecules may be involved as reducing and capping agents during the biosynthesis process [62]. Fouda et al. [63] reported that the peel extract of *Punica granatum* mediated the synthesis of bioactive ZnONPs. The author added the aqueous peel extract of *Punica granatum* into the zinc acetate solution and confirmed the biosynthesis of ZnONPs by visual observation of color change [63]. Fruit extract of *Myrica esculenta* was used by Lal et al. [23] for the rapid and eco-friendly synthesis of ZnONPs. Urge et al., 2023 [2] successfully synthesized ZnONPs using the bulb extract of *Allium sativum* and the root extract of *Zingiber officinale*. They identified various functional groups associated with the formation of ZnONPs [2]. Alotaibi et al. (2022) [64] demonstrated the biosynthesis of ZnONPs using the leaf extract of *Gardenia thailandica* within 1 h of reaction and found spherical-shaped ZnONPs with a 37.4 nm average size. The leaf extract of *Carica papaya* was used for rapid and green synthesis of bioactive ZnONPs [65]. Menazea et al. (2021) [66] used the peel extract of orange for the rapid and facile synthesis of cubic-shaped ZnONPs. Suručić et al. (2020) [67] synthesized ZnONPs using flower extract of *Geranium robertianum*. Plant extract contains various biomolecules such as enzymes, proteins, amino acids, flavonoids, terpenoids and phenolic compounds that play significant roles during the biosynthesis of ZnONPs as reducing and capping agents. Table 2 summarizes the plant-mediated biosynthesis of ZnONPs and their potential antimicrobial applications.

Table 2. Plant-mediated biosynthesis and potential antimicrobial applications of ZnONPs.

Plant	Used Part	Optimum Synthesis Conditions (Salt Concentration, Temperature, Incubation Time)	Size (nm, Nanoparticles/Crystallite)	Shape	Target Pathogens	Reference
Punica granatum	Peel extract	5 mM Zinc acetate, room temperature for overnight	10–45	Spherical	*Staphylococcus aureus*, *Bacillus subtilis*, *Pseudomonas aeruginosa*, *Escherichia coli*, *Candida albicans*	[63]
Cassia siamea	Leaf extract	1.0 mM zinc nitrate, heated for 3 to 4 h	13 (Average)	Spherical, oval, spheroidal	*Pseudomonas aeruginosa*, *Chromobacterium violaceum*	[14]
Cinnamon and bay	Leaves	Zinc salt, room temperature for 24 h	~10, 18.5 and ~30 (Average)	Spherical	*Staphylococcus aureus*, *Staphylococcus epidermidis*, *Escherichia coli*, *Klebsiella pneumoniae*	[9]
Allium sativum, *Zingiber officinale*	Bulb extract, root extract	Zinc acetate solution, 50 °C for 2 h	19.8, 21.9 and 23.9 (Average)	Wurtzite	*Escherichia coli*, *Pseudomonas putida*, *Staphylococcus aureus*, *Streptococcus pyogenes*	[2]
Pisonia Alba	Leaf extract	0.1 M zinc acetate, 70 °C for 2 h	Aggregated	NA	*Staphylococcus aureus*, *Klebsiella pneumoniae*	[36]
Sargassum muticum	Plant extract	5 mM zinc nitrate, 70 °C for 20 min and room temperature for 2 h	15–50	Wurtzite hexagonal	*Bacillus flexus*, *Bacillus filamentosus*, *Acinetobacter baumannii*, *Pseudomonas stutzeri*	[68]
Punica granatum peel and coffee ground	Plant extract	10 mM zinc acetate, 1 h at 70 °C	118.6, 115.7 and 111.2 (Average)	Nanorod	*Pseudomonas aeruginosa*, *Staphylococcus aureus*, *Klebsiella pneumoniae*, *Enterobacter aerogenes*	[69]

Table 2. *Cont.*

Plant	Used Part	Optimum Synthesis Conditions (Salt Concentration, Temperature, Incubation Time)	Size (nm, Nanoparticles/Crystallite)	Shape	Target Pathogens	Reference
Myrica esculenta	Fruits extract	0.5 M zinc acetate, 40 °C for 2 h	31.7 (Average)	NA	*Fusarium oxysporum, Staphylococcus aureus, Pseudomonas aeruginosa, Rosellinia necatrix, Escherichia coli*	[23]
Gardenia thailandica triveng	Leaves	Zinc acetate solution, 70 °C for 30 min, room temperature for 1 h	37.4 (Average)	Spherical	*Pseudomonas aeruginosa* clinical isolates	[64]
Cocos nucifera	Extract	1 M zinc nitrate, 4 h at ambient temperature	28–59	Rock shaped	*S. aureus, E. coli, B. subtilis, K. pneumoniae*	[70]
Clitoria ternatea	Flower extract	0.1 M zinc nitrate, 4 h at 80 °C	40–81	Rod	*S. aureus, E. coli*	[71]
Carica papaya	Leaf extract	0.1 M Zinc acetate, 4 h at 80 °C	15–50	Semi-spherical	*Rosellinia necatrix, Sclerotinia sclerotiorum, Fusarium* spp.	[65]
Tagetes erecta	Flower extract	1.5 mM zinc nitrate, 24 h at 60 °C	30–50	Spherical	*E. coli, S. aureus*	[72]
Spinacea oleracea	Extract	Aqueous zinc acetate solution, 24 h at 60 °C	13.0 (Average)	granular	*Pseudomonas aeruginosa*	[73]
Salvia officinalis	Leaf extract	0.1 M zinc nitrate, 4 h at 50 °C	26.1 (Average)	Wurtzite hexagonal	*Candida albicans* isolates	[62]
Orange	Peel extract	1 M zinc nitrate, 2 h at room temperature	20–60	cubic	*Pseudomonas aeruginosa, B. subtilis*	[66]
Phoenix dactylifera	Waste	5 g zinc nitrate in 50 mL of extract, 30 min at room temperature	30 (Average)	Spherical	*Streptococcus pyogenes, Pseudomonas aeruginosa, Staphylococcus aureus*	[38]
Brassica rapa	Leaf extract	Zinc nitrate solution, 4 h at 80 °C	27.5 (Average)	Irregular	*Micrococcus luteus, Enterobacter aerogenes*	[74]
Red Paprika	Aqueous plant extract	2 M Zinc acetate, 6 h at room temperature	70–80	Rod	*S. enterica.*	[75]
Aloe barbadense	Leaf extract	10 mM zinc nitrate, 60 °C	44 (Average)	Quasi-hexagonal	*Bacillus subtilis, Bacillus licheniformis, Klebsiella pneumonia, Escherichia coli, Candida albicans, Aspergillus niger*	[76]
Geranium robertianum	Flower extract	10 mM zinc acetate, 2 h at room temperature	40 (Average)	Irregular	*Escherichia coli, Pseudomonas aeruginosa, Acinetobacter baumannii, Staphylococcus aureus isolates*	[67]
Ocimum americanum	Plant extract	1 mM zinc nitrate, 1 h at 60 °C	21 (Average)	Spherical	*B. cereus, Staphylococcus aureus, Klebsiella pneumonia, Vibrio parahaemolyticus, Pseudomonas aeruginosa, Escherichia coli, Salmonella typhi, Candida albicans, Xanthomonas citri, Aspergillus parasiticus*	[77]
Azadirachta indica	Leaves	Zinc nitrate solution, boiled at 350 ± 10 °C for 4 min	9–38	Hexagonal	*Klebsiella aerogenes* and *Staphylococcus aureus*	[78]
Cannabis sativa	Leaf	Zinc acetate solution, 80 °C for 12 h	34–38	Spherical	*Escherichia coli, Klebsiella pneumonia, MRSA, Pseudomonas aeruginosa, Salmonella typhi, Staphylococcus aureus*	[79]
Carica papaya	Latex	Zinc nitrate solution, 37 °C for 36 h	11–26	Hexagonal	*Pseudomonas aeruginosa* and *Staphylococcus aureus* compared to *Klebsiella aerogenes* and *Pseudomonas desmolyticum*	[80]

Table 2. *Cont.*

Plant	Used Part	Optimum Synthesis Conditions (Salt Concentration, Temperature, Incubation Time)	Size (nm, Nanoparticles/Crystallite)	Shape	Target Pathogens	Reference
Dolichos lablab L.	Leaf	Zinc acetate solution, incubated 70 °C for 1 h	29 (Average)	Hexagonal	*Bacillus pumilus* and *Sphingomonas paucimobilis*	[81]
Tabernaemontana divaricata	Green leaf	Zinc nitrate solution, 80 °C until precipitation.	20–50	Spherical	*Salmonella paratyphi*, *Escherichia coli* and *Staphylococcus aureus*	[41]
Moringa oleifera (drumstick)	Leaves	Zinc acetate solution, 24 °C for 1 h	52 (Average)	Hexagonal wurtzite	*Bacillus subtilis* and *Escherichia coli*	[82]
Mussaenda frondosa	Leaf/stem	Zinc nitrate solution, 400 °C for 10–30 min	5–20	Spherical	*Staphylococcus aureus* and *Bacillus subtilis*	[83]
Phyllanthus emblica	Plant extract	Zinc chloride solution, 90 °C for 2 h	Aggregated	square-shaped	*S. pyogenes*, *S. aureus*, *S. typhi* and *E. coli*	[84]
Plectranthus amboinicus	Plant extract	Zinc sulfate solution, room temperature for 2 h	Aggregated	Irregular aggregated nanoflakes	*S. aureus* and *E. coli*	[85]

3. Critical Parameters for Rapid and Stable Biosynthesis of ZnONPs

Different parameters significantly affect the rapid and stable synthesis of ZnONPs. Several critical parameters have been identified for the rapid and stable synthesis of ZnONPs, including the concentration of the plant extract and metal salt, incubation time, temperature, pH and stirring rate. The optimal conditions for each parameter may vary depending on the specific plant extract or microbial species and metal salt used. However, some general trends have been observed, such as higher concentrations of plant extracts and metal salts leading to larger yields of nanoparticles, longer incubation times leading to larger particle sizes and higher temperatures leading to faster reaction rates [86–88]. The pH of the reaction also significantly affects the rate of ZnONP formation [62,89].

3.1. Factors Influencing the Mass Production of ZnONPs

The mass production of ZnONPs can be affected by several parameters, including the concentration of plant extracts and metal salts, incubation time, temperature, and pH. Higher concentrations of plant extracts and metal salts generally lead to larger yields of nanoparticles, although there may be an optimal concentration beyond which further increases have little effect. Longer incubation times generally lead to larger particle sizes, which can affect the stability and biocompatibility of the nanoparticles. Higher temperatures can lead to faster reaction rates and larger yields of nanoparticles but may also promote agglomeration and reduce the stability of the particles. The pH can also affect the rate of particle formation, with more acidic or alkaline conditions generally leading to faster reaction rates [62,89,90].

3.2. Factors Influencing the Shape and Size of Synthesized ZnONPs

The shape and size of synthesized ZnONP nanoparticles can be influenced by several factors, including the concentration of plant extracts and metal salts, pH, temperature and stirring rate. Higher concentrations of plant extracts and metal salts generally lead to larger particles, while more acidic or alkaline conditions may promote the formation of rod-shaped particles. pH is an important factor for the biosynthesis of ZnONPs and could alter the shape and size of the synthesized nanoparticles [39,91]. Higher temperatures and faster stirring rates can also promote the formation of smaller particles with more uniform shapes. However, other factors, such as the type of plant extract or microbial species and metal salt used, can also play a role in determining the final size and shape of the nanoparticles [47,92,93].

4. Characterization of Biosynthesized ZnONPs

The use of various analytical techniques such as UV-visible spectrophotometry, XRD, SEM, TEM, FTIR, DLS and zeta potential analyzer analysis in the characterization of biosynthesized ZnONPs has been extensively reported in the literature. These techniques provide valuable information on the physical and chemical properties of nanoparticles, including their size, shape, surface charge, crystallinity and surface functional groups. For instance, UV-visible spectrophotometry is commonly used to determine the optical properties of ZnONPs, including their absorption spectra and bandgap energy. In ZnO, like in any other semiconductor, there is a valence band (VB) and a conduction band (CB) separated by a bandgap of a few eV. The ZnO absorption peaks at the transitions between VB and CB. Under irradiation, when enough energy is provided, an electron can be promoted from VB to CB, which will be recorded by a spectrophotometer as an absorption band/peak. The energy value of this peak is related to the value of the bandgap. Recombination of the excited electron from CB with the hole from VB will produce the fluorescent emission at about 380 nm, which is called exciton recombination. The slight variation of the absorption peak appears due to the different intermediary electronic levels generated by impurities or lattice defects [44]. XRD analysis provides information on the crystalline structure and phase purity of nanoparticles. The crystal size of the biosynthesized ZnONPs is generally calculated on the basis of XRD analysis [44]. SEM and TEM techniques are used to visualize the morphology, size and shape of nanoparticles. In both TEM and DLS, the size of nanoparticles and particle size distribution can be determined. While in TEM, the shape and crystallinity can also be determined, in DLS, the obtained size is usually larger due the presence of a solvent layer on the nanoparticle surface. DLS and a zeta potential analyzer provide information on the particle size distribution and surface charge, respectively.

FTIR analysis provides information on the functional groups present on the nanoparticle surface. The quantity of organics from plant or microbial extracts that are adsorbed on the ZnONP surface can be evaluated by thermal analysis. The chemical composition of produced ZnONP samples was also evaluated by using X-ray photoelectron spectroscopy (XPS) [36]. Several studies have reported the use of these techniques to characterize green-synthesized ZnONPs for various applications. For example, Faisal et al. [15] used UV-visible spectrophotometry, XRD, SEM, EDX and FTIR to characterize the *Paraclostridium benzoelyticum*-bacterium-mediated biosynthesized ZnONPs and investigate their antibacterial, antidiabetic, anti-inflammatory and antiarthritic activities. In another study, Supraja et al. [94] used FTIR, DLS and zeta potential analyzer analysis to characterize *Alstonia scholaris* stem-bark-extract-mediated ZnONPs and evaluate their antimicrobial efficacy. Abomuti et al. [62] used UV-visible spectrophotometry, Raman spectroscopy, SEM, TEM, XRD and FTIR to characterize the biosynthesized ZnONPs using leaf extract of *Salvia officinalis* and investigate their antimicrobial activity against *Candida albicans* isolates. TEM analysis revealed the wurtzite hexagonal shape of synthesized ZnONPs (Figure 3a), and the average size was 26.14 nm (Figure 3b). An SEM image revealed the aggregated form of synthesized ZnONPs and explored some rough, clumsy materials surrounding the ZnONPs (Figure 3c). EDX analysis confirmed the majority of ZnONPs present in the samples. Additional carbon peaks in the EDX spectrum suggested the presence of biomolecules such as vitamins, amino acids, polyphenols, flavonoids and saponins (Figure 3d).

The FTIR spectrum also showed various biomolecules such as polyphenols and other biomolecules present in both aqueous leaf extract of *S. officinalis* and the synthesized ZnONPs, which suggested that these biomolecules are responsible for the synthesis and stabilization of ZnONPs and their biological activities (Figure 4a–c) [62].

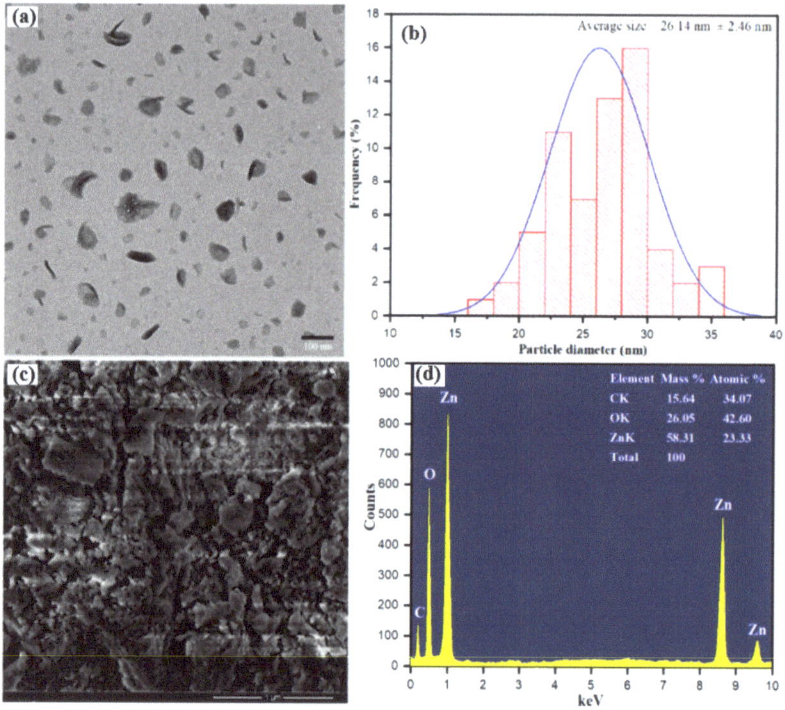

Figure 3. (**a**) Transmission electron microscope (TEM) scale bar: 100 nm; (**b**) particle size distribution histogram; (**c**) scanning electron microscopy (SEM) scale bar: 1 µm; (**d**) the EDX spectra of biosynthesized ZnONPs using leaf extract of *Salvia officinalis*. This figure has been reprinted with permission from Ref. [62], copyright 2021, MDPI.

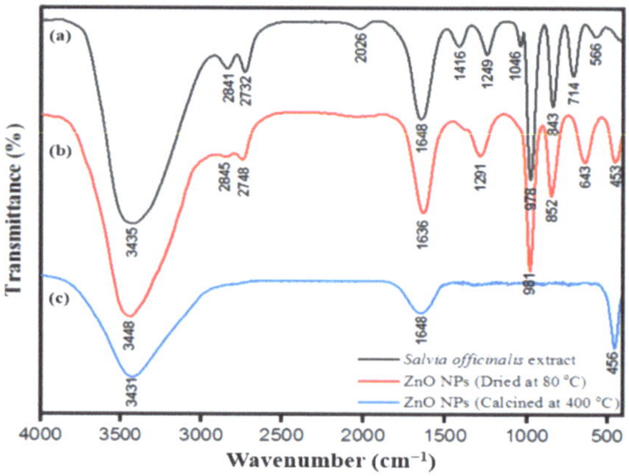

Figure 4. FTIR spectra of (**a**) aqueous leaf extract of *S. officinalis*, (**b**) ZnONPs dried at 80 °C, and (**c**) ZnONPs calcinated at 400 °C. This figure has been reprinted with permission from Ref. [62], copyright 2021, MDPI.

Other studies have reported the use of these techniques to investigate the antimicrobial and antioxidant properties of green-synthesized ZnONPs for various applications. Sonia et al. [95] used UV-visible spectrophotometry, XRD, SEM and DLS to characterize biosynthesized ZnONPs and evaluate their antimicrobial and antioxidant potential for use in a cold-cream formulation. Barsainya and Singh [96] used XRD, SEM and TEM to characterize *Pseudomonas aeruginosa*-mediated ZnONPs and investigate their broad-spectrum antimicrobial effects. Overall, the use of various analytical techniques in the characterization of biosynthesized ZnONPs has provided valuable insights into their physical and chemical properties, enabling researchers to optimize their synthesis and tailor their properties for specific applications. Table 3 summarizes the different characterization techniques used for biosynthesized ZnONPs.

Table 3. Different characterization techniques used for biosynthesized ZnONPs.

Characterization Technique	Principle	Advantage	Reference
UV-visible spectrophotometry	Measures absorbance of light	Rapid and nondestructive	[97]
X-ray diffraction (XRD)	Measures crystal structure and size	Provides detailed crystallographic information	[62]
Scanning electron microscope (SEM)	Provides surface morphology and size	High resolution imaging	[98]
Transmission electron microscope (TEM)	Provides detailed information on size, shape and structure	High resolution imaging and analysis of individual particles	[62]
Fourier transform infrared spectroscopy (FTIR)	Measures functional groups on the nanoparticle surface	Provides information on surface chemistry	[97]
Dynamic light scattering (DLS)	Measures particle size distribution	Rapid and nondestructive	[97]
Zeta potential analyzer	Measures the surface charge of particles in solution	Provides information on particle stability	[97]

5. Antimicrobial Applications and Mechanisms of Biosynthesized ZnONPs

In recent years, there has been a growing interest in the development and utilization of nanomaterials for various applications, particularly in the field of antimicrobial research. Among these nanomaterials, ZnONPs have emerged as a promising candidate due to their unique physicochemical properties and potent antimicrobial activity. ZnONPs have been extensively studied for their ability to inhibit the growth of a wide range of microorganisms, including bacteria, fungi and viruses [24,42,62,99–104]. ZnONPs have potential applications in various fields, including food, agriculture, pharmaceuticals and biotechnology [43]. In the food and agriculture industries, ZnONPs have been shown to have potential applications as a food preservative and to enhance the antifungal activity of endophytic *Bacillus* sp. Fcl1. The extracts prepared from the *Bacillus* sp. Fcl1 cultured in the presence of ZnONPs had an increased production of lipopeptide surfactin derivatives and iturin, which are known for their antimicrobial properties [105]. In the medical field, ZnONPs have shown promise as antimicrobial agents for the treatment of various infections, including skin and wound infections, respiratory tract infections, and urinary tract infections. They have demonstrated broad-spectrum activity against both Gram-positive and Gram-negative bacteria, including multidrug-resistant strains. Furthermore, ZnONPs have been explored for their antifungal activity against pathogenic fungi, such as the *Candida* species, and have shown potential as antiviral agents against a range of viruses, including herpes simplex virus and influenza virus [106,107]. In the pharmaceutical industry, ZnONPs have been investigated for their potential use as a new antimicrobial agent to combat antibiotic-resistant bacteria. ZnONPs exhibited antimicrobial activity against methicillin-resistant *Staphylococcus aureus* (MRSA) and vancomycin-resistant *Enterococcus faecalis* (VRE) [108].

ZnONPs have also been investigated for their potential use in wound healing. The incorporation of ZnONPs into chitosan hydrogels improved their antimicrobial activity against *Staphylococcus aureus* and *Pseudomonas aeruginosa*. The use of ZnONPs in wound dressings could be a promising approach to preventing infections and promoting wound healing. In agriculture, ZnONPs have been utilized as antimicrobial agents for crop protection and disease management. They have been shown to effectively inhibit the growth of plant pathogens, including bacteria and fungi, offering an eco-friendly alternative to conventional pesticides. Additionally, the use of ZnONPs in food packaging materials has gained attention due to their antimicrobial properties, which can help extend the shelf life of perishable food products by inhibiting the growth of spoilage microorganisms. Moreover, ZnONPs have been investigated for their potential in environmental remediation, particularly in water treatment, where they can effectively eliminate waterborne pathogens and provide a sustainable approach for disinfection [40,109–112]. Studies have shown that the antimicrobial activity of ZnO nanoparticles is size-dependent, with smaller particles exhibiting higher antimicrobial activity due to their increased surface area and higher reactivity [113]. In addition, the shape of ZnONPs also plays a crucial role in their antimicrobial activity, with rod-shaped particles exhibiting higher activity than spherical particles [114].

The green synthesis approach utilizes plant extracts, microbes and waste biomaterials as reducing and stabilizing agents, thus reducing the use of hazardous chemicals and energy consumption during the synthesis process. Studies have shown that green synthesis methods produce ZnONPs with superior antimicrobial activity compared to those synthesized using chemical methods. For example, ZnONPs synthesized using aqueous extracts of *Heritiera fomes* and *Sonneratia apetala* mangrove plant species showed significant antimicrobial activity against *E. coli*, *S. aureus* and *B. subtilis* [92]. Similarly, *Alstonia scholaris* stem-bark-extract-mediated ZnONPs demonstrated significant antimicrobial activity against *P. aeruginosa*, *S. aureus* and *B. subtilis* [94]. There are many recent reports on the biosynthesis of ZnONPs using plants and microbes and their potential utilization to control drug-resistant pathogenic microorganisms (Tables 1 and 2). Abomuti et al. [62] reported the biosynthesis of ZnONPs using leaf extract of *Salvia officinalis* and evaluated their antimicrobial activity against pathogenic *Candida albicans* isolates. They found that the biosynthesized ZnONPs strongly suppressed the growth of *C. albicans* isolates and showed a strong zone of inhibition (Figure 5). Faisal et al. [15] reported on the *Paraclostridium benzoelyticum*-bacterium-mediated extracellular synthesis of ZnONPs and evaluated their antimicrobial activity against *Helicobacter suis*, *H. felis*, *H. bizzozeronii* and *H. salomonis*. The biosynthesized ZnONPs strongly inhibited the growth of the tested pathogenic bacteria.

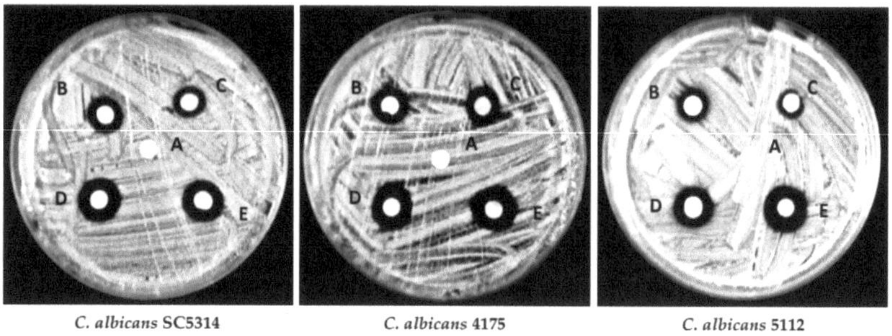

Figure 5. Zones of inhibition around discs impregnated with 1% DMSO (A), 2 μg/mL amphotericin B (B), $\frac{1}{2}$ MIC of ZnONPs (C), MIC of ZnONPs (D), and MFC of ZnONPs (E) against different *Candida albicans* isolates. This figure has been reprinted with permission from Ref. [62], copyright 2021, MDPI.

ZnONPs have gained significant attention as promising antimicrobial agents due to their unique physicochemical properties and broad-spectrum activity against various microorganisms. The antimicrobial mechanisms of ZnONPs involve a combination of physical, chemical and biological processes that collectively contribute to their efficacy in inhibiting the growth and survival of microorganisms [107,111,115]. One of the primary mechanisms by which ZnONPs exert their antimicrobial activity is through the generation of reactive oxygen species (ROS). ZnONPs can undergo redox reactions and produce

ROS, such as superoxide radicals (O^{2-}), hydrogen peroxide (H_2O_2) and hydroxyl radicals (OH·). These ROS are highly reactive and can cause oxidative stress in microbial cells by damaging cellular components, including lipids, proteins and nucleic acids. The accumulation of ROS disrupts normal cellular functions, leading to cell membrane damage, protein denaturation and DNA/RNA degradation, ultimately resulting in microbial cell death [111,116,117]. Moreover, ZnONPs possess a high surface-area-to-volume ratio, which enhances their contact with microbial cells and facilitates physical interactions. The small size of ZnONPs allows them to penetrate microbial cell membranes and enter the cytoplasm. Once inside the cell, ZnONPs can interact with intracellular components, such as enzymes and proteins, disrupting their structure and function. This disruption further contributes to the inhibition of microbial growth and proliferation [111,115,118]. Another important antimicrobial mechanism of ZnONPs is their ability to disrupt the integrity and permeability of microbial cell membranes. ZnONPs can interact with the lipid bilayer of the cell membrane, leading to membrane destabilization and increased membrane permeability. This disruption of the cell membrane integrity compromises the structural integrity of microorganisms and leads to leakage of cellular contents, loss of vital ions and ultimately cell death [111,115,119]. Furthermore, ZnONPs have been found to interfere with microbial enzyme activity. Certain enzymes, such as ATPases and respiratory chain enzymes, are crucial for microbial metabolism and energy production. ZnONPs can inhibit the activity of these enzymes, disrupting the energy balance and metabolic processes of microorganisms. This interference with enzyme activity further contributes to the antimicrobial effects of ZnONPs [111,120]. Table 4 summarizes the modes of action of biosynthesized ZnONPs against different pathogenic microbes.

Abomuti et al. [62] applied plant-mediated biosynthesized ZnONPs to treat the pathogenic *C. albicans* isolates and found that the biosynthesized ZnONPs damaged the cell wall and cell membrane of *C. albicans* and inhibited the production of ergosterol, which lead to the death of the cell (Figure 6).

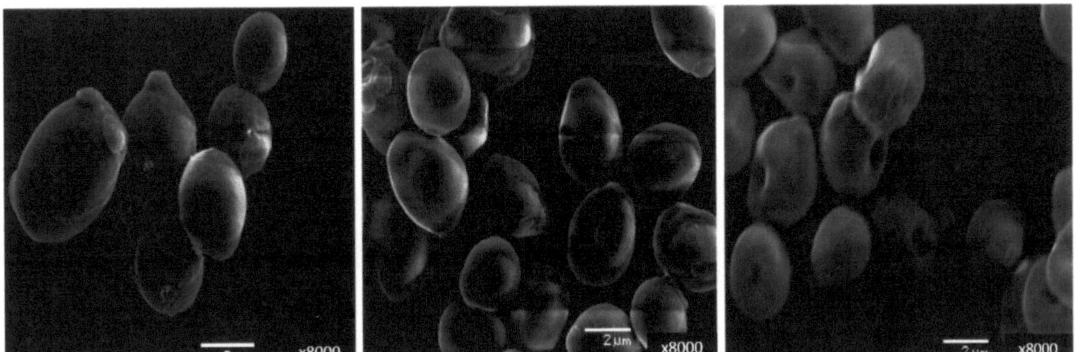

(A) (B) (C)

Figure 6. Scanning electron micrographs (SEM) of *C. albicans* SC5314: (**A**) represents untreated control cells, whereas (**B**,**C**) represent the cells exposed to MIC and MFC of biosynthesized ZnONPs, respectively. This figure has been reprinted with permission from Ref. [62], copyright 2021, MDPI.

According to Ahmed et al. [42], bacterial-mediated biosynthesized ZnONPs effectively control the growth of pathogenic microorganisms *B. glumae* and *B. gladioli*. They reported that synthesized ZnONPs damaged the cell membrane, proteins, ribosome and cytoplasmic materials of *B. glumae* and *B. gladioli*, produced reactive oxygen species and were involved in the leakage of genetic materials, resulting in cell death (Figure 7).

Table 4. Modes of action of green synthesized ZnONPs against pathogenic microbes.

Treated Pathogenic Microbes	Mode of Action	References
H. suis, H. felis, H. bizzozeronii, H. salomonis	Lead to the damage of cell wall, cell membrane and DNA, mitochondrial dysfunction, apoptosis, generation of reactive oxygen species and, finally, cell death.	[15]
S. aureus, E. coli, B. subtilis, P. aeruginosa, C. albicans.	Inhibit different metabolic functions including cell metabolisms, transportation, enzyme activity, etc.; generate reactive oxygen species and lead to the death of cell.	[44]
S. aureus, E. coli, E. faecalis, S. enteritidis, K. pneumoniae, P. aeruginosa, A. baumannii, S. typhimurium, C. albicans	Damage of cell membrane and DNA, leakage of intracellular molecules, denaturation of enzymes and proteins, inhibition of protein synthesis, generation of reactive oxygen species.	[121]
Burkholderia glumae, B. gladioli	Damage cell membrane, proteins, ribosome, and cytoplasmic materials; produce reactive oxygen species and cause leakage of genetic materials, resulting cell death.	[42]
E. coli, Salmonella sp., *S. aureus, S. epidermidis*	Damage the cell membrane, cause leakage of intracellular materials and generate reactive oxygen species, which lead to the death of the cell.	[13]
S. aureus, K. pneumoniae	Generation of reactive oxygen species, DNA damage, protein denaturation and mitochondrial dysfunction.	[36]
P. aeruginosa, C. violaceum	Attach to cell membrane, break membrane permeability, release Zn ions, generate reactive oxygen species.	[14]
E. coli, P. putida, S. aureus, S. pyogenes	Interact with cell membrane, produce reactive oxygen species, damage cell wall, DNA, protein and iron.	[2]
B. flexus, B. filamentosus, A. baumannii, P. stutzeri	Damage of cell wall, inhibition of cellular metabolism and respiration, destruction of DNA and inactivation of protein.	[68]
C. albicans	Disrupt and deform the cell wall and cell membrane and inhibit the production of ergosterol, which lead to cell death.	[62]
S. pyogenes, P. aeruginosa, S. aureus	Production of significant oxygen reactive species including hydroxyl radicals, superoxides and hydrogen peroxide.	[38]
F. oxysporum, S. aureus, P. aeruginosa, R. necatrix, E. coli	Damage cell membrane, generate reactive oxygen species, damage DNA, denature protein, cause ribosomal destabilization and mitochondrial dysfunction, which lead to the death of cell.	[23]

It is important to note that the antimicrobial mechanisms of ZnONPs can vary depending on the type of microorganism and the specific conditions. While ZnONPs exhibit broad-spectrum antimicrobial activity, some microorganisms may exhibit varying degrees of susceptibility due to differences in cell wall composition, membrane structure or defense mechanisms. In conclusion, ZnONPs possess multiple antimicrobial mechanisms that collectively contribute to their effectiveness in inhibiting the growth and survival of microorganisms. These mechanisms include the generation of reactive oxygen species, physical interactions, disruption of cell walls and cell membranes, damage of DNA, interference with microbial enzyme activity, protein denaturation, ribosomal destabilization and mitochondrial dysfunction. Understanding the antimicrobial mechanisms of ZnONPs is crucial for the development of novel antimicrobial strategies and the optimization of their application in various fields, including medicine, food industry, agriculture and environmental remediation.

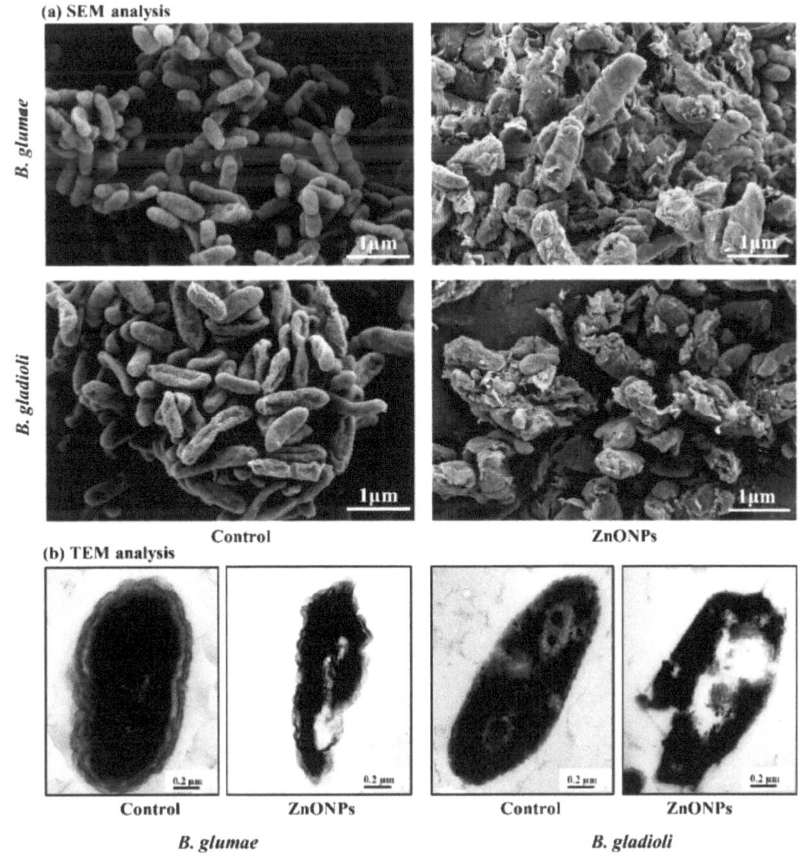

Figure 7. SEM (**a**) and TEM (**b**) images of rice bacterial pathogen *B. glumae* and *B. gladioli* cells after 8 h treatment with (50 μg mL^{-1}) and without (control) biogenic ZnONPs. This figure has been reprinted with permission from Ref. [42], copyright 2021, MDPI.

6. Conclusions and Future Prospects

The use of green synthesis methods for the production of ZnONPs has emerged as a promising approach to achieve enhanced antimicrobial activity with reduced environmental impact. Biosynthesis of ZnONPs using microbes and plants is a facile, non-toxic, cost-effective and eco-friendly method. In this review, the biosynthesis of ZnONPs using microbes and plants has been comprehensively reviewed. The antimicrobial applications and mechanisms of the biosynthesized ZnONPs against various pathogenic microorganisms have also been highlighted. Plant extracts, microbial biomass or culture supernatant contain various biomolecules including enzymes, amino acids, proteins, vitamins, alkaloids, flavonoids, etc., which serve as reducing, capping and stabilizing agents during the safe, facile and rapid biosynthesis of ZnONPs. The antimicrobial activity of ZnONPs is attributed to several mechanisms, including physical damage to microbial cell walls and cell membranes, production of reactive oxygen species and inhibition of microbial enzyme activity. As ZnONPs are edible and safe for utilization, ZnONPs could be potentially utilized in different food industries to control foodborne pathogens, as well as in many other sectors such as health care and agriculture to effectively control different pathogenic microorganisms. ZnONPs also exhibit antioxidant and wound-healing properties, making them suitable for use in cosmetics and dermatological formulations.

In conclusion, the antimicrobial applications of ZnONPs hold great promise for the development of new antimicrobial agents to combat the growing threat of antimicrobial resistance. ZnONPs have potential applications in various fields, including food, agriculture, pharmaceuticals and biotechnology. It is worth mentioning that the safety and potential toxicity of ZnONPs are important considerations for their practical applications. While ZnONPs have demonstrated significant antimicrobial activity, their potential adverse effects on human health and the environment should be thoroughly evaluated. Proper characterization of ZnONPs, including size, shape and surface modifications, is crucial for understanding their interactions with biological systems and optimizing their antimicrobial efficacy while minimizing potential toxic effects.

Author Contributions: Conceptualization, M.A.H.; writing—original draft preparation, M.A.H., M.A.I.A., M.A. and M.S.R.; writing—review and editing, M.A.H., M.M.R., M.A.K.P., S.R.B. and S.A. All authors have read and agreed to the published version of the manuscript.

Funding: This research received no external funding.

Institutional Review Board Statement: Not applicable.

Informed Consent Statement: Not applicable.

Data Availability Statement: Not applicable.

Conflicts of Interest: The authors declare no conflict of interest.

References

1. Pezzoni, M.; Catalano, P.N.; Pizarro, R.A.; Desimone, M.F.; Soler-Illia, G.; Bellino, M.G.; Costa, C.S. Antibiofilm effect of supramolecularly templated mesoporous silica coatings. *Mater. Sci. Eng. C Mater. Biol. Appl.* **2017**, *77*, 1044–1049. [CrossRef]
2. Urge, S.K.; Dibaba, S.T.; Gemta, A.B. Green Synthesis Method of ZnO Nanoparticles using Extracts of *Zingiber officinale* and Garlic Bulb (*Allium sativum*) and Their Synergetic Effect for Antibacterial Activities. *J. Nanomater.* **2023**, *2023*, 7036247.
3. Kumar, R.; Vinoth, S.; Baskar, V.; Arun, M.; Gurusaravanan, P. Synthesis of zinc oxide nanoparticles mediated by *Dictyota dichotoma* endophytic fungi and its photocatalytic degradation of fast green dye and antibacterial applications. *S. Afr. J. Bot.* **2022**, *151*, 337–344. [CrossRef]
4. Akter, S.; Huq, M.A. Biologically rapid synthesis of silver nanoparticles by *Sphingobium* sp. MAH-11^T and their antibacterial activity and mechanisms investigation against drug-resistant pathogenic microbes. *Artif. Cells Nanomed. Biotechnol.* **2020**, *48*, 672–682. [CrossRef]
5. Bachheti, R.K.; Fikadu, A.; Bachheti, A.; Husen, A. Biogenic fabrication of nanomaterials from flower-based chemical compounds, characterization and their various applications: A review. *Saudi J. Biol. Sci.* **2020**, *27*, 2551–2562. [CrossRef]
6. Huq, M.A.; Ashrafudoulla, M.; Rahman, M.M.; Balusamy, S.R.; Akter, S. Green Synthesis and Potential Antibacterial Applications of Bioactive Silver Nanoparticles: A Review. *Polymers* **2022**, *14*, 742. [CrossRef]
7. Motelica, L.; Ficai, D.; Oprea, O.; Ficai, A.; Trusca, R.-D.; Andronescu, E.; Holban, A.M. Biodegradable Alginate Films with ZnO Nanoparticles and Citronella Essential Oil—A Novel Antimicrobial Structure. *Pharmaceutics* **2021**, *13*, 1020. [CrossRef]
8. Suba, S.; Vijayakumar, S.; Vidhya, E.; Punitha, V.N.; Nilavukkarasi, M. Microbial mediated synthesis of ZnO nanoparticles derived from *Lactobacillus* spp.: Characterizations, antimicrobial and biocompatibility efficiencies. *Sens. Int.* **2021**, *2*, 100104. [CrossRef]
9. Ghdeeb, N.J.; Hussain, N.A. Antimicrobial Activity of ZnO Nanoparticles Prepared Using a Green Synthesis Approach. *Nano Biomed. Eng.* **2023**, *15*, 14–20. [CrossRef]
10. Huq, M.A.; Ashrafudoulla, M.; Parvez, M.A.K.; Balusamy, S.R.; Rahman, M.M.; Kim, J.H.; Akter, S. Chitosan-Coated Polymeric Silver and Gold Nanoparticles: Biosynthesis, Characterization and Potential Antibacterial Applications: A Review. *Polymers* **2022**, *14*, 5302. [CrossRef]
11. Huq, M.A.; Akter, S. Bacterial mediated rapid and facile synthesis of silver nanoparticles and their antimicrobial efficacy against pathogenic microorganisms. *Materials* **2021**, *14*, 2615. [CrossRef] [PubMed]
12. Venkatasubbu, G.D.; Baskar, R.; Anusuya, T.; Seshan, C.A.; Chelliah, R. Toxicity mechanism of titanium dioxide and zinc oxide nanoparticles against food pathogens. *Colloids Surf. B Biointerfaces* **2016**, *148*, 600–606. [CrossRef] [PubMed]
13. Yusof, H.M.; Rahman, N.A.; Mohamad, R.; Zaidan, U.H.; Samsudin, A.A. Biosynthesis of zinc oxide nanoparticles by cell-biomass and supernatant of *Lactobacillus plantarum* TA4 and its antibacterial and biocompatibility properties. *Sci. Rep.* **2020**, *10*, 19996. [CrossRef]
14. Khan, M.A.; Lone, S.A.; Shahid, M.; Zeyad, M.T.; Syed, A.; Ehtram, A.; Elgorban, A.M.; Verma, M.; Danish, M. Phytogenically Synthesized Zinc Oxide Nanoparticles (ZnO-NPs) Potentially Inhibit the Bacterial Pathogens: In Vitro Studies. *Toxics* **2023**, *11*, 452. [CrossRef]

15. Faisal, S.; Abdullah; Rizwan, M.; Ullah, R.; Alotaibi, A.; Khattak, A.; Bibi, N.; Idrees, M. Paraclostridium Benzoelyticum Bacterium-Mediated Zinc Oxide Nanoparticles and Their In Vivo Multiple Biological Applications. *Oxid. Med. Cell. Longev.* **2022**, *2022*, 5994033.
16. Motelica, L.; Vasile, B.-S.; Ficai, A.; Surdu, A.-V.; Ficai, D.; Oprea, O.-C.; Andronescu, E.; Jinga, D.C.; Holban, A.M. Influence of the Alcohols on the ZnO Synthesis and Its Properties: The Photocatalytic and Antimicrobial Activities. *Pharmaceutics* **2022**, *14*, 2842. [CrossRef] [PubMed]
17. Tayel, A.A.; El-Tras, W.F.; Moussa, S.; El-Baz, A.F.; Mahrous, H.; Salem, M.F.; Brimer, L. Antibacterial action of zinc oxide nanoparticles against foodborne pathogens. *J. Food Saf.* **2011**, *31*, 211–218. [CrossRef]
18. Elemike, E.E.; Onwudiwe, D.C.; Fayemi, O.E.; Botha, T.L. Green synthesis and electrochemistry of Ag, Au, and Ag–Au bimetallic nanoparticles using golden rod (*Solidago canadensis*) leaf extract. *Appl. Phys. A* **2019**, *125*, 42. [CrossRef]
19. Guzmán, M.G.; Dille, J.; Godet, S. Synthesis of silver nanoparticles by chemical reduction method and their antibacterial activity. *Int. J. Chem. Biomol. Eng.* **2009**, *2*, 104–111.
20. Pauzi, N.; Zain, N.M.; Yusof, N.A.A. Microwave-assisted synthesis of ZnO nanoparticles stabilized with gum arabic: Effect of microwave irradiation time on ZnO nanoparticles size and morphology. *Bull. Chem. React. Eng. Catal.* **2019**, *14*, 182–188. [CrossRef]
21. Iravani, S.; Korbekandi, H.; Mirmohammadi, S.V.; Zolfaghari, B. Synthesis of silver nanoparticles: Chemical, physical and biological methods. *Res. Pharm. Sci.* **2014**, *9*, 385.
22. Jamkhande, P.G.; Ghule, N.W.; Bamer, A.H.; Kalaskar, M.G. Metal nanoparticles synthesis: An overview on methods of preparation, advantages and disadvantages, and applications. *J. Drug Deliv. Sci. Technol.* **2019**, *53*, 101174. [CrossRef]
23. Lal, S.; Verma, R.; Chauhan, A.; Dhatwalia, J.; Guleria, I.; Ghotekar, S.; Thakur, S.; Mansi, K.; Kumar, R.; Kumari, A.; et al. Antioxidant, antimicrobial, and photocatalytic activity of green synthesized ZnO-NPs from *Myrica esculenta* fruits extract. *Inorg. Chem. Comm.* **2022**, *141*, 109518. [CrossRef]
24. Abdelhakim, H.K.; El-Sayed, E.R.; Rashidi, F.B. Biosynthesis of Zinc Oxide Nanoparticles with Antimicrobial, Anticancer, Antioxidant and Photocatalytic Activities by the Endophytic *Alternaria tenuissima*. *J. Appl. Microbiol.* **2020**, *128*, 1634–1646. [CrossRef] [PubMed]
25. Akter, S.; Lee, S.-Y.; Siddiqi, M.Z.; Balusamy, S.R.; Ashrafudoulla, M.; Rupa, E.J.; Huq, M.A. Ecofriendly synthesis of silver nanoparticles by *Terrabacter humi* sp. nov. and their antibacterial application against antibiotic-resistant pathogens. *Int. J. Mol. Sci.* **2020**, *21*, 9746. [CrossRef] [PubMed]
26. Du, J.; Singh, H.; Yi, T.H. Antibacterial, anti-biofilm and anticancer potentials of green synthesized silver nanoparticles using benzoin gum (*Styrax benzoin*) extract. *Bioprocess Biosyst. Eng.* **2020**, *39*, 1923–1931. [CrossRef]
27. Wang, X.; Lee, S.-Y.; Akter, S.; Huq, M.A. Probiotic-mediated biosynthesis of silver nanoparticles and their antibacterial applications against pathogenic strains of *Escherichia coli* O157:H7. *Polymers* **2022**, *14*, 1834. [CrossRef]
28. Ashrafudoulla, M.; Mizan, M.F.R.; Park, S.H.; Ha, S.D. Current and future perspectives for controlling Vibrio biofilms in the seafood industry: A comprehensive review. *Crit. Rev. Food Sci. Nutr.* **2021**, *61*, 1827–1851. [CrossRef]
29. Hamida, R.M.; Ali, M.A.; Goda, D.A.; Khalilad, M.I.; Redhwan, A. Cytotoxic effect of green silver nanoparticles against ampicillin-resistant *Klebsiella pneumoniae*. *RSC Adv.* **2020**, *10*, 21136–21146. [CrossRef]
30. Huq, M.A.; Akter, S. Biosynthesis, characterization and antibacterial application of novel silver nanoparticles against drug resistant pathogenic *Klebsiella pneumoniae* and *Salmonella* Enteritidis. *Molecules* **2021**, *26*, 5996. [CrossRef]
31. Ashrafudoulla, M.; Mizan, M.F.R.; Park, H.; Byun, K.H.; Lee, N.; Park, S.H.; Ha, S.D. Genetic Relationship, Virulence Factors, Drug Resistance Profile and Biofilm Formation Ability of *Vibrio parahaemolyticus* Isolated from Mussel. *Front. Microbiol.* **2019**, *10*, 513. [CrossRef]
32. Afshari, A.; Baratpour, A.; Khanzade, S.; Jamshidi, A. *Salmonella* Enteritidis and *Salmonella* Typhimorium identification in poultry carcasses. *Iran. J. Microbiol.* **2018**, *10*, 45–50. [PubMed]
33. Huq, M.A.; Akter, S. Characterization and Genome Analysis of *Arthrobacter bangladeshi* sp. nov., Applied for the Green Synthesis of Silver Nanoparticles and Their Antibacterial Efficacy against Drug-Resistant Human Pathogens. *Pharmaceutics* **2021**, *13*, 1691. [CrossRef] [PubMed]
34. Huq, M.A. Biogenic silver nanoparticles synthesized by *Lysinibacillus xylanilyticus* MAHUQ-40 to control antibiotic-resistant human pathogens vibrio parahaemolyticus and salmonella typhimurium. *Front. Bioeng. Biotechnol.* **2020**, *8*, 1407. [CrossRef]
35. Barani, M.; Masoudi, M.; Mashreghi, M.; Makhdoumi, A.; Eshghi, H. Cell-free extract assisted synthesis of ZnO nanoparticles using aquatic bacterial strains: Biological activities and toxicological evaluation. *Int. J. Pharm.* **2021**, *606*, 120878. [CrossRef] [PubMed]
36. MuthuKathija, M.; Badhusha, M.S.M.; Rama, V. Green synthesis of zinc oxide nanoparticles using *Pisonia alba* leaf extract and its antibacterial activity. *Appl. Surf. Sci. Adv.* **2023**, *15*, 100400. [CrossRef]
37. Chowdhury, M.A.H.; Ashrafudoulla, M.; Mevo, S.I.U.; Mizan, M.F.R.; Park, S.H.; Ha, S.D. Current and future interventions for improving poultry health and poultry food safety and security: A comprehensive review. *Compr. Rev. Food Sci. Food Saf.* **2023**, *22*, 1555–1596. [CrossRef]
38. Rambabu, K.; Bharath, G.; Banat, F.; Show, P.L. Green synthesis of zinc oxide nanoparticles using *Phoenix dactylifera* waste as bioreductant for effective dye degradation and antibacterial performance in wastewater treatment. *J. Hazard. Mater.* **2021**, *402*, 123560. [CrossRef]

39. Gomaa, E.Z. Microbial Mediated Synthesis of Zinc Oxide Nanoparticles, Characterization and Multifaceted Applications. *J. Inorg. Organomet. Polym.* **2022**, *32*, 4114–4132. [CrossRef]
40. Singh, A.; Singh, N.B.; Afzal, S.; Singh, T.; Hussain, I. Zinc oxide nanoparticles: A review of their biological synthesis, antimicrobial activity, uptake, translocation and biotransformation in plants. *J. Mater. Sci.* **2018**, *53*, 185–201. [CrossRef]
41. Raja, A.; Ashokkumar, S.; Pavithra-Marthandam, R.; Jayachandiran, J.; Khatiwada, C.P.; Kaviyarasu, K.; Ganapathi Raman, R.; Swaminathan, M. Eco-friendly preparation of zinc oxide nanoparticles using Tabernaemontana divaricata and its photocatalytic and antimicrobial activity. *J. Photochem. Photobiol. B Biol.* **2018**, *181*, 53–58. [CrossRef] [PubMed]
42. Ahmed, T.; Wu, Z.; Jiang, H.; Luo, J.; Noman, M.; Shahid, M.; Manzoor, I.; Allemailem, K.S.; Alrumaihi, F.; Li, B. Bioinspired Green Synthesis of Zinc Oxide Nanoparticles from a Native *Bacillus cereus* Strain RNT6: Characterization and Antibacterial Activity against Rice Panicle Blight Pathogens *Burkholderia glumae* and *B. gladioli*. *Nanomaterials* **2021**, *11*, 884. [CrossRef] [PubMed]
43. Yusof, H.M.; Mohamad, R.; Zaidan, U.H.; Abdul Rahman, N.A. Microbial synthesis of zinc oxide nanoparticles and their potential application as an antimicrobial agent and a feed supplement in animal industry: A review. *J. Anim. Sci. Biotechnol.* **2019**, *10*, 57.
44. Abdo, A.M.; Fouda, A.; Eid, A.M.; Fahmy, N.M.; Elsayed, A.M.; Khalil, A.M.A.; Alzahrani, O.M.; Ahmed, A.F.; Soliman, A.M. Green Synthesis of Zinc Oxide Nanoparticles (ZnO-NPs) by *Pseudomonas aeruginosa* and Their Activity against Pathogenic Microbes and Common House Mosquito, *Culex pipiens*. *Materials* **2021**, *14*, 6983. [CrossRef] [PubMed]
45. Jayabalan, J.; Mani, G.; Krishnan, N.; Pernabas, J.; Devadoss, J.M.; Jang, H.T. Green Biogenic Synthesis of Zinc Oxide Nanoparticles Using *Pseudomonas putida* Culture and Its In Vitro Antibacterial and Anti-Biofilm Activity. *Biocatal. Agric. Biotechnol.* **2019**, *21*, 101327. [CrossRef]
46. Jayaseelan, C.; Rahuman, A.A.; Kirthi, A.V.; Marimuthu, S.; Santhoshkumar, T.; Bagavan, A.; Gaurav, K.; Karthik, L.; Rao, K.V.B. Novel microbial route to synthesize ZnO nanoparticles using Aeromonas hydrophila and their activity against pathogenic bacteria and fungi. *Spectrochim. Acta Part A Mol. Biomol. Spectrosc.* **2012**, *90*, 78–84. [CrossRef] [PubMed]
47. Saravanan, M.; Gopinath, V.; Chaurasia, M.K.; Syed, A.; Ameen, F.; Purushothaman, N. Green synthesis of anisotropic zinc oxide nanoparticles with antibacterial and cytofriendly properties. *Microb. Pathog.* **2018**, *115*, 57–63. [CrossRef]
48. Taran, M.; Rad, M.; Alavi, M. Biosynthesis of TiO2 and ZnO nanoparticles by *Halomonas elongata* IBRC-M 10214 in different conditions of medium. *Bioimpacts* **2018**, *8*, 81–89. [CrossRef]
49. Król, A. Mechanism study of intracellular zinc oxide nanocomposites formation. *Colloids Surf.* **2018**, *553*, 349–358. [CrossRef]
50. Mishra, M.; Paliwal, J.; Singh, S.; Ethiraj, S.; Mohanashrinivasan, V. Studies on the inhibitory activity of biologically synthesized and characterized ZnO nanoparticles using L.sporogens against *Staphylococcus aureus*. *J. Pure Appl. Microbiol.* **2013**, *7*, 1263–1268.
51. Kundu, D.; Hazra, C.; Chatterjee, A.; Chaudhari, A.; Mishra, S. Extracellular biosynthesis of zinc oxide nanoparticles using Rhodococcus pyridinivorans NT2: Multifunctional textile finishing, biosafety evaluation and in vitro drug delivery in colon carcinoma. *J. Photochem. Photobiol. B Biol.* **2014**, *140*, 194–204. [CrossRef] [PubMed]
52. Rajabairavi, N.; Raju, C.S.; Karthikeyan, C.; Varutharaju, K.; Nethaji, S.; Hameed, A.S.H.; Shajahan, A. Biosynthesis of Novel Zinc Oxide Nanoparticles (ZnO NPs) Using Endophytic Bacteria *Sphingobacterium thalpophilum*. In *Recent Trends in Materials Science and Applications*; Ebenezar, J., Ed.; Springer: Cham, Switzerland, 2017; pp. 245–254.
53. Rauf, M.A.; Owais, M.; Rajpoot, R.; Ahmad, F.; Khan, N.; Zubair, S. Biomimetically synthesized ZnO nanoparticles attain potent antibacterial activity against less susceptible S. aureus skin infection in experimental animals. *RSC Adv.* **2017**, *7*, 36361–36373. [CrossRef]
54. Balraj, B.; Senthilkumar, N.; Siva, C.; Krithikadevi, R.; Julie, A.; Potheher, I.V.; Arulmozhi, M. Synthesis and characterization of Zinc Oxide nanoparticles using marine *Streptomyces* sp. with its investigations on anticancer and antibacterial activity. *Res. Chem. Intermed.* **2017**, *43*, 2367–2376. [CrossRef]
55. Moghaddam, A.B.; Moniri, M.; Azizi, S.; Rahim, R.A.; Ariff, A.B.; Saad, W.Z.; Namvar, F.; Navaderi, M. Biosynthesis of ZnO Nanoparticles by a New *Pichia kudriavzevii* Yeast Strain and Evaluation of Their Antimicrobial and Antioxidant Activities. *Molecules* **2017**, *22*, 872. [CrossRef]
56. Chauhan, R.; Reddy, A.; Abraham, J. Biosynthesis of silver and zinc oxide nanoparticles using *Pichia fermentans* JA2 and their antimicrobial property. *Appl. Nanosci.* **2015**, *5*, 63–71. [CrossRef]
57. Rajan, A.; Cherian, E.; Gurunathan, D.B. Biosynthesis of zinc oxide nanoparticles using *Aspergillus fumigatus* JCF and its antibacterial activity. *Int. J. Mod. Sci. Technol.* **2016**, *1*, 52–57.
58. Kalpana, V.N.; Kataru, B.A.S.; Sravani, N.; Vigneshwari, T.; Panneerselvam, A.; Devi Rajeswari, V. Biosynthesis of zinc oxide nanoparticles using culture filtrates of *Aspergillus niger*: Antimicrobial textiles and dye degradation studies. *OpenNano* **2018**, *3*, 48–55. [CrossRef]
59. Gurunathan, D.B.; Jagadeesan, C.; Fahad, K.; Praveen, A. Mycological synthesis, characterization and antifungal activity of zinc oxide nanoparticles. *Asian J. Pharm. Technol.* **2013**, *3*, 142–146.
60. Fagier, M.A. Plant-Mediated Biosynthesis and Photocatalysis Activities of Zinc Oxide Nanoparticles: A Prospect towards Dyes Mineralization. *J. Nanotechnol.* **2021**, *2021*, 6629180. [CrossRef]
61. Li, X.; Xu, H.; Chen, Z.-S.; Chen, G. Biosynthesis of Nanoparticles by Microorganisms and Their Applications. *J. Nanomater.* **2011**, *2011*, 270974. [CrossRef]
62. Abomuti, M.A.; Danish, E.Y.; Firoz, A.; Hasan, N.; Malik, M.A. Green Synthesis of Zinc Oxide Nanoparticles Using *Salvia officinalis* Leaf Extract and Their Photocatalytic and Antifungal Activities. *Biology* **2021**, *10*, 1075. [CrossRef] [PubMed]

63. Fouda, A.; Saied, E.; Eid, A.M.; Kouadri, F.; Alemam, A.M.; Hamza, M.F.; Alharbi, M.; Elkelish, A.; Hassan, S.E.-D. Green Synthesis of Zinc Oxide Nanoparticles Using an Aqueous Extract of *Punica granatum* for Antimicrobial and Catalytic Activity. *J. Funct. Biomater.* **2023**, *14*, 205. [CrossRef] [PubMed]
64. Alotaibi, B.; Negm, W.A.; Elekhnawy, E.; El-Masry, T.A.; Elharty, M.E.; Saleh, A.; Abdelkader, D.H.; Mokhtar, F.A. Antibacterial activity of nano zinc oxide green-synthesised from *Gardenia thailandica* triveng. Leaves against *Pseudomonas aeruginosa* clinical isolates: In vitro and in vivo study. *Artif. Cells Nanomed. Biotechnol.* **2022**, *50*, 96–106. [CrossRef]
65. Dulta, K.; Koşarsoy Ağçeli, G.; Chauhan, P.; Jasrotia, R.; Chauhan, P.K. Ecofriendly Synthesis of Zinc Oxide Nanoparticles by *Carica papaya* Leaf Extract and Their Applications. *J. Clust. Sci.* **2022**, *33*, 603–617. [CrossRef]
66. Menazea, A.A.; Ismail, A.M.; Samy, A. Novel Green Synthesis of Zinc Oxide Nanoparticles Using Orange Waste and Its Thermal and Antibacterial Activity. *J. Inorg. Organomet. Polym.* **2021**, *31*, 4250–4259. [CrossRef]
67. Suručić, R.; Šmitran, A.; Gajić, D.; Božić, L.; Antić, M.; Topić-Vučenović, V.; Umičević, N.; Antunović, V.; Jelić, D. Phytosynthesis of zinc oxide nanoparticles with acetonic extract of flowers of *Geranium robertianum* L. (Geraniaceae). *J. Hyg. Eng. Des.* **2020**, *615*, 28.
68. Subramanian, H.; Krishnan, M.; Mahalingam, A. Photocatalytic dye degradation and photoexcited anti-microbial activities of green zinc oxide nanoparticles synthesized via Sargassum muticum extracts. *RSC Adv.* **2022**, *12*, 985–997. [CrossRef]
69. Abdelmigid, H.M.; Hussien, N.A.; Alyamani, A.A.; Morsi, M.M.; AlSufyani, N.M.; Kadi, H.A. Green Synthesis of Zinc Oxide Nanoparticles Using Pomegranate Fruit Peel and Solid Coffee Grounds vs. Chemical Method of Synthesis, with Their Biocompatibility and Antibacterial Properties Investigation. *Molecules* **2022**, *27*, 1236. [CrossRef]
70. Ramesh, R.; Parasaran, M.; Mubashira, G.T.F.; Flora, C.; Khan, F.L.A.; Almaary, K.S.; Elbadawi, Y.B.; Chen, T.-W.; Kanimozhi, K.; Bashir, A.; et al. Biogenic synthesis of ZnO and NiO nanoparticles mediated by fermented *Cocos nucifera*. (L) Deoiled cake extract for antimicrobial applications towards gram positive and gram negative pathogens. *J. King Saud. Univ. Sci.* **2022**, *34*, 101696–101704. [CrossRef]
71. Alahmdi, M.I.; Khasim, S.; Vanaraj, S.; Panneerselvam, C.; Mahmoud, M.A.A.; Mukhtar, S.; Alsharif, M.A.; Zidan, N.S.; Abo-Dya, N.E.; Aldosari, O.F. Green Nanoarchitectonics of ZnO Nanoparticles from *Clitoria ternatea* Flower Extract for In Vitro Anticancer and Antibacterial Activity: Inhibits MCF-7 Cell Proliferation via Intrinsic Apoptotic Pathway. *J. Inorg. Organomet. Polym.* **2022**, *32*, 2146–2159. [CrossRef]
72. Ilangovan, A.; Venkatramanan, A.; Thangarajan, P.; Saravanan, A.; Rajendran, S.; Kaveri, K. Green Synthesis of Zinc Oxide Nanoparticles (ZnO NPs) Using Aqueous Extract of *Tagetes Erecta* Flower and Evaluation of Its Antioxidant, Antimicrobial, and Cytotoxic Activities on HeLa Cell Line. *Curr. Biotechnol.* **2021**, *10*, 61–76. [CrossRef]
73. Djouadi, A.; Derouiche, S. Spinach mediated synthesis of zinc oxide nanoparticles: Characterization, In vitro biological activities study and in vivo acute toxicity evaluation. *Curr. Res. Green Sustain. Chem.* **2021**, *4*, 100214. [CrossRef]
74. Khan, M.I.; Fatima, N.; Shakil, M.; Tahir, M.B.; Riaz, K.N.; Rafique, M.; Iqbal, T.; Mahmood, K. Investigation of in-vitro antibacterial and seed germination properties of green synthesized pure and nickel doped ZnO nanoparticles. *Phys. B Condens. Matter* **2021**, *601*, 412563. [CrossRef]
75. Vijayakumar, S.; González-Sánchez, Z.I.; Malaikozhundan, B.; Saravanakumar, K.; Divya, M.; Vaseeharan, B.; Durán-Lara, E.F.; Wang, M.-H. Biogenic Synthesis of Rod Shaped ZnO Nanoparticles Using Red Paprika (*Capsicum annuum* L. var. grossum (L.) Sendt) and Their in Vitro Evaluation. *J. Clust. Sci.* **2021**, *32*, 1129–1139. [CrossRef]
76. Batool, M.; Khurshid, S.; Qureshi, Z.; Daoush, W.M. Adsorption, antimicrobial and wound healing activities of biosynthesised zinc oxide nanoparticles. *Chem. Pap.* **2021**, *75*, 893–907. [CrossRef]
77. Kumar, N.H.K.; Mohana, N.C.; Nuthan, B.R.; Ramesha, K.P.; Rakshith, D.; Geetha, N.; Satish, S. Phyto-mediated synthesis of zinc oxide nanoparticles using aqueous plant extract of *Ocimum americanum* and evaluation of its bioactivity. *SN Appl. Sci.* **2019**, *1*, 651. [CrossRef]
78. Madan, H.R.; Sharma, S.C.; Udayabhanu; Suresh, D.; Vidya, Y.S.; Nagabhushana, H.; Rajanaik, H.; Anantharaju, K.S.; Prashantha, S.C.; Sadananda-Maiya, P. Facile green fabrication of nanostructure ZnO plates, bullets, flower, prismatic tip, closed pine cone: Their antibacterial, antioxidant, photoluminescent and photocatalytic properties. *Spectrochim. Acta Part A Mol. Biomol. Spectrosc.* **2016**, *152*, 404–416. [CrossRef]
79. Chauhan, A.; Verma, R.; Kumari, S.; Sharma, A.; Shandilya, P.; Li, X.; Batoo, K.M.; Imran, A.; Kulshrestha, S.; Kumar, R. Photocatalytic dye degradation and antimicrobial activities of Pure and Ag-doped ZnO using Cannabis sativa leaf extract. *Sci. Rep.* **2020**, *10*, 7881. [CrossRef]
80. Sharma, S.C. ZnO nano-flowers from Carica papaya milk: Degradation of Alizarin Red-S dye and antibacterial activity against *Pseudomonas aeruginosa* and *Staphylococcus aureus*. *Optik* **2016**, *127*, 6498–6512. [CrossRef]
81. Kahsay, M.H.; Tadesse, A.; RamaDevi, D.; Belachew, N.; Basavaiah, K. Green synthesis of zinc oxide nanostructures and investigation of their photocatalytic and bactericidal applications. *RSC Adv.* **2019**, *9*, 36967–36981. [CrossRef]
82. Pal, S.; Mondal, S.; Maity, J.; Mukherjee, R. Synthesis and Characterization of ZnO Nanoparticles using *Moringa oleifera* Leaf Extract: Investigation of Photocatalytic and Antibacterial Activity. *Int. J. Nanosci. Nanotechnol.* **2018**, *14*, 111–119.
83. Jayappa, M.D.; Ramaiah, C.K.; Kumar, M.A.P.; Suresh, D.; Prabhu, A.; Devasya, R.P.; Sheikh, S. Green synthesis of zinc oxide nanoparticles from the leaf, stem and in vitro grown callus of *Mussaenda frondosa* L.: Characterization and their applications. *Appl. Nanosci.* **2020**, *10*, 3057–3074. [CrossRef] [PubMed]

84. Khalid, A.; Ahmad, P.; Khandaker, M.U.; Modafer, Y.; Almukhlifi, H.A.; Bazaid, A.S.; Aldarhami, A.; Alanazi, A.M.; Jefri, O.A.; Uddin, M.; et al. Biologically Reduced Zinc Oxide Nanosheets Using Phyllanthus emblica Plant Extract for Antibacterial and Dye Degradation Studies. *J. Chem.* **2023**, *2023*, 3971686. [CrossRef]
85. Chandrasekar, L.P.; Sethuraman, B.D.; Subramani, M.; Mohandos, S. Green synthesised ZnO nanoparticles from Plectranthus amboinicus plant extract: Removal of Safranin-O and Malachite green dyes & anti-bacterial activity. *Int. J. Environ. Anal. Chem.* **2023**, 1–18. [CrossRef]
86. Ahmed, S.; Chaudhry, S.A.; Ikram, S. A review on biogenic synthesis of ZnO nanoparticles using plant extracts and microbes: A prospect towards green chemistry. *J. Photochem. Photobiol. B Biol.* **2017**, *166*, 272–284. [CrossRef]
87. Gur, T.; Meydan, I.; Seckin, H.; Bekmezci, M.; Sen, F. Green synthesis, characterization and bioactivity of biogenic zinc oxide nanoparticles. *Environ. Res.* **2022**, *204*, 111897. [CrossRef]
88. Iqbal, J.; Abbasi, B.A.; Yaseen, T.; Zahra, S.A.; Shahbaz, A.; Shah, S.A.; Uddin, S.; Ma, X.; Raouf, B.; Kanwal, S.; et al. Green synthesis of zinc oxide nanoparticles using *Elaeagnus angustifolia* L. leaf extracts and their multiple in vitro biological applications. *Sci. Rep.* **2021**, *11*, 20988. [CrossRef]
89. Chikkanna, M.M.; Neelagund, S.E.; Rajashekarappa, K.K. Green synthesis of zinc oxide nanoparticles (ZnO NPs) and their biological activity. *SN Appl. Sci.* **2019**, *1*, 117. [CrossRef]
90. Yazdanian, M.; Rostamzadeh, P.; Rahbar, M.; Alam, M.; Abbasi, K.; Tahmasebi, E.; Tebyaniyan, H.; Ranjbar, R.; Seifalian, A.; Yazdanian, A. The potential application of green-synthesized metal nanoparticles in dentistry: A comprehensive review. *Bioinorg. Chem. Appl.* **2022**, *2022*, 2311910. [CrossRef]
91. Verma, A.; Mehata, M.S. Controllable synthesis of silver nanoparticles using Neem leaves and their antimicrobial activity. *J. Radiat. Res. Appl. Sci.* **2016**, *9*, 109–115. [CrossRef]
92. Thatoi, P.; Kerry, R.G.; Gouda, S.; Das, G.; Pramanik, K.; Thatoi, H.; Patra, J.K. Photo-mediated green synthesis of silver and zinc oxide nanoparticles using aqueous extracts of two mangrove plant species, *Heritiera fomes* and *Sonneratia apetala* and investigation of their biomedical applications. *J. Photochem. Photobiol. B Biol.* **2016**, 3, 163. [CrossRef] [PubMed]
93. Vimala, K.; Sundarraj, S.; Paulpandi, M.; Vengatesan, S.; Kannan, S. Green synthesized doxorubicin loaded zinc oxide nanoparticles regulates the Bax and Bcl-2 expression in breast and colon carcinoma. *Process Biochem.* **2014**, *49*, 160–172. [CrossRef]
94. Supraja, N.; Prasad, T.; Gandhi, A.D.; Anbumani, D.; Kavitha, P.; Babujanarthanam, R. Synthesis, characterization and evaluation of antimicrobial efficacy and brine shrimp lethality assay of *Alstonia scholaris* stem bark extract mediated ZnONPs. *Biochem. Biophys. Rep.* **2018**, *14*, 69–77. [CrossRef] [PubMed]
95. Sonia, S.; Ruckmani, K.; Sivakumar, M. Antimicrobial and antioxidant potentials of biosynthesized colloidal zinc oxide nanoparticles for a fortified cold cream formulation: A potent nanocosmeceutical application. *Mater. Sci. Eng. C* **2017**, *79*, 581–589.
96. Manjari, B.; Singh, D.P. Green synthesis of zinc oxide nanoparticles by *Pseudomonas aeruginosa* and their broad-spectrum antimicrobial effects. *J. Pure Appl. Microbiol.* **2018**, *12*, 2123–2134.
97. Al-Kurdy, M.J.; Al-Khuzaie, M.G.A.; Abbas, G.A.; Al Dulaimi, Z.M.H. Green synthesis and characterization of zinc oxide nanoparticles using black currant extracts. *AIP Conf. Proc.* **2023**, *1*, 2776.
98. Narayanan, K.B.; Sakthivel, N. Phytosynthesis of gold nanoparticles using leaf extract of *Coleus amboinicus* Lour. *Mater. Charact.* **2010**, *61*, 1232–1238. [CrossRef]
99. Darvish, M.; Ajji, A. Effect of Polyethylene Film Thickness on the Antimicrobial Activity of Embedded Zinc Oxide Nanoparticles. *ACS Omega* **2021**, *6*, 26201–26209. [CrossRef]
100. Halbus, A.F.; Horozov, T.S.; Paunov, V.N. Surface-Modified Zinc Oxide Nanoparticles for Antialgal and Antiyeast Applications. *ACS Appl. Nano Mater.* **2020**, *3*, 440–451. [CrossRef]
101. Sun, Q.; Li, J.; Le, T. Zinc Oxide Nanoparticle as a Novel Class of Antifungal Agents: Current Advances and Future Perspectives. *J. Agric. Food Chem.* **2018**, *66*, 11209–11220. [CrossRef]
102. Morowvat, M.H.; Kazemi, K.; Jaberi, M.A.; Amini, A.; Gholami, A. Biosynthesis and Antimicrobial Evaluation of Zinc Oxide Nanoparticles Using Chlorella vulgaris Biomass against Multidrug-Resistant Pathogens. *Materials* **2023**, *16*, 842. [CrossRef]
103. Bahari, N.; Hashim, N.; Abdan, K.; Md Akim, A.; Maringgal, B.; Al-Shdifat, L. Role of Honey as a Bifunctional Reducing and Capping/Stabilizing Agent: Application for Silver and Zinc Oxide Nanoparticles. *Nanomaterials* **2023**, *13*, 1244. [CrossRef] [PubMed]
104. Li, W.; You, Q.; Zhang, J. Green synthesis of antibacterial LFL-ZnO using *L. plantarum* fermentation liquid assisted by ultrasound-microwave. *J. Alloys Compd.* **2023**, *947*, 169697. [CrossRef]
105. Ravi, A.; Nandayipurath, V.V.T.; Rajan, S.; Salim, S.A.; Khalid, N.K.; Aravindakumar, C.T.; Krishnankutty, R.E. Effect of zinc oxide nanoparticle supplementation on the enhanced production of surfactin and iturin lipopeptides of endophytic *Bacillus* sp. Fcl1 and its ameliorated antifungal activity. *Microb. Pathog.* **2020**, *149*, 104528. [CrossRef] [PubMed]
106. Mishra, P.K.; Mishra, H.; Ekielski, A.; Talegaonkar, S.; Vaidya, B. Zinc oxide nanoparticles: A promising nanomaterial for biomedical applications. *Drug Discov. Today* **2017**, *22*, 1825–1834. [CrossRef]
107. Jin, S.-E.; Jin, H.-E. Antimicrobial Activity of Zinc Oxide Nano/Microparticles and Their Combinations against Pathogenic Microorganisms for Biomedical Applications: From Physicochemical Characteristics to Pharmacological Aspects. *Nanomaterials* **2021**, *11*, 263. [CrossRef]

108. Kim, Y.S.; Kim, J.S.; Cho, H.S.; Rha, D.S.; Kim, J.M.; Park, J.D.; Choi, B.S.; Lim, R.; Chang, H.K.; Chung, Y.H.; et al. Twenty-eight-day oral toxicity, genotoxicity, and gender-related tissue distribution of silver nanoparticles in Sprague-Dawley rats. *Inhal. Toxicol.* **2008**, *20*, 575–583. [CrossRef]
109. Espitia, P.J.P.; Soares, N.F.F.; Coimbra, J.S.R.; De Andrade, N.J.; Cruz, R.S.; Medeiros, E.A.A. Zinc Oxide Nanoparticles: Synthesis, Antimicrobial Activity and Food Packaging Applications. *Food Bioprocess Technol.* **2012**, *5*, 1447–1464. [CrossRef]
110. Kalpana, V.N.; Devi Rajeswari, V. A Review on Green Synthesis, Biomedical Applications, and Toxicity Studies of ZnO NPs. *Bioinorg. Chem. Appl.* **2018**, *2018*, 3569758. [CrossRef]
111. Sirelkhatim, A.; Mahmud, S.; Seeni, A.; Kaus, N.H.M.; Ann, L.C.; Bakhori, S.K.M.; Hasan, H.; Mohamad, D. Review on Zinc Oxide Nanoparticles: Antibacterial Activity and Toxicity Mechanism. *Nano-Micro Lett.* **2015**, *7*, 219–242. [CrossRef]
112. Kumar, R.; Umar, A.; Kumar, G.; Nalwa, H.S. Antimicrobial properties of ZnO nanomaterials: A review. *Ceram. Int.* **2017**, *43*, 3940–3961. [CrossRef]
113. Sportelli; Chiara, M.; Picca, R.A.; Cioffi, N. Recent advances in the synthesis and characterization of nano-antimicrobials. *TrAC Trends Anal. Chem.* **2016**, *84*, 131–138. [CrossRef]
114. Halbus, A.F.; Tommy, S. Colloid particle formulations for antimicrobial applications. *Adv. Colloid Interface Sci.* **2017**, *249*, 134–148. [CrossRef] [PubMed]
115. Raghupathi, K.R.; Koodali, R.T.; Manna, A.C. Size-dependent bacterial growth inhibition and mechanism of antibacterial activity of zinc oxide nanoparticles. *Langmuir* **2011**, *27*, 4020–4028. [CrossRef] [PubMed]
116. Xie, Y.; He, Y.; Irwin, P.L.; Jin, T.; Shi, X. Antibacterial activity and mechanism of action of zinc oxide nanoparticles against *Campylobacter jejuni*. *Appl. Environ. Microbiol.* **2011**, *77*, 2325–2331. [CrossRef]
117. Lipovsky, A.; Nitzan, Y.; Gedanken, A.; Lubart, R. Antifungal activity of ZnO nanoparticles--the role of ROS mediated cell injury. *Nanotechnology* **2011**, *22*, 105101. [CrossRef]
118. Arakha, M.; Saleem, M.; Mallick, B.C.; Jha, S. The effects of interfacial potential on antimicrobial propensity of ZnO nanoparticle. *Sci. Rep.* **2015**, *5*, 9578. [CrossRef]
119. Da-Silva, B.L.; Abuçafy, M.P.; Manaia, E.B.; Oshiro, J.A., Jr.; Chiari-Andréo, B.G.; Pietro, R.C.R.; Chiavacci, L.A. Relationship between structure and antimicrobial activity of zinc oxide nanoparticles: An overview. *Int. J. Nanomed.* **2019**, *14*, 9395. [CrossRef]
120. Jeyabharathi, S.; Chandramohan, S.; Naveenkumar, S.; Sundar, K.; Muthukumaran, A. Synergistic effects of herbal zinc oxide nanoparticles (ZnONPs) and its anti-hyperglycemic and anti-bacterial effects. *Mater. Today Proc.* **2021**, *36*, 390–396. [CrossRef]
121. Obeizi, Z.; Benbouzid, H.; Ouchenane, S.; Yılmaz, D.; Culha, M.; Bououdina, M. Biosynthesis of Zinc Oxide Nanoparticles from Essential Oil of *Eucalyptus globulus* with Antimicrobial and Anti-Biofilm Activities. *Mater. Today Commun.* **2020**, *25*, 225164972. [CrossRef]

pharmaceutics

MDPI

Review

Antibiotic-Loaded Gold Nanoparticles: A Nano-Arsenal against ESBL Producer-Resistant Pathogens

Syed Mohd Danish Rizvi [1,2,*], Amr Selim Abu Lila [1,2,*], Afrasim Moin [1,2], Talib Hussain [2,3], Mohammad Amjad Kamal [4,5,6,7], Hana Sonbol [8] and El-Sayed Khafagy [9,10]

1 Department of Pharmaceutics, College of Pharmacy, University of Ha'il, Ha'il 81442, Saudi Arabia
2 Molecular Diagnostic & Personalized Therapeutic Unit, University of Ha'il, Ha'il 81442, Saudi Arabia
3 Department of Pharmacology and Toxicology, College of Pharmacy, University of Ha'il, Ha'il 81442, Saudi Arabia
4 Institutes for Systems Genetics, Frontiers Science Center for Disease-Related Molecular Network, West China Hospital, Sichuan University, Chengdu 610065, China
5 King Fahd Medical Research Center, King Abdulaziz University, Jeddah 21589, Saudi Arabia
6 Department of Pharmacy, Faculty of Allied Health Sciences, Daffodil International University, Dhaka 1207, Bangladesh
7 Enzymoics, Novel Global Community Educational Foundation, 7 Peterlee Place, Hebersham, NSW 2770, Australia
8 Department of Biology, College of Science, Princess Nourah bint Abdulrahman University, Riyadh 11671, Saudi Arabia
9 Department of Pharmaceutics, College of Pharmacy, Prince Sattam Bin Abdulaziz University, Al-kharj 11942, Saudi Arabia
10 Department of Pharmaceutics and Industrial Pharmacy, Faculty of Pharmacy, Suez Canal University, Ismailia 41522, Egypt
* Correspondence: sm.danish@uoh.edu.sa (S.M.D.R.); a.abulila@uoh.edu.sa (A.S.A.L.)

Citation: Rizvi, S.M.D.; Lila, A.S.A.; Moin, A.; Hussain, T.; Kamal, M.A.; Sonbol, H.; Khafagy, E.-S. Antibiotic-Loaded Gold Nanoparticles: A Nano-Arsenal against ESBL Producer-Resistant Pathogens. *Pharmaceutics* **2023**, *15*, 430. https://doi.org/10.3390/pharmaceutics15020430

Academic Editors: Aura Rusu and Valentina Uivarosi

Received: 7 December 2022
Revised: 21 January 2023
Accepted: 26 January 2023
Published: 28 January 2023

Abstract: The advent of new antibiotics has helped clinicians to control severe bacterial infections. Despite this, inappropriate and redundant use of antibiotics, inadequate diagnosis, and smart resistant mechanisms developed by pathogens sometimes lead to the failure of treatment strategies. The genotypic analysis of clinical samples revealed that the rapid spread of extended-spectrum β-lactamases (ESBLs) genes is one of the most common approaches acquired by bacterial pathogens to become resistant. The scenario compelled the researchers to prioritize the design and development of novel and effective therapeutic options. Nanotechnology has emerged as a plausible groundbreaking tool against resistant infectious pathogens. Numerous reports suggested that inorganic nanomaterials, specifically gold nanoparticles (AuNPs), have converted unresponsive antibiotics into potent ones against multi-drug resistant pathogenic strains. Interestingly, after almost two decades of exhaustive preclinical evaluations, AuNPs are gradually progressively moving ahead toward clinical evaluations. However, the mechanistic aspects of the antibacterial action of AuNPs remain an unsolved puzzle for the scientific fraternity. Thus, the review covers state-of-the-art investigations pertaining to the efficacy of AuNPs as a tool to overcome ESBLs acquired resistance, their applicability and toxicity perspectives, and the revelation of the most appropriate proposed mechanism of action. Conclusively, the trend suggested that antibiotic-loaded AuNPs could be developed into a promising interventional strategy to limit and overcome the concerns of antibiotic-resistance.

Keywords: antibiotic resistance; bacterial pathogens; ESBLs; gold nanoparticles; nano-therapeutics

1. Introduction

Bacterial pathogens produce a class of enzymes known as extended-spectrum β-lactamases (ESBLs) that impart an enhanced resistance towards conventional antibiotics [1]. They are considered a serious clinical concern due to their role in increasing the mortality and morbidity rate in infected patients [2,3]. ESBL producers are involved in urinary tract infections, intra-abdominal infections, respiratory tract infections, and bacteremia [4]. They disarm the cephalosporin class of antibiotics by acting on the β-lactam ring, and substantially affect the therapeutic regime of the infected patient [5]. In addition, ESBLs might show resistance towards other classes of antibiotics (such as tetracyclines, aminoglycosides, trimethoprim, cotrimoxazole, and quinolones) as well, which further diminishes the therapeutic options for the clinicians [6]. However, enhanced mortality in these cases was often linked with inadequate diagnosis and inappropriate antibiotic therapy [7]. In fact, close genotypic observation revealed that ESBL genes have a tendency to transpose between the different pathogens, which eventually leads to resistant infection outbreaks.

The COVID-19 pandemic has given a strong lesson to the entire world to never neglect an impending threat, whether it is small or large. Regrettably, the warning raised by eminent scientists and the WHO about antibiotic resistance has been neglected for decades. Indeed, scientists have speculated antibiotic resistance as the next major issue after the COVID pandemic, and the WHO has listed antimicrobial resistance as one of the three most significant health threats to the worldwide population in the twenty-first century. According to the WHO, most of the resistance issue arises due to the inappropriate application of antibiotics. Thus, a better therapeutic strategy with applicable antibiotic stewardship programs is urgently warranted. The failure of conventional antibiotics, either by ESBLs or by other resistance mechanisms, demands the quest for ameliorated therapeutic options. Moreover, treating infections with the lowest possible dose could be the best possible approach for effective infection control [8]. Interestingly, nanomaterials could provide a plausible approach to deliver antibiotics effectively to resistant pathogens. The nanomaterials provide a large surface area-to-volume ratio that facilitates the binding of a number of ligands (antibiotic molecules) to prepare multivalent nanoparticles against bacterial pathogens [9,10]. In addition, nanomaterials themselves exhibit antibacterial properties via hindering the formation of biofilms, triggering reactive oxygen generation, and interacting with the cell wall, DNA, and proteins of a bacterial cell. As nanomaterials do not have a defined mode of action like antibiotics, they can be very useful for tackling resistance in bacterial pathogens [11]. One such nanomaterial that has been extensively explored against resistant bacterial pathogens is gold nanoparticles (AuNPs). Due to their distinctive properties, AuNPs have been used for other biomedical applications as well, such as diagnostics, colorimetric sensing, photo-therapy, bioimaging, and gene delivery [12,13]. Furthermore, AuNP synthesis does not require complex approaches; it usually involves the addition of a metal (AuCl4 salt) precursor with an appropriate reducing and stabilizing agent [14]. AuNPs bio-synthesis could be performed by using the extracts of plants and micro-organisms [15]. However, the successful grafting of an antibiotic molecule(s) onto the surface of AuNPs involves various strategies such as physical absorption, electrostatic interactions, coupling reactions, and Au -S or -N interactions [16].

AuNPs have been applied to deliver a variety of antibiotics in the past, such as ampicillin, ceftriaxone, cefotaxime, vancomycin, cefoxitin, delafloxacin, ciprofloxacin, levofloxacin, cefixime, cefotetan, colistin, amoxicillin, kanamycin, imipenem, meropenem, cefaclor, daptomycin, streptomycin, gentamycin, rifampicin, penicillin G, polymyxin B, gatifloxacin, norfloxacin, cephalexin, cefadroxil, and cefradine. These studies exhibited that the antibacterial potential of antibiotic-coated/or -conjugated AuNPs was significantly enhanced in comparison to the antibiotics alone (without AuNPs) against the tested bacterial pathogens [16–33]. Interestingly, some of these studies were conducted against highly resistant ESBL producer bacterial pathogens. In fact, AuNPs converted the unresponsive antibiotic into potent antibiotic gold nano-formulation against resistant ESBL strains. The use of AuNPs has certain advantages, such as how their synthesis and fabrication are easier, they are an excellent delivery tool for antibiotics, they lower the antibiotic dosage due to synergism, and they show broad spectrum activity (Figure 1).

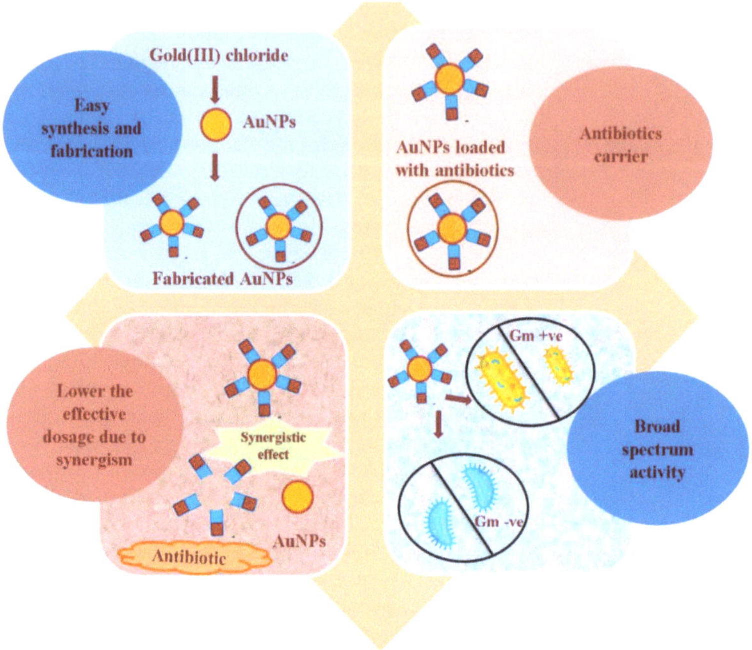

Figure 1. Advantages of AuNPs as a carrier of antibiotics.

However, the major bottlenecks in the clinical transformation of these findings are a lack of information on mechanistic and toxicity aspects. The present review aimed to cover all the viewpoints pertinent to the applicability of antibiotic-loaded AuNPs against ESBL- producing strains. Moreover, the review is subdivided into the following sections to provide a gist from the plethora of information without compromising the intellectual insight of the topic.

- Antibiotic-loaded AuNPs as magic bullets to overcome resistance
- Plausible antibacterial mechanism of AuNPs
- Clinical translation status and Toxicity aspects of AuNP-based drug delivery system
- Future prospects of antibiotic-loaded AuNPs
- Challenges associated with antibiotic-loaded AuNPs

2. Antibiotic-Loaded AuNPs as Magic Bullets to Overcome Resistance

AuNPs are inorganic nanomaterials that have been widely applied in different biomedical applications due to their unique attributes [34]. In addition, AuNPs could be easily synthesized by different chemical/physical or green synthesis approaches [35]. The core of any AuNP synthesis approach includes the reduction of Au+ to Au0 by the reductant, and further stabilization with a capping agent. During chemical synthesis, chemicals are used as a reducing agent; however, in green synthesis, micro-organisms, plant extracts, and enzymes are used instead of chemicals to reduce and stabilize AuNPs [36]. Due to the localized surface plasmon resonance (or oscillations of conduction electrons after irradiation with light) of AuNPs, different colors (light pink to dark purple) can be observed that can be further correlated with shape, size, and aggregation [37–45]. This property of AuNPs assists the researchers in selecting the appropriate nano-formulation for further analysis. However, the grafting of an antibiotic molecule(s) makes AuNPs a useful tool to deliver antibiotics effectively to the targeted bacterial pathogens. Recently, Khandelwal et al. [16] extensively reviewed several approaches of grafting (conjugating or coating) antibiotics onto AuNPs. In short, antibiotic attachment to AuNPs involves electrostatic interaction, coupling reaction, physical absorption, and Au-S or -N interaction [16]. Khandelwal and his team identified that sodium borohydride, trisodium citrate, hydrazine, certain micro-organisms, and enzymes were often used as reducing agents for the reduction of chloroauric acid into AuNPs (Figure 2a); further, antibiotics were used to cap/or stabilize the synthesized AuNPs to obtain the desired antibiotic nano-formulation.

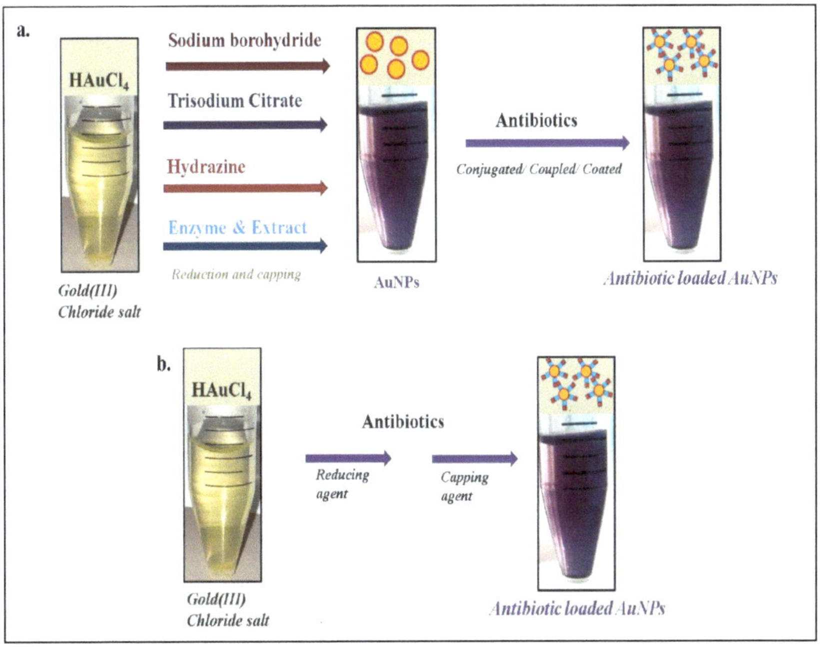

Figure 2. Various approaches used for the synthesis of antibiotic-loaded AuNPs. (**a**) Two or multi-step approach, (**b**) a single-step approach.

In the past, sodium borohydride has been used as a reducing agent for the synthesis of ampicillin, vancomycin, streptomycin, neomycin, gentamicin, and kanamycin AuNPs. However, conjugation for ampicillin was through Au-S interaction, and the authors reported that AuNPs were initially stabilized via citrate molecules, which were further replaced by a thioether moiety of ampicillin by mixing the AuNPs with ampicillin for 24 h [46]. In another study, chitosan was used as a stabilizing agent for AuNPs before preparing AuNP-stabilized vancomycin-loaded liposomes [47]. In addition, bovine serum albumin-capped AuNPs were used to prepare streptomycin, neomycin, gentamicin, and kanamycin conjugated AuNPs by physical adsorption via drop-wise addition of antibiotics in AuNPs solution [48]. On the other hand, trisodium citrate has also been explored as a reducing agent for the synthesis of ciprofloxacin, gentamicin, streptomycin, and neomycin AuNPs. Ciprofloxacin was conjugated with citrate-capped AuNPs through Au-N interaction, herein, N atom of –NH moiety of piperazine group of ciprofloxacin bound strongly onto the surface of AuNPs [49]. Similarly, gentamicin also conjugated with citrate capped-AuNPs via Au-N interactions, where the N atom of the amino group of gentamicin participated in AuNPs surface interaction [50]. Furthermore, citrate-capped AuNPs were mixed and stirred with streptomycin and neomycin to physically adsorb antibiotics on the surface of AuNPs [51]. All the above-discussed antibiotics were conjugated onto the surface of AuNPs without the use of any coupling agent, while a coupling agent such as EDC (1-ethyl-3-(-3-dimethylaminopropyl) carbodiimide) has been applied to attach gentamicin and cefotaxime to the surface of AuNPs. For gentamicin attachment through

EDC, the AuNPs were initially prepared by using hydrazine as a reducing agent followed by capping with glutathione [52], whereas for cefotaxime attachment via EDC, AuNPs were synthesized using bromelain enzyme as a reducing as well as capping agent [29].

Interestingly, in some reports, antibiotics themselves acted as reducing as well as capping agents (Figure 2b), such as bromelain, which eventually converted a two-step process into a facile one-step process [24–27]. An illustrative representation of the antibacterial action of revived antibiotics (after loading to AuNPs) is shown in Figure 3. This one-step strategy has actually eased the burden of the researchers working in the field of antibiotic nano-formulation and decreases the chances of doubts/errors in antibacterial results, as there is no probability of residual harmful chemicals/reducing agents (sodium borohydride, trisodium citrate, hydrazine) in the nano-formulation.

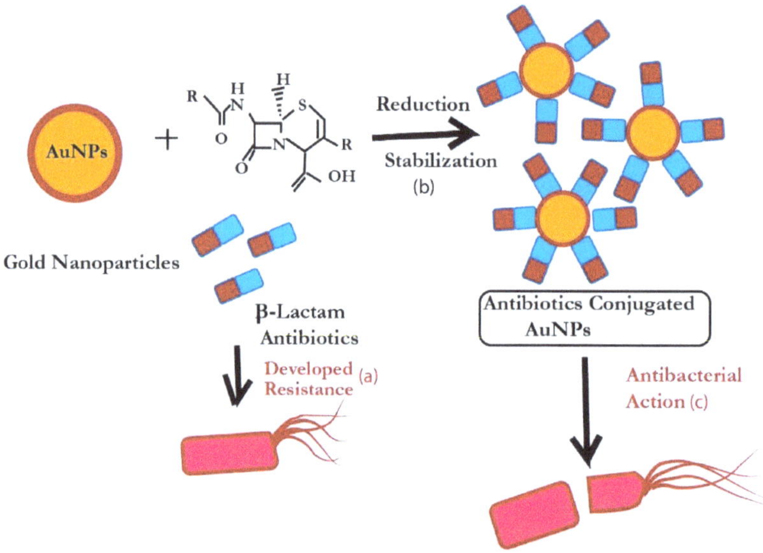

Figure 3. Schematic description of revival of β-lactam antibiotics by AuNPs. (**a**) Bacterial pathogens develop resistance towards β-lactam antibiotics; (**b**) AuNPs were synthesized using the same ineffective β-lactam antibiotic as reducing and stabilizing agent; (**c**) β-lactam antibiotic after loading to AuNPs become potent against the same β-lactam resistant bacterial pathogen.

Before moving forward, it is important to discuss the influence of the sizes and shapes of AuNPs on their antibacterial activity. AuNPs could be developed in different sizes and shapes [14,53–56]. However, sizes from 5 to 70 nm are considered to possess better antibacterial properties than bigger-sized AuNPs [24–29,53]. On the other hand, most of the researchers reported the spherical shape of AuNPs as the most potent antibacterial [24–29,53], but AuNPs can be polygonal-, star-, and flower-shaped as well [54]. In contrast, one report [54] suggested that gold nanoflowers were more active and safer than spherical-shaped AuNPs.

To attain a perfect size and shape, manipulation can be performed in experimental conditions such as pH, temperature, and concentration of reducing and capping agents. Low or acidic pH is usually considered unfavorable for AuNP synthesis, as it forms unstable and aggregating bigger AuNPs. A pH between 6 and 10 is considered most appropriate for AuNP synthesis [57]. Some of the methodologies required boiling or high temperature for AuNP synthesis, but the modification of temperature conditions could influence the size of AuNPs. In some reports, it was suggested that an increase in temperature would eventually increase the size of AuNPs [14]. In fact, temperature's influence on size depends on the type of methodology followed for the AuNP synthesis. The concentration of the reducing agent also influences the size of AuNPs; an increase in the concentration of bromelain and trypsin as reducing agents markedly increases the size of synthesized AuNPs [14,58]. Conclusively, it can be suggested that pH, if kept near to physiological pH, is better, the temperature has to be kept appropriate according to the protocol (sometimes protein is applied during synthesis and high temperature can denature it), and the amount of the reducing agent should be kept as low as possible according to the protocol.

There are numerous reports on the use of AuNPs for antibiotic delivery that are cumulated in Table 1.

Table 1. Antibiotic-loaded AuNPs against different bacterial pathogens.

Nanomaterial	Size and Shape	Targeted Bacteria	Efficacy	Remarks	Ref.
Vancomycin-AuNPs	Polygonal	*Vancomycin-resistant Enterococci*	MIC_{50} of Vancomycin-AuNPs was 2 μg/mL, which was significantly lower than free vancomycin	AuNPs developed have the ability of photothermal killing by irradiation	[17]
Ampicillin-AuNPs	25–50 nm and spherical	*S. aureus, E. coli, B. subtilis, Flavobacteria devorans*	4- and 16-fold increase in activity of ampicillin-AuNPs against amp-resistant and amp-sensitive strains, respectively	Ampicillin-mediated AuNP synthesis, where β−lactam ring remains intact for its action after attachment	[18]
Colistin-AuNPs	5 nm and spherical	*E. coli*	6-times reduction in MIC concentration compared to free colistin	Anionic AuNPs were used to deliver colistin that showed activity at very low dose compared to colistin alone	[20]
Azithromycin/ Streptomycin with AuNPs	20–40 nm and spherical	Clinical *Staphylococcus* spp.	Significant improvement in antibacterial activity in comparison to free antibiotics	Synergistic effect was observed after combining AuNPs with antibiotics	[21]
Ciprofloxacin-AuNPs	10–20 nm and spherical	MDR *K. pneumoniae* MDR *E. coli*	Synergistic antibacterial effect	Bacterial efflux pump is targeted along with usual antibacterial action	[22,23]
Cefotaxime-AuNPs	65 nm and spherical	*E. coli, K. oxytoca, S. aureus, P. aeruginosa*	Marked reduction in MIC concentration was observed against all the tested strains in comparison to free cefotaxime	Cefotaxime-mediated AuNP synthesis, where more than 80% of cefotaxime was loaded and showed potent activity against both gm + ve and gm -ve bacteria	[24]
Ceftriaxone-AuNPs	21 nm and spherical	*E. coli, S. aureus, S. abony, K. pneumoniae*	Significantly (2-fold) better potential against the tested strains in comparison to free ceftriaxone	Ceftriaxone-mediated AuNP synthesis, where 79% of ceftriaxone was loaded and showed potent activity against both gm +ve and gm -ve bacteria	[25]
Cefoxitin-AuNPs	2–12 nm and spherical	ESBL +ve *E. coli, K. pneumoniae*	Marked potency against cefoxitin-resistant strains of *E. coli* and *K. pneumoniae*	Cefoxitin-mediated AuNP synthesis, where 70% of cefoxitin was loaded and showed potent activity against uropathogenic resistant gram -ve strains	[26]

Table 1. *Cont.*

Nanomaterial	Size and Shape	Targeted Bacteria	Efficacy	Remarks	Ref.
Delafloxacin -AuNPs	16 nm and spherical	*E. coli*, *P. aeruginosa S. aureus* *B. subtilis*	Potent antibacterial activity against all the tested gram +ve and -ve strains in comparison to free delafloxacin	Delafloxacin-mediated AuNP synthesis, where around 90% of delafloxacin was loaded and showed more potent activity against gram -ve strains as compared to gram +ve strains	[27]
Cefaclor-AuNPs	22 nm and spherical	*S. aureus*, *E. coli*	Marked increase in potency against both the tested strains	Cefaclor-mediated AuNP synthesis, where AuNPs form pores in the cell wall and ample cefaclor was available for its antibacterial action	[28]
Cefotaxime-AuNPs	17.55 nm And spherical	CTX-M-15 positive *E. coli*, *K. pneumoniae*	Increased potency against CTX-M-15 positive resistant bacterial strains	Cefotaxime was conjugated on bromelain synthesized AuNPs with the help of coupling agent EDC and showed potent activity against resistant gram -ve strains	[29]
Imipenem/Meropenem-AuNPs	35–200 nm	*K.pneumoniae*, *P.mirabilis*, *A. baumanii*	Marked augmentation in antibacterial activity against all the tested strains	Carbapenem antibiotics were loaded on citrate stabilized AuNPs, and reduced the MIC of Imipenem by 4-fold and meropenem by 3-fold	[30]
Amoxicillin-AuNPs	33.9 nm	*Methicillin-resistant S. aureus*	Enhanced potency against MRSA, and less cytototoxicy in in vivo study	Amoxicillin was loaded on herbal synthesized AuNPs and showed potency to overcome β-lactamase-mediated resistance in MRSA	[31]
Vancomycin-AuNPs and Vancomycin AgNPs	11 nm	*Methicillin-resistant S. aureus*	2.4- to 4.8-fold increase in antibacterial activity of AgNPs than AuNPs against MRSA	Vancomycin AgNPs were more effective than vancomycin AuNPs against MRSA	[32]
Daptomycin-AuNPs	80 nm	*E. coli*, *S. aureus*	Antibacterial inhibition rates were 64% and 52% for *S. aureus* and *E. coli*, respectively	Near-infra-red radiation caused significant photothermal inhibition of bacterial growth	[33]

However, the next section elaborates on some of the major findings on antibiotic-loaded AuNPs. The formulation of Au–silica core–shell mesoporous NPs along with silica mesoporous NPs in conjugation with amoxicillin were evaluated for the bactericidal potential against methicillin-resistant *S. aureus* (MRSA), *E. coli*, and *P. aeruginosa*. Both the stated nanocarriers played an imperative role in delivering antibiotics to the bacteria. Approximately a decline of 10 times and 20 times was reported in the effective quantity of amoxicillin against *P. aeruginosa* by using Au–silica core–shell mesoporous and silica mesoporous NPs, respectively [59]. In another study, doxycycline was conjugated with PEGylated-AuNPs, and MIC values were reduced remarkably from 32 μg/mL to 2 μg/mL against *S. aureus*, *E. faecalis*, and *E. faecium* [60].

The single-step process to synthesize AuNPs was applied in an investigation to avert the interference of reducing chemicals by using antibiotics (kanamycin, ampicillin, and streptomycin) as reducing and capping agents. The MIC concentrations of antibiotics-capped AuNPs and free antibiotics were evaluated against *S. aureus*, *E. coli*, and *M. luteus*. MIC was markedly reduced in the case of aminoglycosides after coating to AuNPs. MIC value of streptomycin was reduced from 14 to 7 μg/mL and 22 to 17 μg/mL against *E. coli* and *M. luteus*, respectively, after loading onto AuNPs. However, MIC values of kanamycin were reduced from 30 to 12 μg/mL, 32.5 to 23 μg/mL, and 9 to 5.8 μg/mL against *E. coli*, *M. luteus*, and *S. aureus*, respectively. In fact, a marked decline of 60% was observed in the case of kanamycin-loaded AuNPs in comparison to kanamycin alone [61]. Ampicillin-AuNPs in this report not showing any significance might be due to its fast precipitation from the suspension. In contrast, Chavan and his team used ampicillin (where ampicillin acted as a reducing and stabilizing agent) to produce ampicillin-capped AuNPs, and showed potent activity against an ampicillin-resistant strain of *E. coli* [18]. Additionally, ampicillin was once coupled on chitosan-capped AuNPs; it showed a 2-fold (50%) reduction in MIC values as compared to ampicillin alone against *S. aureus*, *E. coli*, and *K. mobilis* [62]. Recently, other researchers have also applied the one-step synthesis approach to produce cefaclor-, cefotaxime-, delafloxacin-, vancomycin-, and ceftriaxone-loaded AuNPs and observed marked differences in MIC against the resistant bacterial pathogens [24–26,63].

Fayaz and team attached vancomycin to fungal (*Trichoderma viride*) bio-synthesized AuNPs, and compared its activity with vancomycin alone against vancomycin-resistant *S. aureus*, *S. aureus*, and *E. coli* [64]. Vancomycin after attachment to AuNPs showed a reduction in MIC values from 175 to 40 μg/mL, 2 to 1.5 μg/mL, and 50 to 8 μg/mL against *E. coli*, *S. aureus*, and vancomycin-resistant *S. aureus*, respectively. In another study, vancomycin-capped AuNPs were synthesized and explored for their activity against vancomycin-resistant strains (*E. coli*, *E. faecalis*, and *E. faecium*). There is a significant decrease observed in MIC, i.e., shifted from 128 μg/mL to 2 μg/mL [65]. Like the fungal biosynthesis approach, *Rosa damascenes* petal extract was also reported for AuNPs biosynthesis, and the AuNPs were subsequently conjugated with ceftriaxone (Cef-AuNPs). The efficacies of these synthesized nanoparticles were further evaluated for their anticancer (against human breast cancer cells) and bactericidal effects (against ESBL-producing bacteria). It was found that Cef-AuNPs exhibited relatively low anticancer effects; however, conjugation of ceftriaxone on AuNPs restored the activity of ceftriaxone in otherwise resistant bacterial cells [66]. In addition, Pradeepa et al. reported the biosynthesis of AuNPs with exopolysaccharide isolated from *Lactobacillus plantarum*, and their subsequent functionalization with ceftriaxone, ciprofloxacin, cefotaxime, and levofloxacin. These AuNPs exhibited considerable bactericidal effects against multi-drug resistant *S. aureus*, *E. coli*, and *K. pneumoniae*. Among all nano-formulations, the ciprofloxacin-conjugated AuNPs were most active against *E. coli* and *K. pneumoniae*, whereas levofloxacin-conjugated AuNPs were potent against S. aureus [22]. All the antibiotics (alone) tested have MIC values of more than 10 μg/mL; however, MIC values were markedly reduced when they were grafted on AuNPs. Here, levofloxacin-loaded AuNPs were most effective against *S. aureus* (MIC: 0.562 μg/mL), ciprofloxacin-loaded AuNPs were most effective against *K. pneumoniae* (MIC: 0.281 μg/mL) and *E. coli* (MIC: 0.140 μg/mL), and ceftriaxone-loaded AuNPs were most potent against *K. pneumoniae* (MIC: 0.281 μg/mL) [22].

Most of the antibiotics discussed above belong to the β-lactams family, and can be correlated with ESBL-associated resistance, as shown in Table 1. However, some of the studies have mentioned the use of genetically identified ESBL-positive strains for antibacterial analysis. Shaikh et al. conjugated cefotaxime on bromelain enzyme-synthesized AuNPs and tested it on ESBL (CTX-M) positive strains of *E. coli* and *K. pneumoniae* [29]. Importantly, the strains tested were totally resistant to cefotaxime, and acquired sensitivity towards cefotaxime once it was loaded on AuNPs. In simple terms, AuNPs restored the potential of unresponsive cefotaxime. Here, MIC of cefotaxime after loading onto AuNPs was estimated to be 1 and 2 μg/mL against *E. coli* and *K. pneumoniae*, respectively. Recently, Alafnan et al. also applied cefoxitin-loaded AuNPs against ESBL positive cefoxitin-resistant strains of *E. coli* and *K. pneumoniae*, and observed a prominent shift of MIC from 19.5 to 1.5 μg/mL and 23 μg/mL to 2.5 μg/mL against *E. coli* and *K. pneumoniae*, respectively [26].

All these interesting reports confirmed the potency of AuNPs as a tool to combat bacterial resistance, and prompted the deciphering of the plausible mechanism of action of these antibiotic-loaded AuNPs. However, this section mainly pinpointed that antibiotics, once loaded or attached to AuNPs, become significantly active against the bacterial pathogen that was earlier resistant to the same antibiotic. This was evident from a marked decrease in MIC values against resistant pathogens. In some reports, bacterial pathogens were completely resistant at the tested concentration of antibiotic; however, once the antibiotics loaded on AuNPs at the same concentration become resuscitated, they become potent antibacterials. In addition, the methods applied for the synthesis of these nano-antibiotics were quite simple and convenient. Thus, it could be stated that the nano-conversion of antibiotics through AuNPs could revive ineffective antibiotics into potent ones.

3. Plausible Antibacterial Mechanism of AuNPs

The ability of AuNPs to interact with various biomolecules of the bacterial cell provides an added advantage to the antibiotic that is loaded onto them. In simple terms, AuNPs not only ease the entry of antibiotics into the bacterial pathogen, but also provide synergistic effects. There are several investigations that prove the synergism concept. In one study, *Garcinia mangostana* extract was used to bio-synthesize AuNPs, which was further conjugated with antibiotics. Biosynthesized AuNPs (without any antibiotic) did not show any significant antibacterial activity against *Pseudomonas* spp. and *Staphylococcus* spp. However, AuNPs conjugated with streptomycin and azithromycin exhibited enhanced bactericidal efficacy (33.3% and 34.8%, respectively) against *Staphylococcus* spp., as compared to free streptomycin and azithromycin. On the other hand, the conjugation of azithromycin and penicillin with AuNPs augmented their bactericidal efficacy (50% and 75%, respectively) against *Pseudomonas* spp. [67]. Furthermore, it was also reported that AuNPs in combination with antibiotics such as Clavulanate/Amoxy were effective at lower concentrations compared to the effective concentration required by Clavulanate/Amoxy or AuNPs alone [68]. AuNPs can exert their bactericidal effects by different mechanisms, and at the same time, effectively delivers a sufficient amount of antibiotic to perform their antibacterial action. An important aspect of the antibacterial action of AuNPs is that it is not properly defined. This is one sought-after advantage as bacteria usually develop resistance against a particular mechanism of action, and the development of resistance against AuNPs is quite impossible due to their undefined multivalent mode of action.

There are four major mechanisms followed by bacterial pathogens to acquire resistance: i.e., reducing the uptake of antibiotics, effluxing antibiotics once they enter, antibiotics inactivation, and modifying antibiotic targets [69]. ESBL enzymes are mainly linked with the inactivation of antibiotics by breaking the β-lactam ring. However, reports suggested their close association with efflux pumps and reduced uptake [70–73] as well. Thus, ESBL producer bacterial pathogens can acquire resistance by three out of the four well-established mechanisms. Importantly, AuNPs can directly/or indirectly work on all these mechanisms of resistance (Figure 4). Moreover, the antibacterial action of AuNPs on each resistance mechanism has been discussed in the section below.

3.1. Reduction in the Antibiotic Uptake by ESBLs Producing Bacterial Pathogens

Usually, the β-lactam antibiotics enter bacterial pathogens through the porin channels [74–77]. However, bacterial pathogens modify the porin channels to reduce the uptake of β-lactam antibiotics. In a recent study, different ESBL types (TEM-1, SHV-1, CTX-M-15, OXA-48, and VIM-1) were reported in clinical pathogenic strains of *E. coli* and *K. pneumoniae*. In addition, the authors investigated the role of porins (outer membrane proteins) in these ESBL-positive strains. The porin analysis confirmed that about 95.7% and 93.3% of strains of *K. pneumoniae* and *E. coli* either modified or lost their porins. Moreover, the genetic analysis revealed the reason as mutation (frameshift), which eventually translated small-size truncated porin proteins [78]. In a similar study, the role of porins was examined for ESBL-positive strains of *K. pneumoniae* and *E. coli*, and cephalosporins (ceftazidime and cefoxitin) resistance was strongly correlated with the loss of type Omp-K35 porins [79]. In 2008, Martínez-Martínez reviewed the correlation between cell permeability and ESBLs. The author discussed the role of two porin proteins (Omp-K35 and Omp-K36) in ESBL-positive strains of *K. pneumoniae*. Interestingly, the loss of both these proteins was involved in the resistance of β-lactam antibiotics (cephalosporins, carbapenems, and ertapenem) as well as a non-β-lactam antibiotic (fluoroquinolones) [80]. Here, the role of AuNPs is to deliver the antibiotic efficiently to the target pathogens by crossing the cell barrier.

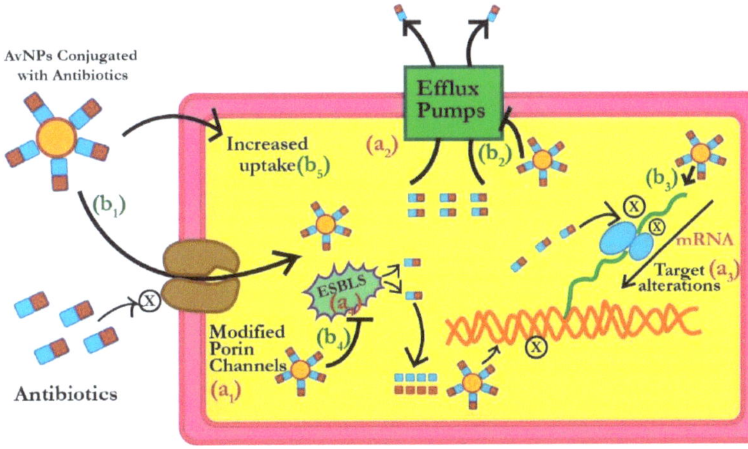

Figure 4. Comparison between (**a**) *bacterial resistance mechanism* and (**b**) *plausible mechanism of action of AuNPs to overcome resistance*. (**a1**) Modification of porins to hinder the entry of antibiotics, whereas (**b1**) same antibiotics, once loaded to AuNPs, gain easy entry into the bacterial pathogen; (**a2**) efflux of antibiotics from bacteria to outside of the cell, whereas (**b2**) inhibition of efflux pumps/decreasing expression of efflux pump genes by AuNPs; (**a3**) alteration of antibiotic target site, whereas, (**b3**) indirect/direct targeting of bacterial biomolecules by AuNPs; (**a4**) Antibiotic inactivating enzymes (ESBLs), whereas (**b4**) saturation of enzymes or direct damage to the enzyme structure by AuNPs. In addition, (**b5**) AuNPs can directly interact with the cell barriers, causing perforation and cell lysis.

Tailored AuNPs have the ability to disrupt the cell membrane integrity and permeability. AuNPs could initially interact with the outer membrane proteins and lipopolysaccharides, and be deposited on the cell surface of the pathogens [28,81]. Further, they can slowly be translocated inside through porin channels or diffuse through the cell membrane [28,82,83]. An earlier investigation has clearly outlined the efficacy of AuNPs in instigating the disruption of bacterial cell membranes, which subsequently results in bacterial death [84,85]. Indeed, Zhao et al. investigated the potential of 4, 6-diamino-2-pyrimidinethiol (DAPT) capped AuNPs against *E. coli*. They observed that free DAPT is devoid of any antibacterial effects; however, when *E. coli* was exposed to DAPT-AuNPs, approximately 70% of the *E. coli* cells exhibited enhanced membrane permeability. Contrastingly, only 5% of the *E. coli* cells were found to be positive for such alteration of permeability in the control group. In addition, exposure to DAPT-AuNPs led to similar effects on *P. aeruginosa*. Moreover, it was observed that DAPT-AuNPs also facilitated the formation of vesicles from the outer membrane of bacterial cells. Eventually, the investigators concluded that DAPT-AuNPs exerted their bactericidal effects by altering the concentration of magnesium ions and subsequently chelating them [85,86]. Another report outlined that the divergent pattern of AuNPs aggregation was responsible for the lysis of *B. subtilis* and *E. coli* [86]. This observation was also supported by the study of Adhikari et al., where they concluded that increasing AuNPs concentration could concomitantly increase the alteration of bacterial cell permeability [87]. In one study, vancomycin alone could not pervade the outer membrane of *E. coli*; however, when added to AuNPs, it showed a promising antibacterial effect [88]. The authors suggested that AuNPs were able to perforate the cells by altering the permeability and stability of the cell membrane, thus allowing vancomycin to be efficiently delivered to the pathogen.

3.2. Efflux of Antibiotics by ESBLs Producing Bacterial Pathogens

Once the antibiotic enters the bacterial cells, they use efflux pumps to reduce the antibiotic load. Interestingly, efflux pumps have shown a correlation to ESBL-producing strains [70]. Maurya and his team [70], while working on ESBL-positive clinical isolates of *K. pneumoniae*, observed the overexpression of efflux pumps (belonging to the RND family) in the tested strains. They concluded that ESBLs were not the only factor against β-lactam antibiotics; efflux pumps also effectively participate in developing resistance. Another investigation also confirmed these findings by applying an efflux pump inhibitor on an ESBL-positive strain. MIC values for cefotaxime, ceftazidime, and amoxy-clavulanic acid were markedly reduced after using the efflux pump inhibitor on resistant *K. pneumoniae* [89]. It is noteworthy to mention that AuNPs can be applied against the efflux pumps as well. Recently, Dorri et al. [90] observed the effect of AuNPs on the efflux pump genes of *Pseudomonas aeruginosa*. They elucidated that AuNPs could reduce the expression of several efflux pumps on the bacterial cell surface by downregulating MexA and MexB efflux pump genes. On the other hand, Khare and his team [23] observed the significant synergistic effect of embelin-capped chitosan-AuNPs along with ciprofloxacin on the efflux pumps of *P. aeruginosa* and *E. coli*.

3.3. Inactivation of Antibiotics by ESBLs Producing Bacterial Pathogens

ESBL enzymes are known for the inactivation of β-lactam antibiotics. Once β-lactam antibiotics enter the ESBL-producing pathogens, ESBL enzymes disarm them by hydrolyzing the β-lactam ring. There are several reports that showed β-lactam antibiotics, once attached to AuNPs, become potent in ESBL-producing resistant strains [Table 1]. However, this change in potency against resistant strains is due to the synergistic effect of AuNPs and β-lactam antibiotics attached to them. Here, two interesting facts about the AuNP-based β-lactam antibiotic delivery system have to be noted: (1) After capping or conjugation, the active part of the antibiotic (β-lactam ring) remains intact and exposed on the AuNPs surface [16,28,91]. (2) Due to the large surface area-to-volume ratio of AuNPs, an ample amount of β-lactam antibiotic molecules can be loaded on them [92,93]. Based on these above findings, the authors proposed that the bacterial pathogens received a sufficient quantity of β-lactam antibiotic that could saturate the ESBLs, and at the same time, antibiotic molecules that remain untouched by ESBLs might start their usual action on cell wall synthesis. In addition, AuNPs have the inherent ability to alter the structure and function of enzymes via interacting with them [94–98]; thus, it might be speculated that AuNPs could interact with ESBLs enzyme directly and disrupt their function.

Apart from AuNPs' interaction with bacterial enzymes/proteins, they have the ability to directly interact with bacterial DNA as well. AuNPs have been reported to enhance bacterial DNA fragmentation by 19.68% in *E. coli*, and showed an apoptotic-like cell death mechanism [99–101]. In addition, AuNPs could increase the expression of a caspase-like protein in *E. coli* that eventually induces ROS and SOS responses, leading to bacterial apoptosis [101]. In fact, some of the authors suggested that increased ROS generation by AuNPs might be responsible for antibacterial potential [39,102]. Contrarily, it has been suggested that instead of ROS generation, AuNPs can cause redox imbalance by reducing glutathione, and cause damage to the bacterial antioxidant system [101]. Thus, AuNPs have the ability to attack the pathogen by alternate pathways, even if the bacterial pathogen has modified the antibiotic target site.

This section deals with the mechanistic aspect of the antibacterial action of antibiotic-loaded AuNPs. The reports revealed that AuNPs not only deliver the antibiotic successfully to the resistant pathogen, but work in synergy with the antibiotic to increase the antibacterial effect. In addition, after the loading of antibiotics onto the AuNPs, the resistance mechanism of the pathogens could be overcome in various ways. In fact, AuNPs could work smartly on each antibiotic resistance mechanism of bacterial pathogens to provide the maximum antibacterial effect. Bacterial pathogens have the ability to develop resistance against the defined mechanism of action of any antimicrobial agent with time; thus, the multi-targeting ability of AuNPs or undefined mechanism of action could be considered a blessing in disguise. The present review tried to propose the best plausible mechanism of action of AuNPs (or antibiotic-loaded AuNPs) based on previous investigations. However, the work on the exact mechanism of action of antibiotic-loaded AuNPs is still obscure and needs to be deciphered.

4. Clinical Translation Status and Toxicity Aspects of AuNP-Based Drug Delivery System

4.1. Clinical Translation Status

Before discussing the clinical translation status, glimpses of some recent global market trends about AuNPs need to be shared. The global market of AuNPs has reached about USD 4.4 billion in the year 2021, and is further expected to reach around USD 8 billion by the year 2027 [103,104]. Several companies such as Sigma-Aldrich, Goldsol, Cytodiagnostics, NanoHybrids, ParticleWorks, BBI Solutions, and Metalor Technologies are applying AuNPs for various purposes [105]. These market trends directly suggest that AuNPs have enormous potential if utilized appropriately. AuNP-based Verigene® system has already obtained approval and is used for genotyping different genes in DNA samples [106]. There are so many clinical trials going on to establish an AuNP-based therapeutic system. Some are in Phase I, such as pro-insulin functionalized on AuNPs (C19-A3 AuNP), T-cell priming cocktails of dengue virus peptides functionalized on AuNPs (naNO-DENGUE), TNF functionalized on PEGylated AuNPs (CYT-6091), and T-cell priming cocktails of coronavirus peptides functionalized on AuNPs (naNO-COVID); however, CNM-Au8 (AuNP in drinkable bicarbonate solution) is in Phase II of clinical trials [NCT04935801]. These AuNPs are applied in different diseases, such as C19-A3 AuNP in autoimmune diabetes, naNO-DENGUE in dengue fever, CYT-6091 in tumors, naNO-COVID in COVID-19, and CNM-Au8 in neurodegenerative diseases [NCT00356980]. There are some other examples as well, such as AuroShell (for different cancer types), NU-0129 (for glioblastoma), and Nanoshell (for atherosclerotic plaques), that are undergoing different stages of clinical trials [107]. Although antibiotic-conjugated AuNPs have not undergone clinical trials, there is a strong probability that they will soon be applied in various antibacterial preparations. However, the lack of investigations on the toxicity aspects of AuNPs and doubt about their fate in the human body are considered major obstacles to the successful conversion of lab-bench findings into bedside medications. The next section covers the toxicity aspects of AuNPs.

4.2. Toxicity Aspects

The scientific literature surveyed in the present review indicated that in the majority of investigations, AuNPs were found to be relatively less toxic chemically. Nevertheless, certain reports have also outlined the potential toxicity of these AuNPs, which is critically governed by the charge, shape, surface chemistry, and size of the synthesized AuNPs. A previously published report elucidated that AuNPs conjugated with ligands, namely $Ph_2PC_6H_4SO_3Na$ and $P(C_6H_4SO_3Na)_3$, showed cytotoxic effects against different cells. It was further shown that smaller AuNPs exhibited approximately 60-fold enhanced cytotoxic effects compared to 15 nm size AuNPs. During an extended study, the same research group demonstrated that AuNPs capped with triphenylphosphine mono-sulfonate (size of 1.4 nm) induced the production of reactive oxygen species (ROS), which subsequently augmented inflammatory mediators resulting in the onset of mitochondria-mediated apoptotic cell death in human cervical carcinoma HeLa cells [108]. Indeed, a report from a different lab also showed that AuNPs having a size of 1.4 nm exhibited high binding affinities towards the DNA of normal as well as cancer cells [109].

Studies by Mironava et al. made it evident that AuNPs having a radius of 13 nm–45 nm fail to enter either the mitochondria or nucleus of human-derived dermal fibroblast cells. Furthermore, their report also indicated that AuNPs within the stated range are localized within the cytoplasmic vacuoles, and AuNPs of around 45 nm instigated increased cellular damage owing to their different uptake and release mechanisms in the cytoplasm [110]. Contrastingly, the shape of AuNPs also plays an important role in regulating drug delivery. It has been demonstrated that spherical AuNPs are more efficiently absorbed than rod-shaped AuNPs [111]. Another important aspect regulating nanoparticle-mediated drug delivery is the charge of nanoparticles. Goodman et al. explicitly showed that nanoparticles bearing a positive charge exert enhanced cytotoxic effects in comparison with negatively charged nanoparticles [112]. In addition, some reports have indicated that the surface chemistry of AuNPs is a more effective mediator of AuNPs toxicity than the charge of AuNPs (alone). This notion is also supported by a study where it was observed that positively charged poly(diallyldimethyl ammonium chloride)-coated AuNPs were more bio-compatible with the cell membrane in comparison to positively charged cetyl trimethylammonium bromide coated AuNPs [113].

Interestingly, some literature has outlined the importance of AuNPs' size and charge in regulating their biodistribution and absorption in different animal models. Several studies concluded that small AuNPs with a negative charge exhibit the highest absorption rate, and thus have distribution in an array of organs within the animals [112–115]. In addition, it has become evident that the shape and capping of AuNPs have also affected their bio-distribution in animal models [115,116]. In contrast, studies have reported the accumulation of AuNPs in the liver and spleen irrespective of their surface chemistry and charge [116,117]. In fact, kidney homeostasis was also affected by exposure to AuNPs. AuNPs also induce size-dependent damaging effects in renal cells where smaller particles have substantial damage in comparison to large particles [116–118]. Moreover, it is now well-established that the route of administration of AuNPs could influence the cytotoxic effects in model animals. It was previously reported that the toxic effects of AuNPs were aggravated after oral and intraperitoneal administration in comparison to administration via the tail vein [119].

It is to be noted that AuNPs genotoxicity has been evaluated in Zebra fish models, and administration of positively charged N,N,N-trimethylammoniumethane thiol stabilized AuNPs instigated disruption in development and pigmentation of the eyes that was concomitantly followed by impaired behavioral attributes with distinctive neuronal damage [120]. Moreover, a previous report has substantiated that AuNPs having a size of 15 nm were competent in inducing phenotypic mutations within generations of *Drosophila melanogaster*, thereby indicating that mutagenic effects of AuNPs can be further transmitted to progenies [121,122]. It is thus evident that there are a large number of contradicting reports available in the scientific database regarding the toxicity of AuNPs; therefore, it is difficult to generalize their important toxicity issues. The investigations reported in the present review indicated some evident issues regarding AuNPs toxicity; nevertheless, it also showed that the toxicity of AuNPs depends collectively on the preparatory methods and physiochemical attributes of AuNPs. Moreover, before concluding any holistic inferences, more elaborative investigations are further warranted for an in-depth understanding of mechanisms regulating the changes in physiochemical aspects of AuNPs within a living system.

This section summarizes the clinical translation status and toxicity aspects of AuNPs. Companies are investing in AuNPs for different applications, and clinical trials are going-on in different phases. Most of the clinical trials have been conducted on fabricated AuNPs against non-infectious diseases, and some are conducted for viral infections. To date, antibiotic-loaded AuNPs have not reached any of the phases of clinical trials. Nevertheless, the results of fabricated AuNPs clinical trials have provided some strong optimism for AuNP-based therapy. Toxicity, biodistribution, and targeting are major obstacles in any drug development process. It is evident from the reports that AuNPs toxicity and distribution majorly depend on the fabrication or modification of the surface. However, antibiotic-loaded AuNPs have not been thoroughly studied for toxicity and biodistribution. Thus, the toxicity of antibiotic-loaded AuNPs could be considered one of the translational gaps in AuNP-based nano-antibiotic development.

5. Future Prospects of Antibiotic-Loaded or -Conjugated Gold Nanoparticles

Till now, this review has substantially compiled and discussed the published research and progress pertinent to antibiotic-loaded AuNPs. However, the question still remains the same: 'Could AuNPs be clinically applied to tackle the superbugs threatening our life?'. The answer to this question will not just be confined to simply saying yes or no. It has been clearly discussed in the above sections that AuNPs are versatile in their ways of interactions with bacteria and their cellular components, and further, their control over their resistance mechanisms. Interestingly, there are various reports suggesting AuNPs' potential as an efficient tool to deliver antibiotics to the pathogen and significantly reduce its effective MIC concentration. However, the mode of action of antibiotic-loaded AuNPs still needs to be fully deciphered and validated. In addition, a substantial focus has to be shifted to deciphering the safety of AuNP-based antibiotic delivery systems. In fact, long-term in vitro and in vivo biosafety experiments have to be designed to translate and guide the successful transformation of research findings into clinical applications. Standardization of experimentations is another area that requires significant improvement in order to perform comparative studies. Nevertheless, it is also a fact that AuNPs are presenting new hope in the current scenario, where clinicians have become helpless against resistant bacterial infections due to the lack of availability of effective therapeutic options. It is strongly anticipated that AuNP-based therapeutic options against antibiotic-resistant pathogens have the capability to overcome resistance from society if utilized in an effective manner.

6. Challenges Associated with Antibiotic-Loaded or -Conjugated Gold Nanoparticles

It is quite clear from the earlier sections that AuNPs could be easily fabricated and loaded with the desired antibiotic(s) by various approaches. In addition, their complete characterization before and after the loading of antibiotics has become convenient nowadays. Moreover, there is a plethora of research that confirmed antibiotic-loaded AuNPs as smart and effective antibacterial agents against resistant pathogens. However, there are still certain challenges that have to be overcome before considering them as the best arsenal against resistant pathogens. The major challenges are as follows: (1) the safety of antibiotic-loaded AuNPs; (2) large-scale production and processing; and (3) cost-effectiveness over antibiotic treatment.

There are several clinical trials going on to evaluate the potential of AuNP-based therapy, but none of them are on antibiotic-loaded AuNPs. The safety profile of antibiotic-loaded AuNPs is not fully investigated, and animal model evaluation studies are still undergoing. More biodistribution and pharmacokinetics studies on these antibiotic-loaded AuNPs have to be designed, as it has been observed that AuNPs have a tendency to aggregate at the site of inoculation. In addition, mistargeting is one of the aspects linked with nanoparticles; hence, this point also needs to be considered while designing antibiotic-loaded AuNPs.

The scenario of large-scale production of nanomedicine is quite different from the laboratory level. Large-scale production requires cost-effective approaches, large equipment, skilled technicians, and a quality control/assurance unit. Although many big industries have started investing in AuNPs for various applications in the last decade, pharma giants also need to step up and show interest in the development of nano-antibiotics from antibiotic-loaded AuNPs. In addition, different approaches for the conversion of these AuNPs from lab scale to industrial scale in the best possible way have to be developed.

The most important question is the cost effectiveness of AuNP-based antibiotics compared to available antibiotic options. AuNP development is itself a costly affair; hence, ways need to be developed to reduce the cost of AuNP-based nano-antibiotics formulation.

Earlier, Zhang et al. [123] nicely reviewed the antimicrobial activity of AuNPs, and covered some aspects of the antimicrobial activity of AuNPs in combination with antibiotics. However, the present review provided detailed information specifically on antibiotic-loaded or conjugated-AuNPs. The review covered the synthesis aspect, provided an opinion on the best possible way of synthesis, tried to cover almost all antibiotic-loaded AuNPs to date, designed the plausible mechanism of action based on the literature, experiences, and understanding, suggested the mechanism to overcome resistance in pathogens, and discussed the bottlenecks for clinical translation and future prospects. All the information pertinent to the above-mentioned topics from July 2001 to November 2022 has been collected, reviewed, interpreted, and summarized on one platform exclusively for antibiotic-loaded AuNPs. In fact, these aspects make the review quite different from the earlier reviews conducted on AuNPs.

7. Conclusions

The advent of nanotechnology has seen a surge in its advancement and usage to cater to the growing need for clinical interventions, primarily in cases of infectious diseases due to the increasing global prevalence of antibiotic resistance. Undoubtedly, conjugation/coating of several antibiotics onto AuNPs has demonstrated elevated antibacterial efficacy against resistant bacterial pathogens. Indeed, simple alteration in the attributes of AuNPs has allowed the investigators to develop novel antibacterial formulations that could plausibly be applied in clinical settings. The mechanistic aspect of the antibacterial action of AuNPs revealed that AuNPs could help to mitigate each and every perspective of antibacterial resistance. Importantly, preclinical findings on AuNPs are gradually moving towards clinical evaluations, and R&D sections of big industries are showing keen interest in these updates. Still, mechanistic details of its action, its fate inside the human body, and biosafety are the segments that need special attention. However, AuNPs are one of the most promising hopes against antibiotic resistance that require proper exploration to be translated from bench to bedside.

Author Contributions: Conceptualization, S.M.D.R. and A.S.A.L.; validation, A.M., T.H., and H.S.; formal analysis, M.A.K.; resources, H.S.; writing—original draft preparation, S.M.D.R., A.S.A.L., and A.M.; writing—review and editing, T.H., M.A.K., H.S., and E.-S.K.; visualization, E.-S.K.; supervision, S.M.D.R.; project administration, A.S.A.L.; funding acquisition, S.M.D.R. All authors have read and agreed to the published version of the manuscript.

Funding: This research has been funded by the Scientific Research Deanship at the University of Ha'il, Saudi Arabia, through project number MDR-22 008.

Institutional Review Board Statement: Not applicable.

Informed Consent Statement: Not applicable.

Data Availability Statement: Not applicable.

Acknowledgments: This research has been funded by Scientific Research Deanship at the University of Ha'il-Saudi Arabia through project number MDR-22 008.

Conflicts of Interest: The authors declare no conflict of interest.

References

1. Shah, A.A.; Hasan, F.; Ahmed, S.; Hameed, A. Characteristics, epidemiology and clinical importance of emerging strains of Gram-negative bacilli producing extended-spectrum beta-lactamases. *Res. Microbiol.* **2004**, *155*, 409–421. [CrossRef] [PubMed]
2. Dhillon, R.H.; Clark, J. ESBLs: A Clear and Present Danger? *Crit. Care Res. Pract.* **2012**, *2012*, 625170. [CrossRef] [PubMed]
3. Laxminarayan, R.; Duse, A.; Wattal, C.; Zaidi, A.K.M.; Wertheim, H.F.L.; Sumpradit, N.; Vlieghe, E.; Hara, G.L.; Gould, I.M.; Goossens, H.; et al. Antibiotic resistance—The need for global solutions. *Lancet Infect. Dis.* **2013**, *13*, 1057–1098. [CrossRef] [PubMed]
4. Rodríguez-Baño, J.; Pascual, A. Clinical significance of extended-spectrum beta-lactamases. *Expert Rev. Anti Infect. Ther.* **2008**, *6*, 671–683. [CrossRef] [PubMed]
5. Ventola, C.L. The antibiotic resistance crisis: Part 2: Management strategies and new agents. *Pharm. Ther.* **2015**, *40*, 344–352.

6. Chaudhuri, A.; Martinez-Martin, P.; Kennedy, P.G.; Andrew Seaton, R.; Portegies, P.; Bojar, M.; Steiner, I. EFNS guideline on the management of community-acquired bacterial meningitis: Report of an EFNS Task Force on acute bacterial meningitis in older children and adults. *Eur. J. Neurol.* **2008**, *15*, 649–659. [CrossRef]
7. Teklu, D.S.; Negeri, A.A.; Legese, M.H.; Bedada, T.L.; Woldemariam, H.K.; Tullu, K.D. Extended-spectrum beta-lactamase production and multi-drug resistance among Enterobacteriaceae isolated in Addis Ababa, Ethiopia. *Antimicrob. Resist. Infect. Control* **2019**, *8*, 39. [CrossRef]
8. Morgan, D.J.; Okeke, I.N.; Laxminarayan, R.; Perencevich, E.N.; Weisenberg, S. Non-prescription antimicrobial use worldwide: A systematic review. *Lancet Infect. Dis.* **2011**, *11*, 692–701. [CrossRef]
9. Soliman, W.E.; Khan, S.; Rizvi, S.M.D.; Moin, A.; Elsewedy, H.S.; Abulila, A.S.; Shehata, T.M. Therapeutic Applications of Biostable Silver Nanoparticles Synthesized Using Peel Extract of Benincasa hispida: Antibacterial and Anticancer Activities. *Nanomaterials* **2020**, *10*, 1954. [CrossRef]
10. Al Saqr, A.; Khafagy, E.S.; Alalaiwe, A.; Aldawsari, M.F.; Alshahrani, S.M.; Anwer, M.K.; Khan, S.; Lila, A.S.A.; Arab, H.H.; Hegazy, W.A.H. Synthesis of Gold Nanoparticles by Using Green Machinery: Characterization and In Vitro Toxicity. *Nanomaterials* **2021**, *11*, 808. [CrossRef]
11. Sánchez-López, E.; Gomes, D.; Esteruelas, G.; Bonilla, L.; Lopez-Machado, A.L.; Galindo, R.; Cano, A.; Espina, M.; Ettcheto, M.; Camins, A.; et al. Metal-Based Nanoparticles as Antimicrobial Agents: An Overview. *Nanomaterials* **2020**, *10*, 292. [CrossRef]
12. Rizvi, S.M.D.; Hussain, T.; Ahmed, A.B.F.; Alshammari, T.M.; Moin, A.; Ahmed, M.Q.; Barreto, G.E.; Kamal, M.A.; Ashraf, G.M. Gold nanoparticles: A plausible tool to combat neurological bacterial infections in humans. *Biomed. Pharmacother.* **2018**, *107*, 7–18. [CrossRef] [PubMed]
13. Kong, F.Y.; Zhang, J.W.; Li, R.F.; Wang, Z.X.; Wang, W.J.; Wang, W. Unique Roles of Gold Nanoparticles in Drug Delivery, Targeting and Imaging Applications. *Molecules* **2017**, *22*, 1445. [CrossRef] [PubMed]
14. Khan, S.; Rizvi, S.M.D.; Avaish, M.; Arshad, M.; Bagga, P.; Khan, M.S. A novel process for size controlled biosynthesis of gold nanoparticles using bromelain. *Mater. Lett.* **2015**, *159*, 373–376. [CrossRef]
15. Camas, M.; Sazak Camas, A.; Kyeremeh, K. Extracellular Synthesis and Characterization of Gold Nanoparticles Using Mycobacterium sp. BRS2A-AR2 Isolated from the Aerial Roots of the Ghanaian Mangrove Plant, Rhizophora racemosa. *Indian J. Microbiol.* **2018**, *58*, 214–221. [CrossRef]
16. Khandelwal, P.; Singh, D.K.; Poddar, P. Advances in the Experimental and Theoretical Understandings of Antibiotic Conjugated Gold Nanoparticles for Antibacterial Applications. *ChemistrySelect* **2019**, *4*, 6719–6738. [CrossRef]
17. Wang, S.G.; Chen, Y.C. Antibacterial gold nanoparticle-based photothermal killing of vancomycin-resistant bacteria. *Nanomedicine* **2018**, *13*, 1405–1416. [CrossRef]
18. Chavan, C.; Kamble, S.; Murthy, A.V.R.; Kale, S.N. Ampicillin-mediated functionalized gold nanoparticles against ampicillin-resistant bacteria: Strategy, preparation and interaction studies. *Nanotechnology* **2020**, *31*, 215604. [CrossRef]
19. Payne, J.N.; Waghwani, H.K.; Connor, M.G.; Hamilton, W.; Tockstein, S.; Moolani, H.; Chavda, F.; Badwaik, V.; Lawrenz, M.B.; Dakshinamurthy, R. Novel synthesis of kanamycin conjugated gold nanoparticles with potent antibacterial activity. *Front. Microbiol.* **2016**, *7*, 607. [CrossRef]
20. Fuller, M.; Whiley, H.; Köper, I. Antibiotic delivery using gold nanoparticles. *SN Appl. Sci.* **2020**, *2*, 1022. [CrossRef]
21. Nishanthi, R.; Malathi, S.; Palani, P. Green synthesis and characterization of bioinspired silver, gold and platinum nanoparticles and evaluation of their synergistic antibacterial activity after combining with different classes of antibiotics. *Mater. Sci. Eng. C* **2019**, *96*, 693–707.
22. Pradeepa; Vidya, S.M.; Mutalik, S.; Udaya Bhat, K.; Huilgol, P.; Avadhani, K. Preparation of gold nanoparticles by novel bacterial exopolysaccharide for antibiotic delivery. *Life Sci.* **2016**, *153*, 171–179. [CrossRef] [PubMed]
23. Khare, T.; Mahalunkar, S.; Shriram, V.; Gosavi, S.; Kumar, V. Embelin-loaded chitosan gold nanoparticles interact synergistically with ciprofloxacin by inhibiting efflux pumps in multidrug-resistant Pseudomonas aeruginosa and Escherichia coli. *Environ. Res.* **2021**, *199*, 111321. [CrossRef]
24. Al Hagbani, T.; Rizvi, S.M.D.; Hussain, T.; Mehmood, K.; Rafi, Z.; Moin, A.; Abu Lila, A.S.; Alshammari, F.; Khafagy, E.S.; Rahamathulla, M.; et al. Cefotaxime Mediated Synthesis of Gold Nanoparticles: Characterization and Antibacterial Activity. *Polymers* **2022**, *14*, 771. [CrossRef] [PubMed]
25. Alshammari, F.; Alshammari, B.; Moin, A.; Alamri, A.; Al Hagbani, T.; Alobaida, A.; Baker, A.; Khan, S.; Rizvi, S.M.D. Ceftriaxone Mediated Synthesized Gold Nanoparticles: A Nano-Therapeutic Tool to Target Bacterial Resistance. *Pharmaceutics* **2021**, *13*, 1896. [CrossRef] [PubMed]
26. Alafnan, A.; Rizvi, S.M.D.; Alshammari, A.S.; Faiyaz, S.S.M.; Lila, A.S.A.; Katamesh, A.A.; Khafagy, E.S.; Alotaibi, H.F.; Ahmed, A.B.F. Gold Nanoparticle-Based Resuscitation of Cefoxitin against Clinical Pathogens: A Nano-Antibiotic Strategy to Overcome Resistance. *Nanomaterials* **2022**, *12*, 3643. [CrossRef]
27. Abu Lila, A.S.; Huwaimel, B.; Alobaida, A.; Hussain, T.; Rafi, Z.; Mehmood, K.; Abdallah, M.H.; Hagbani, T.A.; Rizvi, S.M.D.; Moin, A.; et al. Delafloxacin-Capped Gold Nanoparticles (DFX-AuNPs): An Effective Antibacterial Nano-Formulation of Fluoroquinolone Antibiotic. *Materials* **2022**, *15*, 5709. [CrossRef]
28. Rai, A.; Prabhune, A.; Perry, C.C. Antibiotic mediated synthesis of gold nanoparticles with potent antimicrobial activity and their application in antimicrobial coatings. *J. Mater. Chem.* **2010**, *20*, 6789–6798. [CrossRef]

29. Shaikh, S.; Rizvi, S.M.D.; Shakil, S.; Hussain, T.; Alshammari, T.M.; Ahmad, W.; Tabrez, S.; Al-Qahtani, M.H.; Abuzenadah, A.M. Synthesis and Characterization of Cefotaxime Conjugated Gold Nanoparticles and Their Use to Target Drug-Resistant CTX-M-Producing Bacterial Pathogens. *J. Cell Biochem.* **2017**, *118*, 2802–2808. [CrossRef]
30. Shaker, M.A.; Shaaban, M.I. Formulation of carbapenems loaded gold nanoparticles to combat multi-antibiotic bacterial resistance: In vitro antibacterial study. *Int. J. Pharm.* **2017**, *525*, 71–84. [CrossRef]
31. Kalita, S.; Kandimalla, R.; Sharma, K.K.; Kataki, A.C.; Deka, M.; Kotoky, J. Amoxicillin functionalized gold nanoparticles reverts MRSA resistance. *Mater. Sci. Eng. C Mater. Biol. Appl.* **2016**, *61*, 720–727. [CrossRef]
32. Hur, Y.E.; Park, Y. Vancomycin-Functionalized Gold and Silver Nanoparticles as an Antibacterial Nanoplatform Against Methicillin-Resistant Staphylococcus aureus. *J. Nanosci. Nanotechnol.* **2016**, *16*, 6393–6399. [CrossRef] [PubMed]
33. Wang, J.; Zhang, J.; Liu, K.; He, J.; Zhang, Y.; Chen, S.; Ma, G.; Cui, Y.; Wang, L.; Gao, D. Synthesis of gold nanoflowers stabilized with amphiphilic daptomycin for enhanced photothermal antitumor and antibacterial effects. *Int. J. Pharm.* **2020**, *580*, 119231. [CrossRef] [PubMed]
34. Navya, P.N.; Daima, H.K. Rational engineering of physicochemical properties of nanomaterials for biomedical applications with nanotoxicological perspectives. *Nano Converg.* **2016**, *3*, 1. [CrossRef]
35. Samanta, S.; Agarwal, S.; Nair, K.K.; Harris, R.A.; Swart, H. Biomolecular assisted synthesis and mechanism of silver and gold nanoparticles. *Mater. Res. Express* **2019**, *6*, 82009. [CrossRef]
36. Sengani, M.; Grumezescu, A.M.; Rajeswari, V.D. Recent trends and methodologies in gold nanoparticle synthesis—A prospective review on drug delivery aspect. *OpenNano* **2017**, *2*, 37–46. [CrossRef]
37. Jans, H.; Huo, Q. Gold nanoparticle-enabled biological and chemical detection and analysis. *Chem. Soc. Rev.* **2012**, *41*, 2849–2866. [CrossRef] [PubMed]
38. Burda, C.; Chen, X.; Narayanan, R.; El-Sayed, M.A. Chemistry and properties of nanocrystals of different shapes. *Chem. Rev.* **2005**, *105*, 1025–1102. [CrossRef] [PubMed]
39. Li, N.; Zhao, P.; Astruc, D. Anisotropic Gold Nanoparticles: Synthesis, Properties, Applications, and Toxicity. *Angew. Chem. Int. Ed.* **2014**, *53*, 1756–1789. [CrossRef]
40. Arvizo, R.R.; Bhattacharyya, S.; Kudgus, R.A.; Giri, K.; Bhattacharya, R.; Mukherjee, P. Intrinsic therapeutic applications of noble metal nanoparticles: Past, present and future. *Chem. Soc. Rev.* **2012**, *41*, 2943–2970. [CrossRef] [PubMed]
41. Langille, M.R.; Personick, M.L.; Zhang, J.; Mirkin, C.A. Defining Rules for the Shape Evolution of Gold Nanoparticles. *J. Am. Chem. Soc.* **2012**, *134*, 14542–14554. [CrossRef] [PubMed]
42. Ding, L.; Yao, C.; Yin, X.; Li, C.; Huang, Y.; Wu, M.; Wang, B.; Guo, X.; Wang, Y.; Wu, M. Size, Shape, and Protein Corona Determine Cellular Uptake and Removal Mechanisms of Gold Nanoparticles. *Small* **2018**, *14*, 1801451. [CrossRef] [PubMed]
43. Huang, X.; Jain, P.K.; El-Sayed, I.H.; El-Sayed, M.A. Gold nanoparticles: Interesting optical properties and recent applications in cancer diagnostics and therapy. *Nanomedicine* **2007**, *2*, 681–693. [CrossRef] [PubMed]
44. Singh, D.K.; Jagannathan, R.; Khandelwal, P.; Abraham, P.M.; Poddar, P. In situ synthesis and surface functionalization of gold nanoparticles with curcumin and their antioxidant properties: An experimental and density functional theory investigation. *Nanoscale* **2013**, *5*, 1882–1893. [CrossRef] [PubMed]
45. Ghosh, S.K.; Pal, T. Interparticle Coupling Effect on the Surface Plasmon Resonance of Gold Nanoparticles: From Theory to Applications. *Chem. Rev.* **2007**, *107*, 4797–4862. [CrossRef]
46. Brown, A.N.; Smith, K.; Samuels, T.A.; Lu, J.; Obare, S.O.; Scott, M.E. Nanoparticles functionalized with ampicillin destroy multiple-antibiotic-resistant isolates of Pseudomonas aeruginosa and Enterobacter aerogenes and methicillin-resistant Staphylococcus aureus. *Appl. Environ. Microbiol.* **2012**, *78*, 2768–2774. [CrossRef]
47. Pornpattananangkul, D.; Zhang, L.; Olson, S.; Aryal, S.; Obonyo, M.; Vecchio, K.; Huang, C.M.; Zhang, L. Bacterial toxin-triggered drug release from gold nanoparticle-stabilized liposomes for the treatment of bacterial infection. *J. Am. Chem. Soc.* **2011**, *133*, 4132–4139. [CrossRef]
48. Rastogi, L.; Kora, A.J.; Arunachalam, J. Highly stable, protein capped gold nanoparticles as effective drug delivery vehicles for amino-glycosidic antibiotics. *Mater. Sci. Eng. C* **2012**, *32*, 1571–1577. [CrossRef]
49. Tom, R.T.; Suryanarayanan, V.; Reddy, P.G.; Baskaran, S.; Pradeep, T. Ciprofloxacin-protected gold nanoparticles. *Langmuir* **2004**, *20*, 1909–1914. [CrossRef]
50. Ahangari, A.; Salouti, M.; Saghatchi, F. Gentamicin-gold nanoparticles conjugate: A contrast agent for X-ray imaging of infectious foci due to Staphylococcus aureus. *IET Nanobiotechnol.* **2016**, *10*, 190–194. [CrossRef]
51. Grace, A.N.; Pandian, K. Antibacterial efficacy of aminoglycosidic antibiotics protected gold nanoparticles—A brief study. *Colloids Surf. A Physicochem. Eng. Asp.* **2007**, *297*, 63–70. [CrossRef]
52. Perni, S.; Prokopovich, P. Continuous release of gentamicin from gold nanocarriers. *RSC Adv.* **2014**, *4*, 51904–51910. [CrossRef]
53. Shamaila, S.; Zafar, N.; Riaz, S.; Sharif, R.; Nazir, J.; Naseem, S. Gold Nanoparticles: An Efficient Antimicrobial Agent against Enteric Bacterial Human Pathogen. *Nanomaterials* **2016**, *6*, 71. [CrossRef] [PubMed]
54. Penders, J.; Stolzoff, M.; Hickey, D.J.; Andersson, M.; Webster, T.J. Shape-dependent antibacterial effects of non-cytotoxic gold nanoparticles. *Int. J. Nanomed.* **2017**, *12*, 2457. [CrossRef] [PubMed]
55. Osonga, F.J.; Akgul, A.; Yazgan, I.; Akgul, A.; Eshun, G.B.; Sakhaee, L.; Sadik, O.A. Size and Shape-Dependent Antimicrobial Activities of Silver and Gold Nanoparticles: A Model Study as Potential Fungicides. *Molecules* **2020**, *25*, 2682. [CrossRef] [PubMed]

56. Zhu, S.; Shen, Y.; Yu, Y.; Bai, X. Synthesis of antibacterial gold nanoparticles with different particle sizes using chlorogenic acid. *R Soc. Open Sci.* **2020**, *7*, 191141. [CrossRef] [PubMed]
57. Pourali, P.; Benada, O.; Pátek, M.; Neuhöferová, E.; Dzmitruk, V.; Benson, V. Response of Biological Gold Nanoparticles to Different pH Values: Is It Possible to Prepare Both Negatively and Positively Charged Nanoparticles? *Appl. Sci.* **2021**, *11*, 11559. [CrossRef]
58. Khan, S.; Rizvi, S.M.; Saeed, M.; Srivastava, A.K.; Khan, M.A. Novel Approach for the synthesis of gold nanoparticles using Trypsin. *Adv. Sci. Lett.* **2014**, *20*, 1061–1065. [CrossRef]
59. Marcelo, G.A.; Duarte, M.P.; Oliveira, E. Gold@mesoporous silica nanocarriers for the effective delivery of antibiotics and by-passing of β-lactam resistance. *SN Appl. Sci.* **2020**, *2*, 1354. [CrossRef]
60. Haddada, M.B.; Jeannot, K.; Spadavecchia, J. Novel Synthesis and Characterization of Doxycycline-Loaded Gold Nanoparticles: The Golden Doxycycline for Antibacterial Applications. *Part. Part. Syst. Charact.* **2019**, *36*, 1800395. [CrossRef]
61. Saha, B.; Bhattacharya, J.; Mukherjee, A.; Ghosh, A.; Santra, C.; Dasgupta, A.K.; Karmakar, P. In Vitro Structural and Functional Evaluation of Gold Nanoparticles Conjugated Antibiotics. *Nanoscale Res. Lett.* **2007**, *2*, 614–622. [CrossRef]
62. Chamundeeswari, M.; Sobhana, S.S.; Jacob, J.P.; Kumar, M.G.; Devi, M.P.; Sastry, T.P.; Mandal, A.B. Preparation, characterization and evaluation of a biopolymeric gold nanocomposite with antimicrobial activity. *Biotechnol. Appl. Biochem.* **2010**, *55*, 29–35. [CrossRef] [PubMed]
63. Hagbani, T.A.; Yadav, H.; Moin, A.; Lila, A.S.A.; Mehmood, K.; Alshammari, F.; Khan, S.; Khafagy, E.S.; Hussain, T.; Rizvi, S.M.D.; et al. Enhancement of Vancomycin Potential against Pathogenic Bacterial Strains via Gold Nano-Formulations: A Nano-Antibiotic Approach. *Materials* **2022**, *15*, 1108. [CrossRef] [PubMed]
64. Mohammed Fayaz, A.; Girilal, M.; Mahdy, S.A.; Somsundar, S.S.; Venkatesan, R.; Kalaichelvan, P.T. Vancomycin bound biogenic gold nanoparticles: A different perspective for development of anti VRSA agents. *Process Biochem.* **2011**, *46*, 636–641. [CrossRef]
65. Esmaeillou, M.; Zarrini, G.; Ahangarzadeh Rezaee, M.; Shahbazi Mojarrad, J.; Bahadori, A. Vancomycin Capped with Silver Nanoparticles as an Antibacterial Agent against Multi-Drug Resistance Bacteria. *Adv. Pharm. Bull.* **2017**, *7*, 479–483. [CrossRef]
66. Song, Y.-Z.; Zhu, A.-F.; Song, Y.; Cheng, Z.-P.; Xu, J.; Zhou, J.-F. Experimental and theoretical study on the synthesis of gold nanoparticles using ceftriaxone as a stabilizing reagent for and its catalysis for dopamine. *Gold Bull.* **2012**, *45*, 153–160. [CrossRef]
67. Nishanthi, R.; Palani, P. Green synthesis of gold nanoparticles from the rind extract of Garcinia mangostana and its synergistic effect with antibiotics against human pathogenic bacteria. In Proceedings of the 2016 IEEE 16th International Conference on Nanotechnology (IEEE-NANO), Sendai, Japan, 22–25 August 2016; pp. 431–434.
68. Al-Khafaji, M.H.; Hashim, M.H. The synergistic effect of biosynthesized gold nanoparticles with antibiotic against clinical isolates. *J. Biotechnol. Res. Cent.* **2019**, *13*, 58–62. [CrossRef]
69. Reygaert, W.C. An overview of the antimicrobial resistance mechanisms of bacteria. *AIMS Microbiol.* **2018**, *4*, 482–501. [CrossRef]
70. Maurya, N.; Jangra, M.; Tambat, R.; Nandanwar, H. Alliance of Efflux Pumps with β-Lactamases in Multidrug-Resistant Klebsiella pneumoniae Isolates. *Microb. Drug Resist.* **2019**, *25*, 1155–1163. [CrossRef]
71. Yasufuku, T.; Shigemura, K.; Shirakawa, T.; Matsumoto, M.; Nakano, Y.; Tanaka, K.; Arakawa, S.; Kinoshita, S.; Kawabata, M.; Fujisawa, M. Correlation of overexpression of efflux pump genes with antibiotic resistance in Escherichia coli Strains clinically isolated from urinary tract infection patients. *J. Clin. Microbiol.* **2011**, *49*, 189–194. [CrossRef]
72. Yedekci, S.; Erac, B.; Limoncu, M.H. Detection of the efflux pump-mediated quinolone resistance in ESBL positive Escherichia coli and Klebsiella pneumoniae isolates by phe-Arg-beta naphthylamide. *Turk. J. Pharm. Sci.* **2012**, *9*, 67–74.
73. Tsai, Y.K.; Fung, C.P.; Lin, J.C.; Chen, J.H.; Chang, F.Y.; Chen, T.L.; Siu, L.K. Klebsiella pneumoniae outer membrane porins OmpK35 and OmpK36 play roles in both antimicrobial resistance and virulence. *Antimicrob. Agents Chemother.* **2011**, *55*, 1485–1493. [CrossRef] [PubMed]
74. James, C.E.; Mahendran, K.R.; Molitor, A.; Bolla, J.M.; Bessonov, A.N.; Winterhalter, M.; Pagès, J.M. How beta-lactam antibiotics enter bacteria: A dialogue with the porins. *PLoS ONE* **2009**, *4*, e5453. [CrossRef]
75. Nitzan, Y.; Deutsch, E.B.; Pechatnikov, I. Diffusion of beta-lactam antibiotics through oligomeric or monomeric porin channels of some gram-negative bacteria. *Curr. Microbiol.* **2002**, *45*, 446–455. [CrossRef]
76. Prajapati, J.D.; Kleinekathöfer, U.; Winterhalter, M. How to Enter a Bacterium: Bacterial Porins and the Permeation of Antibiotics. *Chem. Rev.* **2021**, *121*, 5158–5192. [CrossRef]
77. Dé, E.; Baslé, A.; Jaquinod, M.; Saint, N.; Malléa, M.; Molle, G.; Pagès, J.M. A new mechanism of antibiotic resistance in Enterobacteriaceae induced by a structural modification of the major porin. *Mol. Microbiol.* **2001**, *41*, 189–198. [CrossRef] [PubMed]
78. Khalifa, S.M.; Abd El-Aziz, A.M.; Hassan, R.; Abdelmegeed, E.S. β-lactam resistance associated with β-lactamase production and porin alteration in clinical isolates of E. coli and K. pneumoniae. *PLoS ONE* **2021**, *16*, e0251594. [CrossRef] [PubMed]
79. Ananthan, S.; Subha, A. Cefoxitin resistance mediated by loss of a porin in clinical strains of Klebsiella pneumoniae and Escherichia coli. *Indian J. Med. Microbiol.* **2005**, *23*, 20–23. [CrossRef] [PubMed]
80. Martínez-Martínez, L. Extended-spectrum beta-lactamases and the permeability barrier. *Clin. Microbiol. Infect.* **2008**, *14* (Suppl. S1), 82–89. [CrossRef] [PubMed]
81. Verma, A.; Uzun, O.; Hu, Y.; Hu, Y.; Han, H.-S.; Watson, N.; Chen, S.; Irvine, D.J.; Stellacci, F. Surface-structure-regulated cell-membrane penetration by monolayer-protected nanoparticles. *Nat. Mater.* **2008**, *7*, 588–595. [CrossRef]

82. Chen, J.; Hessler, J.A.; Putchakayala, K.; Panama, B.K.; Khan, D.P.; Hong, S.; Mullen, D.G.; Dimaggio, S.C.; Som, A.; Tew, G.N.; et al. Cationic nanoparticles induce nanoscale disruption in living cell plasma membranes. *J. Phys. Chem. B* **2009**, *113*, 11179–11185. [CrossRef] [PubMed]
83. Białas, N.; Sokolova, V.; van der Meer, S.B.; Knuschke, T.; Ruks, T.; Klein, K.; Westendorf, A.M.; Epple, M. Bacteria (E. coli) take up ultrasmall gold nanoparticles (2 nm) as shown by different optical microscopic techniques (CLSM, SIM, STORM). *Nano Select* **2022**, *3*, 1407–1420. [CrossRef]
84. Linklater, D.P.; Baulin, V.A.; Le Guével, X.; Fleury, J.B.; Hanssen, E.; Nguyen, T.H.; Juodkazis, S.; Bryant, G.; Crawford, R.J.; Stoodley, P.; et al. Antibacterial action of nanoparticles by lethal stretching of bacterial cell membranes. *Adv. Mater.* **2020**, *32*, 2005679. [CrossRef] [PubMed]
85. Giri, K.; Yepes, L.R.; Duncan, B.; Parameswaran, P.K.; Yan, B.; Jiang, Y.; Bilska, M.; Moyano, D.F.; Thompson, M.; Rotello, V.M.; et al. Targeting bacterial biofilms via surface engineering of gold nanoparticles. *RSC Adv.* **2015**, *5*, 105551–105559. [CrossRef]
86. Zhao, Y.; Tian, Y.; Cui, Y.; Liu, W.; Ma, W.; Jiang, X. Small molecule-capped gold nanoparticles as potent antibacterial agents that target Gram-negative bacteria. *J. Am. Chem. Soc.* **2010**, *132*, 12349–12356. [CrossRef]
87. Adhikari, M.D.; Goswami, S.; Panda, B.R.; Chattopadhyay, A.; Ramesh, A. Membrane-directed high bactericidal activity of (gold nanoparticle)-polythiophene composite for niche applications against pathogenic bacteria. *Adv. Healthc. Mater.* **2013**, *2*, 599–606. [CrossRef] [PubMed]
88. You, Q.; Zhang, X.; Wu, F.-G.; Chen, Y. Colorimetric and test stripe-based assay of bacteria by using vancomycin-modified gold nanoparticles. *Sens. Actuators B Chem.* **2019**, *281*, 408–414. [CrossRef]
89. Mobasseri, G.; Lin, T.K.; Teh, C.S.J. Association of Efflux Pump and OMPs with Antibiotic Susceptibility Among ESBL-Producing Klebsiella Pneumoniae Clinical Strains in Malaysia. *Res. Sq.* **2021**. [CrossRef]
90. Dorri, K.; Modaresi, F.; Shakibaie, M.R.; Moazamian, E. Effect of gold nanoparticles on the expression of efflux pump mexA and mexB genes of Pseudomonas aeruginosa strains by Quantitative real-time PCR. *Pharmacia* **2022**, *69*, 125–133. [CrossRef]
91. Miller, L.M.; Silver, C.D.; Herman, R.; Duhme-Klair, A.-K.; Thomas, G.H.; Krauss, T.F.; Johnson, S.D. Surface-Bound Antibiotic for the Detection of β-Lactamases. *ACS Appl. Mater. Interfaces* **2019**, *11*, 32599–32604. [CrossRef]
92. Ghosh, P.; Han, G.; De, M.; Kim, C.K.; Rotello, V.M. Gold nanoparticles in delivery applications. *Adv. Drug Deliv. Rev.* **2008**, *60*, 1307–1315. [CrossRef] [PubMed]
93. Brown, S.D.; Nativo, P.; Smith, J.A.; Stirling, D.; Edwards, P.R.; Venugopal, B.; Flint, D.J.; Plumb, J.A.; Graham, D.; Wheate, N.J. Gold nanoparticles for the improved anticancer drug delivery of the active component of oxaliplatin. *J. Am. Chem. Soc.* **2010**, *132*, 4678–4684. [CrossRef] [PubMed]
94. Wu, Z.; Zhang, B.; Yan, B. Regulation of enzyme activity through interactions with nanoparticles. *Int. J. Mol. Sci.* **2009**, *10*, 4198–4209. [CrossRef]
95. Chatterjee, T.; Das, G.; Ghosh, S.; Chakrabarti, P. Effect of gold nanoparticles on the structure and neuroprotective function of protein L-isoaspartyl methyltransferase (PIMT). *Sci. Rep.* **2021**, *11*, 1–3. [CrossRef]
96. Ramalingam, V. Multifunctionality of gold nanoparticles: Plausible and convincing properties. *Adv. Colloid Interface Sci.* **2019**, *271*, 101989. [CrossRef]
97. Shaikh, S.; Nazam, N.; Rizvi, S.M.; Ahmad, K.; Baig, M.H.; Lee, E.J.; Choi, I. Mechanistic insights into the antimicrobial actions of metallic nanoparticles and their implications for multidrug resistance. *Int. J. Mol. Sci.* **2019**, *20*, 2468. [CrossRef]
98. Tao, C. Antimicrobial activity and toxicity of gold nanoparticles: Research progress, challenges and prospects. *Lett. Appl. Microbiol.* **2018**, *67*, 537–543. [CrossRef]
99. Li, Q.; Mahendra, S.; Lyon, D.Y.; Brunet, L.; Liga, M.V.; Li, D.; Alvarez, P.J.J. Antimicrobial nanomaterials for water disinfection and microbial control: Potential applications and implications. *Water Res.* **2008**, *42*, 4591–4602. [CrossRef]
100. Tian, E.K.; Wang, Y.; Ren, R.; Zheng, W.; Liao, W. Gold nanoparticle: Recent progress on its antibacterial applications and mechanisms. *J. Nanomater.* **2021**, *2021*, 1–18. [CrossRef]
101. Lee, H.; Lee, D.G. Gold nanoparticles induce a reactive oxygen species-independent apoptotic pathway in Escherichia coli. *Colloids Surf. B Biointerfaces* **2018**, *167*, 1–7. [CrossRef]
102. Ahmed, F.; Faisal, S.M.; Ahmed, A.; Husain, Q. Beta galactosidase mediated bio-enzymatically synthesized nano-gold with aggrandized cytotoxic potential against pathogenic bacteria and cancer cells. *J. Photochem. Photobiol. B* **2020**, *209*, 111923. [CrossRef] [PubMed]
103. Global Newswire. Available online: https://www.globenewswire.com/news-release/2022/10/13/2534150/0/en/Global-Gold-Nanoparticles-.Market-to-Reach-7-6-Billion-by-2027.html (accessed on 23 November 2022).
104. IMARC. Available online: https://www.imarcgroup.com/gold-nanoparticles-market (accessed on 23 November 2022).
105. Allied Market Research. Available online: https://www.alliedmarketresearch.com/gold-nanoparticles-market-A08997 (accessed on 23 November 2022).
106. FDA. Available online: https://www.accessdata.fda.gov/cdrh_docs/pdf7/k070804.pdf (accessed on 23 November 2022).
107. Zhang, R.; Kiessling, F.; Lammers, T.; Pallares, R.M. Clinical translation of gold nanoparticles. *Drug Deliv. Transl. Res.* **2022**, *13*, 1–8. [CrossRef] [PubMed]
108. Pan, Y.; Neuss, S.; Leifert, A.; Fischler, M.; Wen, F.; Simon, U.; Schmid, G.; Brandau, W.; Jahnen-Dechent, W. Size-dependent cytotoxicity of gold nanoparticles. *Small* **2007**, *3*, 1941–1949. [CrossRef]

109. Tsoli, M.; Kuhn, H.; Brandau, W.; Esche, H.; Schmid, G. Cellular uptake and toxicity of Au55 clusters. *Small* **2005**, *1*, 841–844. [CrossRef]
110. Mironava, T.; Hadjiargyrou, M.; Simon, M.; Jurukovski, V.; Rafailovich, M.H. Gold nanoparticles cellular toxicity and recovery: Effect of size, concentration and exposure time. *Nanotoxicology* **2010**, *4*, 120–137. [CrossRef] [PubMed]
111. Zhao, Y.; Wang, Y.; Ran, F.; Cui, Y.; Liu, C.; Zhao, Q.; Gao, Y.; Wang, D.; Wang, S. A comparison between sphere and rod nanoparticles regarding their in vivo biological behavior and pharmacokinetics. *Sci. Rep.* **2017**, *7*, 4131. [CrossRef] [PubMed]
112. Goodman, C.M.; McCusker, C.D.; Yilmaz, T.; Rotello, V.M. Toxicity of Gold Nanoparticles Functionalized with Cationic and Anionic Side Chains. *Bioconjugate Chem.* **2004**, *15*, 897–900. [CrossRef]
113. Hauck, T.S.; Ghazani, A.A.; Chan, W.C. Assessing the effect of surface chemistry on gold nanorod uptake, toxicity, and gene expression in mammalian cells. *Small* **2008**, *4*, 153–159. [CrossRef]
114. Alkilany, A.M.; Nagaria, P.K.; Hexel, C.R.; Shaw, T.J.; Murphy, C.J.; Wyatt, M.D. Cellular uptake and cytotoxicity of gold nanorods: Molecular origin of cytotoxicity and surface effects. *Small* **2009**, *5*, 701–708. [CrossRef]
115. Zhang, G.; Yang, Z.; Lu, W.; Zhang, R.; Huang, Q.; Tian, M.; Li, L.; Liang, D.; Li, C. Influence of anchoring ligands and particle size on the colloidal stability and in vivo biodistribution of polyethylene glycol-coated gold nanoparticles in tumor-xenografted mice. *Biomaterials* **2009**, *30*, 1928–1936. [CrossRef]
116. Chen, Y.S.; Hung, Y.C.; Liau, I.; Huang, G.S. Assessment of the In Vivo Toxicity of Gold Nanoparticles. *Nanoscale Res. Lett.* **2009**, *4*, 858–864. [CrossRef] [PubMed]
117. De Jong, W.H.; Hagens, W.I.; Krystek, P.; Burger, M.C.; Sips, A.J.; Geertsma, R.E. Particle size-dependent organ distribution of gold nanoparticles after intravenous administration. *Biomaterials* **2008**, *29*, 1912–1919. [CrossRef] [PubMed]
118. Sonavane, G.; Tomoda, K.; Makino, K. Biodistribution of colloidal gold nanoparticles after intravenous administration: Effect of particle size. *Colloids Surf. B Biointerfaces* **2008**, *66*, 274–280. [CrossRef] [PubMed]
119. Alkilany, A.M.; Murphy, C.J. Toxicity and cellular uptake of gold nanoparticles: What we have learned so far? *J. Nanopart. Res.* **2010**, *12*, 2313–2333. [CrossRef] [PubMed]
120. Bar-Ilan, O.; Albrecht, R.M.; Fako, V.E.; Furgeson, D.Y. Toxicity assessments of multisized gold and silver nanoparticles in zebrafish embryos. *Small* **2009**, *5*, 1897–1910. [CrossRef]
121. Pompa, P.P.; Vecchio, G.; Galeone, A.; Brunetti, V.; Sabella, S.; Maiorano, G.; Falqui, A.; Bertoni, G.; Cingolani, R. In Vivo toxicity assessment of gold nanoparticles in Drosophila melanogaster. *Nano Res.* **2011**, *4*, 405–413. [CrossRef]
122. Vecchio, G.; Galeone, A.; Brunetti, V.; Maiorano, G.; Rizzello, L.; Sabella, S.; Cingolani, R.; Pompa, P.P. Mutagenic effects of gold nanoparticles induce aberrant phenotypes in Drosophila melanogaster. *Nanomedicine* **2012**, *8*, 1–7. [CrossRef]
123. Zhang, Y.; Shareena Dasari, T.P.; Deng, H.; Yu, H. Antimicrobial activity of gold nanoparticles and ionic gold. *J. Environ. Sci. Health Part C* **2015**, *33*, 286–327. [CrossRef]

pharmaceutics

MDPI

Article

Bacteriocin-Nanoconjugates (Bac10307-AgNPs) Biosynthesized from *Lactobacillus acidophilus*-Derived Bacteriocins Exhibit Enhanced and Promising Biological Activities

Arif Jamal Siddiqui [1,*], Mitesh Patel [2], Mohd Adnan [1], Sadaf Jahan [3], Juhi Saxena [4], Mohammed Merae Alshahrani [5], Abdelmushin Abdelgadir [1], Fevzi Bardakci [1], Manojkumar Sachidanandan [6], Riadh Badraoui [1,7], Mejdi Snoussi [1,8] and Allal Ouhtit [9,*]

1 Department of Biology, College of Science, University of Ha'il, Ha'il P.O. Box 2440, Saudi Arabia
2 Department of Biotechnology, Parul Institute of Applied Sciences and Centre of Research for Development, Parul University, Vadodara 391760, India
3 Department of Medical Laboratory Sciences, College of Applied Medical Sciences, Majmaah University, Al Majmaah 11952, Saudi Arabia
4 Department of Biotechnology, University Institute of Biotechnology, Chandigarh University, Gharuan, NH-95, Ludhiana-Chandigarh State Hwy, Punjab 140413, India
5 Department of Clinical Laboratory Sciences, Faculty of Applied Medial Sciences, Najran University, 1988, Najran 61441, Saudi Arabia
6 Department of Oral Radiology, College of Dentistry, University of Ha'il, Ha'il P.O. Box 2440, Saudi Arabia
7 Section of Histology-Cytology, Medicine Faculty of Tunis, University of Tunis El Manar, La Rabta-Tunis 1017, Tunisia
8 Laboratory of Genetics, Biodiversity and Valorization of Bio-Resources (LR11ES41), University of Monastir, Higher Institute of Biotechnology of Monastir, Avenue Tahar Hadda, BP74, Monastir 5000, Tunisia
9 Department of Biological and Environmental Sciences, College of Arts and Sciences, Qatar University, Doha P.O. Box 2713, Qatar
* Correspondence: ar.siddiqui@uoh.edu.sa (A.J.S.); alouht@yahoo.co.uk (A.O.); Tel.: +966-557399031 (A.J.S.); +974-44037572 (A.O.)

Abstract: The proteinaceous compounds produced by lactic acid bacteria are called bacteriocins and have a wide variety of bioactive properties. However, bacteriocin's commercial availability is limited due to short stability periods and low yields. Therefore, the objective of this study was to synthesize bacteriocin-derived silver nanoparticles (Bac10307-AgNPs) extracted from *Lactobacillus acidophilus* (*L. acidophilus*), which may have the potential to increase the bioactivity of bacteriocins and overcome the hurdles. It was found that extracted and purified Bac10307 had a broad range of stability for both temperature (20–100 °C) and pH (3–12). Further, based on Sodium dodecyl-sulfate polyacrylamide gel electrophoresis (SDS–PAGE) analysis, its molecular weight was estimated to be 4.2 kDa. The synthesized Bac10307-AgNPs showed a peak of surface plasmon resonance at 430 nm λmax. Fourier transform infrared (FTIR) confirmed the presence of biological moieties, and transmission electron microscopy (TEM) coupled with Energy dispersive X-Ray (EDX) confirmed that AgNPs were spherical and irregularly shaped, with a size range of 9–20 nm. As a result, the Bac10307-AgNPs displayed very strong antibacterial activity with MIC values as low as 8 µg/mL for *Staphylococcus aureus* (*S. aureus*) and *Pseudomonas aeruginosa* (*P. aeruginosa*), when compared to Bac10307 alone. In addition, Bac10307-AgNPs demonstrated promising in vitro antioxidant activity against 2,2-diphenyl-1-picrylhydrazyl (DPPH) (IC_{50} = 116.04 µg/mL) and in vitro cytotoxicity against human liver cancer cells (HepG2) (IC_{50} = 135.63 µg/mL), more than Bac10307 alone (IC_{50} = 139.82 µg/mL against DPPH and 158.20 µg/mL against HepG2). Furthermore, a protein–protein molecular docking simulation study of bacteriocins with target proteins of different biological functions was also carried out in order to ascertain the interactions between bacteriocins and target proteins.

Keywords: bacteria; *L. acidophilus*; silver nanoparticles; cancer; bacteriocins; TEM; protein target

Citation: Siddiqui, A.J.; Patel, M.; Adnan, M.; Jahan, S.; Saxena, J.; Alshahrani, M.M.; Abdelgadir, A.; Bardakci, F.; Sachidanandan, M.; Badraoui, R.; et al. Bacteriocin-Nanoconjugates (Bac10307-AgNPs) Biosynthesized from *Lactobacillus acidophilus*-Derived Bacteriocins Exhibit Enhanced and Promising Biological Activities. *Pharmaceutics* **2023**, *15*, 403. https://doi.org/10.3390/pharmaceutics15020403

Academic Editors: Aura Rusu and Valentina Uivarosi

Received: 6 November 2022
Revised: 6 January 2023
Accepted: 9 January 2023
Published: 25 January 2023

1. Introduction

Lactobacillus is a genus of bacteria known as a probiotic and has been recognized as a vital part of human health and well-being since the 18th century. One of the lactobacilli species, *Lactobacillus acidophilus*, has been studied extensively since it was discovered in 1890 and has gained more attention than any of the others [1]. Research has documented that the organism is an intestinal resident of the human body since its inoculation, which is why it is being commercially available as a dietary supplement as well as in many dairy products [2]. As a result of further research carried out over the past century, it has been reported that individuals who consume products containing *L. acidophilus* have a number of significant health benefits. From this perspective, it can be viewed as having the potential to benefit the host by enhancing lactose digestion, treating diarrhea, improving blood lipid chemistry, boosting immunity, and potentially killing cancer cells [3]. In fact, species of *L. acidophilus* are specially equipped with the producing capabilities of bacteriocins and bacteriocins, such as the compounds lactacin B, lactacin F, acidocin A, and acidocin B, which are at the core of many industrial and medicinal applications [4,5].

The bacteriocins are a miscellaneous group of proteinaceous compounds produced by different types of bacteria that usually exhibit antibacterial activity against pathogenic bacteria belonging to different genera [6]. There are various uses of bacteriocins in the healthcare sector including as biopreservatives for food and as an antibacterial agent for use in biomedical applications, which have attracted the attention of researchers [7,8]. However, to date, nisin and pediocin PA-1 are the only two antimicrobial peptides approved by the Food and Drug Administration (FDA) for use as biopreservatives [9]. Even though various researchers all over the world have characterized and studied a large number of bacteriocins, there are a number of limitations associated with their application, including degradation by proteases, narrow antimicrobial spectrum, restricted production, high dosage needed at the same time, etc. [10].

In the last few years, the combination of nanotechnology with biotechnology has become one of the most important areas of research and development in the medical and pharmaceutical industries due to its potential impact. This technology has also emerged as a promising solution for overcoming some of the limitations of bacteriocins that have been mentioned above, as well as providing a ray of hope for the future. It is well known that nanoparticles synthesized through biological processes are environment-friendly and safe to be used. There have been a number of studies conducted in recent years on the application of metallic nanoparticles, specifically silver nanoparticles (AgNPs), which are highly conductive, magnetic, thermal, and possess different biological properties [11,12]. The bioactive potential of bacteriocin and silver nanoparticles have been reported, which includes antimicrobial, antioxidant, and anticancer potentials. Therefore, in order to increase the bioactivity of bacteriocins, nanotechnology can be useful for conjugating bacteriocins with metal nanoparticles, which may have the potential to increase the bioactivity of bacteriocins [9]. In the present study, bacteriocin Bac10307 was extracted and purified from *L. acidophilus*, and its physicochemical properties were characterized. The synthesis of Bac10307-AgNPs, their characterization via different biophysical methods, and evaluation of their in vitro bioactive potential (antibacterial, antioxidant and cytotoxicity against cancer cells) was carried out. Moreover, the bioactive potential of the reported bacteriocins of *L. acidophilus* were further assessed via in silico molecular docking analysis.

2. Materials and Methods

2.1. Bacterial Strains and Growth Conditions

A standard bacterial strain of *L. acidophilus* MTCC-10307 was obtained from the Microbial Type Culture Collection (IMTECH, Chandigarh, India). Bacteria were grown and maintained on MRS (De Man, Rogosa and Sharpe) agar plates (HiMedia®, Mumbai, India). The pure strain was kept at 4 °C for future use.

2.2. *Extraction and Purification of Bacteriocin from L. acidophilus*

The active culture of *L. acidophilus* was inoculated into MRS broth and incubated at 30 °C for 24–48 h. After incubation, a supernatant was collected using the centrifugation of the grown culture at 10,000 rpm for 15 min at 4 °C. In order to neutralize the effect of organic acid in the collected supernatant, the pH of the supernatant was adjusted to 6.0 by using 1N NaOH solution, and later the filtration of the neutralized supernatant was performed using 0.22 μm membrane filter. Then, a partial purification step involved infusing the collected supernatant with ammonium sulfate salt in the 80% saturation range and continuous stirring on ice, followed by incubating at 4 °C overnight to precipitate proteins. In the next steps, the pellets were collected via centrifugation at 10,000 rpm at 4 °C for 15 min. Then, the obtained pellet was resuspended in a phosphate buffer solution (0.02 M) with pH 7.0. The collected pellet represented crude bacteriocins. The crude bacteriocins were dialyzed overnight at 4 °C against the same buffer to remove salt and other impurities. Lastly, the antibacterial properties of the collected bacteriocins were assessed against different strains of bacteria [13].

2.3. *Analysis of Antibacterial Activity of Partially Purified Bacteriocin-Bac10307*

2.3.1. Bacterial Strains and Growth Conditions

The antibacterial activity of partially purified bacteriocin Bac10307 was carried out against different bacterial pathogens such as, *Staphylococcus aureus* (MTCC96), *Pseudomonas aeruginosa* (MTCC741), *Bacillus subtilis* (MTCC121) and *Escherichia coli* (MTCC 9537). A sterile MHB (HiMedia®, Mumbai, India) was used to grow and maintain all strains of bacteria, which were incubated at 30 °C for 24 h in a shaking condition (120 rpm).

2.3.2. Agar Well Diffusion Assay

The agar well diffusion assay was carried out as an initial test. After growing the bacterial strains overnight in MHB, adjustment in the turbidity of culture was carried out using sterile normal saline solution matching the 0.5 McFarland standard (10^8 CFU/mL). In the following step, 100 μL of each bacterial culture was distributed evenly on the plates, and using a sterile cork borer, wells were made at the center of the plates. Each well was inoculated with 50 μL of the partially purified bacteriocin Bac10307 solution, chloramphenicol (50 μg/mL), and sterile distilled water. Incubation of the plates was carried out at 37 °C for 24 h. As a sign of antibacterial activity, a zone of inhibition was observed [14].

2.4. *Assessment of Stability of Bacteriocin-Bac10307*

The Bac10307 were examined for stability against a variety of physicochemical factors [15].

2.4.1. Impact of Temperatures

The effect of temperatures ranging from 20 to 100 °C on bacteriocin Bac10307 activity was evaluated by incubating bacteriocin Bac10307 at the respective temperatures for 20 min [16]. An antibacterial activity via agar well diffusion assay was performed in order to analyze the effects of temperature on bacteriocin Bac10307 bioactivity.

2.4.2. Impact of pH

The effect of different pH (2–10) on bacteriocin Bac10307 activity was evaluated by incubating bacteriocin Bac10307 at respective pH [17]. In order to adjust the pH of the bacteriocin culture solution, 1N HCl and 1N NaOH solution was used. An antibacterial activity via well diffusion assay was performed in order to analyze the effects of temperature on bacteriocin Bac10307 bioactivity.

2.4.3. Impact of Enzymes

An examination of the effects of various proteolytic enzymes, such as proteinase-K, trypsin, and α-amylase, on bacteriocin Bac10307 activity was evaluated by incubating bacteriocin Bac10307 with the respective enzymes [18]. Each enzyme (1 mg/mL) in separate batches was mixed with the extracted bacteriocin Bac10307 and incubated at 37 °C for 2 h. For the purpose of denaturing the enzyme, further heating was performed on the mixture was performed at 95 °C for 10 min at the end of the incubation procedure. Using the well diffusion assay, the antibacterial activity of bacteriocin was assessed.

2.5. Molecular Mass Determination of Bacteriocin Bac10307 Using SDS–PAGE

The sodium dodecyl sulfate–polyacrylamide gel electrophoresis (SDS–PAGE) was used for the analysis of extracted bacteriocin Bac10307 to determine the molecular mass [19]. Coomassie Brilliant Blue R-250 stain was used to stain the gels after electrophoresis. A protein ladder (245–3.5 kDa) was used to determine the molecular weights of bacteriocin-Bac10307.

2.6. Synthesis of Bacteriocin-10307-AgNPs

Using a method described by Sidhu and Nehra (2021) [20], bacteriocin-derived silver nanoparticles were synthesized. Filter-sterilized solutions of $AgNO_3$ (2 mM) were mixed with partially purified bacteriocin-10307 (5:45 mL) at room temperature for 1 h under UV light. Afterwards, the mixture was centrifuged for 30 min at 12,000 rpm to stop the reaction and remove unbound metal ions and bacteriocin-10307. After centrifugation, the supernatant discarded carefully, and the pellet was twice rinsed in ethanol and resuspended in sterile de-ionized water. As a result of this process, AgNPs were obtained with Bac10307, and as a consequence, they were referred to as Bac10307-AgNPs.

2.7. Characterization of Bac10307-AgNPs

The characterization of Bac10307-AgNPs was carried out via UV–vis spectrophotometry, transmission electron microscopy (TEM), energy-dispersive X-ray spectroscopy (EDX), and Fourier-transform infrared (FT-IR) spectroscopy.

2.7.1. UV–Vis Spectrophotometer

The formation of Bac10307-AgNPs was initially characterized by spectrophotometric analysis. In order to determine the UV–visible spectra of the synthesized Bac10307-AgNPs, the spectra were scanned in a range of wavelengths between 400 and 700 nm with a resolution of 1 nm via a UV–vis spectrophotometer (Shimadzu, Japan) [21].

2.7.2. Transmission Electron Microscopy (TEM) and Energy-Dispersive X-Ray (EDX)

The size and shape of the synthesized Bac10307-AgNPs were characterized by using TEM (Tecnai 20, Philips, Holland). For analysis, Bac10307-AgNPs were equally stained with phosphotungistic acid solution (0.5%) and then fixed on copper grids, dried, and then imaged with a CCD camera in a TEM [22]. Then, EDX analysis (INCA, Oxford Instruments, UK) of the Bac10307-AgNPs was carried out at 20 KeV to accurately define the elemental constitution of the formed particles.

2.7.3. Fourier-Transform Infrared (FT-IR) Analysis

The infrared absorbance of Bac10307-capped AgNPs were measured by using a FTIR spectrophotometer (Bruker®, Billerica, MA, USA) in the spectral range of 400 to 4000 cm^{-1}. The FTIR analysis enabled us to deduce that there are functional groups that play a role in stabilizing and reducing synthesized nanoparticles [23].

2.8. Screening of Antibacterial Activity of Bac10307-AgNPs

2.8.1. Agar Well Diffusion Assay

In order to evaluate the antibacterial activity of Bac10307-AgNPs and AgNPs synthesized via the Brust method against different bacterial pathogens, the agar well diffusion assay was carried out using the method describe above [14].

2.8.2. Assessment of Minimum Inhibitory Concentration (MIC)

In order to determine the MIC value of Bac10307-AgNPs against test bacterial strains, a broth dilution method was employed [24]. An inoculum was prepared by taking an active culture of each bacterium and growing it in MHB for overnight. In 96-well plates (100 μL per well), synthesized Bac10307-AgNPs were diluted two-fold, ranging from 256.0 to 2.0 μg/mL. Following this, 20 μL of each bacterial culture (10^8 CFU/mL) was added and incubated for 24 h at 37 °C. In the next step, MICs were determined by measuring the concentrations at which observable growth was inhibited. The positive control contained only bacteria inoculated without any synthesized Bac10307-AgNPs in the culture, while the negative control contained only the media.

2.9. *Screening of In Vitro Antioxidant Activity of Bac10307-AgNPs*

In order to measure the capability of Bac10307 and Bac10307-AgNPs to scavenge free radicals, the antioxidant activity was measured against DPPH as a measure of their scavenging activity. Then, 10 μL of different concentrations of Bac10307 and Bac10307-AgNPs (2–256 μg/mL) was added to 200 μL of the 0.1 mM DPPH solution in a 96-well plate. The blank consists of 200 μL of DMSO and 10 μL of a compound at various concentrations. The plates were incubated in the dark for a period of 30 min. A microplate reader (iMark, BioRad, USA) was used to measure the decolorization at 495 nm at the end of the incubation. A reaction mixture containing 20 μL of deionized water was used as a control mixture. With respect to the control, the scavenging activity was expressed as a % inhibition [25].

$$\text{DPPH Scavenging activity} = ((\text{Abs Control} - \text{Abs Sample})/\text{AbsControl}) \times 100$$

2.10. *Screening of In Vitro Cytotoxicity Assay (MTT Assay) of Bac10307-AgNPs*

In order to determine the cytotoxic activity of Bac10307 and Bac10307-AgNPs, they were tested on Hep-G2 cells derived from human liver cancer. Dulbecco's Modified Eagle's Medium (DMEM) (MP Biomedicals, Eschwege, Germany) was used to grow Hep-G2 cells in flasks (25 cm^2) at 37 °C in humidified atmospheres with 5% CO_2 supplemented with 10% fetal bovine serum and 10,000 units/mL penicillin and 5 mg/mL streptomycin antibiotic solution (Hi-Media, Mumbai, India). When cells achieved 80% confluency, they were seeded at a density of 10^4 cells per well in 96-well plates and incubated under the same conditions. Following the staining of the cells with Trypan Blue (Hi-Media®, Mumbai, India) (0.4%), the viability of the cells was investigated using a hemocytometer. After that, the cells were exposed to various concentrations of Bac10307 and Bac10307-AgNPs (2–256 μg/mL) for 48 h. Afterwards, the plate was removed from the incubator, and the media containing Bac10307 and Bac10307-AgNPs were aspirated. Thereafter, 200 μL of medium containing 10% MTT reagent (MP Biomedicals, Eschwege, Germany) was added to each well, and the plates were again incubated at 37 °C for an additional 3 h under a humidified atmosphere (5% CO_2). To dissolve the formazan crystals, 100 μL of DMSO (Merck, Darmstadt, Germany) was added in the following step after the medium was removed. In order to measure the amount of formazan crystal in the sample, an ELISA reader (EL10A, Biobase, China) was used to measure the absorbance at the 570 nm and 630 nm wavelengths. Using the dose–response curve for the respective cell line, the percentage of growth inhibition (IC_{50}) was determined by subtracting the background and blank. The positive control used for this assay was the cisplatin [26].

2.11. *Molecular Docking (MD) Assays*

Crystal structures of different target proteins, such as DNA gyrase B (PDB: 6F86.pdb) for antibacterial activity, NADPH oxidase for antioxidant activity (PDB: 2CDU.pdb), and VEGFR2 (PDB: 2OH4.pdb) for anticancer activity, were fetched from the Protein Data Bank (RCSBPDB). Following the retrieval of protein crystal structures, reported bacteriocins of *L. acidophilus*, such as acidocin A, acidocin B, and lactacin F, were predicted from the AlphaFold protein structure database. The ClusPro protein–protein docking server (https:

//cluspro.bu.edu, accessed on 17 October 2022) was used for the simulation of molecular docking [27–29]. To confirm the binding position between bacteriocins and the target proteins, the docking results were visualized in the PyMOL version 2.5.2 and Discovery Studio version 21.1.0.20298.

2.12. Statistical Analysis

All the results are expressed as mean ± SD of the number of experiments performed. A significance test was carried out among the treatments by two-way ANOVA followed by Bonferroni post tests at $p < 0.05$. Statistical analysis was conducted with software GraphPad Prism 8.0.

3. Results

3.1. Bacteriocin-Bac10307: Extraction, Purification, and Antibacterial Activity Analysis

The isolation and purification of bacteriocin Bac10307 was carried out from the *L. acidophilus* bacteria. Among the tested pathogenic test strains that were used as a part of this study, bacteriocin Bac10307 exhibited antibacterial properties against all the tested strains viz. *S. aureus*, *P. aeruginosa*, *B. subtilis*, and *E. coli*, which indicates that Bac10307 demonstrates antibacterial activity against Gram-positive as well as Gram-negative bacteria. There was a maximum zone of inhibition observed for *S. aureus*, followed by *B. subtilis*, *P. aeruginosa*, and *E. coli* (Figure 1).

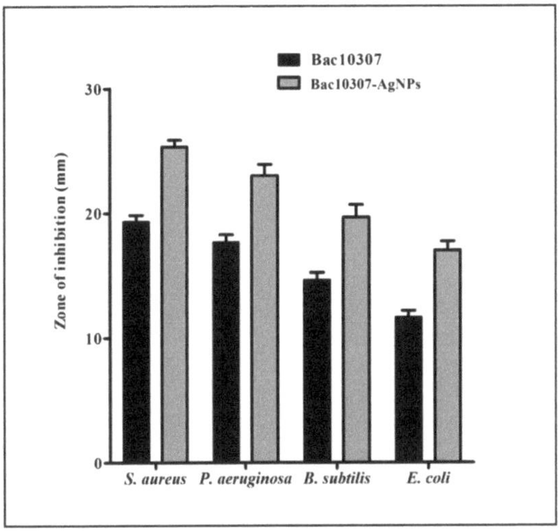

Figure 1. Antibacterial activity (zone of inhibition) of Bac10307 and Bac10307-capped AgNPs against *S. aureus*, *P. aeruginosa*, *B. subtilis*, and *E. coli*. The test was carried out in triplicate, and the data represent the mean ± SD, n = 3.

3.2. Characterization of Purified Bacteriocin-Bac10307

In a study to evaluate the effect of temperature on the antibacterial activity of Bac10307, results showed that Bac10307 was stable at temperatures ranging from 20 to 100 °C. A high level of antibacterial response was observed at temperatures between 30 °C and 40 °C, followed by a slight decline in antibacterial activity as temperatures rose from 30 to 100 °C (Figure 2A). Although the antimicrobial potential of the culture had decreased, it still exhibited high temperature stability despite the decrease in the zone of inhibition.

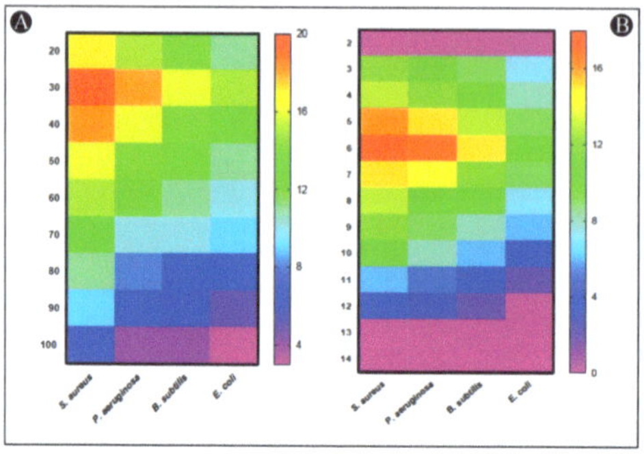

Figure 2. Effect of (**A**) temperature, and (**B**) pH on the activity of Bac10307 extracted from *L. acidophilus*.

From the results of a study conducted to assess how pH affects the antibacterial activity of Bac10307, it showed antibacterial activity between pH ranges of 3 to 12 except against *E. coli*. It was observed that Bac10307 maintained the highest antibacterial activity at pH 6, thus showing the highest stability at this pH as well (Figure 2B).

From the results of the study conducted to assess whether the antibacterial effect was entirely a result of the purified Bac10307, rather than any other molecular moiety present, it has been found that, after treating Bac10307 with proteinase-K and trypsin, antibacterial activity was completely lost, while activity remained unchanged in the presence of α-amylase.

According to the SDS–PAGE gel electrophoresis analysis, the purified bacteriocin Bac10307 has a molecular weight around 4.2 kDa, along with few faint bands in the lane (Figure 3A).

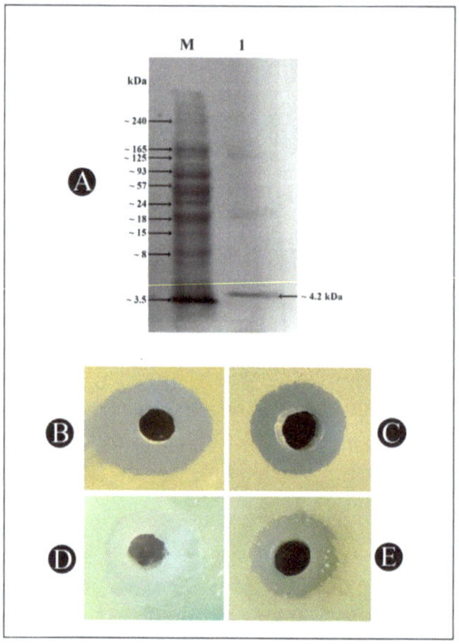

Figure 3. (**A**) Determination of molecular weight of bacteriocin by SD-SPAGE. Lane M contains the molecular-weight marker. Lane 1 contains bacteriocin from *L. acidophilus*. (**B**) Zone of inhibition of antibacterial activity of Bac10307-AgNPs against *S. aureus*, (**C**) zone of inhibition of antibacterial activity of Bac10307-AgNPs against *P. aeruginosa*, (**D**) zone of inhibition of antibacterial activity of Bac10307-AgNPs against *B. subtilis*, (**E**) zone of inhibition of antibacterial activity of Bac10307-AgNPs against *E. coli*.

3.3. Synthesis and Characterization of Bac10307-AgNPs

Following the characterization of Bac10307, the synthesis of Bac10307-AgNPs was carried out. As a result of the addition of Bac10307 to the $AgNO_3$ solution, a color change was observed from light yellow to reddish brown, which provided an indication that Bac10307-AgNPs were synthesized. Different analytical techniques were used for the purpose of determining the size, morphology, and stability of the synthesized Bac10307-AgNPs. The UV–visible spectroscopy analysis revealed the absorption spectrum had a peak maximum at 430 nm, indicating that synthesized Bac10307-AgNPs were successfully synthesized (Figure 4A).

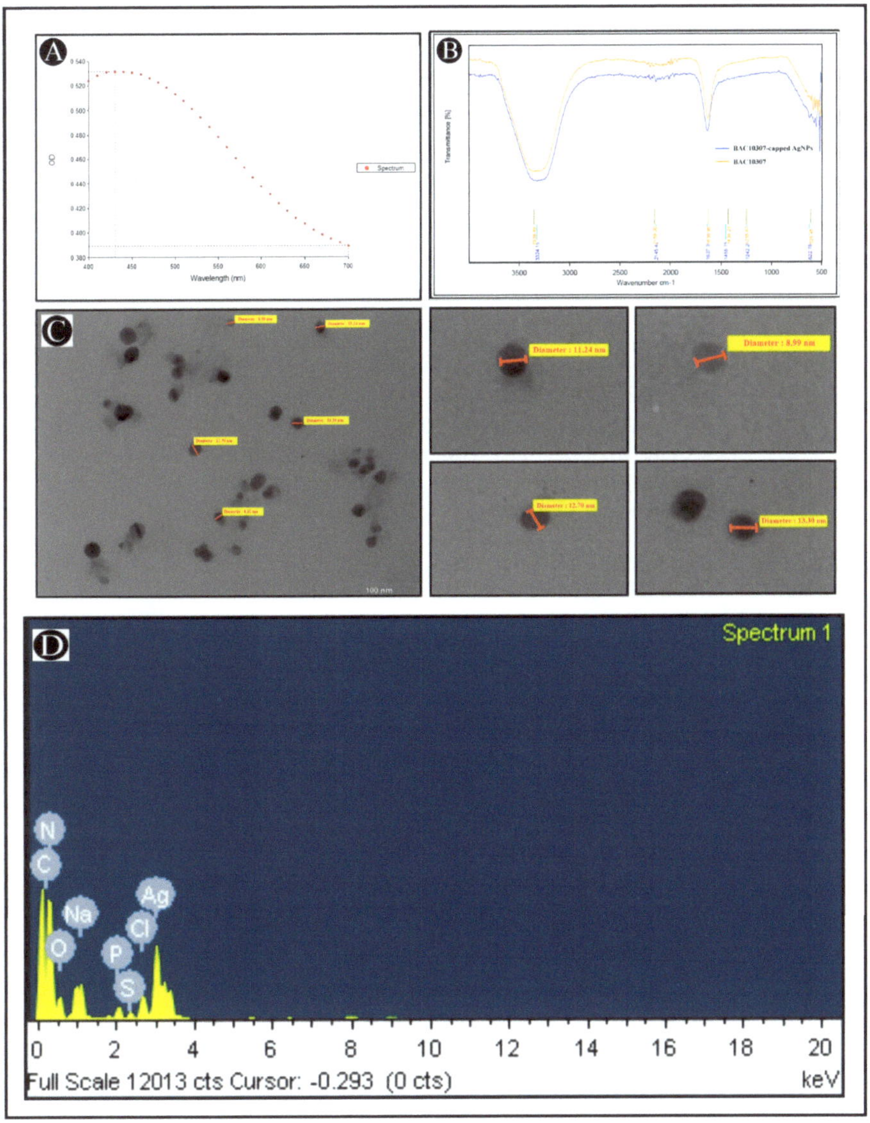

Figure 4. Characterization of Bac10307-AgNPs. (**A**). UV-visible absorption spectra of synthesized Bac10307-AgNPs. (**B**). FT-IR pattern of Bac10307 and Bac10307-AgNPs. (**C**). Morphological analysis of synthesized Bac10307-AgNPs with variable diameter using TEM analysis. (**D**). EDX analysis.

It is known that AgNPs exhibit an absorption peak between 400 and 500 nm in the UV–visible spectrum. Generally, AgNPs appear to have an absorption band due to the free electrons in them, which are caused by their mutual vibration of light wave incidences, resulting in a Surface Plasmon Resonance (SPR) absorption band. The synthesized AgNPs were also subjected to spectroscopic measurements two weeks after synthesis, and the spectroscopic data displayed no significant variation in the spectroscopic results, which was an indication that the synthesized AgNPs were stable over time.

For the identification of functional groups involved during the synthesis of AgNPs, a FTIR study was conducted. In light of the findings of this study, it appears that the structure of Bac10307 did not undergo any major changes as a result of its affiliation with AgNPs during the synthesis process. In addition, an almost similar spectrum was observed for Bac10307-AgNPs as for Bac10307 (Figure 4B). The peaks for Bac10307-AgNPs were observed at 3339.49, 2159.00, 1636.95, 1434.23, and 1255.67 cm^{-1}. These peaks indicate the presence of OH and NH_2 groups, C≡C stretch of alkynes, C–O and C–N stretching and peptide linkage in amides, and C–H stretching.

In the TEM analysis, Bac10307-AgNPs were shown to be spherical nanoparticles with irregular shapes of various sizes and their dispersion was good without any obvious agglomeration. In terms of size, the AgNPs synthesized were between 9 and 20 nm (Figure 4C). In addition, an EDX analysis was carried out to determine the overall composition of elements in the reaction mixture of extracted bacteriocin and silver nitrate after the reactions had been completed. The results revealed a strong signal in the silver region at 3 KeV and confirms the formation of silver nanoparticles along with other elements (Figure 4D).

3.4. Antibacterial Activity of Bac10307 and Synthesized Bac10307-AgNPs

As compared to Bac10307 alone, Bac10307-AgNPs displayed enhancement in the activity. Antibacterial activity of the synthesized Bac10307-AgNPs was 1.35-, 1.31-, 1.34-, and 1.54-fold greater than Bac10307 (Figure 1). As a next step, MIC and MBC analysis was further carried out in the presence of increasing dilutions of Bac10307-AgNPs. A visual analysis as well as measurements of the growth pattern at 600 nm was performed. The values of MIC were 8 μg/mL for *S. aureus* and *P. aeruginosa*, 16 μg/mL for *B. subtilis*, and 64 μg/mL for *E. coli*, and MBC values were observed to be two times higher than the MIC values (Table 1).

Table 1. Antibacterial activity of synthesized Bac10307 and Bac10307-AgNPs.

Test Organisms	**Zone of Inhibition (mm)**			**MIC (μg/mL) Bac10307-AgNPs**	**MBC (μg/mL) Bac10307-AgNPs**
	Bac10307	**AgNPs**	**Bac10307- AgNPs**		
S. aureus	19.66	11.66	25.33	8	16
P. aeruginosa	17.33	10.33	23.00	8	16
B. subtilis	14.66	8.33	19.66	16	32
E. coli	11.66	7.66	17.00	64	128

3.5. In Vitro Antioxidant Activity of Synthesized Bac10307-AgNPs

A study of the antioxidant potential of synthesized Bac10307-AgNPs has been conducted to assess their inhibitory effect on DPPH free radicals. As a result, the synthesized Bac10307-AgNPs were observed to exhibit dose-dependent free radical scavenging activity against DPPH (IC_{50} = 116.04 μg/mL) viz. increase in concentration (2–256 μg/mL) enhanced the antioxidant potentiality more than Bac10307 alone did (IC_{50} = 139.82 μg/mL) (Figure 5A).

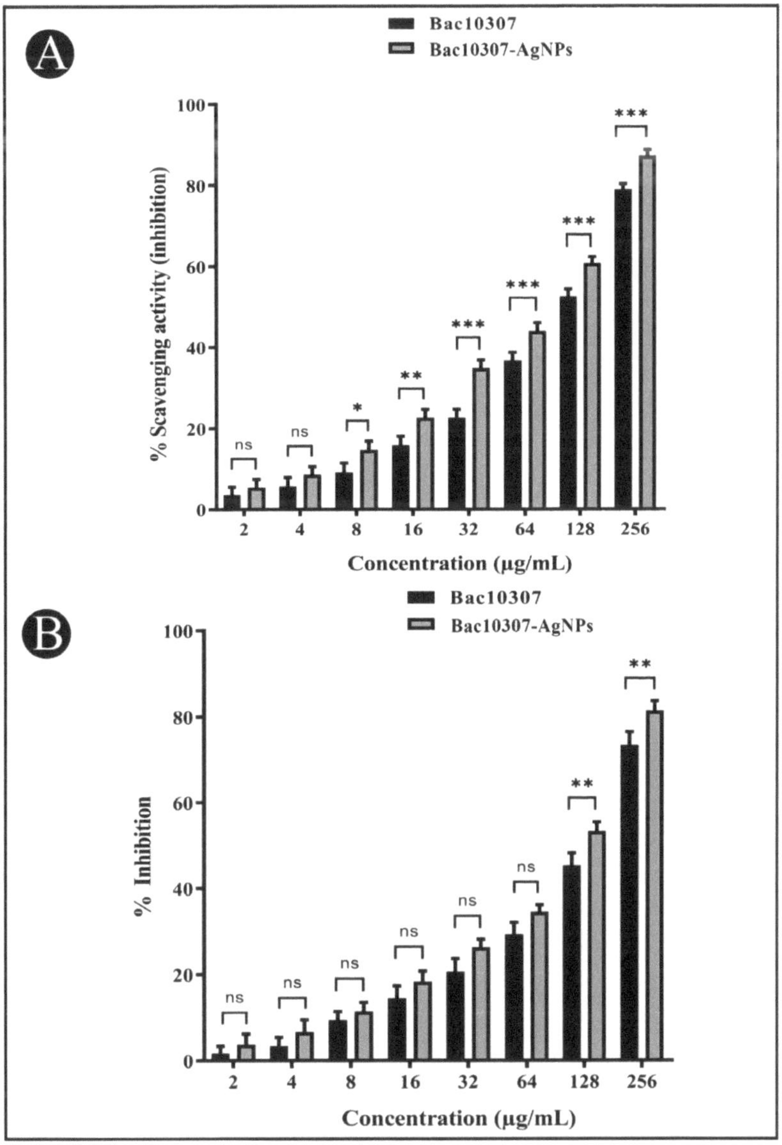

Figure 5. (**A**). Antioxidant activity of Bac10307 and Bac10307-AgNPs against DPPH free radicals. (**B**) Cytotoxicity of Bac10307 and Bac10307-AgNPs against HepG2 cancer cells. The test was carried out in triplicate, and the data represent the mean ± SD, n = 3. Significance; ns > 0.05, * $p < 0.05$, ** $p < 0.01$, *** $p < 0.001$.

3.6. In Vitro Cytotoxicity of Synthesized Bac10307-AgNPs

Potential cytotoxic properties of synthesized Bac10307-AgNPs was evaluated via MTT assay against human liver cancer cells (Hep-G2). The results indicated that Bac10307-AgNPs inhibited the proliferation of Hep-G2 cancer cells (IC_{50} = 135.63 µg/mL) more than Bac10307 alone did (IC_{50} = 158.20 µg/mL) in a dose-dependent manner (Figures 5B and 6A–D).

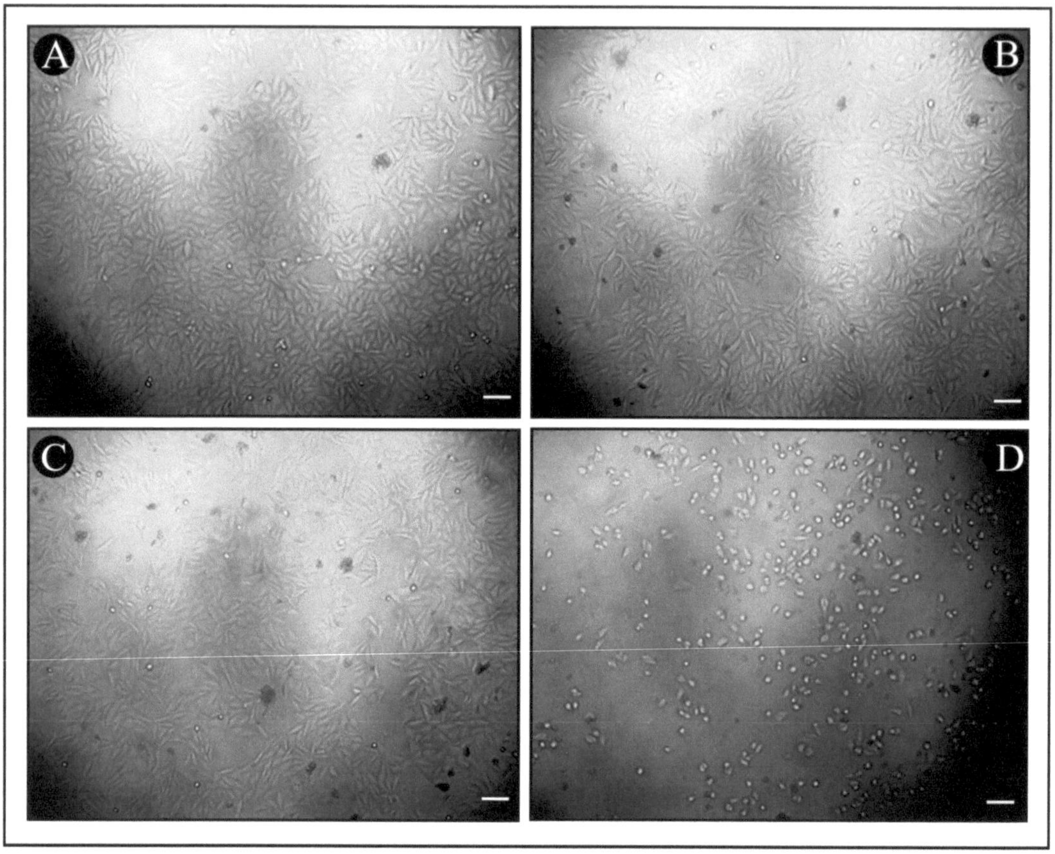

Figure 6. Morphological analysis of HepG2 cells under inverted microscope after treatment with different concentrations of Bac10307-AgNPs with morphological changes. (**A**) Untreated, (**B**) 4 µg/mL, (**C**) 64 µg/mL, (**D**) 256 µg/mL (magnification 20×, scale bar 50 µm).

3.7. Molecular Docking Analysis

To predict the protein–protein binding modes and affinities, ClusPro 2.0 was used to pair the bacteriocins of *L. acidophilus* with the selected target proteins. The ClusPro scores are based on searching for the lowest free binding energy for native site. A summary of the results is represented in Table 2. It shows the size of each cluster (number of members), the cluster center's energy score (i.e., its most neighbouring structure), and its lowest energy structure (Supplementary Table S1). ClusPro has been also used to generate molecular docking complexes that can be used to analyze the interactions between the amino acid residues of target proteins and bacteriocins (Figures 7–9).

Table 2. Interacting active site residues of acidocin A with different target proteins.

Proteins	Receptor-Ligand	Interection Type	Distance
2CDU-Acidocin A	A:LYS78:HZ2–A:ASP282:OD2	Salt Bridge;Attractive Charge	1.76041
	A:LYS78:HZ3–A:ASP282:OD1	Salt Bridge;Attractive Charge	1.75112
	A:CYS133:HN–A:HIS81:NE2	Conventional Hydrogen Bond	2.43145
	A:ILE160:HN–A:PHE80:O	Conventional Hydrogen Bond	2.31372
	A:GLY244:HN–A:HIS81:O	Conventional Hydrogen Bond	1.88916
	A:ALA300:HN–A:PHE76:O	Conventional Hydrogen Bond	2.81082
	A:THR301:HN–A:GLY74:O	Conventional Hydrogen Bond	2.55908
	A:ARG305:HH11–A:TRP71:O	Conventional Hydrogen Bond	1.81072
	A:ARG305:HH21–A:TRP71:O	Conventional Hydrogen Bond	1.84157
	A:ARG431:HH12–A:SER3:O	Conventional Hydrogen Bond	2.70789
	A:PHE433:HN–A:ILE5:O	Conventional Hydrogen Bond	2.04607
	A:SER3:HN–A:GLU366:OE1	Conventional Hydrogen Bond	2.29836
	A:SER7:HG–A:PRO432:O	Conventional Hydrogen Bond	1.84543
	A:GLN9:HE22–A:ASP422:OD1	Conventional Hydrogen Bond	2.12445
	A:THR79:HN–A:PRO298:O	Conventional Hydrogen Bond	2.73643
	A:THR79:HG1–A:PRO298:O	Conventional Hydrogen Bond	1.85808
	A:SER41:CB–A:GLY77:O	Conventional Hydrogen Bond	3.70135
	A:ARG431:CD–A:SER3:O	Carbon Hydrogen Bond	3.15632
	A:HIS81:CE1–A:LEU241:O	Carbon Hydrogen Bond	3.13598
	A:LYS187:NZ–A:PHE80	Pi-Cation	3.51826
	A:ARG305:NH1–A:TRP71	Pi-Cation	4.77402
	A:SER7:CA–A:PHE433	Pi-Sigma	3.67277
	A:ILE243:C,O;GLY244:N–A:PHE80	Amide-Pi Stacked	3.93853
	A:ALA300–A:LYS78	Alkyl	4.9093
	A:ILE438–A:ILE5	Alkyl	4.68217
	A:LYS10–A:MET420	Alkyl	4.61562
	A:PHE367–A:ILE2	Pi-Alkyl	5.07639
	A:TRP71–A:VAL304	Pi-Alkyl	5.08256
	A:TRP71–A:ARG305	Pi-Alkyl	4.70863
	A:TRP71–A:ARG305	Pi-Alkyl	4.06273
	A:TRP71–A:ARG308	Pi-Alkyl	5.17719
	A:PHE76–A:LEU330	Pi-Alkyl	4.80412
	A:HIS81–A:PRO117	Pi-Alkyl	4.38714
	A:HIS81–A:LEU132	Pi-Alkyl	5.41817

Table 2. *Cont.*

Proteins	Receptor-Ligand	Interection Type	Distance
6f86-Acidocin A	A:MET1:N–A:ASP210:OD2	Attractive Charge	5.4936
	A:ARG22:HH11–A:LEU59:O	Conventional Hydrogen Bond	1.77015
	A:ARG22:HH21–A:SER58:OG	Conventional Hydrogen Bond	1.72382
	A:TYR26:HH–A:ASP64:OD2	Conventional Hydrogen Bond	1.97086
	A:ASN46:HD22–A:ALA72:O	Conventional Hydrogen Bond	1.98784
	A:ASN46:HD22–A:THR73:O	Conventional Hydrogen Bond	2.63274
	A:ARG76:HH12–A:GLY77:O	Conventional Hydrogen Bond	1.8161
	A:ARG136:HH11–A:PHE76:O	Conventional Hydrogen Bond	2.53417
	A:ARG136:HH11–A:LYS78:O	Conventional Hydrogen Bond	2.17681
	A:ARG136:HH21–A:LYS78:O	Conventional Hydrogen Bond	1.72262
	A:THR180:HG1–A:SER7:OG	Conventional Hydrogen Bond	1.87972
	A:SER3:HN–A:ARG209:O	Conventional Hydrogen Bond	2.36379
	A:SER3:HG–A:ARG209:O	Conventional Hydrogen Bond	1.86756
	A:GLN9:HE21–A:GLU174:OE2	Conventional Hydrogen Bond	2.01259
	A:LYS10:HN–A:GLN128:OE1	Conventional Hydrogen Bond	2.17849
	A:ALA18:HN–A:ASP14:O	Conventional Hydrogen Bond	1.93332
	A:ALA18:HN–A:LYS15:O	Conventional Hydrogen Bond	2.65481
	A:SER21:HN–A:ALA18:O	Conventional Hydrogen Bond	2.35624
	A:GLY23:HN–A:ALA18:O	Conventional Hydrogen Bond	1.89654
	A:LYS24:HZ3–A:TYR26:OH	Conventional Hydrogen Bond	1.63416
	A:TYR26:HN–A:LYS24:O	Conventional Hydrogen Bond	2.39531
	A:LYS62:HZ1–A:TYR26:O	Conventional Hydrogen Bond	2.61388
	A:LYS62:HZ2–A:TYR26:O	Conventional Hydrogen Bond	2.68718
	A:LYS62:HZ3–A:MET25:O	Conventional Hydrogen Bond	1.66846
	A:LEU68:HN–A:LEU98:O	Conventional Hydrogen Bond	2.64427
	A:THR73:HG1–A:ASP49:OD1	Conventional Hydrogen Bond	1.98276
	A:THR79:HG1–A:ARG76:O	Conventional Hydrogen Bond	1.81635
	A:ARG76:CD–A:GLY77:O	Carbon Hydrogen Bond	3.35609
	A:MET4:CA–A:GLU181:OE2	Carbon Hydrogen Bond	3.26235
	A:TRP71:CD1–A:VAL97:O	Carbon Hydrogen Bond	3.75115
	A:GLU50:OE1–A:PHE76	Pi-Anion	3.4452
	A:ALA18–A:ILE61	Alkyl	4.4781
	A:VAL118–A:LEU65	Alkyl	4.41069
	A:LYS62–A:MET25	Alkyl	5.37497
	A:ALA72–A:VAL120	Alkyl	5.07682

Table 2. *Cont.*

Proteins	Receptor-Ligand	Interection Type	Distance
	A:ALA75–A:PRO79	Alkyl	5.06784
	A:ALA75–A:ILE94	Alkyl	4.19361
	A:TYR26–A:LYS62	Pi-Alkyl	4.48685
	A:TYR26–A:LYS24	Pi-Alkyl	4.99044
	A:TRP71–A:VAL97	Pi-Alkyl	4.62974
	A:TRP71–A:VAL97	Pi-Alkyl	5.0319
	A:PHE76–A:ILE78	Pi-Alkyl	5.21439
	A:PHE80–A:ARG76	Pi-Alkyl	4.69087
2OH4-Acidocin A	A:ARG1078:HH11–A:ASP14:OD1	Salt Bridge;Attractive Charge	1.77815
	A:ARG1122:HH22–A:ASP64:OD2	Salt Bridge;Attractive Charge	1.82447
	A:LYS24:HZ1–A:ASP1044:OD1	Salt Bridge;Attractive Charge	2.0004
	A:LYS24:HZ3–A:ASP1044:OD1	Salt Bridge;Attractive Charge	2.03938
	A:ARG55:HH21–A:GLU1112:OE2	Salt Bridge;Attractive Charge	1.89818
	A:LYS56:HZ1–A:GLU1111:OE1	Salt Bridge;Attractive Charge	1.69962
	A:LYS56:HZ3–A:GLU1111:OE2	Salt Bridge;Attractive Charge	1.80997
	A:LYS78:HZ3–A:GLU1156:OE2	Salt Bridge;Attractive Charge	1.71364
	A:ARG1078:NH2–A:ASP14:OD2	Attractive Charge	2.75179
	A:ARG1122:NH1–A:ASP64:OD1	Attractive Charge	4.71658
	A:ARG55:NH1–A:ASP1110:OD2	Attractive Charge	5.55384
	A:ARG55:NH1–A:GLU1112:OE1	Attractive Charge	2.72487
	A:ARG878:HH11–A:TYR27:OH	Conventional Hydrogen Bond	1.773
	A:ARG927:HH11–A:SER38:O	Conventional Hydrogen Bond	3.0835
	A:ARG927:HH21–A:SER38:O	Conventional Hydrogen Bond	1.74776
	A:ILE1023:HN–A:SER21:O	Conventional Hydrogen Bond	1.98064
	A:ARG1025:HH11–A:SER21:O	Conventional Hydrogen Bond	1.79986
	A:ARG1025:HH21–A:SER21:OG	Conventional Hydrogen Bond	1.96334
	A:ARG1025:HH21–A:GLY22:O	Conventional Hydrogen Bond	2.07187
	A:LYS1060:HZ2–A:LYS36:O	Conventional Hydrogen Bond	1.63582
	A:GLY1061:HN–A:THR35:O	Conventional Hydrogen Bond	2.45869
	A:ALA1063:HN–A:THR35:OG1	Conventional Hydrogen Bond	2.01064
	A:LYS1108:HZ1–A:ILE49:O	Conventional Hydrogen Bond	2.21003
	A:LYS1108:HZ3–A:GLY51:O	Conventional Hydrogen Bond	1.71447
	A:ARG1115:HH12–A:LYS56:O	Conventional Hydrogen Bond	1.81567
	A:ARG1116:HH11–A:GLN57:OE1	Conventional Hydrogen Bond	1.89055
	A:ARG1116:HH21–A:GLN57:OE1	Conventional Hydrogen Bond	1.9005
	A:ARG1116:HH22–A:SER58:O	Conventional Hydrogen Bond	2.01369
	A:ARG1122:HE–A:ASP64:OD1	Conventional Hydrogen Bond	2.45807

Table 2. *Cont.*

Proteins	Receptor-Ligand	Interection Type	Distance
	A:GLY1143:HN–A:ASP64:OD2	Conventional Hydrogen Bond	2.04712
	A:LYS24:HZ1–A:HIS1024:NE2	Conventional Hydrogen Bond	2.30731
	A:LYS24:HZ2–A:HIS1024:O	Conventional Hydrogen Bond	1.64274
	A:HIS33:HN–A:ASP1050:O	Conventional Hydrogen Bond	2.89181
	A:THR35:HG1–A:ARG1059:O	Conventional Hydrogen Bond	2.54504
	A:LYS36:HZ1–A:VAL1107:O	Conventional Hydrogen Bond	1.69429
	A:ARG55:HN–A:GLU1112:OE1	Conventional Hydrogen Bond	2.65589
	A:LYS56:HN–A:GLU1112:OE1	Conventional Hydrogen Bond	2.47201
	A:GLN57:HN–A:GLU1112:OE1	Conventional Hydrogen Bond	1.99761
	A:SER58:HG–A:GLU1119:OE2	Conventional Hydrogen Bond	1.94121
	A:LEU59:HN–A:GLU1119:OE1	Conventional Hydrogen Bond	2.04219
	A:ILE61:HN–A:GLU1119:O	Conventional Hydrogen Bond	1.97082
	A:GLN63:HE21–A:GLY1120:O	Conventional Hydrogen Bond	2.03591
	A:LEU68:HN–A:ASP1139:OD2	Conventional Hydrogen Bond	2.48216
	A:LYS78:HZ1–A:GLN1163:OE1	Conventional Hydrogen Bond	1.98774
	A:LYS78:HZ2–A:ASN1160:OD1	Conventional Hydrogen Bond	1.69053
	A:SER58:CA–A:GLU1119:OE1	Carbon Hydrogen Bond	2.9455
	A:LYS24:NZ–A:HIS1024	Pi-Cation	3.6145
	A:ASP64:OD2–A:HIS1142	Pi-Anion	4.79084
	A:VAL1058:CG1–A:HIS33	Pi-Sigma	3.82332
	A:LYS1021–A:ILE20	Alkyl	4.85838
	A:ALA1101–A:LEU39	Alkyl	4.05593
	A:PRO1149–A:LEU68	Alkyl	5.33682
	A:HIS1142–A:LEU65	Pi-Alkyl	5.30386
	A:TYR27–A:ALA879	Pi-Alkyl	4.63121
	A:TRP40–A:PRO1105	Pi-Alkyl	4.91592
	A:TRP71–A:PRO1149	Pi-Alkyl	4.42062

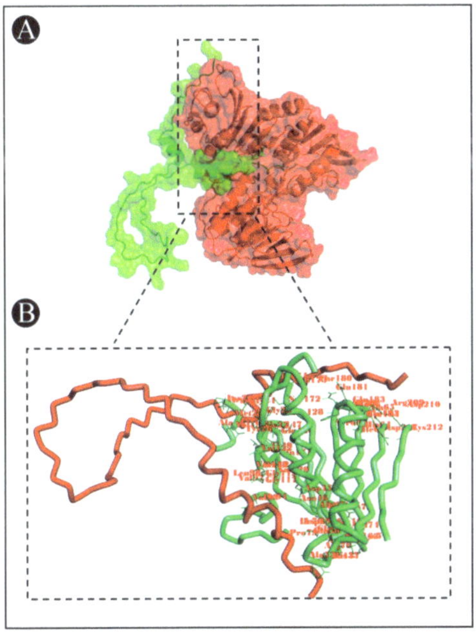

Figure 7. Docking representation of the acidocin A and 2CDU complex. (**A**) The binding interface of the complex, (**B**) the binding interaction between the amino acids.

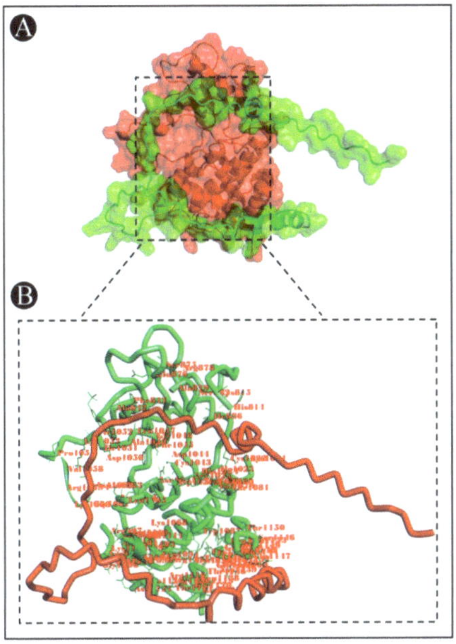

Figure 8. Docking representation of acidocin A and 2OH4 complex. (**A**) The binding interface of the complex, (**B**) the binding interaction between the amino acids.

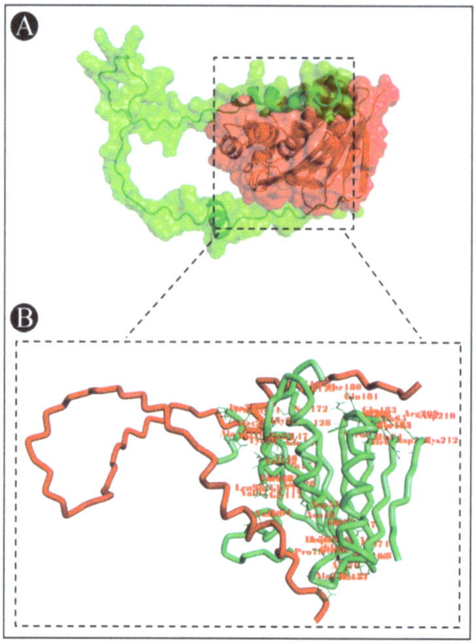

Figure 9. Docking representation of the acidocin A and 6F86 complex. (**A**) The binding interface of the complex, (**B**). the binding interaction between the amino acids.

4. Discussion

The antibacterial activity of bacteriocins makes them a very promising alternative as an additive to the currently used antibiotics combatting the epidemic of different bacterial infections that are sweeping across the globe today. Apart from antimicrobial activity, some of them have also been reported for their multifunctional properties, such as antioxidant and anticancer activity [30–34]. Thus, it is speculated that some of them could constitute a potential source of new biologically active agents in the future. Despite these promising advantages, nisin continues to be the only bacteriocin that is considered safe by the Food and Drug Administration (FDA) and is now used as a food preservative internationally [35]. There are several factors that contribute to the limited availability of bacteriocins in the market as preservatives and antimicrobials, including their high production costs [36], loss of their activity due to proteolytic enzymes [36], their adverse interconnection with other food constituents [37], change in the physical and chemical properties at the time of different food-processing stages [38], insufficient recovery by traditional purification methods of these compounds, and the limited scale of activity detected for most of the tested bacteriocins towards pathogenic bacteria [39]. It has been demonstrated in recent years that optimizing the production conditions, the purification method, the combination with other antimicrobial agents, and the hurdle technology approach can all contribute to solving some of these problems related to bacteriocins [40]. A potential approach to maximizing the effectiveness of bacteriocins is through the use of nanotechnology, which has been shown to be an effective means to overcome the limitations of these peptides [41]. Thus, the purpose of the present study was to elucidate the current applications of nanotechnology in improving the properties and bioactive potential of bacteriocins in order to improve its efficacy.

In the present study, bacteriocin Bac10307 was extracted from *L. acidophilus* and partially purified before being used. A partially purified bacteriocin Bac10307 was observed to possess antibacterial properties against *S. aureus*, *B. subtilis*, *P. aeruginosa*, and *E. coli*, indicating that it exhibits antibacterial properties against both Gram-positive and Gram-negative bacteria. It has also been reported that similar results have been found in a few previous studies. In a study carried out by De Giani et al. (2019) [42], plantsaricin P1053 produced by the *L. plantarum* PBS067 strain was found to show broad spectrum antimicrobial activity against both Gram-positive and Gram-negative bacteria. Similarly, in the study conducted by Danilova et al. (2019) [43], antimicrobial peptides isolated from *L. plantarum* were shown to inhibit the growth of *S. aureus*, *E. coli*, and *P. aeruginosa* in vitro, confirming previous findings.

Among the factors that influence the activity of bacteriocins, temperature is an important one. As shown in the present study, bacteriocin extracted from *L. acidophilus* was quite active even after being exposed to high temperatures, indicating that it is a heat-stable protein. In other studies, Abo-Amer (2007) [44] and Fatima and Mebrouk (2013) [45] have made similar observations that highlight the usefulness of *L. plantarum* bacteriocin as a preservative procedure for food due to its high-temperature tolerance. Similarly, bacteriocin Lac-B23 has been reported to have its antibacterial activity even after being heated for 30 min at 121 °C in order to sustain its antibacterial response [18]. In addition, another study reported that at 50, 70, and 80 °C, the levels of bacteriocins produced by *L. bulgaricus*, *L. acidophilus*, and *L. helveticus* remained constant. In spite of this, the bacteriocins from *L. acidophilus* and *L. bulgaricus* were the only ones still effective at 100 °C [46]. As a result, it can be concluded that each bacteriocin behaves differently depending on the conditions it is exposed to. It should be noted that the bacteriocins obtained in our study were capable of maintaining their activity even at very high temperatures (80–100 °C), thus supporting their potential application in the food industry.

A second factor that affects the antibacterial activity of bacteriocins is pH. During the present study, Bac10307 was found to exhibit antimicrobial activity in the pH range of 3–12 with the highest antimicrobial activity being detected at pH 6. A similar trend has also been reported when optimizing pH values for L23, a novel bacteriocin produced by *L. plantarum*-J23. A pH stability range of 2.0 to 12.0 was observed for the bacteriocin. According to another study, plantsaricin LPL-1, which is produced by *L. plantarum*, was found to be stable in a pH range between 2 and 10, and its antibacterial activity decreased with an increase in pH value until a total loss of activity was observed at pH 11 [15]. The bacteriocin L23 has also been shown to retain 90% of its activity up to pH 7.0 in a previous study [18].

Apart from the effect of temperature and pH, it has been determined that the antibacterial properties of Bac10307 are exclusively due to the protein itself, not by any other molecular moiety following treatment with proteinase-K, trypsin, and α-amylase. Bac10307 did not display any sensitivity towards α-amylase, which indicated that the antibacterial activity of it did not change in the presence of this enzyme. Therefore, we can infer that the presence of hydrogen peroxide and glycoproteins does not have any effect on the antibacterial response. Even though this fact had been noted, the antibacterial activity of the Bac10307 could not recover after treatment with trypsin and proteinase-K, possibly due to the enzymes and their role in destroying the active site of Bac10307 during the process. Based on its sensitivity to both proteolytic enzymes, it was concluded that Bac10307 is a proteinaceous in nature. Previously, Zhang et al., (2018) [18] reported that the bacteriocin Lac-B23 was not sensitive to papain or pepsin, but it lost antimicrobial activity after its treatment with proteinase-K, trypsin, and proteinase-E. Similarly, the antimicrobial activity of the bacteriocin obtained by *L. murinus* AU06 was also completely lost following treatment with chymotrypsin, proteinase K, trypsin, and pepsin [16].

SDS–PAGE gel electrophoresis of the purified Bac10307 was performed, and the molecular mass was determined to be around 4.2 kDa; [47] reported the isolation of sheep raw milk cheese bacteriocin-producing *L. plantarum* strains used in a similar study as ours, and using SDS–PAGE gel electrophoresis and MALDI–TOF analysis, the bacteriocin produced from these strains was determined to have a size of 4.8 kDa. A similar report was published by Song (2009) [48], in which they reported the synthesis of plantaricin ZJ5, which had a molecular mass of 2.5 kDa. It has also been discovered that there are a variety of novel plantaricins discovered from *L. plantarum* in recent years, including the plantaricin ASM1 (5 kDa) [49], plantaricin C19 (3.8 kDa) [50], plantaricin 163 (3.5 kDa) [51], plantaricin Y (4.2 kDa) [52], plantaricin LPL-1 [53], and Lac B-23 [18].

A number of factors have been identified that limit the activity of natural bacteriocins, including the rapid degradation of the bacteriocins within a few days in the environment as well as a high effective concentration accompanied by a low yield [54]. As one of the most successful methods of overcoming most of these problems, nanotechnology can be considered one of the most modern methods. According to Lazzari et al., (2012) [55], the stability of nanoparticles in biological fluids is excellent, in addition to their efficient antimicrobial properties due to the high surface area of the particles. Because of these advantages, it seems like a good idea to incorporate nanotechnology into bacteriocin encapsulation to enhance its properties [56]. As a consequence, using the nanotechnology approach, we produced bacteriocin-derived silver nanoparticles using the bacteriocin extracted from the culture and compared the bioactive potential of the bacteriocin with the nanoparticle formulations. It appears from the results of our study that Bac10307-AgNPs were synthesized, which was confirmed by UV–vis spectroscopy. There is a strong band of absorption at 430 nm that was observed in the synthesized Bac10307-AgNPs as a result of their SPR properties. There is a strong possibility that this was caused by the stimulation of longitudinal plasmon vibrations and the reduction of $AgNO_3$ ions as well [57]. A FT-IR study was conducted in order to determine the functional properties of nanoparticles by identifying the associated functional groups. An analysis of the FT-IR spectrum revealed a number of absorption peaks, including those associated with the OH and NH_2 groups, stretching of alkynes, C–O and C–N stretching and peptide linkage in amides, and C–H stretching. In the analysis of images obtained by the TEM of Bac10307-AgNPs, it can be seen that the majority of the particles were crystalline in nature and irregularly shaped or spherical in shape, with varying sizes. It has been reported in previous studies that the TEM analysis results of the spherical Bac23-capped AgNPs were irregularly shaped and of different sizes [20]. EDX is an analytical technique used to determine the elemental composition of a sample and to characterize its chemical composition, which relies on the interaction of some source of X-ray excitation with the sample. According to the EDAX spectral analysis of Bac10307-AgNPs preparations, there was a strong silver signal that is typical for metallic silver. However, weaker signals related to other atoms were also detected, which can be attributed to the bacteriocin bound to the AgNPs. Based on the results of the antibacterial response, Bac10307-AgNPs showed an enhancement in antibacterial performance compared to Bac10307 and AgNPs alone in terms of antibacterial effectiveness. Taking these results into account, it can be suggested that there may be a synergistic or enhanced effect of bacteriocin and AgNPs. Considering the recent findings, it might be possible to use AgNPs as an adjuvant for the treatment of various infectious diseases caused by Gram-negative and Gram-positive bacteria. Hence, the findings of our study support the claim that AgNPs are capable of exerting significant antibacterial activity, which can be used to enhance the effectiveness of existing antibiotics against Gram-negative and Gram-positive bacteria. Earlier research conducted by few researchers has also indicated that bacteriocin-derived AgNPs increase the antibacterial activity [58–60]. According to Thirumurugan et al., 2013 [60], an increase in activity was observed upon the combination of gold nanoparticles with bacteriocins. Anti-listerial activity also increased when gold nanoparticles were combined with pediocin–LAP conjugates, as reported by Singh et al., 2018 [61]. In addition, Morales-Avila et al., 2017 [62], found that ubiquicidin-conjugated SNPs showed improved antimicrobial activity compared to silver or gold nanoparticles alone in their study. Various free radicals are linked to oxygen, including reactive oxygen species (ROS) and reactive nitrogen species (RNS), which are able to react with molecules other than oxygen. By generating these free radicals, oxidative stress is induced, causing proteins, lipids, and nucleic acids to be damaged. Thus, free radicals are believed to play a role in a wide range of diseases, such as aging, inflammatory diseases (such as arthritis, a variety of respiratory diseases, and vasculitis in adults), neurological disorders (such as Alzheimer's disease, Parkinson's disease), ischemic diseases (stroke, heart attacks, and intestinal ischemia), and various types of cancer [25]. There are certain substances called antioxidants that act as defenses against free radicals. A DPPH assay was used to evaluate the in vitro antioxidant activity of Bac10307-AgNPs, and the results revealed that the Bac10307-AgNPs could scavenge radicals to a larger extent compared with Bac10307 alone.

At the present time, in spite of all the advances in oncology, cancer remains one of the most life-threatening diseases around the world [63]. In the world, liver cancer is ranked as the third-leading cause of death from cancer worldwide. In 2020, an estimated 830,180 people died around the world as a result of this disease [64]. Currently, radiation therapy, chemotherapy, and surgery are the three most common methods for treating cancer. This treatment has a range of side effects that are known to have a negative impact on human health. Therefore, there is a need for the findings of an alternative treatments or compounds which can treat cancer [65]. In this regard, the in-vitro cytotoxic potential of synthesized Bac10307-AgNPs was also investigated in this study for their anticancer potential against liver cancer cells. Based on the cytotoxic activity results of Bac10307-AgNPs, it has been found that they significantly inhibit the viability of liver cancer cells more than Bac10307 alone.

Moreover, the use of computer-aided drug discovery approaches is becoming more prevalent and is becoming one of the most useful tools for detecting medications derived from natural resources. For pharmaceutical and technology research, computational prediction models are essential for guiding the process of selecting the most appropriate methodology. These models have also been applied to the in silico prediction of drug behavior, including pharmacokinetics, pharmacology, and toxicology [66]. As a strategy for developing and testing pharmaceuticals, molecular docking has proven to be an efficient and cost-effective technique at present. Using this approach, it is possible to generate data on the interactions between drugs and receptors. These data can then be used for predicting the binding orientation of drugs to their targets. It has also been demonstrated that, using this method, a molecule can placed non-covalently into the binding site of an object macromolecule which facilitates systematic investigation, resulting in the binding of every ligand to the specific active sites of the object macromolecule [67,68].

The protein–protein docking technique is one of the most popular molecular modelling techniques because it is based on the use of computer algorithms and techniques in order to predict a complex's orientation and position as molecules are arranged together [69]. Using the ClusPro web server, simulations of molecular docking were conducted to determine the possibility of bacteriocin–protein interactions in the present study. The docking events resulted in the formation of stable complexes and the determination of lowest energy. Docking models are ranked by ClusPro in relation to the size of the conformation cluster to which they belong. As part of the docking energy calculation, ClusPro provides two types of docking energy: the core energy of a cluster of conformations and the lowest energy in the cluster as a whole [70]. There are a number of biomolecular applications in which protein–protein docking can be utilized, such as exploration of the conformational properties of enzymes, interactome predictions, recognition of molecules, dimerization of proteins, synthesis of specific probes for target proteins, aggregation of amyloid plaques, prediction of protein interactions, design of disease-fighting peptides, and designing vaccines [71].

Bacterial DNA gyrase is a type IIA DNA topoisomerase that plays a very important role in the replication and transcription processes of bacterial DNA [72]. The NADPH oxidase (nicotinamide adenine dinucleotide phosphate) enzymes are multi-subunit protein complexes. It is a membrane-bound protein whose primary function is to transfer electrons across the plasma membrane to molecular oxygen, producing the superoxide anion and reactive oxygen species (ROS), such as hydrogen peroxide and hydroxyl radicals. Most ROS are produced by the activity of NADPH oxidase, which is the most prevalent ROS production process [73–76]. In addition, in order to promote cancer angiogenesis as well as metastasis, VEGFR2 (vascular endothelial growth factor receptor 2) tyrosine kinase receptor plays an important role. Upon activation by VEGF, which is the ligand of VEGFR2, VEGFR2 appears to promote the formation of new blood vessels in its neighboring tissues, thereby facilitating the delivery of growth factors, nutrients, and oxygen for the proliferation, migration, metastasis, and survival of cancer cells. In many types of cancer, including liver cancer, VEGF- and VEGFR2-mediated metastasis contributes to the aggressive nature of the cancer and leads to high mortality rates [77,78]. Therefore, all three proteins are being considered as highly promising targets for respective biological activity, and the molecular docking study was carried out to examine the binding interactions of known bacteriocins of *L. acidophilus* with them, which confirm our finding of the bacteriocins that possess different biological activity. Furthermore, the results of in silico analysis findings also point to the possible mechanism of action of bacteriocin molecules in terms of targeting specific proteins, and this could be investigated further in order to design bacteriocins that target specific biological activities.

5. Conclusions

In this study, bacteriocin Bac10307 was extracted from the lactic acid bacteria *L. acidophilus*, and a single-step synthesis of Bac10307-AgNPs was performed in order to increase the bioactivity of bacteriocins. After being exposed to a range of temperatures and pH conditions, different levels of bioactivity were retained, and the molecular weight was determined to be 4.2 kDa. As compared to Bac10307 alone, Bac10307-AgNPs displayed better antibacterial activity against Gram-positive and Gram-negative bacteria, in vitro antioxidant activity against DPPH free radicals, and in vitro cytotoxic activity against liver cancer cells (HepG2) due to their small size and greater stability. Consequently, this nano-preparation could be applied efficiently in many practical applications, such as in the food industry or in the medical industry, as long as it is carefully evaluated for its safety before being used. However, the antioxidant and cytotoxic effects of Bac10307 and Bac10307-AgNPs have been observed in vitro in the present study, for which further research is needed to see whether the Bac10307 and Bac10307-AgNP are capable of manifesting similar effects in vivo.

Supplementary Materials: The following supporting information can be downloaded at: https://www.mdpi.com/article/10.3390/pharmaceutics15020403/s1, Table S1: Interacting active site residues of other bacteriocins with different target proteins.

Author Contributions: Conceptualization, A.J.S., M.P. and M.A.; methodology, F.B., M.M.A., J.S., S.J., M.S. (Manojkumar Sachidanandan) and M.S. (Mejdi Snoussi); validation, M.S. (Mejdi Snoussi), A.O., J.S., A.A., M.M.A., M.S. (Manojkumar Sachidanandan) and S.J.; formal analysis, M.A., R.B., F.B., M.P., M.S. (Manojkumar Sachidanandan) and A.O.; investigation, F.B., M.M.A., R.B., J.S., A.O., M.S. (Mejdi Snoussi), A.A. and S.J.; data curation, F.B., M.P., A.A., J.S., M.S. (Manojkumar Sachidanandan) and R.B.; writing—original draft preparation, A.J.S., M.P. and M.A.; writing—review and editing, A.J.S., A.O. and S.J.; visualization, A.A., M.M.A., M.S. (Mejdi Snoussi) and R.B.; supervision, A.J.S. and M.A.; project administration, A.J.S. All authors have read and agreed to the published version of the manuscript.

Funding: This research has been funded by Scientific Research Deanship at University of Ha'il –Ha'il, Saudi Arabia through project number RG-22009.

Institutional Review Board Statement: Not applicable.

Informed Consent Statement: Not applicable.

Data Availability Statement: Not applicable.

Acknowledgments: I would like to thank and appreciate all the support and technical assistance provided by Scientific Research Deanship at University of Ha'il, Ha'il, Saudi Arabia through project number RG-22009.

Conflicts of Interest: The authors declare no conflict of interest.

References

1. Irkitova, A.N.; Matsyura, A.V. Ecological and biological characteristics of *Lactobacillus acidophilus*. *Ukr. J. Ecol.* **2017**, *7*, 214–230. [CrossRef] [PubMed]
2. Villamil, L.; Reyes, C.; Martínez-Silva, M.A. In vivo and in vitro assessment of *Lactobacillus acidophilus* as probiotic for tilapia (*Oreochromis niloticus*, Perciformes: Cichlidae) culture improvement. *Aquac. Res.* **2014**, *45*, 1116–1125. [CrossRef]
3. Remes-Troche, J.M.; Coss-Adame, E.; Valdovinos-Díaz, M.; Gómez-Escudero, O.; Icaza-Chávez, M.E.; Chávez-Barrera, J.A.; Zárate-Mondragón, F.; Velasco, J.A.V.-R.; Aceves-Tavares, G.R.; Lira-Pedrín, M.A.; et al. Lactobacillus acidophilus LB: A useful pharmabiotic for the treatment of digestive disorders. *Ther. Adv. Gastroenterol.* **2020**, *13*, 1756284820971201. [CrossRef] [PubMed]
4. Gaspar, C.; Donders, G.G.; Palmeira-De-Oliveira, R.; Queiroz, J.A.; Tomaz, C.; Martinez-De-Oliveira, J. Bacteriocin production of the probiotic *Lactobacillus acidophilus* KS400. *AMB Express* **2018**, *8*, 153. [CrossRef]
5. Tang, H.W.; Phapugrangkul, P.; Fauzi, H.M.; Tan, J.S. Lactic Acid Bacteria Bacteriocin, an Antimicrobial Peptide Effective Against Multidrug Resistance: A Comprehensive Review. *Int. J. Pept. Res. Ther.* **2022**, *28*, 14. [CrossRef]
6. Silva, S.P.; Ribeiro, S.C.; Teixeira, J.A.; Silva, C.C. Application of an alginate-based edible coating with bacteriocin-producing *Lactococcus* strains in fresh cheese preservation. *LWT* **2022**, *153*, 112486. [CrossRef]
7. Cotter, P.; Hill, C.; Ross, R. Bacteriocins: Developing innate immunity for food. *Nat. Rev. Genet.* **2005**, *3*, 777–788. [CrossRef]
8. El-Gendy, A.O.; Essam, T.M.; Amin, M.A.; Ahmed, S.H.; Nes, I.F. Clinical Screening for Bacteriocinogenic *Enterococcus faecalis* Isolated from Intensive Care Unit Inpatient in Egypt. *J. Microb. Biochem. Technol.* **2013**, *4*, 161–167. [CrossRef]
9. Martín, R.; Escobedo, S.; Martín, C.; Crespo, A.; Quiros, L.M.; Suarez, J.E. Chemotherapy, Surface glycosaminoglycans protect eukaryotic cells against membrane-driven peptide bacteriocins. *Antimicrob. Agents Chemother.* **2015**, *59*, 677–681. [CrossRef]
10. Sidhu, P.K.; Nehra, K. Bacteriocin-nanoconjugates as emerging compounds for enhancing antimicrobial activity of bacteriocins. *J. King Saud. Univ.* **2019**, *31*, 758–767. [CrossRef]
11. Ansari, A.; Zohra, R.R.; Tarar, O.M.; Qader, S.A.U.; Aman, A. Screening, purification and characterization of thermostable, protease resistant Bacteriocin active against methicillin resistant *Staphylococcus aureus* (MRSA). *BMC Microbiol.* **2018**, *18*, 192. [CrossRef]
12. Patil, S.D.; Sharma, R.; Bhattacharyya, T.; Kumar, P.; Gupta, M.; Chaddha, B.S.; Navani, N.K.; Pathania, R. Antibacterial potential of a small peptide from *Bacillus* sp. RPT-0001 and its capping for green synthesis of silver nanoparticles. *J. Microbiol.* **2015**, *53*, 643–652. [CrossRef] [PubMed]
13. Yang, E.; Fan, L.; Jiang, Y.; Doucette, C.; Fillmore, S. Antimicrobial activity of bacteriocin-producing lactic acid bacteria isolated from cheeses and yogurts. *AMB Express* **2012**, *2*, 48. [CrossRef] [PubMed]
14. Patel, M.; Siddiqui, A.J.; Hamadou, W.S.; Surti, M.; Awadelkareem, A.M.; Ashraf, S.A.; Alreshidi, M.; Snoussi, M.; Rizvi, S.M.D.; Bardakci, F.; et al. Inhibition of Bacterial Adhesion and Antibiofilm Activities of a Glycolipid Biosurfactant from *Lactobacillus rhamnosus* with Its Physicochemical and Functional Properties. *Antibiotics* **2021**, *10*, 1546. [CrossRef]
15. Wang, Y.; Shang, N.; Qin, Y.; Zhang, Y.; Zhang, J.; Li, P. The complete genome sequence of *Lactobacillus plantarum* LPL-1, a novel antibacterial probiotic producing class IIa bacteriocin. *J. Biotechnol.* **2018**, *266*, 84–88. [CrossRef] [PubMed]
16. Elayaraja, S.; Annamalai, N.; Mayavu, P.; Balasubramanian, T. Production, purification and characterization of bacteriocin from *Lactobacillus murinus* AU06 and its broad antibacterial spectrum. *Asian Pac. J. Trop. Biomed.* **2014**, *4*, S305–S311. [CrossRef]
17. Miao, J.; Guo, H.; Ou, Y.; Liu, G.; Fang, X.; Liao, Z.; Ke, C.; Chen, Y.; Zhao, L.; Cao, Y. Purification and characterization of bacteriocin F1, a novel bacteriocin produced by *Lactobacillus paracasei* subsp. tolerans FX-6 from Tibetan kefir, a traditional fermented milk from Tibet, China. *Food Control* **2014**, *42*, 48–53. [CrossRef]
18. Zhang, J.; Yang, Y.; Yang, H.; Bu, Y.; Yi, H.; Zhang, L.; Han, X.; Ai, L. Purification and Partial Characterization of Bacteriocin Lac-B23, a Novel Bacteriocin Production by *Lactobacillus plantarum* J23, Isolated from Chinese Traditional Fermented Milk. *Front. Microbiol.* **2018**, *9*, 2165. [CrossRef] [PubMed]
19. Hassan, M.U.; Nayab, H.; Rehman, T.U.; Williamson, M.P.; Haq, K.U.; Shafi, N.; Shafique, F. Characterisation of Bacteriocins Produced by *Lactobacillus* spp. Isolated from the Traditional Pakistani Yoghurt and Their Antimicrobial Activity against Common Foodborne Pathogens. *BioMed Res. Int.* **2020**, *2020*, 8281623. [CrossRef] [PubMed]
20. Sidhu, P.K.; Nehra, K. Purification and characterization of bacteriocin Bac23 extracted from *Lactobacillus plantarum* PKLP5 and its interaction with silver nanoparticles for enhanced antimicrobial spectrum against food-borne pathogens. *LWT* **2021**, *139*, 110546. [CrossRef]
21. Adnan, M.; Patel, M.; Reddy, M.N.; Alshammari, E. Formulation, evaluation and bioactive potential of *Xylaria primorskensis* terpenoid nanoparticles from its major compound xylaranic acid. *Sci. Rep.* **2018**, *8*, 1740. [CrossRef]
22. Awadelkareem, A.M.; Al-Shammari, E.; Elkhalifa, A.O.; Adnan, M.; Siddiqui, A.J.; Patel, M.; Khan, M.I.; Mehmood, K.; Ashfaq, F.; Badraoui, R. Biosynthesized Silver Nanoparticles from *Eruca sativa* Miller Leaf Extract Exhibits Antibacterial, Antioxidant, Anti-Quorum-Sensing, Antibiofilm, and Anti-Metastatic Activities. *Antibiotics* **2022**, *11*, 853. [CrossRef]
23. Adnan, M.; Siddiqui, A.J.; Ashraf, S.A.; Snoussi, M.; Badraoui, R.; Alreshidi, M.; Elasbali, A.M.; Al-Soud, W.A.; Alharethi, S.H.; Sachidanandan, M. Polyhydroxybutyrate (PHB)-Based Biodegradable Polymer from *Agromyces indicus*: Enhanced Production, Characterization, and Optimization. *Polymers* **2022**, *14*, 3982. [CrossRef] [PubMed]

24. Wiegand, I.; Hilpert, K.; Hancock, R.E.W. Agar and broth dilution methods to determine the minimal inhibitory concentration (MIC) of antimicrobial substances. *Nat. Protoc.* **2008**, *3*, 163–175. [CrossRef]
25. Awadelkareem, A.M.; Al-Shammari, E.; Elkhalifa, A.E.O.; Adnan, M.; Siddiqui, A.J.; Snoussi, M.; Khan, M.I.; Azad, Z.R.A.A.; Patel, M.; Ashraf, S.A. Phytochemical and In Silico ADME/Tox Analysis of *Eruca sativa* Extract with Antioxidant, Antibacterial and Anticancer Potential against Caco-2 and HCT-116 Colorectal Carcinoma Cell Lines. *Molecules* **2022**, *27*, 1409. [CrossRef]
26. Reddy, M.N.; Adnan, M.; Alreshidi, M.M.; Saeed, M.; Patel, M. Evaluation of Anticancer, Antibacterial and Antioxidant Properties of a Medicinally Treasured Fern *Tectaria coadunata* with its Phytoconstituents Analysis by HR-LCMS. *Anti-Cancer Agents Med. Chem.* **2020**, *20*, 1845–1856. [CrossRef] [PubMed]
27. Kozakov, D.; Beglov, D.; Bohnuud, T.; Mottarella, S.E.; Xia, B.; Hall, D.R.; Vajda, S. How good is automated protein docking? *Proteins Struct. Funct. Bioinform.* **2013**, *81*, 2159–2166. [CrossRef]
28. Kozakov, D.; Hall, D.R.; Xia, B.; Porter, K.A.; Padhorny, D.; Yueh, C.; Beglov, D.; Vajda, S. The ClusPro web server for protein–protein docking. *Nat. Protoc.* **2017**, *12*, 255–278. [CrossRef] [PubMed]
29. Desta, I.T.; Porter, K.A.; Xia, B.; Kozakov, D.; Vajda, S. Performance and Its Limits in Rigid Body Protein-Protein Docking. *Structure* **2020**, *28*, 1071–1081.e3. [CrossRef]
30. Lagos, R.; Tello, M.; Mercado, G.; García, V.; Monasterio, O. Antibacterial and antitumorigenic properties of microcin E492, a pore-forming bacteriocin. *Curr. Pharm. Biotechnol.* **2009**, *10*, 74–85. [CrossRef]
31. Guzmán-Rodríguez, J.J.; Ochoa-Zarzosa, A.; López-Gómez, R.; López-Meza, J.E. Plant Antimicrobial Peptides as Potential Anticancer Agents. *BioMed Res. Int.* **2015**, *2015*, 735087. [CrossRef]
32. Deslouches, B.; Steckbeck, J.D.; Craigo, J.K.; Doi, Y.; Burns, J.L.; Montelaro, R.C. Engineered Cationic Antimicrobial Peptides To Overcome Multidrug Resistance by ESKAPE Pathogens. *Antimicrob. Agents Chemother.* **2015**, *59*, 1329–1333. [CrossRef]
33. Agrawal, S.; Acharya, D.; Adholeya, A.; Barrow, C.; Deshmukh, S.K. Nonribosomal Peptides from Marine Microbes and Their Antimicrobial and Anticancer Potential. *Front. Pharmacol.* **2017**, *8*, 828. [CrossRef] [PubMed]
34. Huang, L.; Chen, D.; Wang, L.; Lin, C.; Ma, C.; Xi, X.; Chen, T.; Shaw, C.; Zhou, M. Dermaseptin-PH: A Novel Peptide with Antimicrobial and Anticancer Activities from the Skin Secretion of the South American Orange-Legged Leaf Frog, *Pithecopus (Phyllomedusa) hypochondrialis*. *Molecules* **2017**, *22*, 1805. [CrossRef] [PubMed]
35. Delves-Brougthon, J. Nisin and its uses as a food preservative. *Food Technol.* **1990**, *44*, 100–117.
36. Bradshaw, J.P. Cationic antimicrobial peptides. *BioDrugs* **2003**, *17*, 233–240. [CrossRef]
37. Schilliager, U.; Geisen, R.; Holzapfel, W.H. Potential of antagonistic microganisms and bacteriocins for the biological preservation of food. *Trends Food Sci Tech.* **1997**, *7*, 158–164. [CrossRef]
38. Davidson, P.M.; Sofos, J.N.; Branen, A.L. *Antimicrobials in Food*; CRC Press: Boca Raton, FL, USA, 2005.
39. Riley, M.A.; Wertz, J.E. Bacteriocins: Evolution, Ecology, and Application. *Annu. Rev. Microbiol.* **2002**, *56*, 117–137. [CrossRef]
40. Saraniya, A.; Jeevaratnam, K. Optimization of nutritional and non-nutritional factors involved for production of antimicrobial compounds from *Lactobacillus pentosus* SJ65 using response surface methodology. *Braz. J. Microbiol.* **2014**, *45*, 81–88. [CrossRef] [PubMed]
41. Salmaso, S.; Elvassore, N.; Bertucco, A.; Lante, A.; Caliceti, P. Nisin-loaded poly-l-lactide nano-particles produced by CO_2 anti-solvent precipitation for sustained antimicrobial activity. *Int. J. Pharm.* **2004**, *287*, 163–173. [CrossRef]
42. De Giani, A.; Bovio, F.; Forcella, M.; Fusi, P.; Sello, G.; Di Gennaro, P. Identification of a bacteriocin-like compound from *Lactobacillus plantarum* with antimicrobial activity and effects on normal and cancerogenic human intestinal cells. *AMB Express* **2019**, *9*, 88. [CrossRef] [PubMed]
43. Danilova, T.A.; Adzhieva, A.A.; Danilina, G.A.; Polyakov, N.B.; Soloviev, A.I.; Zhukhovitsky, V.G. Antimicrobial Activity of Supernatant of *Lactobacillus plantarum* against Pathogenic Microorganisms. *Bull. Exp. Biol. Med.* **2019**, *167*, 751–754. [CrossRef]
44. Abo-Amer, A.E. Characterization of a bacteriocin-like inhibitory substance produced by *Lactobacillus plantarum* isolated from Egyptian home-made yogurt. *Sci. Asia.* **2007**, *33*, 313–319. [CrossRef]
45. Djadouni, F.; Kihal, M. Characterization and determination of the factors affecting anti-listerial bacteriocins from Lactobacillus plantarum and *Pediococcus pentosaceus* isolated from dairy milk products. *Afr. J. Food Sci.* **2013**, *7*, 35–44.
46. Moghaddam, M.Z.; Sattari, M.; Mobarez, A.M.; Doctorzadeh, F. Inhibitory effect of yogurt *Lactobacilli bacteriocins* on growth and verotoxins production of enterohemorrhgic *Escherichia coli* O157: H7. *Pak. J. Biol. Sci.* **2006**, *9*, 2112–2116. [CrossRef]
47. Milioni, C.; Martínez, B.; Degl'Innocenti, S.; Turchi, B.; Fratini, F.; Cerri, D.; Fischetti, R. A novel bacteriocin produced by *Lactobacillus plantarum* LpU4 as a valuable candidate for biopreservation in artisanal raw milk cheese. *Dairy Sci. Technol.* **2015**, *95*, 479–494. [CrossRef]
48. Song, J.Y.; Kim, B.S. Rapid biological synthesis of silver nanoparticles using plant leaf extracts. *Bioproc. Biosyst. Eng.* **2009**, *32*, 79–84. [CrossRef]
49. Hata, T.; Tanaka, R.; Ohmomo, S. Isolation and characterization of plantaricin ASM1: A new bacteriocin produced by *Lactobacillus plantarum* A-1. *Int. J. Food Microbiol.* **2010**, *137*, 94–99. [CrossRef]
50. Atrih, A.; Rekhif, N.; Moir, A.; Lebrihi, A.; Lefebvre, G. Mode of action, purification and amino acid sequence of plantaricin C19, an anti-*Listeria* bacteriocin produced by *Lactobacillus plantarum* C19. *Int. J. Food Microbiol.* **2001**, *68*, 93–104. [CrossRef] [PubMed]

51. Hu, M.; Zhao, H.; Zhang, C.; Yu, J.; Lu, Z. Purification and Characterization of Plantaricin 163, a Novel Bacteriocin Produced by *Lactobacillus plantarum* 163 Isolated from Traditional Chinese Fermented Vegetables. *J. Agric. Food Chem.* **2013**, *61*, 11676–11682. [CrossRef]
52. Chen, Y.-S.; Wang, Y.-C.; Chow, Y.-S.; Yanagida, F.; Liao, C.-C.; Chiu, C.-M. Purification and characterization of plantaricin Y, a novel bacteriocin produced by *Lactobacillus plantarum* 510. *Arch. Microbiol.* **2014**, *196*, 193–199. [CrossRef] [PubMed]
53. Wang, Y.; Qin, Y.; Zhang, Y.; Wu, R.; Li, P. Antibacterial mechanism of plantaricin LPL-1, a novel class IIa bacteriocin against *Listeria monocytogenes*. *Food Control* **2019**, *97*, 87–93. [CrossRef]
54. Mills, S.; Ross, R.; Hill, C. Bacteriocins and bacteriophage; a narrow-minded approach to food and gut microbiology. *FEMS Microbiol. Rev.* **2017**, *41*, S129–S153. [CrossRef] [PubMed]
55. Lazzari, S.; Moscatelli, D.; Codari, F.; Salmona, M.; Morbidelli, M.; Diomede, L. Colloidal stability of polymeric nanoparticles in biological fluids. *J. Nanoparticle Res.* **2012**, *14*, 920. [CrossRef]
56. Niaz, T.; Shabbir, S.; Noor, T.; Imran, M. Antimicrobial and antibiofilm potential of bacteriocin loaded nano-vesicles functionalized with rhamnolipids against foodborne pathogens. *LWT* **2019**, *116*, 108583. [CrossRef]
57. Kumar, C.G.; Mamidyala, S.K. Extracellular synthesis of silver nanoparticles using culture supernatant of *Pseudomonas aeruginosa*. *Colloids Surf. B Biointerfaces* **2011**, *84*, 462–466. [CrossRef]
58. Saravana, K.; Annalakshmi, A. Enhancing the antimicrobial activity of nisin by encapsulating on silver nanoparticle synthesized by *Bacillus* sp. *Int. J. Pharma. Biol. Arch.* **2012**, *3*, 406–410.
59. Gomaa, E.Z. Synergistic Antibacterial Efficiency of Bacteriocin and Silver Nanoparticles Produced by Probiotic *Lactobacillus paracasei* Against Multidrug Resistant Bacteria. *Int. J. Pept. Res. Ther.* **2019**, *25*, 1113–1125. [CrossRef]
60. Thirumurugan, A.; Ramachandran, S.; Gowri, A.S. Combined effect of bacteriocin with gold nanoparticles against food spoiling bacteria-an approach for food packaging material preparation. *Int. Food Res. J.* **2013**, *20*, 1909–1912.
61. Singh, A.K.; Bai, X.; Amalaradjou, M.A.R.; Bhunia, A.K. Antilisterial and Antibiofilm Activities of Pediocin and LAP Functionalized Gold Nanoparticles. *Front. Sustain. Food Syst.* **2018**, *2*, 74. [CrossRef]
62. Morales-Avila, E.; Ferro-Flores, G.; Ocampo-García, B.E.; López-Téllez, G.; López-Ortega, J.; Rogel-Ayala, D.G.; Sánchez-Padilla, D. Antibacterial Efficacy of Gold and Silver Nanoparticles Functionalized with the Ubiquicidin (29–41) Antimicrobial Peptide. *J. Nanomater.* **2017**, *2017*, 5831959. [CrossRef]
63. Elkhalifa, A.E.O.; Al-Shammari, E.; Alam, M.J.; Alcantara, J.C.; Khan, M.A.; Eltoum, N.E.; Ashraf, S.A. Okra-derived dietary Carotenoid lutein against Breast Cancer, with an Approach towards Developing a Nutraceutical Product: A Meta-analysis Study. *J. Pharm. Res. Int.* **2021**, *33*, 135–142. [CrossRef]
64. Cao, W.; Chen, H.-D.; Yu, Y.-W.; Li, N.; Chen, W.-Q. Changing profiles of cancer burden worldwide and in China: A secondary analysis of the global cancer statistics 2020. *Chin. Med. J.* **2021**, *134*, 783–791. [CrossRef] [PubMed]
65. Lee, Y.-C.; Lin, H.-H.; Hsu, C.-H.; Wang, C.-J.; Chiang, T.-A.; Chen, J.-H. Inhibitory effects of andrographolide on migration and invasion in human non-small cell lung cancer A549 cells via down-regulation of PI3K/Akt signaling pathway. *Eur. J. Pharmacol.* **2010**, *632*, 23–32. [CrossRef] [PubMed]
66. Loza-Mejía, M.A.; Salazar, J.R.; Sánchez-Tejeda, J.F. In Silico Studies on Compounds Derived from Calceolaria: Phenylethanoid Glycosides as Potential Multitarget Inhibitors for the Development of Pesticides. *Biomolecules* **2018**, *8*, 121. [CrossRef]
67. Lee, K.; Kim, D. In-Silico Molecular Binding Prediction for Human Drug Targets Using Deep Neural Multi-Task Learning. *Genes* **2019**, *10*, 906. [CrossRef]
68. Bharathi, A.; Roopan, S.M.; Vasavi, C.S.; Munusami, P.; Gayathri, G.A.; Gayathri, M. In silico molecular docking and in vitro antidiabetic studies of dihydropyrimido [4,5-a] acridin-2-amines. *BioMed Res. Int.* **2014**, *2014*, 971569. [CrossRef]
69. Comeau, S.R.; Gatchell, D.W.; Vajda, S.; Camacho, C.J. ClusPro: A fully automated algorithm for protein-protein docking. *Nucleic Acids Res.* **2004**, *32*, W96–W99. [CrossRef]
70. Xue, L.C.; Dobbs, D.; Honavar, V. HomPPI: A class of sequence homology based protein-protein interface prediction methods. *BMC Bioinform.* **2011**, *12*, 244. [CrossRef]
71. Hao, T.; Peng, W.; Wang, Q.; Wang, B.; Sun, J. Reconstruction and Application of Protein–Protein Interaction Network. *Int. J. Mol. Sci.* **2016**, *17*, 907. [CrossRef]
72. Alfonso, E.E.; Deng, Z.; Boaretto, D.; Hood, B.L.; Vasile, S.; Smith, L.H.; Chambers, J.W.; Chapagain, P.; Leng, F. Novel and Structurally Diversified Bacterial DNA Gyrase Inhibitors Discovered through a Fluorescence-Based High-Throughput Screening Assay. *ACS Pharmacol. Transl. Sci.* **2022**, *5*, 932–944. [CrossRef] [PubMed]
73. Suh, Y.-A.; Arnold, R.S.; Lassegue, B.; Shi, J.; Xu, X.X.; Sorescu, D.; Chung, A.B.; Griendling, K.K.; Lambeth, J.D. Cell transformation by the superoxide-generating oxidase Mox1. *Nat. Cell Biol.* **1999**, *401*, 79–82. [CrossRef]
74. Dupuy, C.; Ohayon, R.; Valent, A.; Noël-Hudson, M.-S.; Dème, D.; Virion, A. Purification of a Novel Flavoprotein Involved in the Thyroid NADPH Oxidase. *J. Biol. Chem.* **1999**, *274*, 37265–37269. [CrossRef]
75. Bedard, K.; Krause, K.-H. The NOX Family of ROS-Generating NADPH Oxidases: Physiology and Pathophysiology. *Physiol. Rev.* **2007**, *87*, 245–313. [CrossRef] [PubMed]
76. Gao, H.-M.; Zhou, H.; Hong, J.-S. NADPH oxidases: Novel therapeutic targets for neurodegenerative diseases. *Trends Pharmacol. Sci.* **2012**, *33*, 295–303. [CrossRef] [PubMed]

77. Simons, M.; Gordon, E.; Claesson-Welsh, L. Mechanisms and regulation of endothelial VEGF receptor signalling. *Nat. Rev. Mol. Cell Biol.* **2016**, *17*, 611–625. [CrossRef]
78. Yu, J.; Zhang, Y.; Leung, L.-H.; Liu, L.; Yang, F.; Yao, X. Efficacy and safety of angiogenesis inhibitors in advanced gastric cancer: A systematic review and meta-analysis. *J. Hematol. Oncol.* **2016**, *9*, 111. [CrossRef]

pharmaceutics

MDPI

Article

Levofloxacin and Ciprofloxacin Co-Crystals with Flavonoids: Solid-State Investigation for a Multitarget Strategy against *Helicobacter pylori*

Cecilia Fiore [1,2,*], Federico Antoniciello [3,*], Davide Roncarati [3], Vincenzo Scarlato [3], Fabrizia Grepioni [1] and Dario Braga [1]

1 Department of Chemistry "Giacomo Ciamician", University of Bologna, Via Selmi 2, 40126 Bologna, Italy; fabrizia.grepioni@unibo.it (F.G.); dario.braga@unibo.it (D.B.)

2 Department of Applied Science and Technology (DISAT), Politecnico di Torino, Corso Duca degli Abruzzi 24, 10129 Torino, Italy

3 Department of Pharmacy and Biotechnology (FaBiT), University of Bologna, Via Selmi 3, 40126 Bologna, Italy; davide.roncarati@unibo.it (D.R.); vincenzo.scarlato@unibo.it (V.S.)

* Correspondence: cecilia.fiore@polito.it (C.F.); federic.antoniciell2@unibo.it (F.A.); Tel.: +39-051-2094207 (F.A.)

Abstract: In this paper, we address the problem of antimicrobial resistance in the case of *Helicobacter pylori* with a crystal engineering approach. Two antibiotics of the fluoroquinolone class, namely, levofloxacin (LEV) and ciprofloxacin (CIP), have been co-crystallized with the flavonoids quercetin (QUE), myricetin (MYR), and hesperetin (HES), resulting in the formation of four co-crystals, namely, LEV·QUE, LEV·MYR, LEV_2·HES, and CIP·QUE. The co-crystals were obtained from solution, slurry, or mechanochemical mixing of the reactants. LEV·QUE and LEV·MYR were initially obtained as the ethanol solvates LEV·QUE·xEtOH and LEV·MYR·xEtOH, respectively, which upon thermal treatment yielded the unsolvated forms. All co-crystals were characterized by powder X-ray diffraction and thermal gravimetric analysis. The antibacterial performance of the four co-crystals LEV·QUE, LEV·MYR, LEV_2·HES, and CIP·QUE in comparison with that of the physical mixtures of the separate components was tested via evaluation of the minimal inhibitory concentration (MIC) and minimal bactericidal concentration (MBC). The results obtained indicate that the association with the co-formers, whether co-crystallized or forming a physical mixture with the active pharmaceutical ingredients (API), enhances the antimicrobial activity of the fluoroquinolones, allowing them to significantly reduce the amount of API otherwise required to display the same activity against *H. pylori*.

Keywords: co-crystals; crystal engineering; flavonoids; antimicrobials; HP1043; essential transcription factor; *Helicobacter pylori*

Citation: Fiore, C.; Antoniciello, F.; Roncarati, D.; Scarlato, V.; Grepioni, F.; Braga, D. Levofloxacin and Ciprofloxacin Co-Crystals with Flavonoids: Solid-State Investigation for a Multitarget Strategy against *Helicobacter pylori*. *Pharmaceutics* **2024**, *16*, 203. https://doi.org/10.3390/pharmaceutics16020203

Academic Editors: Aura Rusu and Valentina Uivarosi

Received: 15 January 2024
Accepted: 29 January 2024
Published: 30 January 2024

1. Introduction

Helicobacter pylori is a Gram-negative and transmissible pathogen that colonizes the human stomach, causing chronic infections that result in several gastric disorders, such as peptic ulceration, gastric adenocarcinoma, and MALT lymphoma. Most gastric cancer diagnoses are indeed attributable to *H. pylori* infection [1,2]. Like other superbugs, *H. pylori* rapidly develops resistance to the standard therapies, leading to a significant decrease in their efficacy and eradication cure rates between 70 and 50% [3]. Moreover, only a few antibiotics (such as amoxicillin, clarithromycin, metronidazole, tetracycline, levofloxacin, and rifabutin) can be used effectively for the eradication of *H. pylori* in clinical practice, typically when administered to patients in combined therapies with a proton-pump inhibitor (PPI) and/or a bismuth component that brings additional antibiotic effect and mucosal protection against aggressive factors [4,5]. Following the limited choice of effective therapeutics and the extensive use of certain antibiotics in the general population, rapid development of primary antibiotic resistance has been noted in *H. pylori* [3].

The fluoroquinolones levofloxacin and ciprofloxacin show a broad spectrum of activity against Gram-positive and Gram-negative bacteria. Levofloxacin-based regimens to treat *H. pylori* infections are usually triple-therapies including a PPI and amoxicillin [6–9]. It has been observed in recent studies that the efficacy of levofloxacin-containing therapy is decreasing, most likely due to increased primary resistance [3,10]. In order to offer an alternative to the standard therapies for the treatment of *H. pylori* infection, in a few studies, the efficacy of a ciprofloxacin-based regimen has also been explored [11,12].

The World Health Organization (WHO) [13] and the World Gastroenterology Organization (WGO) [14] have included *H. pylori* in their list of "priority pathogens" for which new antibiotics are urgently needed, and with this pressing need for novel therapeutic options, the scientific community's interest in traditional medicine and the use of natural products as sources of novel antibacterial drugs has been reinforced [15].

It is well established that co-crystallization is a viable crystal engineering route to the synthesis of new materials and/or to the enhancement of the properties of active molecules [16,17]. In recent publications, we have shown that the solid-state association of active ingredients, such as ciprofloxacin and antibiotics of the cephalosporin class, with molecular components belonging to the GRAS (Generally Recognized as Safe) family allows us to enhance and/or alter the overall antimicrobial performance of the antibiotics [18,19].

Following the same approach, we now focus on bioactive compounds isolated from natural sources, which have gained interest in the scientific community due to their beneficial effects on human health [20,21]. Flavonoids are a large family of naturally occurring bioactive compounds present in various species and in a wide variety. Plant flavonoids play an important role in the protection against pathogenic microorganisms, such as bacteria, fungi, and viruses [15,22–24].

In order to tackle the antimicrobial resistance (AMR) problem in the case of *H. pylori*, we have explored the effect on the antibiotic activity of the co-crystallization of two antibiotics of the fluoroquinolone class, namely, levofloxacin and ciprofloxacin, with three natural compounds of the flavonoid family: quercetin, myricetin, and hesperetin. Quercetin (QUE) is an important phytochemical, a flavonol, belonging to the flavonoid group of polyphenols. It is widely distributed in various fruits, vegetables, and beverages as well as in flowers, leaves, and seeds [25]. QUE possesses many pharmacological activities such as antioxidant [26,27], anticancer [28,29], anti-inflammatory [30–32], antimicrobial [32–34], etc. Myricetin (MYR) is a flavonoid of the flavone type, present as well in many vegetables, fruits, nuts, berries, and herbs [35]; MYR exhibits antioxidant properties, free radical-scavenging effects, and more beneficial properties [36–42]. Hesperetin (HES) is another flavonoid, of the flavanone class [43]; HES possesses different activities as well, such as antioxidant, anti-inflammatory, antimicrobial, and anticarcinogenic [44–46].

The antibacterial activity and bioavailability of flavonoids are affected by various parameters, such as molecular conformation, hydrophobicity, solubility, etc. [47,48]. The exact mechanisms of the antibacterial effects of flavonoids remain unclear, although several mechanisms of action have been proposed, such as interference with bacterial DNA synthesis, bacterial movement, cytoplasmic membrane permeability, and the inhibition of bacterial metalloenzymes [22,33,49].

As reported for other phytochemicals, the antimicrobial activity of flavonoids appears multifactorial by acting against different molecular targets in the pathogen instead of having one specific action site [22,33].

Bacterial transcriptional and post-transcriptional regulators (TRs and PTRs) have emerged for their significant potential as novel drug targets [50]. Targeting a bacterial TR that controls a cluster of fundamental genes is an example of a specific multitargeting approach with high specificity for the pathogen. HP1043, also referred to as HsrA, is a conserved and essential TR that is involved in the tight regulation of a plethora of housekeeping and essential genes. This regulator is an orphan response regulator that lacks its cognate sensor histidine kinase. Due to its involvement in crucial pathways for the viability of the bacterium, HP1043 is a potentially optimal novel target for antimicrobial drug discovery [50–52]. Recent studies have demonstrated that a group of flavonoids can inhibit HP1043 DNA binding, resulting in antimicrobial activity against *H. pylori* [44,45]. Therefore, the concept of creating a co-crystal of an antibiotic with a flavonoid used as a co-former is one of the first examples of a multitarget approach that involves the essential bacterial TR HP1043.

In this work, we report the preparation and characterization of four co-crystals obtained by combining the fluoroquinolones levofloxacin (LEV) and ciprofloxacin (CIP) with the flavonoids quercetin (QUE), myricetin (MYR), and hesperetin (HES) (see Scheme 1). Co-crystals of LEV with QUE and MYR, invariably obtained as non-stoichiometric EtOH solvates, i.e., LEV·QUE·xEtOH and LEV·MYR·xEtOH, respectively, had to be converted into their stable, unsolvated forms LEV·QUE and LEV·MYR with mild thermal treatment. LEV_2·HES and CIP·QUE, on the contrary, were always obtained as unsolvated co-crystals. The four novel materials were then tested for their potential antimicrobial activity in comparison with the equivalent physical mixtures of APIs and co-formers.

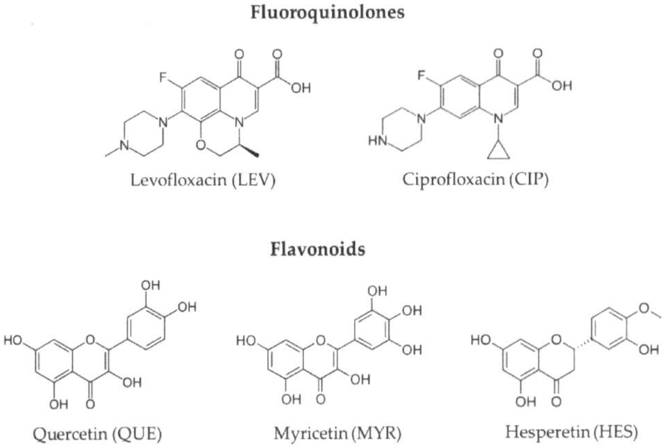

Scheme 1. The two fluoroquinolones (LEV, CIP) and the three flavonoids (QUE, MYR, HES) used in this work.

Solid-state characterization for all the products was performed via powder X-ray diffraction (PXRD) and thermal gravimetric analysis (TGA) (see the Supplementary Materials). Composition and purity of the products were confirmed using 1H NMR spectroscopy (see the Supplementary Materials).

2. Materials and Methods

All reagents and solvents used in this work were purchased from Sigma-Aldrich (Merck, Massachusetts, U.S.) or TCI Europe (TCI Europe N.V., Belgium -Tokyo Chemical Industry, Japan) and used without further purification.

2.1. Synthethic Methodologies

2.1.1. Mechanochemical Synthesis

All the co-crystals were synthesized mechanochemically with liquid-assisted grinding (LAG) [53] with ethanol (100 μL); a Retsch MM200 Mixer Mill (Verder Scientific- Verder Group, Netherlands) was employed, operated for 2 h at a frequency of 25 Hz, with 5 mL agate jars and 2 agate balls (diameter 5 mm). A 1:1 stoichiometry of the reagents was first tried (0.5 mmoL, i.e., 169.12, 159.12, 75.57, 180.68, and 165.67 mg for QUE·$2H_2O$, MYR, HES, LEV·$0.5H_2O$, and CIP, respectively), which yielded the ethanol solvates LEV·QUE·xEtOH, LEV·MYR·xEtOH, and the unsolvated co-crystal CIP·QUE. In the case of the 1:1 reaction of LEV·$0.5H_2O$ with HES, the 2:1 co-crystal LEV_2·HES was invariably obtained together with excess HES. The stoichiometry of the reaction was thus modified into 2:1, yielding quantitatively more LEV_2·HES. All products were left to dry out at room temperature, collected from the jar, and analyzed with PXRD. No dependance on the amount of EtOH used in LAG was observed.

2.1.2. Slurry in Ethanol

The co-crystals LEV·QUE·xEtOH, LEV·MYR·xEtOH, and CIP·QUE were also synthesized via slurry in ethanol (1 mL) of 1:1 stoichiometric mixture (2:1 in the case of the reaction between LEV and HES) of the reactants (same mmol and mg as in the mechanochemical synthesis). The suspensions were kept under stirring in the dark, to prevent a possible degradation of the flavonoids, and at room temperature for 3 days in a 10 mL glass vial closed with a PE pressure plug. The solid products were recovered and analyzed after filtration and drying. As the amount of ethanol detected in the two solids LEV·QUE·xEtOH and LEV·MYR·xEtOH was not constant, as observed in a number of syntheses, the co-crystals were subjected to mild thermal treatment (see below) that converted them to their stable, unsolvated forms, LEV·QUE and LEV·MYR, to be used for the antimicrobial tests.

2.1.3. Crystallization from Solution

Attempts at growing single crystals by synthesis or recrystallization of the solid products from ethanol either resulted in the formation of polycrystalline powders or, in the case of the solvated co-crystals, of poorly diffracting single crystals, due to rapid loss of ethanol even during short-time X-ray data acquisitions.

2.2. Solid-State Characterization

2.2.1. Powder X-ray Diffraction

Room-temperature powder X-ray diffraction patterns were collected using Bragg–Brentano geometry on a PANalytical X'Pert Pro (Malvern Panalytical-Spectris, Malvern, UK) automated diffractometer equipped with an X'Celerator detector (Malvern Panalytical-Spectris, Malvern, UK), using Cu Kα radiation (λ = 1.5418 Å) without a monochromator in the 3–40° 2θ range (continuous scan mode, step size: 0.033°; time/step: 30 s; Soller slit: 0.04 rad; anti-scatter slit: $\frac{1}{2}$; divergence slit: $\frac{1}{4}$; 40 mA × 40 kV).

2.2.2. Variable-Temperature Powder X-ray Diffraction (VT-PXRD)

For all the co-crystals discussed in this work, powder X-ray diffractograms were collected in the 3–40° 2θ range, in open air using Bragg–Brentano geometry, with a PANalytical X'Pert PRO automated diffractometer, equipped with an X'Celerator detector, using Cu Kα radiation without a monochromator and an Anton Paar TTK 450 (Anton Paar, Graz, Austria) system for measurements at controlled temperature.

2.2.3. Thermogravimetric Analysis (TGA)

TGA measurements for all co-crystals were performed using a Perkin-Elmer TGA7 (Perkin-Elmer-Medtech, Shelton, CT, USA) instrument in the temperature range 30–300 °C under a N_2 gas flow, at a heating rate of 10 °C min^{-1}.

2.3. Solution ^1H NMR Characterization

^1H NMR spectroscopy was performed to ascertain stoichiometry and purity of the co-crystals. All the NMR spectra for starting materials and products discussed in this work were recorded with a Varian MR400 (Varian-Scientific Instruments, Palo Alto, CA, USA), operating at the frequency of 400 MHz on proton, equipped with PFG (Pulse Field Gradient) ATB (AutoSwitchable Broadband) Probes.

2.4. Antimicrobial Activity Tests against Helicobacter pylori

The co-crystals LEV·QUE, LEV·MYR, LEV_2·HES, and CIP·QUE were subjected to antimicrobial testing against *H. pylori*. The antimicrobial activity was assessed using the broth microdilution method according to CLSI and EUCAST guidelines. All solutions/suspensions were tested in parallel, using *H. pylori* G27 and *H. pylori* 26695 strains with different standard methods to determine their minimal inhibitory concentrations (MICs) and minimal bactericidal concentrations (MBCs). Drugs, flavonoids, and co-crystals were tested in 11 progressive concentrations ranging from 512 to 0.5 μg/mL. Compound solutions/suspensions were all prepared following the same procedure: 20 mg of analyte in 10 mL of physiological solution (0.9% NaCl) to a final concentration of 2 mg/mL; physical mixtures were prepared simply by mixing drug dispersions/solution and flavonoid dispersions in stoichiometric ratios. The antibacterial assay was carried out using a 96-well microtiter plate; the first column of wells was filled with 100 μL of 2× Brucella broth supplemented with 10% fetal bovine serum (FBS), and the subsequent columns were filled with 100 μL of 1× Brucella broth supplemented with 5% FBS. Then, 100 μL of sample solution/dispersion were added in the first column, obtaining a concentration of 1 mg/mL. The two-fold serial dilutions were obtained by taking 100 μL from column 1 and mixing it with 1× broth in column 2 and then proceeding in the same way from column 2 to well 3, and so on. The volume withdrawn from the last column was discarded, leaving 100 μL in all the wells. Afterwards, 100 μL of bacteria diluted in the same supplemented broth medium were added to each well to a final concentration of 1.0×10^5 CFU/mL. The whole procedure resulted in 1:2 serial dilutions ranging from 512 to 0.5 μg/mL from well 1 to well 11. Negative controls were used to verify that the compound solutions/suspensions were not contaminated, while a positive control was added to check for bacterial growth and fitness. The positive control was used as a comparison to evaluate the MIC and the MBC. Plates were incubated in a CO_2-controlled incubator (9% CO_2) at 37 °C and examined visually after 72 h. MIC values were defined as the lowest concentration of compound that inhibited the visible growth of bacteria after 72 h of incubation. For MBC determinations, 10 μL aliquots of diluted bacterial cultures around the MIC were spotted on Brucella broth agar supplemented with 5% FBS and incubated for 48 h in a 9% CO_2 environment at 37 °C. MBC was defined as the lowest concentration of compound that prevented the growth of ≥99.9% of *H. pylori*. Each experiment was performed in triplicate to confirm the results.

3. Results and Discussion

3.1. Co-Crystallization of Levofloxacin with Quercetin, Myricetin, and Hesperetin

As mentioned above, the co-crystallization of levofloxacin with quercetin or myricetin results in the 1:1 solvated co-crystals LEV·QUE·xEtOH and LEV·MYR·xEtOH. Recrystallization attempts always yielded tiny crystals of insufficient quality for single crystal X-ray diffraction; attempts at fast data collections failed, even at low temperature, due to the rapid loss of ethanol under the X-ray radiation.

In order to obtain stable co-crystals LEV·QUE and LEV·MYR, suitable for antimicrobial tests, the solvated co-crystals were desolvated using mild thermal treatment. The desolvation process was followed by variable temperature powder X-ray diffraction (VT-PXRD). Modifications in the powder patterns of the two ethanolates can already be appreciated at 80 °C and at 30 °C for LEV·QUE·xEtOH and LEV·MYR·xEtOH, respectively. The heating process was stopped at 120 °C, which ensured complete desolvation of both co-crystals.

Figures 1 and 2 show a comparison of the powder patterns, all collected at room temperature, for reagents, solvated products, and unsolvated co-crystals resulting from the VT-PXRD process. It is interesting to observe that the two unsolvated co-crystals LEV·QUE and LEV·MYR appear to be isostructural.

At variance with the 1:1 stoichiometry observed in the case of LEV·QUE and LEV·MYR, the co-crystallization of levofloxacin with hesperetin invariably yielded a 2:1 stoichiometric product (LEV_2·HES). Figure 3 shows a comparison of the powder patterns for the two reagents and the co-crystal LEV_2·HES.

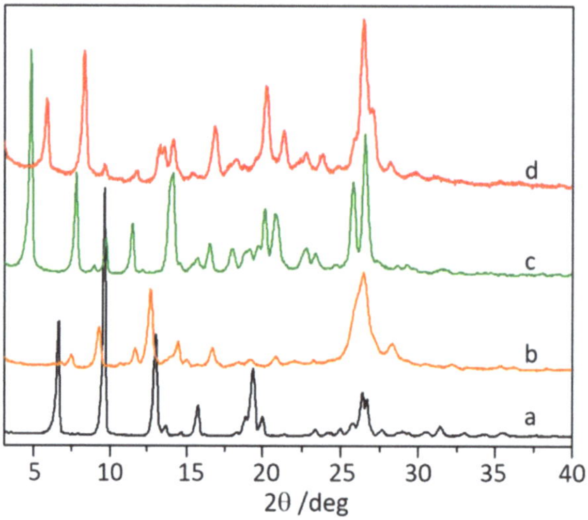

Figure 1. From bottom to top: PXRD patterns at room temperature for LEV·0.5H_2O (a, black), QUE·2H_2O (b, orange), LEV·QUE·xEtOH as obtained from ball milling (c, green), and LEV·QUE obtained using VT-PXRD (d, red).

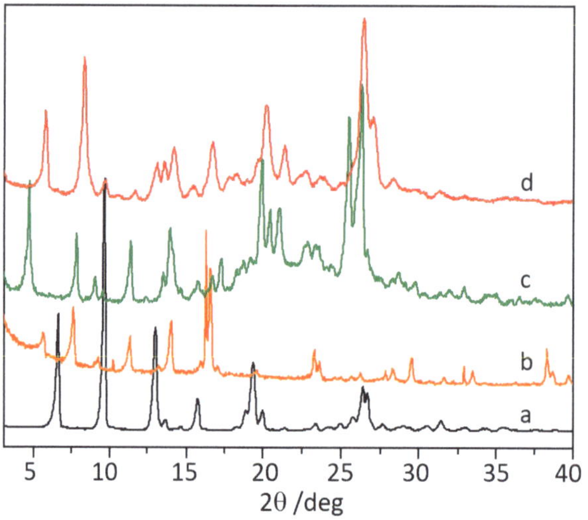

Figure 2. From bottom to top: PXRD patterns at room temperature for LEV·0.5H_2O (a, black), MYR (b, orange), LEV·MYR·xEtOH as obtained from ball milling (c, green), and LEV·MYR obtained using VT-PXRD (d, red).

The comparisons in Figures 1–3 allow us to see that mixing LEV with QUE, MYR, or HES leads to new compounds and not to physical mixtures of the starting materials, which would result in an overlay of the diffraction patterns of the reagents.

TGA measurements, confirming the presence of solvent in the co-crystals of LEV with QUE and MYRz, as obtained from the synthesis, and the unsolvated nature of the LEV_2·HES co-crystal, and ^{1}H NMR spectroscopic analyses that confirm chemical composition and stoichiometry for the LEV·QUE, LEV·MYR, and LEV_2·HES co-crystals used for the antimicrobial tests, can be found in the Supplementary Materials, together with a comparison of the powder patterns for the products of the ball milling and slurry co-crystallization processes.

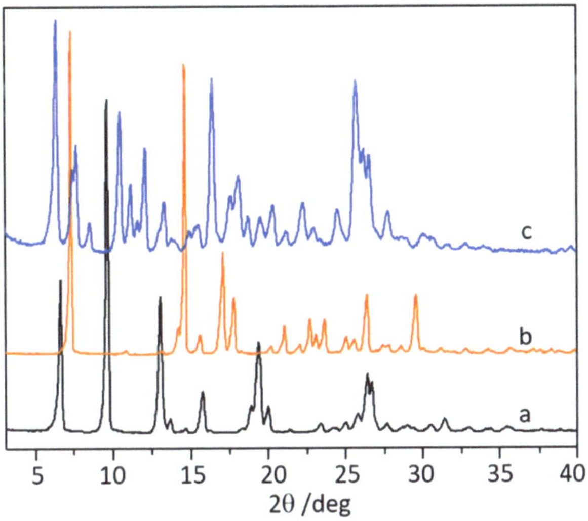

Figure 3. From bottom to top: PXRD patterns of LEV·0.5H_2O (a, black), HES (b, orange), and the LEV_2·HES product from slurry (c, blue).

3.2. Co-Crystallization of Ciprofloxacin with Quercetin

Co-crystallization of ciprofloxacin (CIP) with the three flavonoids was successful only in the case of quercetin, yielding the novel crystalline compound CIP·QUE (See Figure 4. PXRD patterns). Due to the large difference in the solubility of CIP and QUE, the co-crystal could only be obtained via ball-milling and slurry, not from solution.

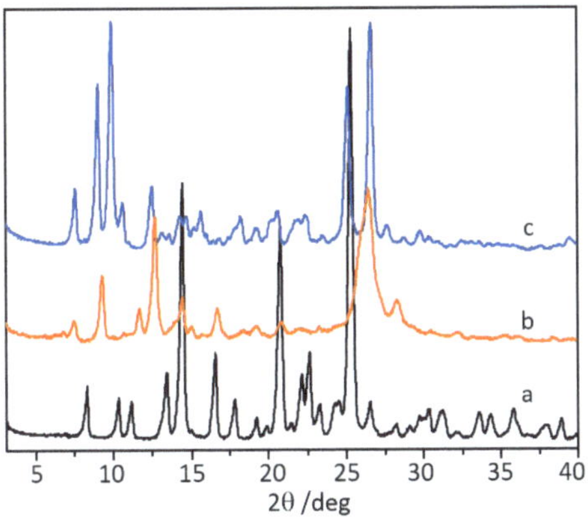

Figure 4. From bottom to top: PXRD patterns of CIP (a, black), QUE·2H_2O (b, orange), and CIP·QUE product as obtained from slurry (c, blue).

TGA measurement, confirming the unsolvated nature of the CIP·QUE co-crystal, and ^{1}H NMR spectroscopic analysis that confirms the co-crystal chemical composition and stoichiometry can be found in the Supplementary Materials.

3.3. Antimicrobial Activity

The MIC and MBC values for each entity considered in this work are reported in Table 1 and graphically represented in Figure 5. Under the experimental conditions used, the MIC values obtained for both LEV_2·HES and LEV·QUE co-crystals and the antibiotic alone were identical for the *H. pylori* G27 strain. LEV_2·HES and CIP·QUE co-crystals exhibited equivalent antibacterial activity to their respective antibiotics alone against *H. pylori* 26695 strain. Nevertheless, there was a significant difference between the two data sets as the co-crystals contained significantly less of the antibiotic levofloxacin. Specifically, the co-crystal suspensions of levofloxacin and quercetin (LEV·QUE), levofloxacin and hesperetin (LEV_2·HES), and ciprofloxacin and quercetin (CIP·QUE) contained, respectively, 50%, 33%, and 50% fewer antibiotics, in terms of moles of levofloxacin or ciprofloxacin. Remarkably, there was no significant difference between the co-crystal suspensions and the physical mixtures having the same relative molar amounts. These results may indicate that physical co-crystallization of the two chemicals occurred during the antimicrobial assays or that the antibiotics' interaction mechanisms with the cellular membrane were altered due to the presence of flavonoids. On the other hand, the co-crystal and physical mixture containing myricetin (LEV·MYR, LEV + MYR) resulted in a lower antimicrobial effect in both strains, as seen in the higher MIC and MBC values. Notably, the flavonoids, namely, hesperetin, myricetin, and quercetin, demonstrated a considerably low antibacterial activity, incomparable to that of antibiotics or suspensions, with MIC values from 128 to 512 μg/mL.

Table 1. Minimal inhibitory and bactericidal concentration (in brackets) values for co-crystals (indicated as ANTIBIOTIC·FLAVONOID), physical mixtures (indicated as ANTIBIOTIC + FLAVONOID), and single compounds. *H. pylori* G27 and *H. pylori* 26695 strains were used to perform antimicrobial assays. Data shown are median values of three independent experiments.

	MIC [μg/mL] (MBC)	
Compounds	***H. pylori* Strains**	
	G27	**26695**
LEV_2·HES	1 (2)	0.5 (1)
2LEV + HES	1 (2)	0.5 (1)
LEV·MYR	4 (8)	2 (4)
LEV + MYR	4 (8)	4 (8)
LEV·QUE	1 (2)	1 (2)
LEV + QUE	1 (2)	1 (2)
LEV	1 (2)	0.5 (1)
CIP·QUE	2 (4)	1 (2)
CIP + QUE	2 (4)	2 (2)
CIP	2 (2)	1 (2)
HES	128 (256)	128 (256)
MYR	256 (512)	256 (512)
QUE	512 (512)	256 (512)

Overall, we concluded that for *H. pylori*, the combination of flavonoids with an antibiotic capable of forming co-crystals may be a new and advanced approach to reduce the total amount of antibiotic used for treatment while maintaining the same antimicrobial efficacy. This result is in line with the recommendations and guidelines of the WHO [13] and the WGO [14] to reduce the use of antibiotics to prevent or at least slow the emergence and spread of antibiotic-resistant pathogenic strains.

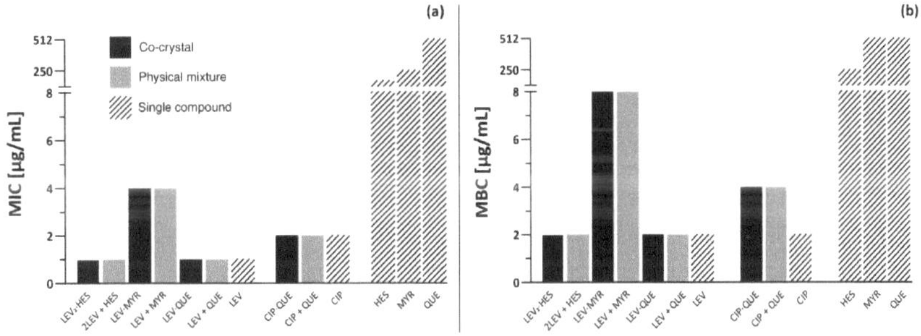

Figure 5. Histogram representation of the minimal inhibitory (**a**) and bactericidal (**b**) for *H. pylori* G27. Data shown are median values of three independent experiments.

4. Conclusions

In the need for alternatives to the common drug discovery process, to reduce costs, time, and energy investments, co-crystallization and supramolecular aggregation techniques are offering us a viable and eco-friendly route to design and prepare novel pharmaceutical materials with desired modified properties [19,54–56].

In this work, we have reported the preparation and characterization of a series of co-crystals obtained by co-crystallizing via solid-state solvent-free methodologies two antibiotics of the fluoroquinolone class, namely, levofloxacin and ciprofloxacin with the flavonoids quercetin, myricetin, and hesperetin. As a result, we prepared and characterized four novel co-crystals, namely, LEV·QUE, LEV·MYR, LEV_2·HES, and CIP·QUE. LEV·QUE and LEV·MYR were obtained by desolvation of the corresponding xEtOH solvates. LEV·QUE, LEV·MYR, LEV_2·HES, and CIP·QUE were then tested against two different strains of *H. pylori*, a bacterium included in the list of "priority pathogens", according to the WHO and WGO [14,57]. Interestingly, the high MICs observed for the flavonoids against *H. pylori* G27 and 26695 strains under experimental conditions are in contrast with data presented in other studies [44,45]. Nonetheless, our approach led to an unexpected but worth reporting outcome. Indeed, while no significant difference in the antimicrobial activity was observed between the co-crystal suspensions and the physical mixtures used as comparison reference, the antimicrobial efficacy of the antibiotics was improved. Our research reveals that the combination of CIP and LEV with flavonoids, whether as co-crystals or as physical mixtures, yields equivalent results in MIC and MBC but permits the use of a reduced antibiotic dose (between half and two thirds in moles). Moreover, the fact that the co-crystal and the physical mixture perform equally well may indicate that, under the experimental conditions, either the antibiotics LEV and CIP form aggregates with flavonoids that have similar properties to the co-crystals or their presence enables a different mechanism of interaction with bacterial cell membranes, improving the overall efficacy.

The antimicrobial activity tests suggest that there may be an additive or synergistic effect between the antibiotics LEV and CIP, interfering with the bacterial DNA replication, and the flavonoids HES and QUE, targeting the *H. pylori* TR HP1043, whether as physical mixtures or co-crystals. Although the proposed multitarget approach may have major advantages in reducing the amount of antibiotics required, further investigation is needed to confirm this hypothesis.

Supplementary Materials: The following supporting information can be downloaded at: https://www.mdpi.com/article/10.3390/pharmaceutics16020203/s1. Figure S1: Comparison of the experimental PXRD patterns for LEV·QUE·xEtOH as obtained from ball milling (a, green) and slurry (b, blue); Figure S2: Comparison of the experimental PXRD patterns for LEV·MYR·xEtOH as obtained from ball milling (a, green) and slurry (b, blue); Figure S3: Comparison of the experimental PXRD patterns for LEV2·HES as obtained from ball milling (a, green) and slurry (b, blue); Figure S4:

Comparison of the experimental PXRD patterns for CIP·QUE as obtained from ball milling (a, green) and slurry (b, blue); Figure S5: TGA trace for LEV·QUE·xEtOH; Figure S6: TGA trace for LEV·MYR·xEtOH; Figure S7: TGA trace for LEV2·HES; Figure S8: TGA trace for CIP·QUE; Figure S9: ^{1}H NMR Levofloxacin; Figure S10: ^{1}H NMR Quercetin; Figure S11: ^{1}H NMR Myricetin; Figure S12: ^{1}H NMR Hesperetin; Figure S13: ^{1}H NMR Ciprofloxacin; Figure S14: ^{1}H NMR LEV·QUE·xEtOH; Figure S15: ^{1}H NMR LEV·QUE; Figure S16: ^{1}H NMR LEV·MYR·xEtOH; Figure S17: ^{1}H NMR LEV·MYR; Figure S18: ^{1}H NMR LEV2·HES; Figure S19: ^{1}H NMR CIP·QUE.

Author Contributions: Conceptualization, D.B., C.F., F.A. and D.R.; methodology, C.F., F.A. and F.G.; formal analysis, D.B., C.F., F.A. and F.G.; investigation, D.B., C.F. and F.A.; writing—original draft preparation, C.F. and F.A.; writing—review and editing, D.B., C.F., F.A., D.R., V.S. and F.G.; visualization, C.F. and F.A.; supervision, D.B., D.R. and V.S.; funding acquisition, D.B., V.S., D.R. and F.G. All authors have read and agreed to the published version of the manuscript.

Funding: This research was funded by MUR, project "Nature Inspired Crystal Engineering" (PRIN2020) to D.B., MUR grant PRIN 2020YXFSW5 to V.S., and from Alma Mater Studiorum—University of Bologna to D.B., V.S., D.R., and F.G.

Institutional Review Board Statement: Not applicable.

Informed Consent Statement: Not applicable.

Data Availability Statement: The data presented in this study are all available in the main text.

Acknowledgments: The assistance of Stefano Grilli (Department of Chemistry "Giacomo Ciamician", Alma Mater Studiorum—University of Bologna) with the ^{1}H NMR spectroscopy measurements is gratefully acknowledged.

Conflicts of Interest: The authors declare no conflicts of interest.

References

1. Dunn, B.E.; Cohen, H.; Blaser, M.J. Helicobacter Pylori. *Clin. Microbiol. Rev.* **1997**, *10*, 720–741. [CrossRef]
2. McColl, K.E.L. Clinical Practice. Helicobacter Pylori Infection. *N. Engl. J. Med.* **2010**, *362*, 1597–1604. [CrossRef]
3. Tshibangu-Kabamba, E.; Yamaoka, Y. Helicobacter Pylori Infection and Antibiotic Resistance—From Biology to Clinical Implications. *Nat. Rev. Gastroenterol. Hepatol.* **2021**, *18*, 613–629. [CrossRef] [PubMed]
4. Yang, H.; Guan, L.; Hu, B. Detection and Treatment of Helicobacter Pylori: Problems and Advances. *Gastroenterol. Res. Pract.* **2022**, *2022*, e4710964. [CrossRef] [PubMed]
5. Hooi, J.K.Y.; Lai, W.Y.; Ng, W.K.; Suen, M.M.Y.; Underwood, F.E.; Tanyingoh, D.; Malfertheiner, P.; Graham, D.Y.; Wong, V.W.S.; Wu, J.C.Y.; et al. Global Prevalence of Helicobacter Pylori Infection: Systematic Review and Meta-Analysis. *Gastroenterology* **2017**, *153*, 420–429. [CrossRef] [PubMed]
6. Nista, E.C.; Candelli, M.; Cremonini, F.; Cazzato, I.A.; Di Caro, S.; Gabrielli, M.; Santarelli, L.; Zocco, M.A.; Ojetti, V.; Carloni, E.; et al. Levofloxacin-Based Triple Therapy vs. Quadruple Therapy in Second-Line Helicobacter Pylori Treatment: A Randomized Trial. *Aliment. Pharmacol. Ther.* **2003**, *18*, 627–633. [CrossRef] [PubMed]
7. Di Caro, S.; Franceschi, F.; Mariani, A.; Thompson, F.; Raimondo, D.; Masci, E.; Testoni, A.; La Rocca, E.; Gasbarrini, A. Second-Line Levofloxacin-Based Triple Schemes for Helicobacter Pylori Eradication. *Dig. Liver Dis.* **2009**, *41*, 480–485. [CrossRef] [PubMed]
8. Gisbert, J.P.; Pérez-Aisa, Á.; Bermejo, F.; Castro-Fernández, M.; Almela, P.; Barrio, J.; Cosme, Á.; Modolell, I.; Bory, F.; Fernández-Bermejo, M.; et al. Second-Line Therapy with Levofloxacin after Failure of Treatment to Eradicate Helicobacter Pylori Infection: Time Trends in a Spanish Multicenter Study of 1000 Patients. *J. Clin. Gastroenterol.* **2013**, *47*, 130–135. [CrossRef] [PubMed]
9. Perna, F.; Zullo, A.; Ricci, C.; Hassan, C.; Morini, S.; Vaira, D. Levofloxacin-Based Triple Therapy for Helicobacter Pylori Re-Treatment: Role of Bacterial Resistance. *Dig. Liver Dis.* **2007**, *39*, 1001–1005. [CrossRef] [PubMed]
10. Drlica, K.; Malik, M. Fluoroquinolones: Action and Resistance. *Curr. Top. Med. Chem.* **2005**, *3*, 249–282. [CrossRef]
11. Forsmark, C.E.; Mel Wilco, C.; Cello, J.P.; Margaretten, W.; Lee, B.; Sachdeeva, M.; Satow, J.; Sande, M.A. Ciprofloxacin in the Treatment of Helicobacter Pylori in Patients with Gastritis and Peptic Ulcer. *J. Infect. Dis.* **1990**, *162*, 998–999. [CrossRef] [PubMed]
12. Dresner, D.; Coyle, W.; Nemec, R.; Peterson, R.; Duntemann, T.; Lawson, J.M. Efficacy of Ciprofloxacin in the Eradication of Helicobacter Pylori. *S. Med. J.* **1996**, *89*, 775–778. [CrossRef] [PubMed]
13. World Health Organisation. *Helicobacter pylori*. Available online: https://monographs.iarc.who.int/wp-content/uploads/2018/06/mono100B-15.pdf (accessed on 13 January 2023).
14. World Gastroenterology Organisation. *Helicobacter Pylori*. Available online: https://www.worldgastroenterology.org/guidelines/helicobacter-pylori (accessed on 13 January 2023).
15. Anand, U.; Nandy, S.; Mundhra, A.; Das, N.; Pandey, D.K.; Dey, A. A Review on Antimicrobial Botanicals, Phytochemicals and Natural Resistance Modifying Agents from Apocynaceae Family: Possible Therapeutic Approaches against Multidrug Resistance in Pathogenic Microorganisms. *Drug Resist. Updat.* **2020**, *51*, 100695. [CrossRef] [PubMed]

16. Qiao, N.; Li, M.; Schlindwein, W.; Malek, N.; Davies, A.; Trappitt, G. Pharmaceutical Co-Crystals: An Overview. *Int. J. Pharm.* **2011**, *419*, 1–11. [CrossRef] [PubMed]
17. Duggirala, N.K.; Perry, M.L.; Almarsson, Ö.; Zaworotko, M.J. Pharmaceutical Co-crystals: Along the Path to Improved Medicines. *Chem. Commun.* **2015**, *52*, 640–655. [CrossRef]
18. Fiore, C.; Baraghini, A.; Shemchuk, O.; Sambri, V.; Morotti, M.; Grepioni, F.; Braga, D. Inhibition of the Antibiotic Activity of Cephalosporines by Co-Crystallization with Thymol. *Cryst. Growth Des.* **2022**, *22*, 1467–1475. [CrossRef]
19. Shemchuk, O.; d'Agostino, S.; Fiore, C.; Sambri, V.; Zannoli, S.; Grepioni, F.; Braga, D. Natural Antimicrobials Meet a Synthetic Antibiotic: Carvacrol/Thymol and Ciprofloxacin Co-crystals as a Promising Solid-State Route to Activity Enhancement. *Cryst. Growth Des.* **2020**, *20*, 6796–6803. [CrossRef]
20. Kosalec, I.; Rai, M. Natural Antimicrobials: An Introduction. In *Promising Antimicrobials from Natural Products*; Springer: Cham, Switzerland, 2022; pp. 3–13. [CrossRef]
21. Rai, M.; Kosalec, I. *Promising Antimicrobials from Natural Products*; Springer: Dordrecht, The Netherlands, 2022. [CrossRef]
22. Havsteen, B.H. The Biochemistry and Medical Significance of the Flavonoids. *Pharmacol. Ther.* **2002**, *96*, 67–202. [CrossRef]
23. Lalani, S.; Poh, C.L. Flavonoids as Antiviral Agents for Enterovirus A71 (EV-A71). *Viruses* **2020**, *12*, 184. [CrossRef]
24. Panche, A.N.; Diwan, A.D.; Chandra, S.R. Flavonoids: An Overview. *J. Nutr. Sci.* **2016**, *5*, e47. [CrossRef]
25. Anand David, A.V.; Arulmoli, R.; Parasuraman, S. Overviews of Biological Importance of Quercetin: A Bioactive Flavonoid. *Pharmacogn. Rev.* **2016**, *10*, 84–89. [CrossRef]
26. Xu, D.; Hu, M.J.; Wang, Y.Q.; Cui, Y.L. Antioxidant Activities of Quercetin and Its Complexes for Medicinal Application. *Molecules* **2019**, *24*, 1123. [CrossRef] [PubMed]
27. Zhang, M.; Swarts, S.G.; Yin, L.; Liu, C.; Tian, Y.; Cao, Y.; Swarts, M.; Yang, S.; Zhang, S.B.; Zhang, K.; et al. Antioxidant Properties of Quercetin. *Adv. Exp. Med. Biol.* **2011**, *701*, 283–289. [CrossRef] [PubMed]
28. Hisaka, T.; Sakai, H.; Sato, T.; Goto, Y.; Nomura, Y.; Fukutomi, S.; Fujita, F.; Mizobe, T.; Nakashima, O.; Tanigawa, M.; et al. Quercetin Suppresses Proliferation of Liver Cancer Cell Lines in Vitro. *Anticancer Res* **2020**, *40*, 4695–4700. [CrossRef] [PubMed]
29. Zhou, J.; Fang, L.; Liao, J.; Li, L.; Yao, W.; Xiong, Z.; Zhou, X. Investigation of the Anti-Cancer Effect of Quercetin on HepG2 Cells in Vivo. *PLoS ONE* **2017**, *12*, e0172838. [CrossRef] [PubMed]
30. González-Segovia, R.; Quintanar, J.L.; Salinas, E.; Ceballos-Salazar, R.; Aviles-Jiménez, F.; Torres-López, J. Effect of the Fl Avonoid Quercetin on Infl Ammation and Lipid Peroxidation Induced by Helicobacter Pylori in Gastric Mucosa of Guinea Pig. *J. Gastroenterol.* **2008**, *43*, 441–447. [CrossRef] [PubMed]
31. Guan, F.; Wang, Q.; Bao, Y.; Chao, Y. Anti-Rheumatic Effect of Quercetin and Recent Developments in Nano Formulation. *RSC Adv.* **2021**, *11*, 7280–7293. [CrossRef] [PubMed]
32. Azeem, M.; Hanif, M.; Mahmood, K.; Ameer, N.; Chughtai, F.R.S.; Abid, U. An Insight into Anticancer, Antioxidant, Antimicrobial, Antidiabetic and Anti-Inflammatory Effects of Quercetin: A Review. *Polym. Bull.* **2022**, *80*, 241–262. [CrossRef] [PubMed]
33. Cushnie, T.P.T.; Lamb, A.J. Antimicrobial Activity of Flavonoids. *Int. J. Antimicrob. Agents* **2005**, *26*, 343–356. [CrossRef]
34. Lenard, N.; Henagan, T.M.; Lan, T.; Nguyen, A.; Bhattacharya, D. Antimicrobial Activity of Quercetin: An Approach to Its Mechanistic Principle. *Molecules* **2022**, *27*, 2494. [CrossRef]
35. Semwal, D.K.; Semwal, R.B.; Combrinck, S.; Viljoen, A. Myricetin: A Dietary Molecule with Diverse Biological Activities. *Nutrients* **2016**, *8*, 90. [CrossRef] [PubMed]
36. Park, K.S.; Chong, Y.; Kim, M.K. Myricetin: Biological Activity Related to Human Health. *Appl. Biol. Chem.* **2016**, *59*, 259–269. [CrossRef]
37. Tong, Y.; Zhou, X.M.; Wang, S.J.; Yang, Y.; Cao, Y.L. Analgesic Activity of Myricetin Isolated from Myrica Rubra Sieb. et Zucc. Leaves. *Arch. Pharmacal. Res.* **2009**, *32*, 527–533. [CrossRef] [PubMed]
38. Ha, T.K.; Jung, I.; Kim, M.E.; Bae, S.K.; Lee, J.S. Anti-Cancer Activity of Myricetin against Human Papillary Thyroid Cancer Cells Involves Mitochondrial Dysfunction–Mediated Apoptosis. *Biomed. Pharmacother.* **2017**, *91*, 378–384. [CrossRef] [PubMed]
39. Yang, Z.J.; Wang, H.R.; Wang, Y.I.; Zhai, Z.H.; Wang, L.W.; Li, L.; Zhang, C.; Tang, L. Myricetin Attenuated Diabetes-Associated Kidney Injuries and Dysfunction via Regulating Nuclear Factor (Erythroid Derived 2)-like 2 and Nuclear Factor-KB Signaling. *Front. Pharmacol.* **2019**, *10*, 647. [CrossRef] [PubMed]
40. Jiang, M.; Zhu, M.; Wang, L.; Yu, S. Anti-Tumor Effects and Associated Molecular Mechanisms of Myricetin. *Biomed. Pharmacother.* **2019**, *120*, 109506. [CrossRef]
41. Gordon, M.H.; Roedig-Penman, A. Antioxidant Activity of Quercetin and Myricetin in Liposomes. *Chem. Phys. Lipids.* **1998**, *97*, 79–85. [CrossRef]
42. Taheri, Y.; Suleria, H.A.R.; Martins, N.; Sytar, O.; Beyatli, A.; Yeskaliyeva, B.; Seitimova, G.; Salehi, B.; Semwal, P.; Painuli, S.; et al. Myricetin Bioactive Effects: Moving from Preclinical Evidence to Potential Clinical Applications. *BMC Complement. Med. Ther.* **2020**, *20*, 1–14. [CrossRef]
43. Srimathi Priyanga, K.; Vijayalakshmi, K. Investigation of Antioxidant Potential of Quercetin and Hesperidin: An in Vitro Approach. *Asian J. Pharm. Clin. Res.* **2017**, *10*, 83–86. [CrossRef]
44. González, A.; Casado, J.; Lanas, Á. Fighting the Antibiotic Crisis: Flavonoids as Promising Antibacterial Drugs Against Helicobacter Pylori Infection. *Front. Cell. Infect. Microbiol.* **2021**, *11*, 671. [CrossRef]
45. González, A.; Salillas, S.; Velázquez-Campoy, A.; Espinosa Angarica, V.; Fillat, M.F.; Sancho, J.; Lanas, Á. Identifying Potential Novel Drugs against Helicobacter Pylori by Targeting the Essential Response Regulator HsrA. *Sci. Rep.* **2019**, *9*, 11294. [CrossRef]

46. Chadha, K.; Karan, M.; Bhalla, Y.; Chadha, R.; Khullar, S.; Mandal, S.; Vasisht, K. Co-crystals of Hesperetin: Structural, Pharmacokinetic, and Pharmacodynamic Evaluation. *Cryst. Growth Des.* **2017**, *17*, 2386–2405. [CrossRef]
47. Manach, C.; Scalbert, A.; Morand, C.; Rémésy, C.; Jiménez, L. Polyphenols: Food Sources and Bioavailability. *Am. J. Clin. Nutr.* **2004**, *79*, 727–747. [CrossRef]
48. Manach, C.; Williamson, G.; Morand, C.; Scalbert, A.; Rémésy, C. Bioavailability and Bioefficacy of Polyphenols in Humans. I. Review of 97 Bioavailability Studies. *Am. J. Clin. Nutr.* **2005**, *81*, 230S–242S. [CrossRef]
49. Mirzoeva, O.K.; Grishanin, R.N.; Calder, P.C. Antimicrobial Action of Propolis and Some of Its Components: The Effects on Growth, Membrane Potential and Motility of Bacteria. *Microbiol. Res.* **1997**, *152*, 239–246. [CrossRef] [PubMed]
50. Roncarati, D.; Scarlato, V.; Vannini, A. Targeting of Regulators as a Promising Approach in the Search for Novel Antimicrobial Agents. *Microorganisms* **2022**, *10*, 185. [CrossRef] [PubMed]
51. Zannoni, A.; Pelliciari, S.; Musiani, F.; Chiappori, F.; Roncarati, D.; Scarlato, V. Definition of the Binding Architecture to a Target Promoter of HP1043, the Essential Master Regulator of Helicobacter Pylori. *Int. J. Mol. Sci.* **2021**, *22*, 7848. [CrossRef] [PubMed]
52. Vannini, A.; Roncarati, D.; D'Agostino, F.; Antoniciello, F.; Scarlato, V. Insights into the Orchestration of Gene Transcription Regulators in Helicobacter Pylori. *Int. J. Mol. Sci.* **2022**, *23*, 13688. [CrossRef]
53. Tan, D.; Loots, L.; Friščić, T. Towards medicinal mechanochemistry: Evolution of milling from pharmaceutical solid form screening to the synthesis of active pharmaceutical ingredients (APIs). *Chem. Commun.* **2016**, *52*, 7760–7781. [CrossRef]
54. Sekhon, B.S. Drug-Drug Co-Crystals. *DARU J. Pharm. Sci.* **2012**, *20*, 45. [CrossRef]
55. Bordignon, S.; Vioglio, P.C.; Priola, E.; Voinovich, D.; Gobetto, R.; Nishiyama, Y.; Chierotti, M.R. Engineering Codrug Solid Forms: Mechanochemical Synthesis of an Indomethacin–Caffeine System. *Cryst. Growth Des.* **2017**, *17*, 5744–5752. [CrossRef]
56. Byrn, S.R.; Pfeiffer, R.R.; Stephenson, G.; Grant, D.J.W.; Gleason, W.B. Solid-State Pharmaceutical Chemistry. *Chem. Mater.* **1994**, *6*, 1148–1158. [CrossRef]
57. Farhadi, F.; Khameneh, B.; Iranshahi, M.; Iranshahy, M. Antibacterial Activity of Flavonoids and Their Structure–Activity Relationship: An Update Review. *Phytother Res.* **2019**, *33*, 13–40. [CrossRef] [PubMed]

pharmaceutics

Article

Synthesis of 6″-Modified Kanamycin A Derivatives and Evaluation of Their Antibacterial Properties

Kseniya Shapovalova [1], Georgy Zatonsky [1], Natalia Grammatikova [1], Ilya Osterman [2,3], Elizaveta Razumova [4], Andrey Shchekotikhin [1] and Anna Tevyashova [1,*]

1 Gause Institute of New Antibiotics, 11 B. Pirogovskaya, 119021 Moscow, Russia; schapowalowa.kseniya2014@yandex.ru (K.S.); gzatonsk@gmail.com (G.Z.); ngrammatikova@yandex.ru (N.G.); shchekotikhin@mail.ru (A.S.)
2 Center of Life Sciences, Skolkovo Institute of Science and Technology, Bolshoy Boulevard 30, bld. 1, 121205 Moscow, Russia; osterman@yandex.ru
3 Center for Translational Medicine, Sirius University of Science and Technology, Olympic Avenue 1, 354340 Sochi, Russia
4 Department of Chemistry, Lomonosov Moscow State University, Leninskie Gory 1, 119991 Moscow, Russia; elizaveta_razumova@list.ru
* Correspondence: chulis@mail.ru

Abstract: Aminoglycosides are one of the first classes of antibiotics to have been used clinically, and they are still being used today. They have a broad spectrum of antimicrobial activity, making them effective against many different types of bacteria. Despite their long history of use, aminoglycosides are still considered promising scaffolds for the development of new antibacterial agents, particularly as bacteria continue to develop resistances to existing antibiotics. We have synthesized a series of 6″-deoxykanamycin A analogues with additional protonatable groups (amino-, guanidino or pyridinium) and tested their biological activities. For the first time we have demonstrated the ability of the tetra-*N*-protected-6″-*O*-(2,4,6-triisopropylbenzenesulfonyl)kanamycin A to interact with a weak nucleophile, pyridine, resulting in the formation of the corresponding pyridinium derivative. Introducing small diamino-substituents at the 6″-position of kanamycin A did not significantly alter the antibacterial activity of the parent antibiotic, but further modification by acylation resulted in a complete loss of the antibacterial activity. However, introducing a guanidine residue led to a compound with improved activity against *S. aureus*. Moreover, most of the obtained 6″-modified kanamycin A derivatives were less influenced by the resistant mechanism associated with mutations of the elongation factor G than the parent kanamycin A. This suggests that modifying the 6″-position of kanamycin A with protonatable groups is a promising direction for the further development of new antibacterial agents with reduced resistances.

Keywords: antimicrobial resistance; aminoglycosides; kanamycin; chemical modification; mode of action; translation inhibition

Citation: Shapovalova, K.; Zatonsky, G.; Grammatikova, N.; Osterman, I.; Razumova, E.; Shchekotikhin, A.; Tevyashova, A. Synthesis of 6″-Modified Kanamycin A Derivatives and Evaluation of Their Antibacterial Properties. *Pharmaceutics* **2023**, *15*, 1177. https://doi.org/10.3390/pharmaceutics15041177

Academic Editors: Aura Rusu and Valentina Uivarosi

Received: 2 March 2023
Revised: 3 April 2023
Accepted: 4 April 2023
Published: 7 April 2023

1. Introduction

The overuse and misuse of antibiotics, both in human medicine and agriculture, has led to a concerning increase in antimicrobial resistance (AMR) [1]. AMR is a significant public health threat that limits our ability to treat infections effectively, leading to longer hospital stays, higher healthcare costs and increased mortality rates. The 2017 WHO report has identified a list of twelve antibiotic-resistant "priority pathogens", nine of which are Gram-negative bacteria [2]. These bacteria are particularly challenging to treat due to their unique outer membrane structures, which limit the effectiveness of many commonly used antibiotics. According to expert estimates, the problem of AMR may worsen as a consequence of the COVID-19 coronavirus infection pandemic, as most of those who became ill were given antimicrobials to prevent or treat bacterial complications [3,4].

Aminoglycosides (AG) (Figure 1) are one of the first classes of antibiotics that were discovered, and they are still relevant today due to their broad-spectrum antimicrobial activity. They are active against gram-positive (G+) and gram-negative bacteria (G−), as well as mycobacteria [5]. AG are commonly used for the treatment of infections caused by G- bacteria, aerobic bacilli and staphylococci. They are often used in combination with other antibiotics such as β-lactams or vancomycin to improve their efficacy. Streptomycin, a member of the AG family, is still used in combination therapy to treat *Mycobacterium tuberculosis* [6]. Other AG such as kanamycin (KANA, **1**) and amikacin (Figure 1) are used as second-line drugs in the treatment of resistant *M. tuberculosis* infections [7].

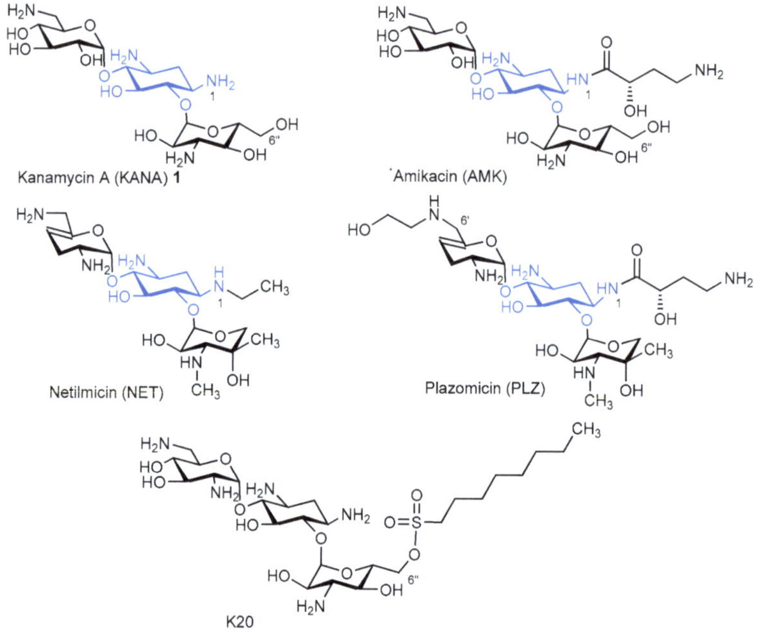

Figure 1. Structures of selected aminoglycoside antibiotics.

The mechanism of action of aminoglycosides is based on inhibition of protein synthesis as a result of binding with the 16S rRNA of the bacterial ribosome 30S-subunit [8,9]. It was demonstrated that different classes of AG might bind to various sites of the 16S rRNA. Nevertheless, the common outcome is a change of a conformation of the A site to one that mimics the closed state induced by the interaction between cognate tRNA and mRNA. This leads to the inhibition of the proofreading capabilities of the ribosome and the promotion of mistranslation, ultimately inhibiting protein synthesis [10]. Additionally, aminoglycoside binding can also affect the translocation process catalyzed by the elongation factor G (EF-G) [11].

Aminoglycoside antibiotics have been widely used since the 1940s, but their effectiveness has been limited by the emergence of bacterial resistance. In addition to resistance, AG can also cause serious side effects, such as kidney damage, hearing loss and vestibular toxicity [12,13]. Since the 1970s, attempts have been made to obtain semi-synthetic aminoglycoside antibiotics; as a result, amikacin (AMK) and netilmicin (NET) were introduced into clinical practice in 1976 and 1981, respectively (Figure 1). More recently, plazomicin (PLZ, Figure 1) has been developed to overcome the resistance mechanisms that have evolved against older aminoglycosides. PLZ is a new generation aminoglycoside that has been designed to evade the most common aminoglycoside-modifying enzymes (AMEs) produced by bacteria. The FDA approved plazomicin in 2018 for the treatment of complicated urinary tract infections, including pyelonephritis, caused by certain gram-negative bacteria. Its approval marked an important step in the rejuvenation of the aminoglycoside class of antibiotics [14,15].

It was established that the major causes of antimicrobial resistance to AG are caused by a reduction in intracellular concentrations of antibiotics by bacterial efflux pumps or through reduced membrane permeability as well as the decreased affinity of the drug for its target bacterial ribosome, either by modifications of the drug or of the ribosome. The most clinically important mechanisms of resistance to AG are due to structural modifications of AGs by AMEs, which recatalyze regioselective modifications of the aminoglycoside molecule, such as *N*-acetylation, *O*-phosphorylation or an attachment of a nucleotide at one of the hydroxyl group of AG. Recently, it has also been demonstrated that some bacterial species, including *Pseudomonas aeruginosa*, *Escherichia coli* and *Acinetobacter baumannii*, quickly develop point mutations in the gene *fusA* (encoding the EF-G protein) when grown in sublethal concentrations of aminoglycosides such as kanamycin, tobramycin and gentamicin [16,17]. These mutations were reported as a novel mechanism of aminoglycoside resistance in the clinical strains of *P. aeruginosa* [18].

It is a valid approach to synthesize new derivatives of aminoglycosides to address the challenges posed by antimicrobial resistance and the limitations of existing antibiotics. Thus, we aimed to synthesize a series of new derivatives of AG in an attempt to find new compounds which possess activity against resistant strains of microorganisms (including strains with characterized mutations in the gene *fusA* (EF-G)) and/or with improved pharmacological properties.

Kanamycin A, one of the first representatives of aminoglycosides and a starting compound for the semi-synthetic antibiotic amikacin [19], was chosen as a starting scaffold for chemical modification. The primary hydroxyl group in the 6″ position was selected for modification due to its availability and potential for selective transformation. Recently, comprehensive reviews have discussed various types of modifications of the aminoglycoside family of antibiotics [5,20]. Among those, different modifications of the primary hydroxyl group in the 6″ position of the antibiotic (AMK, KANA, kanamycin B and tobramycin) (Figure 2) were described, including the introduction of dithiol or azide groups, as well as an obtaining of the thioethers [20].

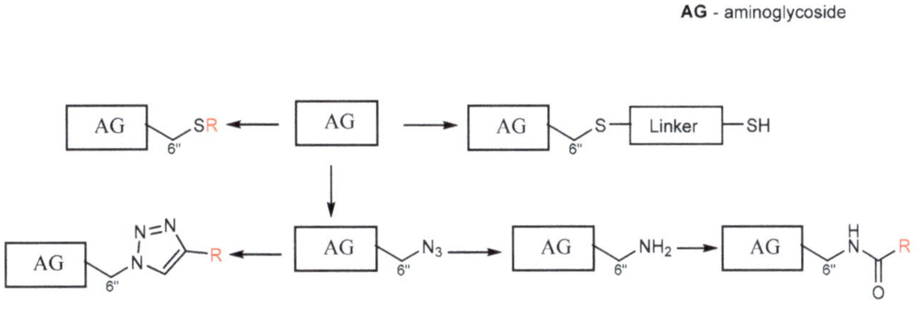

Figure 2. Types of semisynthetic AG derivatives obtained by the chemical transformation of the 6″-hydroxy group.

Furthermore, the replacement of hydroxyl moieties by amines on the cores of various AGs was performed to explore the importance of electrostatic interactions for the binding between RNA and AGs and to identify a common recognition pattern [21]. These results have demonstrated that the presence of several amino groups on an AG core, including the KANA series, correlates with an increase in inhibitory activity, as well as an increase in binding with the 16S rRNA of the bacterial ribosome 30S-subunit [20].

Interestingly, the modification of KANAs at the 6″-position also extended their potential application as antifungal drugs or fungicides for agriculture [22–24]. For example, the KANA derivative K20 (Figure 1) has been shown to exhibit antifungal activity against various fungi, including *Fusarium graminearum*, a pathogen that causes fusariosis in wheat [25,26].

Herein, we describe synthesis of a new series of 6″-modified KANA derivatives bearing additional groups that can be protonated at physiological pH. Varying the structure of the introduced fragment (alkyl amino-, guanidino- heterocyclic and hydroxyalkylamino) was carried out in order to established structure–antimicrobial-activity relationships, including an ability to overcome resistance of microorganisms caused by mutations in the gene *fusA* (EF-G).

2. Materials and Methods

2.1. Chemistry

Kanamycin A was a commercially available product of Abcr GmbH (Karlsruhe, Germany). All other solvents and reagents were commercially available products from Aldrich (Saint Louis, MO, USA) and Merck (Darmstadt, Germany). DMF (dried over $CaCl_2$, then over P_2O_5) and pyridine (dried over KOH, then over $CaCl_2$) were distilled before use.

The course of reactions, purification and extraction procedures, and the identities of the obtained compounds, were monitored by TLC and HPLC methods. TLC was performed on plates with 60F254 silica gel (Merck, Darmstadt, Germany). Kanamycin and its derivatives were visualized on chromatograms in iodine vapor or by a solution of ninhydrin in ethanol or 6N sulfuric acid solution followed by heating. UV-absorbing derivatives were also detected in UV light.

The preparative isolation and purification of the compounds were performed on silica gel columns (Kieselgel G60, 0.040–0.063 mm, Merck, Darmstadt, Germany). For neutralization, DOWEX 50 WX2 (100–200 mesh) ion-exchange resin (SERVA, Heidelberg, Germany) was used. All solutions were dried over sodium sulfate and evaporated in a vacuum at a temperature below 40 °C.

Analytical HPLC was performed on an LC-20AD chromatograph (Shimadzu, Kyoto, Japan) using a UV detector and a Kromasil-100-C18, 4.6250 mm column (Phenemenex, Torrance, CA, USA) at a flow rate of 1 mL/min in systems:

System (A1): A (0.01M H_3PO_4, pH 2.6) and B (MeCN), linear acetonitrile concentration gradient from 20→80% acetonitrile in 30 min, then from 80→20% in 3 min;

System (A2): A ($HCOONH_4$ 0.2%, pH 4.5) and B (MeCN), linear acetonitrile concentration gradient from 40→90% for 30 min, then from 90→40% for 3 min;

System (A3): A (0.01M H_3PO_4, pH 2.6) and B (MeCN), linear acetonitrile concentration gradient from 80→95% for 30 min, then from 95→80% for 3 min;

System (A4): A ($HCOONH_4$ 0.2%, pH 4.5) and B (MeCN), linear acetonitrile concentration gradient from 20→90% for 30 min, then from 90→95% for 5 min, then from 95→95% for 5 min, then from 95→20% for 5 min;

System (A5): A ($HCOONH_4$ 0.2%, pH 8.4) and B (MeCN), linear acetonitrile concentration gradient from 40→90% for 30 min, then from 90→40% for 3 min;

System (A6): A ($HCOONH_4$ 0.2%, pH 8.4) and B (MeCN), linear acetonitrile concentration gradient from 10→60% for 30 min, then from 60→10% for 3 min.

The purities of the intermediates and final compounds were at least 90% by HPLC (for UV-absorbing compounds).

Elemental analysis was performed on the automated PerkinElmer 2400 CHN microanalyzer. High-resolution mass spectra (HR MS) were obtained by electrospray ionization (ESI) on a micrOTOF-Q II instrument (Bruker Daltonics GmbH, Bremen, Germany). The ^{1}H, ^{13}C and ^{15}N NMR spectra were recorded in DMSO-d6 at 25 °C on a Bruker AV III 500 spectrometer (Bruker Biospin AG, Fällanden, Switzerland) at 500.2 MHz, 125.8 MHz and 50.7 MHz for ^{1}H, ^{13}C and ^{15}N, respectively. Signal assignment in NMR spectra was performed using two-dimensional COSY, TOCSY, NOESY, HSQC, HMBC and ^{1}H-^{15}N edHSQC experiments. Standard pulse sequences were used. The ^{1}H and ^{13}C NMR spectra were referenced using either residual DMSO solvent signals (2.50 ppm for DMSO-d6 for ^{1}H spectra and 49.5 ppm for DMSO-d6 for ^{13}C spectra) or signals of internal DSS reference for

D_2O solutions. The ^1H-^{15}N edHSQC spectrum was externally referenced against CH_3NO_2 for ^{15}N.

1,3,6′,3″-Tetra-*N*-Cbz-6″-*O*-(2,4,6-triisopropylbenzenesulfonyl)kanamycin A (**2**)

1st step

The solution of benzylchloroformate (2.40 mL, 16.7 mmol) in acetone (10 mL) was added dropwise at 0 °C to the mixture kanamycin A monosulfate (2.0 g, 3.43 mmol) and saturated water solution of Na_2CO_3 (26.7 mL). The reaction mixture was stirred at 0 °C for 2 h, then at rt for 8 h. The resulting precipitate was filtered off and then suspended in 1M HCl (70 mL) and stirred for 30 min. The precipitate was filtered off, washed with H_2O and dried in a vacuum over P_2O_5. The target 1,3,6′,3″-tetra-*N*-Cbz-kanamycin A was obtained as a white solid (3.44 g, 98% yield) and used without the additional purification at the next stage.

HRMS (ESI): calculated for $[C_{50}H_{61}N_4O_{19}]^+$ = 1021.3930 $[C_{50}H_{64}N_5O_{19}]^+$ = 1038.4196 $[C_{50}H_{60}N_4O_{19}Na]^+$ = 1043.3749, found $[M+H]^+$ = 1021.4185 $[M+NH_4]^+$ = 1038.4467 $[M+Na]^+$ = 1043.4044, R_f ($CHCl_3$:MeOH 10:1) = 0.5, R_t (system A2) = 13.41 min.

^1H NMR (δ, ppm, J/Hz): 1.46–3.56 (m, 7H, cHex), 3.07–4.93 (m, 7H, $CH_{1'\text{-}6'}$), 3.31–4.99 (m, 7H, $CH_{1''\text{-}6''}$), 3.67 (d, 2H, ^3J = 6.1 Hz, -OH-$CH_{CH2'',CH4''}$-), 4.23 (t, 1H, ^3J = 5.6 Hz, -OH-CH_2 $_{CH6''}$-), 4.85–5.18 (m, 8H, -OCH_2), 5.24 (bs, 1H, -OH-CH $_{cHex5}$), 5.34 (d, 1H, ^3J = 5.6 Hz, -OH-$CH_{CH2'\text{-}CH4'}$-), 6.84 (s, 1H, -NH-CH_2 $_{CH6'}$-), 7.01 (s, 1H, -NH-CH_2 $_{CH3''}$-), 7.17 (s, 1H, -NH-CH_{cHex3}-), 7.21–7.42 (m, 20H, 4 × Ph), 7.43 (s, 1H, -NH-CH_{cHex1}-).

^{13}C NMR (δ, ppm, J/Hz): 34.4, 41.7, 49.7, 50.1, 56.5, 60.2, 65.0, 65.3, 67.2, 70.1, 70.6, 70.7, 72.3, 72.7, 72.9, 74.1, 80.4, 84.3, 97.3, 101.1, 127.7, 128.3, 136.8–137.4, 155.6, 155.9, 156.5, 156.6.

2nd step

The 2,4,6-Triisopropylbenzenesulfonylchloride (1.28 g, 4.23 mmol) was added to the solution of 1,3,6′,3″-tetra-*N*-Cbz-kanamycin A (1.0 g, 0.98 mmol) and 4-(*N*,*N*-dimethylamino)pyridine (517 mg, 4.23 mmol) in dry pyridine (15 mL). The reaction mixture was stirred 6 h at room temperature (rt), then an additional amount of 2,4,6-triisopropylbenzenesulfonylchloride (1.28 g, 4.23 mmol) was added and the reaction mixture was stirred at rt for 20 h. An aqueous solution of HCl (1N, 70 mL) and water (100 mL) was added to the reaction mixture. The product was extracted with ethyl acetate (3 × 60 mL) and organic fractions were combined, dried over Na_2SO_4, filtered off and evaporated to dryness. The target compound was purified by the column chromatography on silica gel. The elution was carried out by $CHCl_3$ (200 mL), followed by the mixture $CHCl_3$-CH_3OH (100:3). Fractions which contained the target compound were combined and evaporated to dryness, resulting in **2** (1.12 g, 89% yield) as a light-yellow solid.

HRMS (ESI): calculated for $[C_{65}H_{86}N_5O_{21}S]^+$ = 1304.5536, found $[M+NH_4]^+$ = 1304.5655, R_f ($CHCl_3$:MeOH 100:15) = 0.57, R_t (system A3) = 8.31 min.

^1H NMR (δ, ppm, J/Hz): 1.19–1.21 (m, 18H, 6×-CH_3), 1.41–3.55 (m, 7H, cHex), 3.06–4.89 (m, 7H, $CH_{1'\text{-}6'}$), 3.29–4.97 (m, 7H, $CH_{1''\text{-}6''}$), 3.67 (d, 2H, ^3J = 6.1 Hz, -OH-$CH_{CH2'',CH4''}$-), 3.99–4.06 (m, 3H, -$CH(CH_3)_3$), 4.86–5.11 (m, 8H, -OCH_2), 5.24 (bs, 1H, -OH-CH_{cHex5}), 5.34 (d, 1H, ^3J = 5.6 Hz, -OH-$CH_{CH2'\text{-}CH4'}$-), 6.83 (s, 1H, -NH-CH_2 $_{CH6'}$-), 7.06 (s, 1H, -NH-CH_2 $_{CH3''}$-), 7.18 (s, 1H, -NH-CH_{cHex3}-), 7.25–7.39 (m, 20H, 4 × Ph), 7.34 (s, 1H, -NH-CH_{cHex1}-).

^{13}C NMR (δ, ppm, J/Hz): 23.2, 24.37, 24.45, 29.0, 34.5, 41.6, 49.6, 50.0, 56.6, 65.0, 65.3, 66.4, 67.5, 69.6, 69.7, 70.4, 70.6, 72.2, 72.6, 74.2, 80.0, 84.6, 97.4, 101.2, 123.7, 127.6, 128.2, 137.0, 137.1, 137.2, 150.2, 153.6, 155.5, 155.8, 156.5, 156.6.

1,3, 6′,3″-Tetra-*N*-Boc-6″-*O*-(2,4,6-triisopropylbenzeneosulfonyl)kanamycin A (**3**)

1st step

The solution of di-*tert*-butyldicarbonate (1.5 g, 6.86 mmol) and Et_3N (0.5 mL, 3.43 mmol) in DMSO (12 mL) was added to a suspension of kanamycin A monosulfate (500 mg, 0.86 mmol) and NaOH (34 mg, 0.858 mmol) in H_2O (2 mL). The reaction mixture was stirred at rt for 12 h, then NH_4OH (conc, 5 mL) was added. The obtained solid was filtered over celite, and a cake was washed with H_2O (2 × 20 mL) and ethyl acetate (20 mL). The target compound was eluted from celite with methanol (50 mL) and the obtained solution was evaporated to dryness, resulting in 1,3, 6′,3″-tetra-*N*-Boc-kanamycin A (0.47 g, 62% yield) as white solid which was used without the additional purification at the next stage.

HRMS (ESI): calculated for $[C_{38}H_{68}N_4O_{19}Na]^+$ = 907.4376, found $[M+Na]^+$ = 907.4533, R_f (MeOH:NH_3 7:10) = 0.36.

^{1}H NMR (δ, ppm, J/Hz): 1.36 (s, 9H, 3×-CH_3), 1.37 (s, 9H, 3×-CH_3), 1.38 (s, 18H, 6×-CH_3) 1.38–3.42 (m, 7H, cHex), 3.04–4.88 (m, 7H, $CH_{1'-6'}$), 2.9–4.89 (m, 7H, $CH_{1''-6''}$), 3.69 (d, 2H, ^3J = 6.1 Hz, -OH-$CH_{CH2'',CH4''}$-), 4.21 (t, 1H, ^3J = 5.6 Hz, -OH-$CH_{2\ CH6'''}$-), 5.25 (bs, 1H, -OH-CH_{cHex5}), 5.35 (d, 1H, ^3J = 5.6 Hz, -OH-$CH_{CH2'-CH4'}$-), 6.35 (s, 1H, -NH-$CH_{2CH6'}$-), 6.5 (s, 1H, -NH-$CH_{2\ CH3''}$-), 6.58 (s, 1H, -NH-CH_{cHex3}-), 6.96 (s, 1H, -NH-CH_{cHex1}-).

^{13}C NMR (δ, ppm, J/Hz): 28.1, 28.2, 28.3, 34.7, 41.4, 49.1, 50.0, 55.9, 60.3, 67.5, 70.1, 70.3, 70.5, 72.1, 72.7, 72.9, 75.0, 77.8, 80.4, 83.9, 97.8, 101.1, 154.9, 155.3, 156.1, 156.3.

2nd step

The 2,4,6-Triisopropylbenzenesulfonylchloride (1.74 g, 5.74 mmol) was added to the mixture of 1,3,6′,3″-tetra-*N*-Boc-kanamycin A (1.18 g, 1.33 mmol) and 4-(*N*,*N*-dimethylanimo) pyridine (702 mg, 5.74 mmol) in dry pyridine (30 mL). The reaction mixture was stirred at rt for 6 h, then an additional portion of 2,4,6-triisopropylbenzenesulfonylchloride (1.74 g, 5.74 mmol) was added and the reaction mixture was stirred at rt for 20 h. An aqueous solution of HCl (1N, 70 mL) and H_2O (100 mL) was added to the reaction mixture. The target compound was extracted with ethyl acetate (3 × 60 mL) and the organic fraction was dried over Na_2SO_4, filtered off and concentrated in a vacuum. The product was purified by column chromatography in silica gel and the column was eluted by $CHCl_3$ (150 mL), followed by the mixture of $CHCl_3$-CH_3OH (100:2). Fractions which contained the target compound were combined and evaporated to dryness, resulting in **3** (0.59 g, 39% yield) as a light-yellow solid.

HRMS (ESI): calculated for $[C_{53}H_{91}N_4O_{21}S]^+$ = 1151.5896, found $[M+H]^+$ = 1151.5847, R_f ($CHCl_3$:MeOH 10:1) = 0.31, R_t (system A1) = 9.44 min.

6″-(Piperidin-1-yl)-6″-deoxykanamycin A acetate (**4**)

1st step

Compound **2** (200 mg, 0.156 mmol) was dissolved in dry pyridine (5 mL) and NaI (2 mg, 0.016 mmol) and iPr_2EtN (0.1 mL, 0.77 mmol) were added to the reaction mixture. The reaction mixture was refluxed for 1 h, then cooled to rt and diluted with H_2O (50 mL). The product was extracted with ethyl acetate (3 × 30 mL) and the organic fractions were combined, dried over Na_2SO_4 and evaporated to dryness. The residue was purified by flash-chromatography on silica gel. The elution was carried out by $CHCl_3$ (50 mL), followed by the mixture $CHCl_3$-CH_3OH-NH_4OH (10:3:1). Fractions which contained the target compound were combined and evaporated to dryness, resulting in 1,3,6′,3″-tetra-*N*-Cbz-6″-(pyridin-1-ium)-6″-deoxykanamycin A (167 mg, 98% yield) as a white solid.

HRMS (ESI): calculated for $[C_{55}H_{64}N_5O_{18}]^+$ = 1082.4246, found $[M]^+$ = 1082.4249, R_f ($CHCl_3$:MeOH 100:15) = 0.17, R_t (system A2) = 11.09 min.

^{1}H NMR (δ, ppm, J/Hz): 1.43–3.46 (m, 7H, cHex), 3.1–4.56 (m, 7H, $CH_{1'-6'}$), 3.15–4.95 (m, 7H, $CH_{1''-6''}$), 4.86–5.11 (m, 8H, -OCH_2), 6.78 (t, 1H, ^3J = 4.9 Hz, -NH-$CH_{2\ CH6'}$-), 7.1 (s, 1H, -NH-$CH_{2\ CH3''}$-), 7.14 (s, 1H, -NH-CH_{cHex3}-), 7.25–7.39 (m, 20H, 4×Ph), 7.39 (s, 1H, -NH-CH_{cHex1}-) 8.12 (s, 2H, $Py_{3'}$), 8.58 (s, 1H, $Py_{4'}$), 8.81 (s, 2H, $Py_{2'}$).

^{13}C NMR (δ, ppm, J/Hz): 33.7, 41.2, 49.1, 50.3, 55.9, 61.9, 65.0, 65.3, 68.9, 69.1, 70.2, 70.3, 71.5, 72.2, 73.9, 79.1, 84.7, 98.1, 101.0, 127.1, 127.6, 128.2, 145.0, 145.4, 155.5, 155.8, 156.5, 156.6.

2nd step

1,3,6′,3″-Tetra-*N*-Cbz-6″-(pyridin-1-ium)-6″-deoxykanamycin A (54 mg, 0,05 mmol) was dissolved in CH_3OH (2 mL), then Pd/C (5%, 85 mg) was added and the reaction mixture was acidified to pH 3 by the addition of CH_3COOH. The reaction mixture was vigorously stirred at rt at H_2 flow (1 atm) for 3 h. The catalyst was filtered off via celite; the cake was washed with CH_3OH (5 mL) and H_2O (5 mL), and the combined filtrate was concentrated in a vacuum. The target compound was precipitated by the addition of acetone (10 mL), filtered off and dried in a vacuum over P_2O_5, resulting in compound **4** (25 mg, 58% yield) as a white solid.

Anal. calculated for [$C_{23}H_{44}N_5O_{10}$×5AcOH×5H_2O]: C, 42.12; H, 7.93; N, 7.44, O 42.51. Found: C, 42.10; H, 7.90; N, 7.43.

HRMS (ESI): calculated for [$C_{23}H_{45}N_5O_{10}$]$^+$ = 552.3245, found [M+H]$^+$ = 552.3216, R_f (NH_4OH:iPrOH 10:7) = 0.31, T_{mp} = 201 °C (decomp.). The assignment of the signals in the ^{1}H and ^{13}C NMR spectra is presented in the Table S1.

6″-(Pyridin-1-ium)-6″-deoxykanamycin A trifluoroacetate (**5**)

1st step

Compound **3** (60 mg, 0.052 mmol) was dissolved in dry pyridine (2 mL), then NaI (1 mg, 0.005 mmol) and iPr_2EtN (34 mg, 0.26 mmol) were added to the reaction mixture. The obtained solution was refluxed for 1 h, then cooled to room temperature and diluted with H_2O (40 mL). The product was extracted with ethyl acetate (3 × 15 mL) and the organic fractions were combined, dried over Na_2SO_4, filtered off and evaporated to dryness in a vacuum. The product was purified by flash chromatography on silica gel and the elution was carried by the mixture $CHCl_3$-CH_3OH (10:1, 25 mL) followed by the mixture $CHCl_3$-CH_3OH-NH_4OH (10:5:3). Fractions which contained the target compound were combined and evaporated to dryness in a vacuum, resulting in 1,3,6′,3″-tetra-*N*-Boc-6″-(pyridin-1-ium)-6″-deoxykanamycin A (35 mg, 71% yield) as a white solid.

HRMS (ESI): calculated for [$C_{43}H_{72}N_5O_{18}$]$^+$ = 946.4872, found [M]$^+$ = 946.4979, R_f ($CHCl_3$:MeOH 100:15) = 0.15.

2nd step

Trifluoroacetic acid (0.2 mL, 2.752 mmol) was added dropwise to the solution of 1,3,6′,3″-tetra-*N*-Boc-6″-(pyridin-1-ium)-6″-deoxykanamycin A (30 mg, 0.03 mmol) in CH_2Cl_2 (1 mL). The reaction mixture was stirred at rt for 4 h and then evaporated to dryness in a vacuum. The addition of Et_2O (10 mL) to the residue resulted in the formation of the precipitate, which was filtered off, washed with Et_2O (50 mL) and dried in a vacuum over P_2O_5, resulting in the target compound **5** (23 mg, 63% yield) obtained as a white solid.

HRMS (ESI): calculated for [$C_{23}H_{40}N_5O_{10}$]$^+$ = 546.2775, found [M]$^+$ = 546.2752, R_f (NH_4OH:iPrOH 10:7) = 0.3, T_{mp} = 205 °C (decomp.).

The assignment of the signals in the ^{1}H and ^{13}C spectra is presented in Table S1.

6″-(2-Aminoethylamino)-6″-deoxykanamycin A acetate (**6**)

1st step

6″-(2-Aminoethylamino)-1,3,6′,3″-tetra-*N*-Cbz-6″-deoxykanamycin A (**6a**)

A mixture of compound **2** (805 mg, 0.626 mmol) and ethylenediamine (3.5 mL) was stirred at rt for 24 h, then the reaction mixture was diluted with H_2O (150 mL). The forming precipitate was filtered off, washed with H_2O and dried in a vacuum at 45 °C and then in a vacuum over P_2O_5. The target 6″-(2-aminoethylamino)-1,3,6′,3″-tetra-*N*-Cbz-6″-deoxykanamycin A (**6a**) (612 mg, 92%) was obtained as a light-yellow solid and used without additional purification on the next stage.

HRMS (ESI): calculated for [$C_{52}H_{67}N_6O_{18}$]$^+$ = 1063.4511 [$C_{52}H_{66}N_6O_{18}Na$]$^+$ = 1085.1150 [$C_{52}H_{66}N_6O_{18}K$]$^+$ = 1101.4071, found [M+H]$^+$ = 1063.4506 [M+Na]$^+$ = 1085.1326 [M+K]$^+$ = 1101.4065, R_f ($CHCl_3$:MeOH:HCOOH 13:5:0.1) = 0.45, R_t (System A4) = 17.5 min.

2nd step

6″-(2-Aminoethylamino)-1,3,6′,3″-tetra-*N*-Cbz-6″-deoxykanamycin A (**6a**) (61 mg, 0.057 mmol) was dissolved in CH_3OH (2 mL) and 5% Pd/C (95 mg) was added to the reaction mixture. The CH_3COOH was added to the reaction mixture until pH 3 was reached, and the mixture was vigorously stirred at H_2 flow (1 atm.) for 4 h. The catalyst was filtered off via a celite layer; the cake was washed with CH_3OH (5 mL) and H_2O (5 mL), and the combined filtrate was concentrated in a vacuum. The target compound was precipitated by the addition of acetone (10 mL), filtered off and dried in a vacuum over P_2O_5, resulting in the target compound **6** (32.8 mg, 69%) as a white solid.

Anal. calculated for [$C_{20}H_{42}N_6O_{10}$×5AcOH×3H_2O]: C, 40.91; H, 7.78; N, 9.54, O 41.77. Found: C, 40.91; H, 7.63; N, 9.50.

HRMS (ESI): calculated for [$C_{20}H_{43}N_6O_{10}$]$^+$ = 527.3040, found [M+H]$^+$ = 527.3032, R_f (NH_4OH:iPrOH 10:7) = 0.32, T_{mp} = 181 °C (decomp.).

The assignment of the signals in the ^{1}H and ^{13}C spectra is presented in Table S1.

6′′-(3-Aminopropyl-1-amino)-6′′-deoxykanamycin A acetate (**7**)

1st step

6′′-(3-Aminopropyl-1-amino)-1,3,6′,3′′-tetra-*N*-Cbz-6′′-deoxykanamycin A (**7a**)

A mixture of compound **2** (200 mg, 0.156 mmol) and propan-1,3-diamine (3.5 mL) was stirred at rt for 24 h, then the reaction mixture was diluted with H_2O (100 mL). The forming precipitate was filtered off, washed with H_2O and dried in a vacuum at 45 °C and then in a vacuum over P_2O_5 at rt. The target 6′′-(3-aminopropyl-1-amino)-1,3,6′,3′′-tetra-*N*-Cbz-6′′-deoxykanamycin A (**7a**) (136 mg, 81%) was obtained as a white solid and used without additional purification on the next stage.

HRMS (ESI): calculated for $[C_{53}H_{69}N_6O_{18}]^+$ = 1077.4668, found $[M+H]^+$ = 1077.4667, Rf ($CHCl_3$:MeOH:HCOOH 13:5:0.1) = 0.42, R_t (System A4) = 16.5 min.

2nd step

6′′-(3-Aminopropyl-1-amino)-1,3,6′,3′′-tetra-*N*-Cbz-6′′-deoxykanamycin A (**7a**) (138 mg, 0.129 mmol) was dissolved in CH_3OH (2.5 mL) and 5% Pd/C (180 mg) was added to the reaction mixture. The CH_3COOH was added to the reaction mixture until pH 3 was reached, and the mixture was vigorously stirred at H_2 flow (1 atm.) for 4 h. The catalyst was filtered off via a celite layer; the cake was washed with CH_3OH (5 mL) and H_2O (5 mL), and the combined filtrate was concentrated in a vacuum. The target compound was precipitated by the addition of acetone (10 mL), filtered off and dried in a vacuum over P_2O_5, resulting in the target compound **7** (103 mg, 95%) as a white solid.

Anal. calculated for $[C_{21}H_{44}N_6O_{10} \times 5AcOH \times 1H_2O]$: C, 43.35; H, 7.75; N, 9.78, O 39.12. Found: C, 43.35; H, 7.75; N, 9.78.

HRMS (ESI): calculated for $[C_{21}H_{45}N_6O_{10}]^+$ = 541.3197, found $[M+H]^+$ = 541.3122, R_f (NH_4OH:iPrOH 1:1) = 0.15, T_{mp} = 176 °C (decomp).

The assignment of the signals in the ^{1}H and ^{13}C spectra is presented in Table S1.

6′′-(2-Hydroxyethyl-1-amino)-6′′-deoxykanamycin A trifluoroacetate (**8**)

1st step

1,3,6′,3′′-Tetra-*N*-Boc-6′′-(2-hydroxyethyl-1-amino)-6′′-deoxykanamycin A (**8a**)

A mixture of compound 3 (100 mg, 0.087 mmol) and 2-aminoethanol (1.5 mL) was stirred at rt for 24 h, then the reaction mixture was diluted with H_2O (100 mL). The forming precipitate was filtered off, washed with H_2O and dried in a vacuum at 45 °C and then in a vacuum over P_2O_5 at rt. The target 1,3,6′,3′′-tetra-*N*-Boc-6′′-(2-hydroxyethyl-1-amino)-6′′-deoxykanamycin A (**8a**) (35 mg, 45%) was obtained as a white solid and used without additional purification on the next stage.

HRMS (ESI): calculated for $[C_{40}H_{74}N_5O_{19}]^+$ = 928.4978, found $[M+H]^+$ = 928.4988, R_f ($CHCl_3$:MeOH:HCOOH 7:1:0.3) = 0.28.

^{1}H NMR (δ, ppm, J/Hz): 1.36 (s, 9H, 3×-CH_3), 1.37 (s, 9H, 3×-CH_3), 1.38 (s, 18H, 6×-CH_3), 1.47–3.47 (m, 7H, cHex), 2.90–4.91 (m, 7H, -$CH_{1''-6''}$), 3.0 (s, 2H, -NH-$\underline{CH_2}$-), 3.1–4.92 (m, 7H, -$\underline{CH}_{1'-6'}$), 3.63 (s, 2H, -$\underline{CH_2}$-OH), 6.35 (bt, 1H, ^3J = 4.5 Hz, -$\underline{NH}$-CH_2 $_{CH6'}$-), 6.57 (d, 1H, ^3J = 9.3 Hz, -$\underline{NH}$-CH_2 $_{CH3''}$-), 6.64 (bd, 1H, ^3J = 7.0 Hz, -$\underline{NH}$-CH_{cHex3}-), 6.97 (bs, 1H, -$\underline{NH}$-CH_{cHex1}-).

^{13}C NMR (δ, ppm, J/Hz): 28.1–28.3, 34.5, 41.3, 48.5, 48.9, 49.8, 50.4, 55.6, 56.8, 68.4, 69.5, 69.9, 70.0, 70.5, 72.6, 75.4, 77.4–77.9, 78.0, 80.2, 84.3, 98.6, 101.1, 154.9–156.2.

2nd step

Trifluoroacetic acid (0.2 mL, 2.752 mmol) was added dropwise to a solution of 1,3,6′,3′′-tetra-*N*-Boc-6′′-(2-hydroxyethyl-1-amino)-6′′-deoxykanamycin A (**8a**) (30 mg, 0.032 mmol) in CH_2Cl_2 (2 mL). The reaction mixture was stirred at rt for 24 h and then evaporated to dryness in a vacuum. The addition of acetone (10 mL) to the residue resulted in the formation of a white solid which was filtered off, washed with acetone (3 × 10 mL) and dried in a vacuum over P_2O_5. Finally, 6′′-(2-Hydroxyethylamino)-6′′-deoxykanamycin A (**8**) (10 mg, 27%) was obtained as a white solid in the form of trifluoroacetate.

Anal. calculated for $[C_{20}H_{41}N_6O_{10} \times 5TFA \times 1H_2O]$: C, 32.35; H, 4.34; N, 7.55, F 25.59, O 30.17. Found: C, 32.35; H, 4.60; N, 7.50.

HRMS (ESI): calculated for $[C_{20}H_{42}N_5O_{11}]^+$ = 528.2881, found $[M+H]^+$ = 528.2870, R_f (NH_4OH:iPrOH 1:1) = 0.32, T_{mp} = 186 °C (decomp.).

The assignment of the signals in the ^1H and ^{13}C spectra is presented in Table S1.

6″-((*S*)-7-((2-(4-Amino-2-hydroxybutanamido)ethyl)amino))-6″-deoxykanamycin A acetate (**9**)

1st step

Benzotriazol-1-yloxytripirrolidonophosphonium hexafluorophosphate (PyBoP) (196 mg, 0.39 mmol) was added portionwise to the solution of 6″-(2-aminoethylamino)-1,3,6′,3″-tetra-*N*-Cbz-6″-deoxykanamycin A (**6a**) (200 mg, 0.188 mmol) and (S)-4-(((benzyloxy)carbonyl) amino)-2-hydroxybutanoic acid (143 mg, 0.57 mmol) in DMSO (2 mL). The pH of the reaction mixture was kept ~8 by the addition of Et_3N (~200 µL). The reaction mixture was stirred at rt for 48 h, then H_2O (100 mL) was added. The forming precipitate was filtered off, washed with Et_2O (50 mL), dried and purified by the column chromatography on silica gel. The elution was carried out by the mixture $CHCl_3$:CH_3OH:HCOOH (5:1:0.3). Fractions which contained the target compound were combined and evaporated to dryness, resulting in the target intermediate 6″-((*S*)-7-((2-(4-(benzyloxycarbonyl)amino-2-hydroxybutanamido)ethyl)amino))-1,3,6′,3″-tetra-*N*-Cbz-6″-deoxykanamycin A (164 mg, 67%) as a white solid.

HRMS (ESI): calculated for $[C_{64}H_{80}N_7O_{22}]^+$ = 1298.53, found $[M+H]^+$ = 1298.5398, R_f ($CHCl_3$:MeOH:HCOOH 5:1:0.3) = 0.41, R_t (System A4) = 20.8 min.

^1H NMR (δ, ppm, J/Hz): 1.51–3.56 (m, 7H, cHex), 1.57 (s, 1H, $-CH_{1'}-\underline{CH_{2'}}-$), 1.83 (s, 1H, $-CH_{1'}-\underline{CH_{2'}}-$), 2.65 (s, 2H, $-\underline{CH_2}$-NHCO), 2.66–5.00 (m, 7H, $CH_{1''-6''}$), 3.08–4.98 (m, 7H, $CH_{1'-6'}$), 3.1 (s, 2H, $-CH_{2'}-\underline{CH_{3'}}-$), 3.18 (s, 2H, $-NH-\underline{CH_2}-$), 3.88 (s, 1H, -NHCO-$\underline{CH_{1'}}$-), 4.87–5.09 (m, 10H, $-OCH_2$), 6.83 (t, 1H, ^3J = 4.7 Hz, $-\underline{NH}-CH_{2\,CH6'}-$), 7.02 (d, 1H, ^3J = 9.0 Hz, $-\underline{NH}-CH_{2\,CH3''}-$), 7.18 (d, 1H, ^3J = 8.6 Hz, $-\underline{NH}-CH_{cHex3}-$), 7.22 (t, 1H, ^3J = 5.5 Hz, $-CH_{3'}-\underline{NH}-$), 7.26–7.37 (m, 20H, 4×Ph), 7.41 (s, 1H, $-\underline{NH}-CH_{cHex1}-$), 7.81 (t, 1H, ^3J = 5.3 Hz, $-CH_2-\underline{NH}$-CO).

^{13}C NMR (δ, ppm, J/Hz): 34.3, 34.5, 37.1, 37.6, 41.6, 48.5, 49.6, 49.6, 50.2, 56.4, 64.9, 65.0, 65.1, 69.1, 69.4, 69.9, 70.5, 70.5, 70.7, 72.3, 72.7, 74.3, 80.4, 84.5, 97.4, 101.2, 127.5, 127.6, 128.2, 155.5, 155.9, 156.0, 156.4, 156.5, 164.5.

2nd step

The 6″-((*S*)-7-((2-(4-(Benzyloxycarbonyl)amino-2-hydroxybutanamido)ethyl)amino))-1,3,6′,3″-tetra-*N*-Cbz-6″-deoxykanamycin (150 mg, 0.116 mmol) was dissolved in CH_3OH (3 mL), then 5% Pd/C (200 mg) was added and the reaction mixture was acidified to pH 3 by the addition of CH_3COOH. The reaction mixture was vigorously stirred at rt at H_2 flow (1 atm) for 2 h. The catalyst was filtered off via a celite layer; the cake was washed with CH_3OH (5 mL) and H_2O (5 mL), and the combined filtrate was concentrated in a vacuum. The target compound was precipitated by the addition of acetone (10 mL), filtered off and dried in a vacuum over P_2O_5, resulting in compound **9** in the form of acetate (97 mg, 91% yield) as a white solid.

Anal. calculated for $[C_{24}H_{49}N_7O_{12}\times5AcOH\times1H_2O]$: C, 43.17; H, 7.57; N, 10.36, O 38.9. Found: C, 43.17; H, 7.57; N, 10.36.

HRMS (ESI): calculated for $[C_{24}H_{50}N_7O_{12}]^+$ = 628.3517, found $[M+H]^+$ = 628.3479, R_f (NH_4OH:iPrOH 1:1) = 0.27, T_{mp} = 179 °C (decomp.).

The assignment of the signals in the ^1H and ^{13}C spectra is presented in Table S1.

6″-(2-(3-(1-Hydroxy-1,3-dihydrobenzo[c][1,2]oxaborol-7-yl)-*N*-(ethyl-1-amino)propanamide)-6″-deoxykanamycin acetate (**10**)

1st step

1,3,6′,3″-Tetra-*N*-Cbz-6″-(2-(3-(1-hydroxy-1,3-dihydrobenzo[c][1,2]oxaborol-7-yl)-*N*-(ethyl-1-amino)propanamide)-6″-deoxykanamycin A

PyBoP (98 mg, 0.188 mmol) was added portionwise to the solution of 6″-(2-aminoethylamino)-1,3,6′,3″-tetra-N-Cbz-6″-deoxykanamycin A (**6a**) (100 mg, 0.094 mmol) and 3-(1-hydroxy-1,3-dihydrobenzo[c][1,2]oxaborol-7-yl)propanoic acid (58 mg, 0.282 mmol) in DMSO (2 mL). The pH of the reaction mixture was kept ~8 by the addition of Et_3N (~50 µL). The reaction mixture was stirred at rt for 24 h, then Et_2O (50 mL) was added. The forming precipitate was filtered off, washed with Et_2O (5 × 10 mL) and dried over P_2O_5, and the obtained product was used without additional purification on the next stage (70 mg, 60%).

HRMS (ESI): calculated for $[C_{62}H_{76}BN_6O_{21}]^+$ = 1251.5156, found $[M+H]^+$ = 1251.5124, R_f ($CHCl_3$:MeOH:HCOOH 11.5:3:1.5) = 0.37, R_t (System A5) = 16.0 min

2nd step

The 1,3,6′,3″-Tetra-*N*-Cbz-6″-(2-(3-(1-hydroxy-1,3-dihydrobenzo[c][1,2]oxaborol-7-yl)-*N*-(ethyl-1-amino)propanamide)-6″-deoxykanamycin A (60 mg, 0.048 mmol) was dissolved in CH_3OH (3.5 mL), then 5% Pd/C (85 mg) was added and the reaction mixture was acidified to pH 3 by the addition of CH_3COOH. The reaction mixture was vigorously stirred at rt at H_2 flow (1 atm) for 2 h. The catalyst was filtered off via celite layer; the cake was washed with CH_3OH (5 mL) and H_2O (5 mL), and the combined filtrate was concentrated in a vacuum. The target compound was precipitated by the addition of acetone (10 mL) and was filtered off and dried in a vacuum over P_2O_5, resulting in compound **10** (22 mg, 45% yield) as a white solid.

HRMS (ESI): calculated for $[C_{30}H_{51}BN_6O_{13}]$ = 714.3607, found $[M+H]^{2+}$ = 357.1795, R_f (NH_4OH:iPrOH 10:7) = 0.3, R_t (System A6) = 20.2 min, T_{mp} = 245 °C (decomp.).

The assignment of the signals in the ^1H and ^{13}C spectra is presented in Table S1.

6″-(2-Guanidinoethylamino)-6″-deoxykanamycin A acetate (**11**)

1st step

1,3,6′,3″-Tetra-*N*-Cbz-6″-(2-guanidinoethylamino)-6″-deoxykanamycin A

Ethyldiisopropylamine (EDIA, 80 µL, 0.452 mmol) was added to mixture of 6″-(2-aminoethylamino)-1,3,6′,3″-tetra-*N*-Cbz-6″-deoxykanamycin A (**6a**) (160 mg, 0.151 mmol) and 1*H*-pyrazole-1-carboximidamide hydrochloride (33 mg, 0.25 mmol) in DMF (2 mL). The reaction mixture was stirred at rt for 24 h, then Et_2O (50 mL) was added. The forming precipitate was filtered off, washed with Et_2O (5 × 10 mL) and dried over P_2O_5, and the obtained product was used without additional purification on the next stage (125 mg, 75%).

HRMS (ESI): calculated for $[C_{53}H_{69}N_8O_{18}]^+$ = 1105.4729, found $[M+H]^+$ = 1105.4456, R_f ($CHCl_3$:MeOH:HCOOH 5:1:0.3) = 0.4, R_t (System A4) = 16.9 min.

2nd step

The 1,3,6′,3″-Tetra-*N*-Cbz-6″-(2-guanidinoethylamino)-6″-deoxykanamycin A (125 mg, 0.113 mmol) was dissolved in CH_3OH (4 mL), then 5% Pd/C (190 mg) was added and the reaction mixture was acidified to pH 3 by the addition of CH_3COOH. The reaction mixture was vigorously stirred at rt at H_2 flow (1 atm) for 4 h. The catalyst was filtered off via a celite layer; the cake was washed with CH_3OH (5 mL) and H_2O (5 mL), and the combined filtrate was concentrated in a vacuum. The target compound was precipitated by the addition of acetone (10 mL), filtered off and dried in a vacuum over P_2O_5, resulting in compound **11** (83 mg, 85% yield) as a white solid.

Anal. calculated for $[C_{21}H_{44}N_8O_{10} \times 5AcOH \times 6H_2O]$: C, 38.11; H, 7.84; N, 11.47, O 42.58. Found: C, 38.11; H, 7.84; N, 11.47.

HRMS (ESI): calculated for $[C_{21}H_{45}N_8O_{10}]^+$ = 569.3259, found $[M+H]^+$ = 569.3467, R_f (NH_4OH:iPrOH 1:1) = 0.28, T_{mp} = 202 °C (decomp.).

The assignment of the signals in the ^1H and ^{13}C spectra is presented in Table S1.

6″-(2-Amino-4,5-dihydro-1H-imidazol-1-yl)-1,3,6′,3″-tetra-N-Cbz-6″-deoxykanamycin A trifluoroacetate (**12**)

EDIA (120 µL, 0.66 mmol) was added to a mixture of 6″-(2-aminoethylamino)-1,3,6′,3″-tetra-*N*-Cbz-6″-deoxykanamycin A (**6a**) (234 mg, 0.221 mmol) and *tert*-butyl-(((*tert*-butyloxycarbonyl)amino)(1*H*-pyrazol-1-yl)methylen) carbamate (137 mg, 0.441 mmol) in DMF (4.5 mL). The reaction mixture was stirred at 50 °C for 24 h, then Et_2O (150 mL) was added. The forming precipitate was filtered off, washed with Et_2O (5 × 10 mL) and dried in a vacuum over P_2O_5. The resulting intermediate was further dissolved in CH_2Cl_2 (2 mL) and TFA (0.2 mL, 2.75 mmol) was added dropwise. The reaction mixture was stirred at rt for 24 h and then evaporated to dryness in a vacuum. The target compounds were purified by column chromatography on silica gel. The elution was carried out by the mixture $CHCl_3$:MeOH:HCOOH (10:1.5:0.3). The fractions which contained the individual compounds were combined and evaporated to dryness, resulting in trifluoroacetate of 1,3,6′,3″-tetra-*N*-Cbz-6″-(2-guanidinoethylamino)-6″-deoxykanamycin A (white solid, 25 mg, 25%) and compound **12** in the form of trifluoroacetate (white solid, 20 mg, 23%).

Derivative **12**. HRMS (ESI): calculated for $[C_{53}H_{66}N_7O_{18}]^+$ = 1088.4386, found $[M+H]^+$ = 1088.4459, R_f ($CHCl_3$:MeOH:HCOOH 5:1:0.5) = 0.41, R_t (System A4)= 19.1 min.

^{1}H NMR (δ, ppm, J/Hz): 1.50–3.59 (m, 7H, cHex), 3.06–4.98 (m, 7H, $CH_{1''-6''}$), 3.09–4.86 (m, 7H, $CH_{1'-6'}$), 3.47 (s, 2H, -NH-CH_2-<u>CH_2</u>-), 3.65 (s, 1H, -NH-<u>CH_2</u>-CH_2-), 3.72 (s, 1H), (s, 1H, -NH-<u>CH_2</u>-CH_2-), 4.45–5.1 (m, 8H, -O<u>CH_2</u>), 6.80 (t, 1H, 3J = 4.8 Hz, -<u>NH</u>-$CH_{2\,CH6'}$-), 7.07 (d, 1H, ^{3}J = 9.2 Hz, -<u>NH</u>-$CH_{2\,CH3''}$-), 7.17 (d, 1H, ^{3}J = 8.2 Hz, -<u>NH</u>-CH_{cHex1}-), 7.25–7.40 (m, 20H, 4×Ph), 7.36 (s, 1H, -<u>NH</u>-CH_{cHex3}-), 7.55 (s, 1H, -<u>NH</u>-CH_2-CH_2-), 7.71 (s, 1H, -C-NH_2).

^{13}C NMR (δ, ppm, J/Hz): 34.3, 40.6, 41.5, 45.8, 48.5, 49.6, 50.4, 56.2, 65.1, 65.3, 69.3, 69.7, 70.0, 70.5, 70.7, 72.6, 73.0, 74.4, 79.8, 85.1, 97.9, 101.5, 127.6, 128.2, 136.9, 137.1, 137.2, 156.5, 156.6, 157.6, 157.9, 158.8.

2.2. *Biology*

2.2.1. Microorganisms

The microbial strains were obtained from the working collection of Gause Institute of New Antibiotics (GINA). Control strains of microorganisms included in the study: *S. aureus* ATCC 29213, *E. coli* ATCC 25922, *P. aeruginosa* ATCC 27853 and *M. smegmatis* ATCC 607. Microbial cultures were preserved at a low temperature (−75 °C) in trypticase-soy broth (Becton, Dickinson, France) with 10–15% glycerol added. Storage under these conditions was performed according to CLSI recommendations [27]. Before the experiment, bacterial strains were activated after cryopreservation by seeding on trypticase-soy agar medium (Beckton, Dickinson, France) and incubated at (36 ± 1) °C for 16–24 h. Individual morphologically homogeneous colonies were suspended in sterile physiological solution, and the turbidity of the suspension was set to 0.5 units according to the McFarland standard on the DEN-1 device (Biosan, Riga, Latvia), which corresponds to 1.5 × 10^8 CFU/mL for bacterial cultures.

2.2.2. Sample Preparation

Samples were dissolved in sterile distilled water or dimethyl sulfoxide (DMSO), according to the physicochemical characteristic of the samples studied, to a concentration of 10.000 μg/mL. To obtain working solutions, dilutions ranging from 64–0.5 μg/mL were performed.

2.2.3. Assay Setting

Activity was assessed using minimum inhibitory concentration (MIC) values by the microdilution method in Mueller–Hinton Broth (Beckton and Dickinson, France), according to the procedure recommended for determining the sensitivities of microorganisms to antimicrobial agents [27].

The analysis was performed in 96-well plates (Medpolymer, Moscow, Russia). The inoculum was introduced no later than 15 min after preparation. MIC values were analyzed after 15–18 h of incubation at (36 ± 1) °C. The growth of microorganisms in the presence of the tested samples was compared with the growth control without exposure. MIC was determined by the lowest concentration suppressing the visible growth of microorganisms.

The criterion for the accuracy of the obtained results was the control antibiotic kanamycin A and standard strains: *S. aureus* ATCC 29213, *E. coli* ATCC 25922, for which the MIC values were determined: *S. aureus* ATCC 29213—1–4 μg/mL; *E. coli* ATCC 25922–1–4 μg/mL. The MICs of the reference strains must not exceed the confidence limits given in [27], provided that the assay conditions are standard.

2.2.4. Determination of Antibiotic Activity by the Agar-Diffusion Method

On Petri dishes with solid LB-agar medium (1.5%), an overnight culture of the *E. coli* strain JW5503 [28], and the same strain with a deleted kanamycin resistance cassette removed according to the method described in the publication [29], was applied. After drying, 1 μL of antibiotic at a concentration of 50 mg/mL was applied to Petri dishes and incubated at 37 °C for 18 h. Then, Petri dishes were scanned on a ChemiDoc device (Bio-Rad, Hercules, CA, USA) in channels Cy2, Cy3, Cy5. Antibiotic activity was qualitatively determined by the size of the zone of inhibition.

2.2.5. Determination of the Minimum Inhibitory Concentration

Testing was carried out on 2 strains: *E. coli* JW5503 [28] with a removed kanamycin resistance cassette using the method described in the publication [29] and a strain selected from the above by in vivo selection on kanamycin with substitution P610T. Totals of 200 μL (in rows 2–11) and 400 μL (in the first row) of LB liquid medium containing an overnight culture of 3 strains: JW5503 [28] with a deleted kanamycin resistance cassette, diluted 1000-fold, were added to each well of a 96-well 2 mL plate. Then, 2 μL of 50 μg/mL antibiotic was added to each well of the first row. After that, successive dilutions were carried out within one horizontal row, with the antibiotic concentration decreasing by a factor of 2 at each step. The last 2 rows served as controls: row 12 was the original LB medium without cells and antibiotic, row 11 was the cells without antibiotic. After culturing for 18 h at 37 °C and constant agitation, cells were transferred to a low transparent 96-well plate and optical density A590 was measured using a Victor X5 2030 spectrofluorimeter (Perkin Elmer, Waltham, MA, USA). The concentration of the antibiotic in the first well in the dilution series in which the cells did not grow was the minimum inhibitory concentration. The experiment was repeated three times for each antibiotic.

2.2.6. Determination of Translation Accuracy Using Reporters

To qualitatively determine the accuracy of translation in the presence of antibiotics, the *E. coli* strain JW5503 [28], with a kanamycin resistance cassette removed according to the method described in the publication [29], transformed with pJC27 plasmids, on which the β-galactosidase gene encoded, containing an error in the enzyme active center (E537) [30]: GAA→GAC, and a control without replacement, were used. Thus, active β-galactosidase could be synthesized only in the case of translation error.

Petri dishes (10 cm) with solid medium (20 mL) LB-agar (1.5%) containing chloramphenicol at concentrations of 11.3 μg/mL and 80 μg/mL X-Gal were prepared. A mixture of 3.5 mL of cooled LB-agar medium (0.6%) containing 11.3 μg/mL chloramphenicol and 0.5 mL of liquid cell culture A600~1.0 was applied to these Petri dishes, then the dishes were left until solidified. From 1 to 2 μL of antibiotics at concentrations of 50 mg/mL were applied to the resulting two-layer cell culture mediums and incubated at 37 °C for 18 h. The results were documented using a Samsung Galaxy Tab A71 phone camera. The occurrence of blue staining of indigo, a product of the degradation of the X-Gal substrate by the enzyme, along the edge of the inhibition zone indicates that the antibiotic causes translation errors.

3. Results

3.1. Chemistry

For the synthesis of a series of new 6″-modified KANA derivatives, we employed the common strategy which includes two synthetic steps: (1) the protection of all amino groups with *tert*-butyloxycarbonyl (Boc) or benzyloxycarbonyl (Cbz) groups, followed by (2) the activation of the primary 6″-hydroxyl group by introducing a good leaving group, i.e., triisopropylbenzenesulfonyl (TIBS).

The syntheses of the 6″-substituted kanamycin derivatives **4**–**8** were performed starting from the commercially available monosulfate of KANA (**1**) (Schemes 1 and 2). Tetra-*N*-Cbz-6″-*O*-(2,4,6-triisopropylbenzenesulfonyl)kanamycin A (**2**) was obtained in two steps [31]. First, the amino groups of kanamycin A were protected by Cbz groups by the reaction with CbzCl in the presence of Na_2CO_3 (Scheme 1). Due to the fact that the reaction of tetra-*N*-Cbz-kanamycin A with *p*-toluenesulfonyl chloride was not selective, the sterically hindered sulfonating agent, 2,4,6-triisopropylbenzenesulfonyl chloride (TIBSCl), was used. The reaction was carried out at room temperature in pyridine, resulting in compound **2** in an 87% yield for two steps.

Tetra-*N*-Boc-6″-*O*-(2,4,6-triisopropylbenzenesulfonyl)kanamycin A (**3**) was obtained by a similar procedure: first, the amino groups of KANA were protected by Boc-groups by the reaction with Boc_2O in the presence of NaOH, allowing for an increase in the yield of the target intermediate up to 62% in comparison with the previously described 50% for the two-stages procedure (via the obtaining of the KANA-free base and an introduction of the protective groups) [32]. The reaction of tetra-*N*-Boc-kanamycin A with TIBSCl was carried out at room temperature in pyridine resulting in compound **3** in a 39% yield after a chromatographic purification [33].

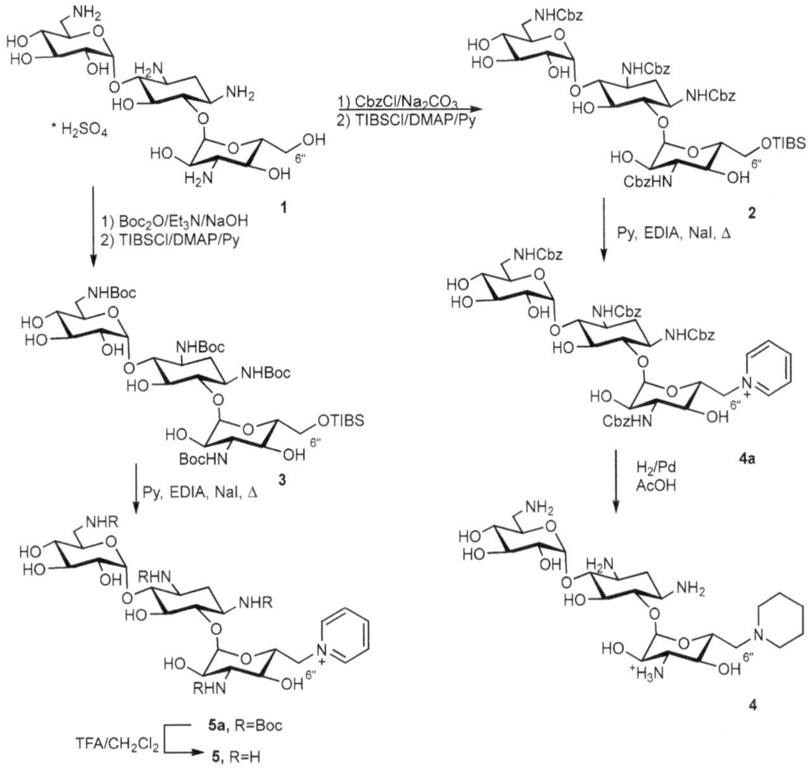

Scheme 1. Synthesis of 6″-modified kanamycin A derivatives **4**, **5** (*corresponding salt, Δ reflux).

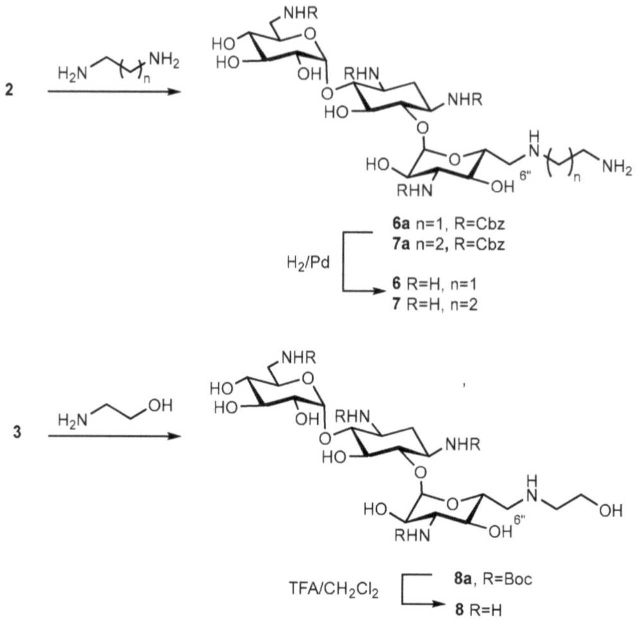

Scheme 2. Synthesis of 6″-modified KANA derivatives **6**–**8**.

Next, the interaction of tetra-*N*-protected 6″-*O*-(2,4,6-triisopropylbenzenesulfonyl) kanamycin A (**2** or **3**) with different *N*-nucleophiles was evaluated. Initially, pyridine was used as a solvent for this reaction; however, the elucidation of the structures of the obtained products by the NMR and ESI MS methods revealed that the main reaction products corresponded to the 1,3,6′,3″-tetra-*N*-Cbz-6″-(pyridine-1-ium)-6″-deoxykanamycin A (**4a**) and 1,3,6′,3″-tetra-*N*-Boc-6″-(pyridine-1-ium)-6″-deoxykanamycin A (**5a**) which were isolated in 98% and 71% yields, respectively. However, the classic method of deprotection of the Cbz-group by hydrogenolysis resulted in the simultaneous reduction of the pyridine ring, and 6″-(piperidin-1-yl)-6″-deoxykanamycin A (**4**) was isolated in the form of acetate in 58% yield. The removal of the *N*-Boc-protective groups by the treatment with trifluoroacetic acid (TFA) proceeded smoothly and resulted in the target 6″-(pyridine-1-ium)-6″-deoxykanamycin A (**5**) which was obtained as trifluoroacetate in a 63% yield.

The next step of the KANA modification involved the reaction of the Cbz-protected intermediate (**2**) with an excess of diamines (ethane-1,2-diamine or propane-1,3-diamine), followed by the deprotection of Cbz-groups by hydrogenolisys (Scheme 2). Corresponding 6″-(2-aminoethylamino)-6″-deoxykanamycin A (**6**) and 6″-(3-aminopropylamino)-6″-deoxykanamycin A (**7**) were isolated as acetates in 63% and 77% yields, respectively. The 6″-(2-hydroxyethylamino)-6″-deoxykanamycin A (**8**) was obtained analogously by the interaction of tetra-*N*-Boc-6″-*O*-(2,4,6-triisopropylbenzenesulfonyl)kanamycin A (**3**) with ethanolamine, followed by Boc-deprotection by the treatment with TFA.

Tetra-*N*-Cbz-protected 6″-(2-aminoethylamino)-6″-deoxykanamycin A (**6a**) was used for the further modification of the primary amino group of the 2-aminoethyl residue (Scheme 3).

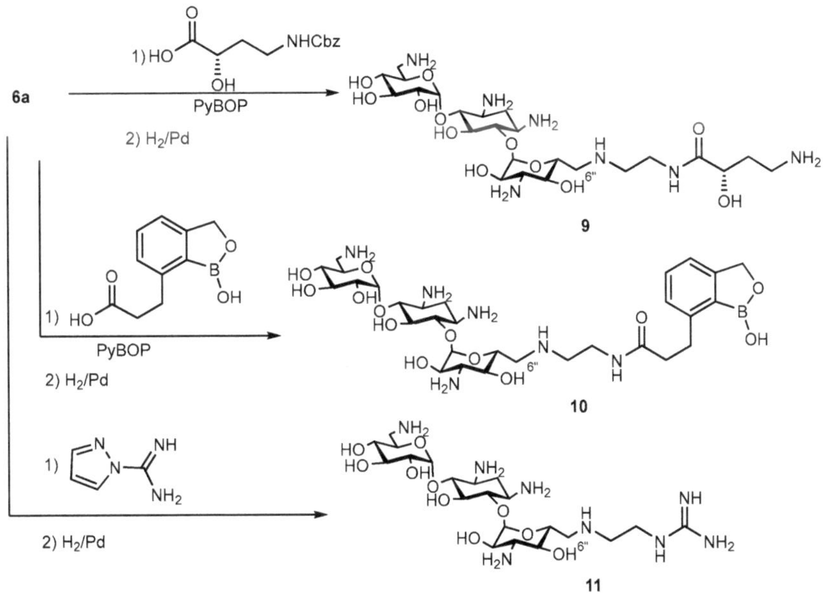

Scheme 3. Modification of tetra-N-Cbz-protected 6″-(2-aminoethylamino)-6″-deoxykanamycin A (**6a**).

The 6″-((*S*)-7-((2-(4-amino-2-hydroxybutanamido)ethyl)amino))- 6″-deoxykanamycin A (**9**) was obtained by the acylation of the intermediate **6a** with (*S*)-4-(((benzyloxy)carbonyl) amino)-2-hydroxybutanoic acid [34] in the presence of the condensing agent benzotriazol-1-yloxytripyrrolidinophosphonium hexafluorophosphate (PyBop)) followed by the amino groups' deprotection by hydrogenolysis (Scheme 3). Compound **9** was isolated in a 61% yield for two steps.

The organoboron moiety is one of the promising pharmacophores in medicinal chemistry [35], and we aimed to investigate the effect of this modification on the pharmacological activity of the natural AGs. As such, a congener **10** in which KANA conjugated with benzoxaborole residue was prepared by the acylation of the intermediate **6a** with 3-(1-hydroxy-1,3-dihydrobenzo[c][1,2]oxaborol-7-yl)propionic acid in the presence of PyBop reagent followed by the Cbz-groups cleavage by hydrogenolysis. The target derivative **10** was isolated as an acetate in a 27% yield counting for two stages.

The 6″-(2-Guanidinoethylamino)-6″-deoxykanamycin A (**11**) was obtained by the guanidation of the intermediate **6a** with 1*H*-pyrazole-1-carboxamide followed by deprotection in 64% yield (Scheme 3). Initially, the di-Boc-derivative of 1*H*-pyrazole-1-carboxamide (*tert*-butyl-((Boc)amino)(1*H*-pyrazol-1-yl)methylene) carbamate [36]) was employed for the synthesis of the target compound **11** (Scheme 4), but the Boc-group cleavage from the intermediate **11a** by the treatment with TFA led to the formation of a mixture of products. The obtained mixture was further separated by the column chromatography method, resulting in the two main compounds which were analyzed by physico-chemical and spectral methods. Along with the target Cbz-protected guanidine derivative **11,** the side imidazoline derivative **12** was isolated from the reaction mixture (Scheme 4). The structure of compound **12** was elucidated using mass spectrometry and NMR spectroscopy data analysis.

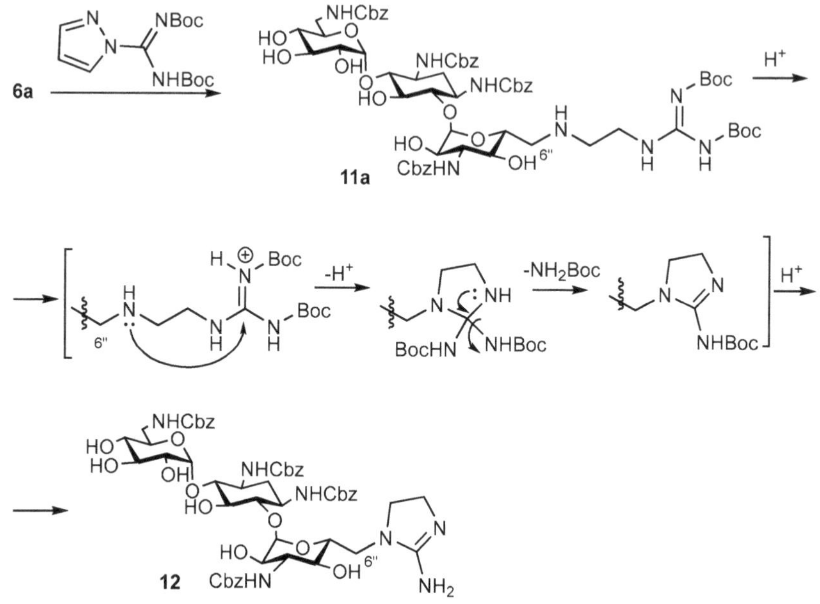

Scheme 4. Interaction of tetra-*N*-Cbz-protected 6″-(2-aminoethylamino)-6″-deoxykanamycin A (**6a**) with *tert*-butyl-((Boc)amino)(1*H*-pyrazol-1-yl)methylene)carbamate followed by N-Boc-deprotection.

The ^{1}H NMR spectrum of compound **12** does not reveal the signals of the Boc-group as well as the signals of NH groups of the guanidine residue. A cyclic structure of the side 6″-group in derivative **12** was proposed based on the ^{1}H-^{13}C HMBC and ^{1}H-^{15}N correlation experiments on direct spin–spin interaction constants with multiplicity edition (^{1}H-^{15}N edHSQC) data (Figures S29 and S30 in the Supporting Information File). A correlation between the signals of the H-6 protons of the 3,6-dideoxy-3,6-diaminoglucose residue and the signal of carbon of the guanidine residue at 158.9 ppm was observed in the HMBC spectrum of compound **12** (See Supporting Information File). This interaction is only possible if the carbon atom of guanidine is located equidistant from both CH_2 groups and this fragment has a cyclic (imidazoline) structure.

Based on these data, the structure of the obtained side product **12** corresponds to 6″-(2-amino-4,5-dihydro-1*H*-imidazol-1-yl)-6″-deoxykanamycin A (Scheme 4). The suggested structure of compound **12** was also supported by ^{1}H and ^{1}H-^{15}N edHSQC NMR spectroscopy data. A broad peak at 7.71 ppm with the integral intensity of two proton units corresponding to the amino group was observed in the ^{1}H NMR spectrum of derivative **12**. The ^{1}H-^{15}N HSQC correlation spectrum also reveals the signal of the NH_2 group, with a negative polarity at −311.2 ppm (See Supporting Information File) along with the signals of the NH amide protons of the Cbz-protecting groups.

HR ESI mass spectrum has the only monoisotopic peak at 1088.4459 Da, which is in complete agreement with the proposed structure of compound **12**. However, the isolated yield of compound **12** was low (~20%), and we were not able to obtain the corresponding deprotected derivative in the amounts sufficient for further biological studies.

The purity of the intermediate and target compounds **4–11** was confirmed by the TLC and/or HPLC methods (for UV-absorbing derivatives) and by the elemental analysis data. Structures were confirmed by the HR ESI mass spectrometry and NMR spectroscopy methods.

3.2. *In Vitro Antimicrobial Activity Studies*

The antibacterial activities of the new KANA derivatives **4–11** were evaluated on a panel of G− and G+ bacterial strains in comparison with the parent KANA (**1**) (Table 1).

Table 1. Antibacterial activity of the new obtained kanamycin derivatives **4–11** in comparison with the KANA (**1**).

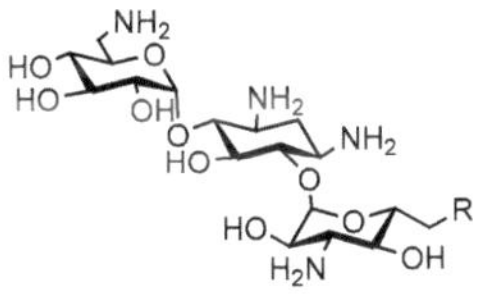

Compound	R	MIC *, µg/mL			
		S. aureus ATCC 29213	*E. coli* ATCC 25922	*P. aeruginosa* ATCC 27853	*M. smegmatis* ATCC 607
1	OH	2	2	>64	0.125–0.25
4	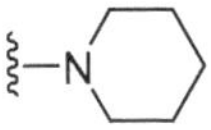	>64	>64	>64	64
5	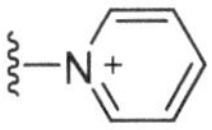	>64	>64	>64	32
6	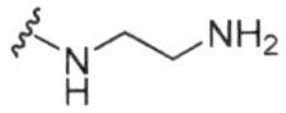	2	4	32	1
7	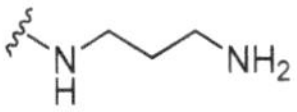	2	8	>64	0.5
8	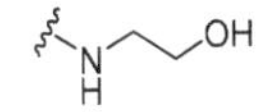	8	32	>64	4
9	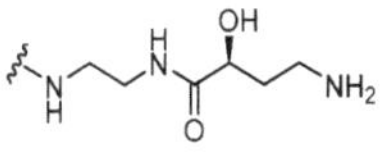	8	32	>64	1
10	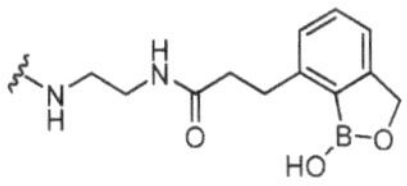	>64	>64	>64	8
11	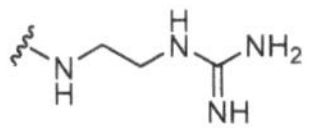	0.5	4	64	0.25

* MIC—minimal inhibitory concentration, MICs are measured as the lowest concentration of agents that prevent any visible growth. The results of the experiments were definitely reproducible. In cases of full coincidence of the data obtained, the MIC is represented as a single number.

The results of the screening demonstrated that none of the tested compounds, including KANA (**1**), were active against the *P. aeruginosa* ATCC 27853 strain (MICs > 32 µg/mL). The introduction of the piperidine or pyridinium residues at the 6″-position of KANA (compounds **4** and **5**) resulted in the significant loss of the antibacterial activity against all tested strains, including *Staphylococcus aureus* ATCC 29213 (G+), *E. coli* ATCC 25922 (G−) and *Mycobacterium smegmatis* ATCC 607 (MICs > 64 µg/mL), suggesting that a bulky cyclic residue might disrupt the interaction of the antibiotic with the target. On the contrary, the presence of the diamino group (compounds **6** and **7**) allowed them to retain antibacterial activity against three of the tested strains (MICs~0.5–4 µg/mL vs. MICs~0.125–4 for **1**). However, further modification of the amino group of compound **6** by (*S*)-4-(((benzyloxy)carbonyl)amino)-2-hydroxybutyric acid (compound **9**) or benzoxaborole residue (compound **10**) resulted in a dramatic decrease of the antibacterial activity in comparison with both KANA (**1**) and compound **6** (MICs~8.5–64 µg/mL for **9** and **10** vs. MICs~0.125–4 for KANA and MICs~1–4 for compound **6**).

The most active among the series of KANA analogues was the guanidine derivative **11**, that demonstrated two-times-less activity in comparison with the parent kanamycin A

(**1**) against *E. coli* ATCC 25922 strain, similar activity against *M. smegmatis* ATCC 607 strain, and was four-times more active than kanamycin A (**1**) against the *S. aureus* ATCC 29213 strain (MICs values zero-point-five and two for compound **11** and KANA, respectively).

Next, we checked if the new derivatives are "sensitive" to the most common mechanism of resistance to aminoglycoside antibiotics, which is based on the work of the aminoglycoside-modifying enzymes (AMEs) [37]. An in-depth evaluation of the antibacterial activities of compounds **7**, **8** and **11** revealed that they were inactive against the kanamycin A-resistant strains *Proteus mirabilis* ESBL 137, *Klebsiella pneumoniae* 1951, *K. pneumoniae* ESBL 126, *E. coli* ESBL 135, *Methicillin resistant S. aureus* 88 (MRSA) and *Staphylococcus epidermidis* C 2001MR (MICs > 64 μg/mL, data not shown). Inactivity against *P. aeruginosa* ATCC 27853 (Table 1) could be explained by the presence of the aminoglycoside-3′-phosphotransferase gene in the genome [38].

An evaluation of the antibacterial activity of the KANA derivatives **4**, **6–11** by the diffusion-in-agar method on *E. coli* BW25113 Δ*tolC* and the same strain bearing the aminogly coside-3′-phosphotransferase gene on a plasmid revealed that tested compounds **4**, **6–11** demonstrated significantly lower potencies against the resistant strain, not surprisingly suggesting that they were substrates for the aminoglycoside-3′-phosphotransferase (Figure S31).

Although the inactivation of the AGs by the modifying enzymes is the most common resistance mechanism, mutations in the gene *fusA* (EF-G) can also be responsible for the resistance to aminoglycosides; P610T EF-G mutations were reported to be distributed in clinically important strains [39,40].

Next, we tested the activity of KANA derivatives **4**, **6–11** against the *fusA* mutant strain with the substitution P610T. Although the tested compounds **4**, **6–11** in general demonstrated lower antibacterial activities (Table 2) in comparison with KANA (**1**), the difference between MICs values against the wild type and the resistant strains was less significant for 6″-modified KANA derivatives than for the parent antibiotic: the MIC/MIC (WT) ratio for the tested compounds **4**, **6–11** was **1–4** vs. **6–12** for KANA, respectively. Thus, one can hypothesize that 6″-modified compounds are less affected by the resistance that occurs as a mutation in the gene of the elongation factor G.

Table 2. Antibacterial activity of the KANA derivatives **4**, **6–11** against *E. coli* BW25113 Δ*tolC* strain and its derivative with mutated *fusA* (P610T).

Compound	*E. coli* BW25113 Δ*tolC*, MIC, μg/mL	*E. coli* BW25113 Δ*tolC* P610T EF-G (P610T), MIC, μg/mL	MIC(P610T)/MIC
KANA (**1**)	5	31	6
Fusidic acid	2	2	1
Erythromycin	2	2	1
4	>250	>250	-
6	63	125	2
7	125	125	1
8	125	500	4
9	125	250	2
10	250	500	2
11	31	63	2

As the mechanism of the antibacterial action of AG is based on the misreading of mRNA and the incorporation of the incorrect amino acids during protein synthesis, our next step included an evaluation of the action of new KANA derivatives on the *E. coli* BW25113 reporter strain which contains the β-galactosidase gene with a mutation in the enzyme active (catalytic) site E537 [30] (Figure 3).

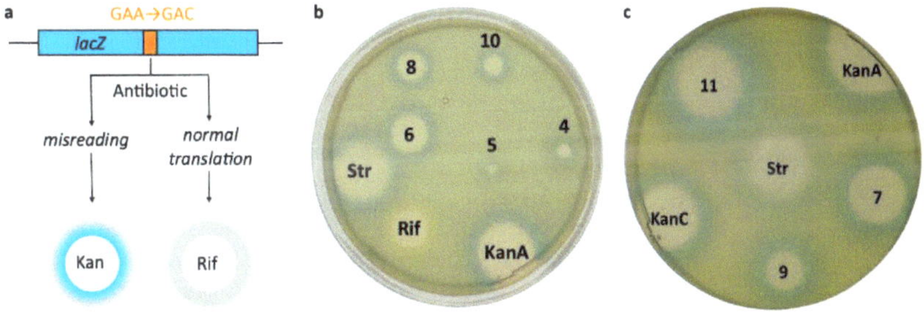

Figure 3. Kanamycin and its derivatives increase the misreading of 537 codon GAC (Asp) of the β-galactosidase gene by GlutRNA. (**a**)—schematic depicting the principle of the method. If an antibiotic causes decoding errors, GAC is decoded as GAA, a β-galactosidase is synthesized which cleaves the X-Gal substrate, causing indigo blue staining. Otherwise, no functional protein is formed. (**b**,**c**)—results of the test for compounds **4**–**11**. KANA—Kanamycin A; KanC—Kanamycin C; Str—Streptomycin; Rif—Rifampicin. Concentration of **4**–**11**, KANA (**c**), KanC, Rif—50 mg/mL; Str, KANA (**b**)—5 mg/mL. Volume of each antibiotic 1 μL. Streptomycin and kanamycins are miscoding inductors, rifampicin affects RNA synthesis and does not induce ribosomal errors. An active β-galactosidase is synthesized only in the case of a translation error, and if the mechanism of action of the antibiotic is associated with the miscoding, we observe indigo blue staining along the edge of the inhibition zone due to the presence of a degradation product of the X-Gal substrate. Figure 3 shows that all tested analogs **4**, **6**–**11** caused a blue coloring of the bacterial lawn, which specifies translation errors in the targeted cells. Thus, according to this data, modifications of the 6″ position of kanamycin A do not prevent the induction of translation errors.

4. Discussion

Aminoglycoside antibiotics, cidal inhibitors of bacterial protein synthesis, have experienced a renaissance during the last two decades. The development of plazomicin, the first new AG approved by the FDA in nearly 40 years, is an example and confirmation of the renewed interest in this "old" class of antibiotics. According to the recent scoping review, plazomicin seems to be a powerful, practical and safe tool for the control and resolution of infections that would not respond with favorable outcomes to the use of classic broad-spectrum antibiotics, but this new antimicrobial drug, to be properly exploited and have its effectiveness maintained over time, should be administered only when necessary, and sparingly [41].

The expansion of the aminoglycoside antibiotic class might help to fill an urgent unmet need in the new antimicrobial drugs effective against the ever-expanding spread of multidrug-resistant pathogens, especially G-negative bacteria [42].

Aiming at finding new active AG derivatives, we studied the modification of the 6″-position of KANA resulting in a series of 6″-deoxykanamycin A analogues bearing an additional basic group that could be ionized at physiological pH (amino-, guanidino or pyridinium).

For the first time, we demonstrated the ability of tetra-*N*-(Boc or Cbz-protected)-6″-*O*-(2,4,6-triisopropylbenzenesulfonyl)kanamycin A to interact with a weak nucleophile such as pyridine, resulting in the formation of the corresponding pyridinium derivative. However, such a modification turned out to be unfavorable for the antibacterial activity of the target compound obtained after the amino group's deprotection. The introduction of the small diamino residues at the 6″-position of KANA did not significantly alter the antibacterial activity of the parent antibiotic; nevertheless, further modification by the acylation reaction resulted in a complete loss of potency, while the introduction of the guanidine residue led to the compound **11** with an improved activity against the *S. aureus* ATCC 29213 strain. Unsurprisingly, the modification of KANA at the 6″-position does not help overcome resistance caused by aminoglycoside-3′-phosphotransferase, i.e., studied transformations of the molecule most likely do not prevent the antibiotic from being phosphorylated at 3′-hydroxy group [38].

Interestingly, we observed that the difference in susceptibility between the *E. coli* ATCC 25922 strain and the BW25113 *E. coli* strain with the Δ*tolC* knockout is less pronounced for KANA (~2 times) and increased significantly for its new analogs **4**, **6–11** (up to 15 times in the case of compound **6**). While the ribosomes and translation factors of both strains are almost identical, the discovered difference could appear because of the difference in the lipopolysaccharides (LPS) and cell wall structures of the outer membranes of the *E. coli* BW25113 ΔtolC and *E. coli* ATCC 25922 strains [43]. Despite their frequent use as therapeutic agents, the mechanisms of aminoglycoside outer-membrane (OM) translocation remain incompletely understood. The self-promoted pathway is a proposed uptake mechanism. Here, divalent cations between LPS molecules are displaced by AGs which leads to brief OM destabilization, thereby enabling OM translocation. LPS—being the major component of the outer leaflet of the OM—plays a central role for the integrity and the selective permeability of the OM [43]. Hence, the difference in activity between the ATCC 25922 and BW25113 *E. coli* strains suggests that the decline might be due to penetration issues, as these strains have different LPS and cell walls, which could provide different sensitivities to antibiotics.

However, the obtained 6″-modified KANA derivatives **4**, **6–11** were less influenced by the resistant mechanism associated with mutations of the elongation factor G than the parent KANA (**1**), suggesting that this direction of the modification is still prospective for the further investigations. AGs inhibit translocation, and recently it has been demonstrated that they trap ribosomes in the conformation, which is not preferable for EF-G binding [44]. The EF-G mutants (P610T) that possess resistance to aminoglycosides probably could bind to ribosome even in the presence of the aminoglycoside. Synthesized 6″-modified KANA derivatives could trap ribosomes in the conformation, which is not preferable for wild-type and mutant EF-G. Further research on the molecular basis of EF-G mutations in aminoglycoside resistance could shed light on these observations.

Supplementary Materials: The following supporting information can be downloaded at: https://www.mdpi.com/article/10.3390/pharmaceutics15041177/s1, Table S1: Assignments of the signals in 1H and 13C NMR spectra of compounds **4–11**; Figures S1 and S2: 1H and 13C NMR spectra of 1,3,6′,3″-tetra-N-Cbz-kanamycin A; Figures S3 and S4: 1H and 13C NMR spectra of 1,3,6′,3″-tetra-N-Boc-kanamycin A; Figures S5 and S6: 1H and 13C NMR spectra of 1,3,6′,3″-tetra-N-Cbz-6″-O-(2,4,6-triisopropylbenzenesulfonyl)kanamycin A (**2**); Figures S7–S28: 1H and 13C NMR spectra of the kanamycin A derivatives **4a**, **4–7**, **8a**, **8**, **9a**, **9–11**; Figure S29: Fragment of the HMBC 1H-13C spectrum of compound **12**; Figure S30: 1H-15N edHSQC spectrum of compound **12**; Figure S31: The antibacterial activity of the kanamycin A derivatives **4**, **6–11** and reference antibiotics.

Author Contributions: Conceptualization, A.T. and A.S.; methodology, A.T.; investigation, K.S., E.R., N.G. and G.Z.; resources, A.S.; writing—original draft preparation, K.S. and E.R.; writing—review and editing, A.T., I.O. and A.S.; supervision, A.T. and I.O.; project administration, A.T. All authors have read and agreed to the published version of the manuscript.

Funding: This research was partly funded by Russian Science Foundation, grant number 21-64-00006 (E.R., work involving studies on mutant strains and studies of the mode of action).

Institutional Review Board Statement: Not applicable.

Informed Consent Statement: Not applicable.

Data Availability Statement: Data are contained within the article and in the Supporting Information File.

Conflicts of Interest: The authors declare no conflict of interest.

Abbreviations

Boc, *tert*-butyloxycarbonyl; Cbz, benzyloxycarbonyl; d, doublet; dd, doublet of doublets; DMF, dimethylformamide; DMSO, dimethylsulfoxide; HPLC, high performance liquid chromatography; HRMS (ESI), high-resolution mass spectrometry with electrospray ionization; IC_{50}, is the amount of a drug which causes the inhibition of growth of the 50% of cells; MIC, minimum inhibitory concentration; NMR, nuclear magnetic resonance; PyBop, benzotriazol-1-yloxypyrrolodinophosphnium hexafluorophosphate; rt, room temperature; s, singlet; TFA, trifluoroacetic acid; TIBS, 2,4,6-triisopropylben zenesulfonyl; TLC, thin layer chromatography; t, triplet.

References

1. Ferri, M.; Ranucci, E.; Romagnoli, P.; Giaccone, V. Antimicrobial Resistance: A Global Emerging Threat to Public Health Systems. *Crit. Rev. Food Sci. Nutr.* **2017**, *57*, 2857–2876. [CrossRef] [PubMed]
2. Pontefract, B.A.; Ho, H.T.; Crain, A.; Kharel, M.K.; Nybo, S.E. Drugs for Gram-Negative Bugs from 2010–2019: A Decade in Review. *Open Forum Infect. Dis.* **2020**, *7*, ofaa276. [CrossRef] [PubMed]
3. Ghosh, S.; Bornman, C.; Zafer, M.M. Antimicrobial Resistance Threats in the Emerging COVID-19 Pandemic: Where do We Stand? *J. Infect. Public Health.* **2021**, *14*, 555–560. [CrossRef] [PubMed]
4. Lai, C.C.; Chen, S.Y.; Ko, W.C.; Hsueh, P.R. Increased Antimicrobial Resistance during the COVID-19 Pandemic. *Int. J. Antimicrob. Agents.* **2021**, *57*, 106324. [CrossRef] [PubMed]
5. Tevyashova, A.N.; Shapovalova, K.S. Potential for the Development of a New Generation of Aminoglycoside Antibiotics. *Pharm. Chem. J.* **2021**, *55*, 860–875. [CrossRef]
6. Menzies, D.; Benedetti, A.; Paydar, A.; Martin, I.; Royce, S.; Pai, M.; Vernon, A.; Lienhardt, C.; Burman, W. Effect of Duration and Intermittency of Rifampin on Tuberculosis Treatment Outcomes: A Systematic Review and Meta-analysis. *PLoS Med.* **2009**, *6*, e1000146. [CrossRef]
7. Brossier, F.; Veziris, N.; Aubry, A.; Jarlier, V.; Sougakoff, W. Detection by Genotype MTBDRsl Test of Complex Resistance Mechanisms to Second-line Drugs and Ethambutol in Multidrug-resistant Mycobacterium Tuberculosis Complex Isolates. *J. Clin. Microbiol.* **2010**, *48*, 1683–1689. [CrossRef]
8. Carter, A.P.; Demons, W.M.; Brodersen, D.E.; Morgan-Warren, R.J.; Wimberly, B.T.; Ramakrishan, V. Functional Insights from the Structure of the 30S Ribosomal Subunit and Its Interactions with Antibiotics. *Nature* **2000**, *407*, 340–348. [CrossRef]
9. Fourmy, D.; Recht, M.I.; Blanchard, S.C.; Puglisi, J.D. Structure of the A Site of Escherichia coli 16 S Ribosomal RNA Complexed with an Aminoglycoside Antibiotic. *Science* **1996**, *274*, 1367–1371. [CrossRef]
10. Jana, S.; Deb, J.K. Molecular Understanding of Aminoglycoside Action and Resistance. *Appl. Microbiol. Biotechnol.* **2006**, *70*, 140–150. [CrossRef]
11. Cabanas, M.J.; Vazquez, D.; Modolell, J. Inhibition of Ribosomal Translocation by Aminoglycoside Antibiotics. *Biochem. Biophys. Res. Commun.* **1978**, *83*, 991–997. [CrossRef] [PubMed]
12. Selimoglu, E. Aminoglycoside-induced Ototoxicity. *Curr. Pharm. Des.* **2007**, *13*, 119–126. [CrossRef] [PubMed]
13. Lopez-Novoa, J.M.; Quiros, Y.; Vicente, L.; Morales, A.I.; Lopez-Hernandez, F.J. New Insights into the Mechanism of Aminoglycoside Nephrotoxicity: An Integrative Point of View. *Kidney Int.* **2011**, *79*, 33–45. [CrossRef]
14. Krause, K.M.; Krause, K.M.; Serio, A.W.; Kane, T.R.; Connolly, L.E. Aminoglycosides: An Overview. *Cold Spring Harb. Perspect. Med.* **2016**, *6*, a027029. [CrossRef]
15. Al-Tawfiq, J.A.; Momattin, H.; Al-Ali, A.Y.; Eljaaly, K.; Tirupathi, R.; Haradwala, M.B.; Areti, S.; Alhumaid, S.; Rabaan, A.A.; Mutair, A.A.; et al. Antibiotics in the Pipeline: A Literature Review (2017–2020). *Infection* **2021**, *50*, 553–564. [CrossRef] [PubMed]
16. Scribner, M.R.; Santos-Lopez, A.; Marshall, C.W.; Deitrick, C.; Cooper, V.S. Parallel Evolution of Tobramycin Resistance across Species and Environments. *MBio* **2020**, *11*, e00932-20. [CrossRef]
17. Ibacache-Quiroga, C.; Oliveros, J.C.; Couce, A.; Blázquez, J. Parallel Evolution of High Level Aminoglycoside Resistance in Escherichia Coli under Low and High Mutation Supply Rates. *Front. Microbiol.* **2018**, *9*, 427. [CrossRef]
18. Bolard, A.; Plésiat, P.; Jeannot, K. Mutations in Gene fusA1 as a Novel Mechanism of Aminoglycoside Resistance in Clinical Strains of Pseudomonas aeruginosa. *Antimicrob. Agents Chemother.* **2018**, *62*, e01835-17. [CrossRef]
19. Kawaguchi, H.; Naito, T.; Nakagawa, S.; Fujisawa, K.I. BB-K8, a New Semisynthetic Aminoglycoside Antibiotic. *J. Antibiot.* **1972**, *25*, 695–708. [CrossRef]
20. Chandrika, N.T.; Garneau-Tsodikova, S. Comprehensive Review of Chemical Strategies for the Preparation of New Aminoglycosides and Their Biological Activities. *Chem. Soc. Rev.* **2018**, *47*, 1189–1249. [CrossRef]
21. Wang, H.; Tor, Y. RNA–Aminoglycoside Interactions: Design, Synthesis, and Binding of "Amino-aminoglycosides" to RNA. *Angew. Chem. Int. Ed.* **1998**, *37*, 109–111. [CrossRef]
22. Subedi, Y.P.; AlFindee, M.N.; Takemoto, J.Y.; Chang, C.W.T. Antifungal Amphiphilic Kanamycins: New Life for an Old Drug. *Med. Chem. Comm.* **2018**, *9*, 909–919. [CrossRef] [PubMed]

23. Subedi, Y.P.; Roberts, P.; Grilley, M.; Takemoto, J.Y.; Chang, C.W.T. Development of Fungal Selective Amphiphilic Kanamycin: Cost-effective Synthesis and Use of Fluorescent Analogs for Mode of Action Investigation. *ACS Infect. Dis.* **2019**, *5*, 473–483. [CrossRef] [PubMed]
24. Subedi, Y.P.; Pandey, U.; Alfindee, M.N.; Montgomery, H.; Roberts, P.; Wight, J.; Nichols, G.; Grilley, M.; Takemoto, J.Y.; Chang, C.W.T. Scalable and Cost-effective Tosylation-mediated Synthesis of Antifungal and Fungal Diagnostic 6″-Modified Amphiphilic Kanamycins. *Eur. J. Med. Chem.* **2019**, *182*, 111639. [CrossRef]
25. Takemoto, J.Y.; Wegulo, S.N.; Yuen, G.Y.; Stevens, J.A.; Jochum, C.C.; Chang, C.W.T.; Kawasakia, Y.; Miller, G.W. Suppression of wheat Fusarium Head Blight by Novel Amphiphilic Aminoglycoside Fungicide K20. *Fungal Biol.* **2018**, *122*, 465–470. [CrossRef]
26. Alfindee, M.N.; Subedi, Y.P.; Grilley, M.M.; Takemoto, J.Y.; Chang, C.W.T. Antifungal Activities of 4″,6″-Disubstituted Amphiphilic Kanamycins. *Molecules* **2019**, *24*, 1882. [CrossRef]
27. Clinical and Laboratory Standards Institute (CLSI). *Methods for Dilution Antimicrobial Susceptibility Tests for bacteria that Grow Aerobically*, 10th ed.; Approved Standard, (M07-A10); Clinical and Laboratory Standards Institute (CLSI): Wayne, PA, USA, 2015.
28. Baba, T.; Ara, T.; Hasegawa, M.; Takai, Y.; Okumura, Y.; Baba, M.; Datsenko, K.A.; Tomita, M.; Wanner, B.L.; Mori, H. Construction of Escherichia coli K-12 In-frame, Single-gene Knockout Mutants: The Keio Collection. *Mol. Syst. Biol.* **2006**, *2*, 2006.0008. [CrossRef]
29. Datsenko, K.A.; Wanner, B.L. One-step Inactivation of Chromosomal Genes in Escherichia Coli K-12 Using PCR Products. *Proc. Natl. Acad. Sci. USA* **2000**, *97*, 6640–6645. [CrossRef]
30. Manickam, N.; Nag, N.; Abbasi, A.; Patel, K.; Farabaugh, P.J. Studies of Translational Misreading in vivo Show that the Ribosome Very Efficiently Discriminates against Most Potential Errors. *RNA* **2014**, *20*, 9–15. [CrossRef]
31. Chen, G.; Pan, P.; Yao, Y.; Chen, Y.; Meng, X.; Li, Z. Regioselective Modification of Amino Groups in Aminoglycosides Based on Cyclic Carbamate Formation. *Tetrahedron* **2008**, *64*, 9078–9087. [CrossRef]
32. Hiraiwa, Y.; Usui, T.; Akiyama, Y.; Maebashi, K.; Minowa, N.; Ikeda, D. Synthesis and Antibacterial Activity of 5-Deoxy-5-Episubstituted Arbekacin Derivatives. *Bioorg. Med. Chem. Lett.* **2007**, *17*, 3540–3543. [CrossRef] [PubMed]
33. Van Schepdael, A.; Delcourt, J.; Mulier, M.; Busson, R.; Verbist, L.; Vanderhaeghe, H.J.; Mingeot-Leclercq, M.P.; Tulkens, P.M.; Claes, P.J. New Derivatives of Kanamycin B Obtained by Modifications and Substitutions in Position 6″. 1. Synthesis and Microbiological Evaluation. *J. Med. Chem.* **1991**, *34*, 1468–1475. [CrossRef] [PubMed]
34. Arıcan, M.O.; Erdogan, S.; Mert, O. Amine-functionalized Polylactide–PEG Copolymers. *Macromolecules* **2018**, *51*, 2817–2830. [CrossRef]
35. Tevyashova, A.N.; Chudinov, M.V. Progress in the Medicinal Chemistry of Organoboron Compounds. *Russ. Chem. Rev.* **2021**, *90*, 451–487. [CrossRef]
36. Castillo-Melendez, J.A.; Golding, B.T. Optimisation of the Synthesis of Guanidines from Amines via Nitroguanidines Using 3, 5-Dimethyl-N-nitro-1H-pyrazole-1-carboxamidine. *Synthesis* **2004**, *10*, 1655–1663. [CrossRef]
37. Becker, B.; Cooper, M.A. Aminoglycoside Antibiotics in the 21st Century. *ACS Chem. Biol.* **2013**, *8*, 105–115. [CrossRef] [PubMed]
38. Hainrichson, M.; Yaniv, O.; Cherniavsky, M.; Nudelman, I.; Shallom-Shezifi, D.; Yaron, S.; Baasov, T. Overexpression And Initial Characterization of The Chromosomal Aminoglycoside 3′-O-Phosphotransferase APH(3′)-Iib from Pseudomonas Aeruginosa. *Antimicrob. Agents Chemother.* **2007**, *51*, 774–776. [CrossRef]
39. Mogre, A.; Sengupta, T.; Veetil, R.T.; Ravi, P.; Seshasayee, A.S.N. Genomic Analysis Reveals Distinct Concentration-dependent Evolutionary Trajectories for Antibiotic Resistance in Escherichia Coli. *DNA Res.* **2014**, *21*, 711–726. [CrossRef]
40. Mogre, A.; Veetil, R.T.; Seshasayee, A.S.N. Modulation of Global Transcriptional Regulatory Networks as a Strategy for Increasing Kanamycin Resistance of the Translational Elongation Factor-G Mutants in Escherichia Coli. *Genes Genomes Genet.* **2017**, *7*, 3955–3966. [CrossRef]
41. Alfieri, A.; Franco, S.D.; Donatiello, V.; Maffei, V.; Fittipaldi, C.; Fiore, M.; Coppolino, F.; Sansone, P.; Pace, M.C.; Passavanti, M.B. Plazomicin against Multidrug-Resistant Bacteria: A Scoping Review. *Life* **2022**, *12*, 1949. [CrossRef]
42. Terren, M.; Taccani, M.; Pregnolato, M. New Antibiotics for Multidrug-Resistant Bacterial Strains: Latest Research Developments and Future Perspectives. *Molecules* **2021**, *26*, 2671. [CrossRef] [PubMed]
43. Ebbensgaard, A.; Mordhorst, H.; Aarestrup, F.M.; Hansen, E.B. The Role of Outer Membrane Proteins and Lipopolysaccharides for the Sensitivity of Escherichia coli to Antimicrobial Peptides. *Front Microbiol.* **2018**, *9*, 2153. [CrossRef] [PubMed]
44. Parajuli, N.P.; Mandava, C.S.; Pavlov, M.Y.; Sanyal, S. Mechanistic Insights into Translation Inhibition by Aminoglycoside Antibiotic Arbekacin. *Nucleic Acids Res.* **2021**, *49*, 6880–6892. [CrossRef] [PubMed]

pharmaceutics

MDPI

Article

Synthesis, Characterization, and Docking Study of Novel Thioureidophosphonate-Incorporated Silver Nanocomposites as Potent Antibacterial Agents

Ahmed I. El-Tantawy [1,*], Elshaymaa I. Elmongy [2,*], Shimaa M. Elsaeed [3], Abdel Aleem H. Abdel Aleem [1], Reem Binsuwaidan [2], Wael H. Eisa [4], Ayah Usama Salman [5], Noura Elsayed Elharony [1] and Nour F. Attia [6]

[1] Department of Chemistry, Faculty of Science, Menoufia University, Shibin El Kom 32511, Egypt; aelgokha@yahoo.com (A.A.H.A.A.); nora7arony@yahoo.com (N.E.E.)
[2] Department of Pharmaceutical Sciences, College of Pharmacy, Princess Nourah bint Abdulrahman University, P.O. Box 84428, Riyadh 11671, Saudi Arabia; rabinsuwaidan@pnu.edu.sa
[3] Department of Analysis and Evaluation, Egyptian Petroleum Research Institute, Cairo 11727, Egypt; shy_saeed@yahoo.com
[4] Spectroscopy Department, Physics Division, National Research Centre (NRC), Cairo 12622, Egypt; wael_karnor@yahoo.com
[5] Department of Botany and Microbiology, Faculty of Science, Menoufia University, Shibin El Kom 32511, Egypt; ayahsalman6060@gmail.com
[6] Gas Analysis and Fire Safety Laboratory, Chemistry Division, National Institute for Standards, 136, Giza 12211, Egypt; drnour2005@yahoo.com
* Correspondence: chemahmed293@gmail.com (A.I.E.-T.); eielmongy@pnu.edu.sa (E.I.E.)

Abstract: Newly synthesized mono- and bis-thioureidophosphonate (MTP and BTP) analogues in eco-friendly conditions were employed as reducing/capping cores for 100, 500, and 1000 mg L^{-1} of silver nitrate. The physicochemical properties of silver nanocomposites (MTP(BTP)/Ag NCs) were fully elucidated using spectroscopic and microscopic tools. The antibacterial activity of the nanocomposites was screened against six multidrug-resistant pathogenic strains, comparable to ampicillin and ciprofloxacin commercial drugs. The antibacterial performance of BTP was more substantial than MTP, notably with the best minimum inhibitory concentration (MIC) of 0.0781 mg/mL towards *Bacillus subtilis*, *Salmonella typhi*, and *Pseudomonas aeruginosa*. Among all, BTP provided the clearest zone of inhibition (ZOI) of 35 ± 1.00 mm against *Salmonella typhi*. After the dispersion of silver nanoparticles (AgNPs), MTP/Ag NCs offered dose-dependently distinct advantages over the same nanoparticle with BTP; a more noteworthy decline by 4098 × MIC to 0.1525×10^{-3} mg/mL was recorded for MTP/Ag-1000 against *Pseudomonas aeruginosa* over BTP/Ag-1000. Towards methicillin-resistant *Staphylococcus aureus* (*MRSA*), the as-prepared MTP(BTP)/Ag-1000 displayed superior bactericidal ability in 8 h. Because of the anionic surface of MTP(BTP)/Ag-1000, they could effectively resist *MRSA* (ATCC-43300) attachment, achieving higher antifouling rates of 42.2 and 34.4% at most optimum dose (5 mg/mL), respectively. The tunable surface work function between MTP and AgNPs promoted the antibiofilm activity of MTP/Ag-1000 by 1.7 fold over BTP/Ag-1000. Lastly, the molecular docking studies affirmed the eminent binding affinity of BTP over MTP—besides the improved binding energy of MTP/Ag NC by 37.8%—towards *B. subtilis*-2FQT protein. Overall, this study indicates the immense potential of TP/Ag NCs as promising nanoscale antibacterial candidates.

Keywords: thioureidophosphonates; silver nanocomposites; antibacterial; bactericidal; antifouling; antibiofilm; molecular docking

Citation: El-Tantawy, A.I.; Elmongy, E.I.; Elsaeed, S.M.; Abdel Aleem, A.A.H.; Binsuwaidan, R.; Eisa, W.H.; Salman, A.U.; Elharony, N.E.; Attia, N.F. Synthesis, Characterization, and Docking Study of Novel Thioureidophosphonate-Incorporated Silver Nanocomposites as Potent Antibacterial Agents. *Pharmaceutics* **2023**, *15*, 1666. https://doi.org/10.3390/pharmaceutics15061666

Academic Editors: Aura Rusu and Valentina Uivarosi

Received: 10 May 2023
Revised: 27 May 2023
Accepted: 31 May 2023
Published: 6 June 2023

1. Introduction

Recently, the emergence of antibiotic-resistant microbes has been seen as a global health concern affecting many people's lives [1]. Regarding bacteria, the overuse of antibiotics, combined with poor health awareness and lack of technological capacity, has significantly increased the ability of bacteria to cross the boundaries of living systems, giving rise to more resistant genes, and raising the incidence of disease and death. Consequently, antimicrobial resistance (AMR) has caused several obstacles in public health care [1–3]. The growth of extracellular polymeric substances (EPS) as protective architectures surrounding bacteria is another sign of bacterial resistance [4]. Thus, finding novel, effective, and long-lasting biofilm preventing and disrupting agents is a key challenge for combating AMR [1,5]. Accordingly, the revival of nanotechnology along with the industrial expansion of antibiotics have lately pushed metal nanoparticles (MNPs) to the forefront of attention [6,7]. Noble MNPs have drawn utmost focus of researchers in several assorted domains with respect to optical [8], catalytic [9], energetic [10], and medical applications [11–13]. The unrivalled surface energy of noble MNPs promotes the generation of new superb physical, chemical, and biological properties such as small particle sizes, light susceptibility, tailored morphology and surface interactions, chemical stability, and biological compatibility [14,15]. Among noble MNPs, silver nanoparticles (AgNPs) surpassed all due to their tunable surface engineering, potent biological activity, multiple inhibition mechanisms, and facile methods of synthesis [16–19]. However, some demerits concerning the antibacterial activity of AgNPs were encountered, such as the possibility of particle agglomeration, elevated cost, developed AMR to AgNPs, and their toxicological effects at high concentrations [20,21]. Therefore, it was imperative to decorate AgNPs on inert surfaces [22] or/and combine them with active materials to avoid agglomeration and provide better antibacterial potency with less toxic effects of free AgNPs [20]. Therefore, alternative approaches are being pursued for the fabrication of AgNP composites by employing graphene [23], polymers [24], plant extract [16], clay [25], polysaccharide [26], and fatty acid [27]. The main disadvantages related to these nanohybrids were incomplete antibacterial efficacy [24], rapid release of active components [28], cost and time-ineffective operation [29], aggregation affinity [30], and higher cytotoxicity [31–33]. On top of this, α-aminophosphonates (α-APs), as a significant class of organophosphorus compounds, were remarkably exploited in several amplified domains [34,35]. Lately, α-APs have captivated researchers' interests in numerous applicable dimensions such as wastewater treatment [36,37], rare earth metal removal [38,39], catalysis [40], sensing [41], flame retardancy [42], agrochemical technology [35,42], and corrosion inhibition [43]. Moreover, α-APs have had unprecedented success in several medical arenas, such as antioxidant, antifungal, anti-HIV agents, antimicrobial, anticancer, antiviral, peptidomimetics, and enzyme inhibitors [34,35,44]. This growing interest was ascribed to their structural analogy to α-amino acids, ease of synthesis, elevated metabolic and chemical stability, high atom economy, bioavailability, structural and functional diversity, insignificant cytotoxicity, and potent biological properties [34,35,45]. Therefore, α-APs were deemed a worthy choice for AgNPs dispersion to bring extra synergistic antibacterial properties as part of a sustainable approach. Remarkably, our group has long been involved in developing different series of phosphonate derivatives in medical applications as antibacterial agents [45,46], urokinase-type plasminogen inhibitors [47], DNA gyrase inhibitors [48], anticancer [49], antifungal agents [49]. This is in addition to designing and synthesizing other potent antibacterial agents for various industrial applications [22,50,51]. Based on the above considerations, two novel thioureidophosphonates (TPs) were synthesized via non-metal green catalyst and incorporated with silver ion precursor giving TP-wrapped silver nanocomposites (TP/Ag NCs). The main objective of the study was to explore the impact of functionalized AgNPs on the antibacterial activity raw TP analogues.

2. Materials and Methods

2.1. Characterization Techniques

The Fourier transform infrared spectroscopy (FT-IR) analysis has been accomplished for all samples on Bruker Alpha II spectrometer, Bremen, Germany, in the wavenumber range 4000–400 cm^{-1}. The (^{1}H-, ^{13}C-, and ^{31}P) nuclear magnetic resonance (NMR) spectra were consecutively recorded at 400, 101, and 162 MHz in DMSO-d_6 using a Bruker Avance III HD, 600 MHz-NMR spectrometer probe, and BBFO cryoprobe (JEOL, Tokyo,

Japan). The elemental analysis of samples (C, H, N, and S) was undertaken for the raw TP derivatives (MTP and BTP) by CHNS Vario EL III Elementar analyzer, Germany. The phosphorus content (%) was estimated via the chemical digestion in sulfuric/nitric solution and photometric measurements at λ_{max} = 410 nm. Melting points (m.p) were recorded using (DMP-600, A and E Lab, London, UK) without correction. The surface images of nanocomposites were obtained using transmission electron microscope (TEM) by JEOL, JEM-2100 Tokyo, Japan. The crystalline properties of nanocomposites were obtained using powder X-ray diffraction (XRD) analysis using Shimadzu 6000 X-ray diffractometer with Cu Kα-radiation (λ = 1.54 nm) at 25 °C in the 2θ range of 10–80° operating at a scan rate of 1 deg/min. X-ray photoelectron spectroscopy (XPS) was conducted using a Perkin Elmer PHI 5600, Perkin Elmer Instruments, Waltham, MA, USA, with analytical zone's diameter of 1 mm and indium sheets for sample deposition using Al Kα X-rays radiation source (200 W). The photometric assays of antibacterial results were measured by (Infinite F50 Robotic absorbance microplate reader) in the wavelength range of 400 to 750 nm. The zeta potential charge of silver nanocomposites was determined via dynamic light scattering using Zetasizer Nano ZS, Malvern Instruments Ltd., Malvern, UK. Scanning electron microscopy (SEM) was performed using JSM 6390 LA, JEOL, Tokyo, Japan, with a 15 KV accelerating voltage.

2.2. Chemicals

Thiourea (99.0%, purity) and triphenyl phosphite (98.0%, purity) were obtained from Macklin (Beijing, China). Terephthalaldehyde (98.0%, purity), pyridinium trifluoromethanesulfonate (98.0%, purity) (as protic ionic liquid), and silver nitrate (99.8%, purity) ($AgNO_3$) were purchased from Aladdin (Beijing, China). Solvents, such as acetonitrile (CH_3CN), ethanol, and methanol were obtained from a commercial supplier (Sigma Aldrich, Cairo, Egypt) and used without further drying and purification. Deionized water was used to prepare all solutions and suspensions.

2.3. Preparation of α-Thioureidophosphonate Cores

The synthesis process included preparation of two different systems of mono and bis thioureidophosphonate (TP) products, where the involved components (thiourea, terephthalaldehyde, and triphenyl phosphite) were dissolved in acetonitrile (CH_3CN, 5 and 10 mL) with the aid of a pyridinium trifluoromethanesulfonate (pyridinium triflate) as a Lewis acid protic ionic liquid-based catalyst. In the meantime, thiourea (1.42 g, 18.62 mmol)/(2.84 g, 37.24 mmol), (2.50 g, 18.61 mmol) terephthalaldehyde, triphenyl phosphite (5.78 g, 18.62 mmol)/(11.55 g, 37.24 mmol), and pyridinium triflate (0.21 g, 5 mole %)/(0.42 g, 5 mole %) in 5 and 10 mL of CH_3CN were progressively incorporated, affording MTP and BTP in a molar ratio of 1:1:1 and 2:1:2, respectively. Further, both solutions were magnetically stirred overnight under ambient conditions and the reaction was monitored via qualitative thin layer chromatography (TLC) using hexane–methylene chloride (3:1) as eluent mixture. Eventually, the final products were filtered off under vacuum, washed with methanol, dried, and kept in a desiccator for 2 days giving MTP and BTP in good yields.

Diphenyl ((4-formylphenyl) (thioureido)methyl) phosphonate, denoted as mono-thioureidophosphonate (MTP):

Light-beige solid, yield: (7.25 g, 91.72%), m.p: 160–163 °C, FT-IR: 3457.74–3311.18 cm^{-1} (NH)str. + (NH_2) str. overlapped, 3057.58 cm^{-1} (C=CH str., benzene ring), 2894.63 cm^{-1} (C H str., aliphatic), 1698.02 cm^{-1} (-CHO, formyl), 1590.99 cm^{-1}, (NH+NH_2) bending, 1525.42 cm^{-1} (>C=C<) phenyl rings, 1488.78 cm^{-1} (>C=S) asym., 1194.69 cm^{-1} (-P=O), 944.95 cm^{-1} (P-O-C), 760.78 cm^{-1} (P–C), and 684.61 cm^{-1} (>C=S) sym. ^{1}H-NMR; δ ppm: 5.50 (d, 1H, P-C–H), 6.63–7.99 (m, Ar-H, 14H), 9.40–9.52 (br, 2H,-NH_2), 9.76 (br. s, 1H, >NH), and 10.04 (s, 1H, -CHO). ^{13}C-NMR (DMSO-d6, 101 MHz); δ ppm: 54.59 and 56.16 ppm (P-C–H), 115.24, 120.22, 120.53, 125.39, 127.96, 128.92, 129.90, 149.80 (Ar-C), 183.84 (>C=S), and 192.73 (-CHO). ^{31}P-NMR (DMSO-d6, 162 MHz); δ 14.08 ppm. Elemental analysis calc.

(%) for $C_{21}H_{19}N_2O_4PS$: C, 59.15; H, 4.49; N, 6.57; P, 7.26; S, 7.52; and O, 15.01; meas. (%): C, 57.85; H, 4.27; N, 6.34; P, 6.97; and S, 6.99.

Tetraphenyl (1,4-phenylenebis(thioureidomethylene)) bis(phosphonate) denoted as bis-thioureidophosphonate (BTP):

Light-yellow solid, yield: (11.75 g, 87.71%), m.p: 135–137 °C, FTIR: 3310.21 cm^{-1} [(NH)str. + (NH_2) str. overlapped], 3057.58 cm^{-1} (C=CH str., benzene ring), 2895.59 cm^{-1} (C–H str., aliphatic), 1591.95 (>NH + -NH_2) bending, 1527.35 cm^{-1} (>C=C<) phenyl rings, 1489.74 cm^{-1} (>C=S) asym., 1195.65 (-P=O), 947.84 (P-O-C), 761.74 cm^{-1} (P–C), and 761.74 cm^{-1} (>C=S) sym. ^{1}H-NMR; δ ppm: 5.93 (s, 2H, P-C–H), 6.54–7.61 (Ar-H, m, 24H), 9.21–9.33 (br. m, 4H, NH_2), and 9.38 ppm (br. s, 2H). ^{13}C-NMR (DMSO- d6, 101 MHz); δ ppm: 54.50 and 56.06 (P-C–H), 115.26, 120.29, 120.86, 125.40, 127.50, 129.33, 129.84, and 149.94 (Ar-C), and 183.83 (>C=S). ^{31}P-NMR (DMSO- d6, 162 MHz); δ ppm: 14.85 ppm. Elemental analysis calc. (%) for $C_{34}H_{32}N_4O_6P_2S_2$: C, 56.82; H, 4.49; N, 7.82; P, 8.62; S, 8.92; and O, 13.36; found: C, 54.97; H,4.36; N, 8.18; P, 8.83; and S, 7.91.

2.4. Synthesis of α-Thioureidophosphonate-Based Silver Nanoparticles

In 250 mL glass beaker, 0.6 g of each raw powder of MTP and BTP were dispersed individually in 150 mL of $AgNO_3$ solution of 100, 500, and 1000 mg L^{-1} concentrations. Then, the prepared solutions were magnetically stirred (200 rpm) for 12 h, at ambient conditions. Afterward, the attained colloidal solutions were centrifuged, and the settled nanoparticles were washed with ethanol/deionized water and then oven-dried at 50 °C for further characterization [52].

2.5. Microorganisms and Media

Nutrient broth, Tryptic soy broth (TSB), and nutrient agar were purchased from Bacto, Australia. Mueller Hilton broth (Becton Dickinson, Sparks, MD, USA), DMSO and iodonitrotetrazolium chloride (INT) were procured from RandM marketing, Essex UK. The reference antibiotics ciprofloxacin, vancomycin hydrochloride, and ampicillin were supplied from Sigma Aldrich, Germany. Standard 96-wells microplate reader, pipette, 96-wells microtiter, 15 mL centrifuge tubes were obtained from Lab supply company, Cairo, Egypt. The crystal violet, glacial acetic acid, and 1× Phosphate-buffer saline were purchased from Thermo Fisher Scientific (Waltham, MA, USA). Clinical isolates of methicillin-resistant *Staphylococcus aureus* (*MRSA*), *Streptococcus mutans* (*S. mutans*), *Bacillus subtilis* (*B. subtilis*), *Pseudomonas aeruginosa* (*P. aeruginosa*), *Salmonella typhi* (*S. typhi*), and *Serratia marcescens* (*S. marcescens*) were acquired from National Research Center, Cairo, Egypt, along with their ATCC references (*MRSA*-ATCC 43300), (*S. mutans*-ATCC 35668), (*B. subtilis*-ATCC 6633), (*P. aeruginosa*-ATCC 27853), (*S. typhi*-ATCC 6539), and (*S. marcescens*-ATCC 13880), respectively.

2.6. Molecular Docking Study

Molecular docking studies were conducted using molecular operating environment (MOE) [53] with the aid of Discovery studio. Four proteins from different microorganisms of Gram-positive and Gram-negative bacteria (*MRSA*, *B. subtilis*, *P. aeruginosa*, and *S. typhi*) were downloaded for modeling study from the protein data bank (PDB codes: 4DKI, 2FQT, 5ZHN and 3ZQE), respectively [54–57]. Ligand and protein structural optimizations were applied by calculating partial charges, 3D protonation, strands correction, followed by energy minimization [58]. The selected docking protocol was induced fit, where the ligand active site was selected as a placement guide. Exclusion of pharmacophore annotations was selected. The gradient for energy minimization was 0.05, and MMFF94X was the force field by default [59].

2.7. Pharmacokinetics In Silico Screening

Pharmacokinetics prediction of the final compounds was performed in silico using the available software preADMET (https://preadmet.bmdrc.kr/) accessed on 20 April 2023.

3. Results and Discussion

3.1. Chemistry

3.1.1. Synthesis and Structural Characterization of Thioureidophosphonate Compounds

Two novel organophosphorus compounds were prepared in a facile one pot Kabachnik–Fields reaction via pyridinium triflate as, a green protic ionic liquid, as a Lewis acid catalyst [36]. Two different molar ratios of 1:1:1 and 2:1:2 were inserted, zeta-potential charge, for the three thiourea, terephthalaldehyde, and triphenyl phosphite reactants, giving mono and bis substituted thioureidophosphonates (MTP and BTP) (Scheme 1). Both reactions were performed in acetonitrile (CH_3CN) as a solvent at room temperature with overnight stirring and followed by TLC using an eluent mixture of hexane–methylene chloride (3:1). Moreover, the attained yields reached around 91.72 and 87.71% for MTP and BTP, successively.

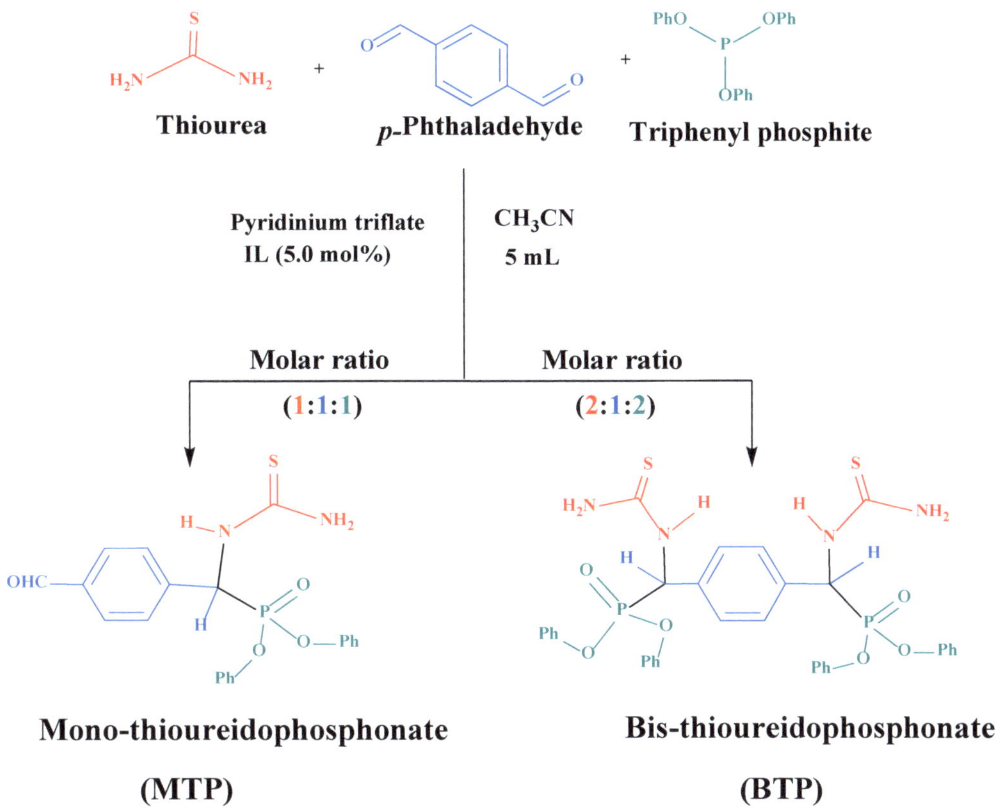

Scheme 1. One pot-three component synthesis of MTP and BTP.

The chemical structures of TPs (MTP and BTP) were fully elucidated through FT-IR spectroscopy, (^{1}H-, ^{13}C-, and ^{31}P) -NMR techniques, and elementary (CHNS) analysis, successively. Referring to the FT-IR spectra of raw MTP and BTP analogues (Figure 1), the absorption bands stretched at $\bar{\nu}$ = 3310/3458, 3058, and 1526 cm^{-1}, indicated to primary/secondary amine (-NH_2/>NH) and aromatic (C–H) and >C=C< bonds, consecutively. The aliphatic bands of C–H, -P=O, and P–C were recorded at $\bar{\nu}$ = 2896, 1196, and 762 cm^{-1}, respectively. Moreover, two peaks were noticed at $\bar{\nu}$ = 945 and 948 cm^{-1}, due to the presence of P–O–C bond in MTP and BTP, respectively. Remarkably, one distinctive vibration band was observed, indicating the stretching of -CHO in MTP compound. Apart from this band observed at $\bar{\nu}$ = 1698 cm^{-1}, the bending vibration of (>NH) was assigned at $\bar{\nu}$ = 1591 cm^{-1}. Furthermore, symmetrical and asymmetrical vibrations of (>C=S) were viewed at $\bar{\nu}$ = 1490 cm^{-1} and $\bar{\nu}$ = 686–687 cm^{-1} for both characterized compounds, successively. Thus, the FT-IR spectroscopic tool reflected the complete formation of raw TP products.

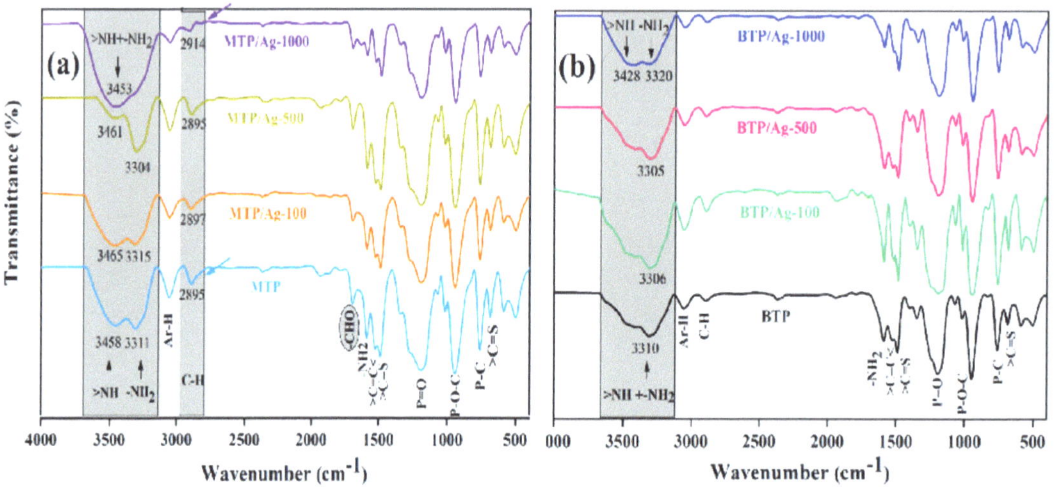

Figure 1. (**a**) FT-IR spectra of Ag NCs of MTP and (**b**) BTP compared to their AgNPs-free cores.

The ^{1}H-NMR spectra were performed in deuterated DMSO, elucidating the formation of both TPs with notably characteristic chemical shifts (δ) values in the aliphatic and aromatic regions. First, the chiral proton of P–C–H appeared at δ = 5.50 ppm (1H, d), while all Ar–H were demonstrated as combined peaks in δ range of 6.63–7.99 ppm (Ar-H, m, 14H). Likewise, the 2^{ry} (>NH) proton was depicted as a broad singlet at δ = 9.76 ppm (br.s, 1H), while the 1^{ry} (-NH_2) protons were observed as a broad doublet at δ = 9.40–9.52 ppm (br, d, 2H). The singlet peak at δ = 10.04 ppm (s, 1H) illustrated the presence of a freely unreacted formyl (-CHO) group, affirming the successful synthesis of MTP (Figure S1a). On the other hand, two chiral centers of P–C–H with a singlet peak were disclosed at δ = 5.93 ppm (s, 2H) in BTP. Further, protons of the five aromatic rings were uncovered as multiplet peaks with lower δ = 6.54–7.61 ppm (m, 24H) in comparison to MTP. Similarly, the two terminal amine groups were noted as a broad multiplet at δ = 9.21–9.33 ppm (br. m, 4H). Lastly, the two secondary amino groups (>NH) were illustrated as a broad singlet peak at δ = 9.38 ppm (Figure S1b). Moreover, ^{13}C-NMR spectra of both TPs conducted in deuterated DMSO. The MTP spectrum gave representative peaks of P–C–H chiral carbon displayed at δ = 54.59 and 56.16 ppm while the aromatic C–Hs were observed at δ = 115.24, 120.22, 120.53, 125.39, 127.96, 128.92, 129.90, and 149.80 ppm. In addition, thiocarbonyl (>C=S) and formyl (-CHO) carbon were shown at δ = 183.84 and 192.73 ppm, sequentially (Figure S1c). Two significant signals of chiral centers in BTP were identified at δ = 54.50 and 56.06 ppm. Furthermore, the aromatic carbon atoms were clarified in eight signals with δ = 115.26, 120.29, 120.86, 125.40, 127.50, 129.33, 129.84, 149.94 ppm, while (>C=S) carbon was noticed at δ = 183.83 ppm (Figure S1d). The phosphorus atoms in MTP and BTP were individually resonated as a single peak at δ = 14.08 and 14.85 ppm, respectively (Figure S1e,f). Additionally, the elemental analysis of the as-prepared TPs manifested the successful reactions between thiourea, terephthalaldehyde, and triphenyl phosphite, individually (Table S1) (Figure S2).

Accordingly, the mechanistic route of the reaction occurred through two major steps: (a) the in situ generation of Schiff base via activation of the formyl group by Lewis acid (LA) catalyst; this facilitated the condensation reaction between thiourea and terephthalaldehyde via nucleophilic addition of a (thiourea) nitrogen lone pair to the electrophilic carbon of the activated carbonyl group of -CHO; (b) the nucleophilic attack of the (triphenyl phosphite) phosphorus atom on the electrophilic carbon of the imine moiety (>C=N-), followed by the extrusion of the phenol molecule through formation of the in situ phosphonium salt and hydroxy phosphite intermediates (Scheme 2) [36].

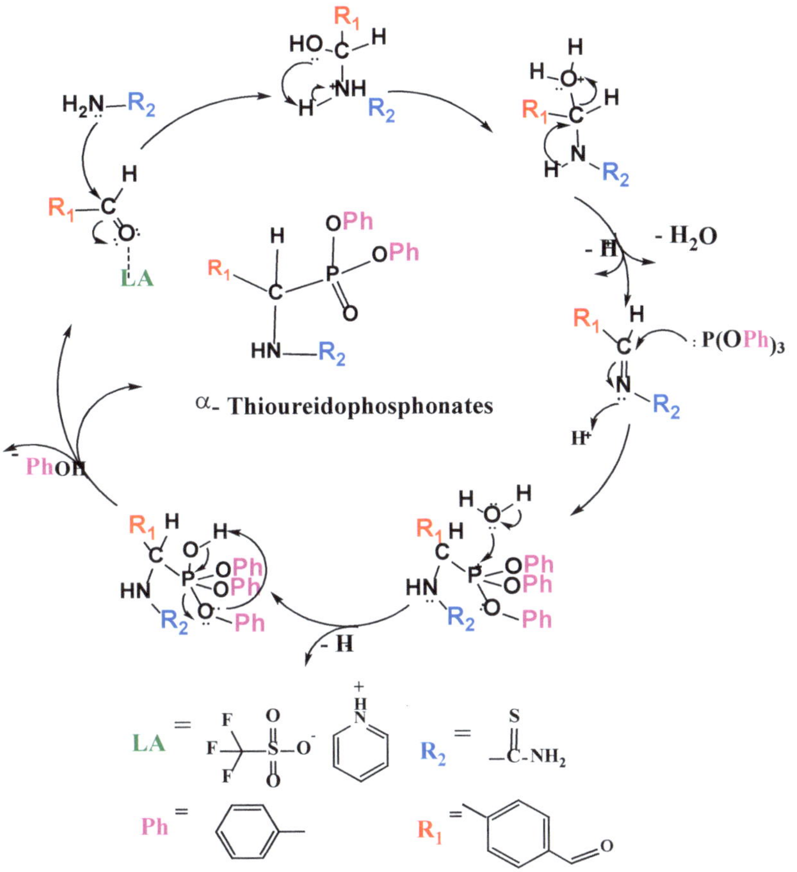

Scheme 2. The proposed mechanism of the one-pot three-component reaction catalyzed by pyridinium triflate as protic ionic liquid.

3.1.2. Fabrication and Structural Elucidation of Thioureidophosphonates Capped Silver Nanoparticles

Well dispersed AgNPs were produced via one-pot synthesis method using thioureidophosphonates (TPs) as dual-functioning reducing and capping agents. This affords spherical AgNPs different dispersion patterns based on the reaction conditions of AgNPs precursor concentrations and the structure of TPs (Figure S3).

The structure and dispersion of AgNPs in the developed nanoscale formulations were fully elucidated using different tools. The FT-IR spectra of MTP incorporated with different molar ratios of silver loading (100, 500, and 1000 mg Ag L^{-1}) illustrated meaningful changes in the characteristic absorption bands of capping agent (MTP) (Figure 1a). Notably, the position of the secondary amine (>NH) of MTP at ν = 3458 cm^{-1} was shifted to ν = 3465, 3461, and 3453 cm^{-1} as for 100, 500, and 1000 mg Ag L^{-1}, respectively. Furthermore, another successive shift occurred from ν = 3311 cm^{-1} to 3315, 3304, and 3453 cm^{-1}, revealing that terminal amine (-NH_2) was also involved in the interaction and reduction of Ag^+ ions in all concentrations of 100, 500, and 1000 mg Ag L^{-1}, respectively. Further, the aliphatic (H-C-P) bond was dramatically shifted from ν = 2895 cm^{-1} to ν = 2914 cm^{-1} in MTP/Ag-1000. On the other side, the FT-IR spectra of BTP and its (100, 500, and 1000) AgNP dispersions displayed similar changes, with a substantial shifting of amine functional groups from ν = 3310 cm^{-1} to ν = 3306, 3305, and (3320–3428) cm^{-1}, consecutively (Figure 1b). Hence, FT-IR technique validated the real contribution of raw TPs in the reduction and capping process and, in turn, the formation of AgNPs (Table S2). Basically, a gradual change in the color of Ag NC solutions was noticed when concentration of dispersed $AgNO_3$ was altered from 100 to 500, and then 1000 mg Ag L^{-1} (Figure S4).

The morphology and dispersion nature of developed silver nanoparticles (AgNPs) were scrutinized using microscopic techniques. Accordingly, the TEM imaging for MTP/Ag-500 displayed good dispersion of spherical AgNPs with an average mean size range of 6.8–20.1 nm (Figure 2a–c). On the other hand, some irregularly spherical and agglomerated AgNPs were observed for BTP/Ag-500 with a mean size range of 5.6–22.6 nm. Remarkably, the non-agglomerated AgNPs on MTP could be ascribed to the smooth morphological structure of MTP facilitating the surface interactions with Ag^+ ions, while the higher density of chelating centers in BTP significantly improved the reduction rate of Ag^+ ions (with deeper color); thus, some smaller AgNPs were attained with the BTP surface (Figure 2d–f). The emergence of aggregated AgNPs could be related to the steric hinderance of BTP structure lowering the capping efficiency [60].

Moreover, the crystallinity of the as-synthesized TPs after AgNPs functionalization was investigated compared to that of raw capping agents using XRD analysis. First, broad XRD patterns were individually centered at 2 theta (2θ) = 21.7° with (110) diffraction phases, reflecting the amorphous structure of both raw MTP and BTP analogues. The emergence of broad patterns stemmed from the strong inter- and intra-molecular hydrogen bonding in raw TP cores [36]. Further, well resolved and sharper diffraction peaks were noticed for both MTP and BTP/Ag-500 at 2θ angles of 37.97°, 43.83°, 64.16°, and 77.49° corresponding to 111, 200, 220, and 311 Bragg peaks of metallic silver in a face-centered cubic (FCC) structure, progressively (Figure 3). Consequently, these results were in agreement with the unit cell structure of silver lines of JCPDS (File No. 04–0783) [61].

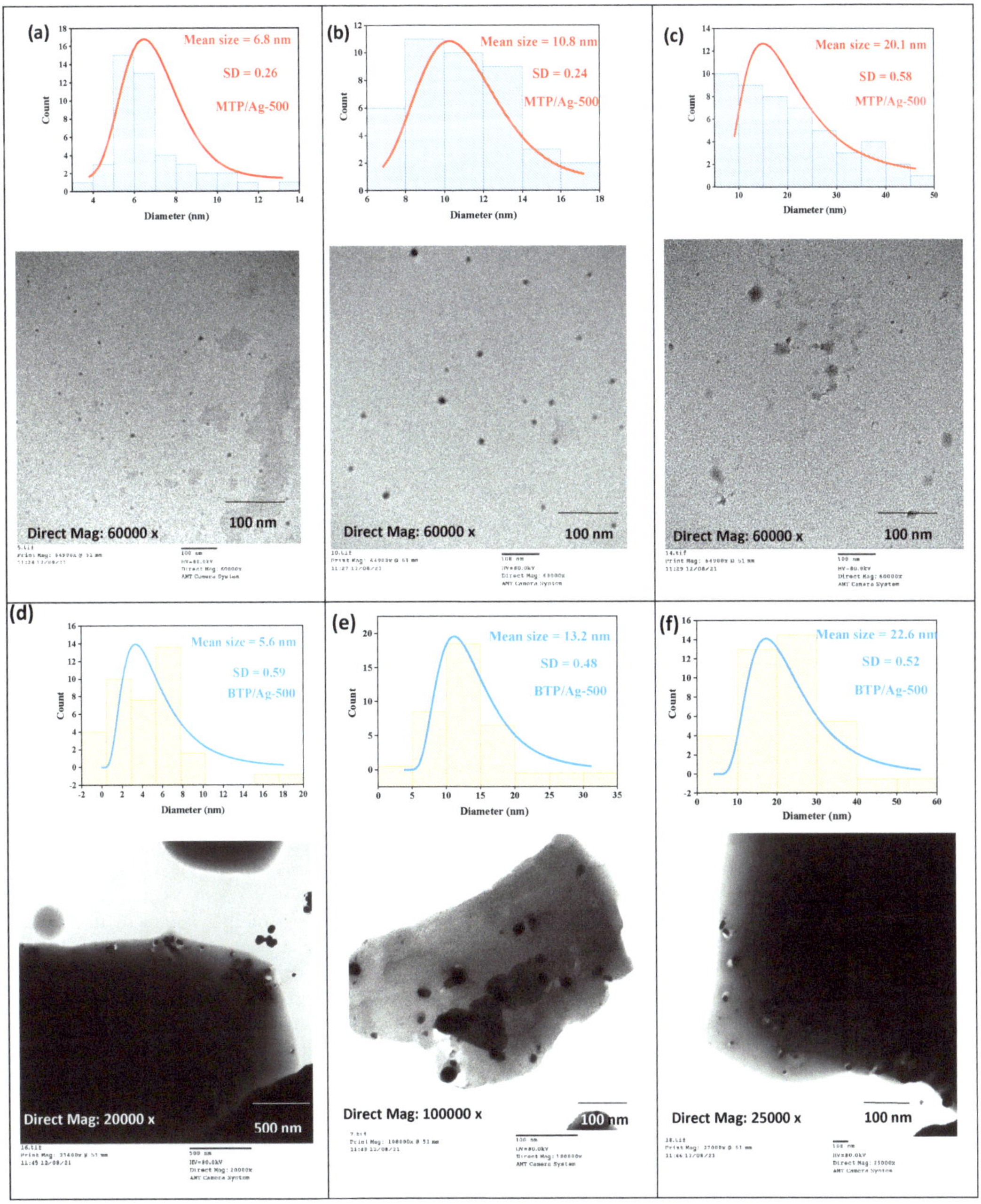

Figure 2. TEM images and size distributions by the histogram in (**a**–**c**) for MTP/Ag-500 NC with 100 nm scale bar, and in (**d**–**f**) for BTP/Ag-500 NC with 500 nm scale bar (**d**) and 100 nm (**e**,**f**), respectively.

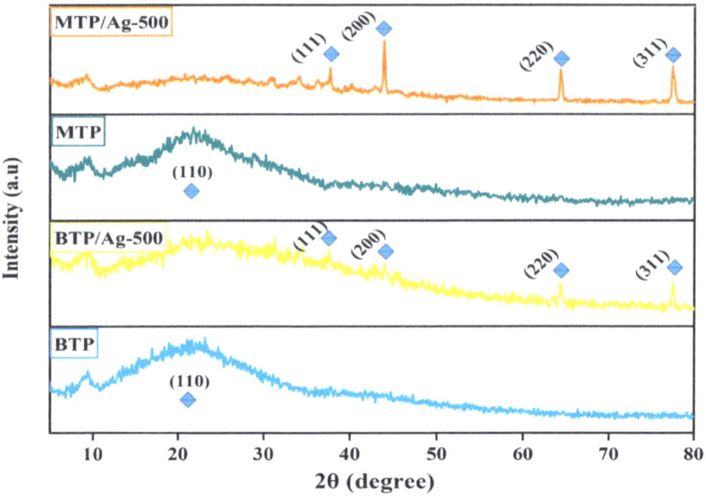

Figure 3. XRD patterns of MTP, MTP/Ag-500, BTP, and BTP/Ag-500 structures.

To validate the most significant changes that occurred to raw functional groups after Ag^+ ions incorporation and formation of AgNPs, X-ray photoelectron spectroscopy analysis (XPS) was carried out for MTP/Ag-500. The XPS results of MTP/Ag-500 were studied based on evaluating the changes in binding energies (BEs), atomic percentages (%), electronic properties, and chemical composition of MTP before and after Ag^+ ion interactions. Five elemental signals of C 1s (at BE: 285.84–287.23 eV), N 1s (400.72–401.63 eV), O 1s (533.02–534.81 eV), P 2p (134.32–134.57 eV), and S 2p (163.19–164.19 eV) were mainly evolved, consecutively (Figures 4a and S5). Regarding the spectrum of MTP/Ag-500 composite, two intensive peaks appeared at BEs of 368.11 and 374.14 eV were ascribed to Ag $3d_{5/2}$ and Ag $3d_{3/2}$ of Ag^0 particles, respectively. In addition, the inset manifested that Ag $3d_{5/2}$ peak was deconvoluted into two peaks observed at 368.02 eV and 368.84 eV, while Ag $3d_{3/2}$ was also divided into two peaks of 374.0 eV and 374.73 eV, respectively (Figure 4b) [62]. However, some other peaks successively emerged at BEs of 366.27, 369.03, and 373.30 eV. They could have originated from the incomplete reduction of Ag^+ ions in the form of Ag^+-N or Ag^+-O. On top of this, the rough calculation results evaluated that around 92.28 atomic % of Ag^+ ions were reduced to Ag^0, proving the prominent ability of MTP functional groups in the interaction and reduction of Ag^+ ions to Ag^0 particles. Moreover, a series of Ag 3s, Ag $3p_{1/2}$, Ag $3p_{3/2}$, Ag 4s, and Ag 4p signals appeared at BEs of 719, 604, 573, 98, and 60 eV, respectively. Thus, the XPS spectrum of the MTP surface exposed to Ag^+ ions was altered to validate the changes in binding and chelation routes. Furthermore, some changes were primarily observed via minor shifts of BEs from (0.04–0.46) eV, besides considerable changes in the atomic percentages (%) of raw elemental functional groups that were estimated from 0.72–25.57%. Basically, these notably affected functional groups were ordered, respectively, in a descending mode according to changes in BEs as follows: C–S ($2p_{1/2}$) > C–C, C–H, and C=C > HC=O and -OH (H_2O) > C–S ($2p_{3/2}$) > P–C and P–O ($2p_{1/2}$) > >NH and -NH_2 > C=S > C–N > π–π* sat, benzene rings, and C=S > C-OH, P–O, and C–O–C > C–O, C–N, C–P, and C=O (Table S3). Furthermore, after Ag^+ ions complexation and formation of additional O–H (from H_2O) on the MTP, the main signal deconvolution assessed that Ag^+ ions may be sorbed in their hydrated form (i.e., their solvated form). In this regard, the changes that occurred in BEs after AgNPs decoration were consistent with the results discussed before.

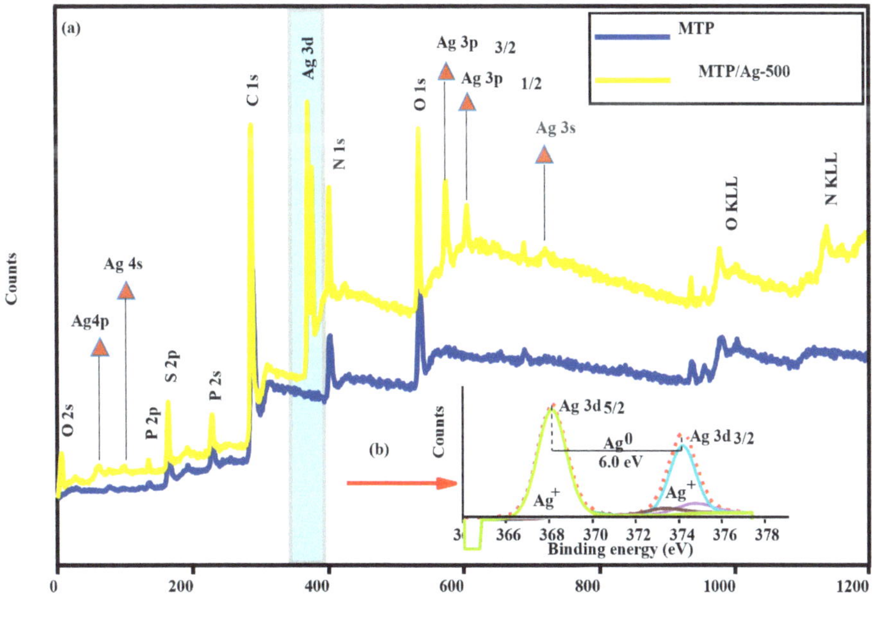

Figure 4. (**a**) XPS spectra of the raw MTP and MTP/Ag-500 nanocomposite and (**b**) the inset figure of Ag3d peak deconvoluted into Ag3d $_{5/2}$ and $_{3/2}$ for MTP/Ag-500.

3.2. Antibacterial Activity

The antibacterial potency of synthesized thioureidophosphonates (TPs) and their fabricated AgNPs-based composites was evaluated against several strains. The antibacterial activity using the agar well diffusion method was conducted against six clinical bacterial strains and their ATCC references of Gram-positive (methicillin-resistant *Staphylococcus aureus* (*MRSA*), *Streptococcus mutans*, and *Bacillus subtilis*) and Gram-negative (*Pseudomonas aeruginosa*, *Salmonella typhi*, and *Serratia marcescens*) bacteria as well. Moreover, zone of inhibition diameters, minimum inhibitory concentration (MIC), minimum bactericidal concentration (MBC), time–kill kinetics, antiadhesion activity, and antibiofilm assay with morphological investigation were assessed for all developed compounds.

3.2.1. Bactericidal Properties

The Killing Action against Gram-Positive Strains

MTP and BTP showed significant resistance against methicillin-resistant *Staphylococcus aureus* (*MRSA*), *Streptococcus mutans* (*S. mutans*), and *Bacillus subtilis* (*B. subtilis*), compared to Ampicillin and Ciprofloxacin as reference antibiotics (Tables 1–3). First, MTP exhibited higher MIC (0.625 mg/mL) than BTP against *MRSA*, reducing MIC values by 5 and 1.2 times compared to Ampicillin and Ciprofloxacin controls, respectively. On the other hand, MIC attained for BTP was equal to 0.3125 mg/mL, which had twofold better antibacterial superiority than MTP against *MRSA*. The antibacterial evaluation was performed against *S. mutans* with respective MIC values of 0.3125 and 0.156 mg/mL for MTP and BTP, while the estimated MIC values towards *B. subtilis* reached 0.3125 and 0.0781 mg/mL. Compared to Ampicillin and Ciprofloxacin, MTP reduced MIC values by 5 times towards *S. mutans*, while the relative decline in MIC reached 12.8 and 5 times against *B. subtilis*, consecutively. BTP had more structural diversity, allowing it to be more powerful than MTP, minimizing MIC values by two and four times against *S. mutans* and *B. subtills*, sequentially. Screening both MTP and BTP against *MRSA* (ATCC-43300) resulted in higher MIC values = 1.25 mg/mL for both analogues. MTP and BTP recorded MICs at lower concentrations of 0.625 and 0.3125 mg/mL against *S. mutans* (ATCC-35668) and *B. subtilis* (ATCC-6633), progressively. The zone of inhibition (ZOI) was measured for each strain with DMSO as a negative control. Including the diameter of each well (6 mm) before treatment, MTP gave ZOIs in a range of 28 ± 1.0, 30 ± 1.00, and 24 ± 1.00 mm, whereas the treatment with BTP increased the ZOIs width towards *MRSA*, *S. mutans*, and *B. subtilis* strains, respectively. Both TPs with MBC/MIC ratio of 2(+) have bactericidal properties, unlike Ampicillin and Ciprofloxacin. TPs loaded with silver nanoparticles (AgNPs) (100, 500, and 1000 mg Ag L^{-1}) were used to investigate the antibacterial properties towards three strains accompanied with a dose-dependent improvement in susceptibility. A clear MIC decline to very minute concentrations was appreciated from 0.156 to 0.1525 × 10^{-3} mg/mL with the three strains. The MIC of MTP significantly dropped by (4 × MIC) after treating *MRSA* and *S. mutans* with MTP/Ag-100. Afterward, MTP/Ag-500 and MTP/Ag-1000 showed increased bactericidal properties against both strains, i.e., 16 and 2049 times sequentially. The treatment of MTP/Ag-(100, 500, and 1000) to *B. subtilis* increased the potential bactericidal activity by 16, 128, and 1024 times, respectively. BTP/Ag-100 showed a more significant decline in MIC values by two and eight times against *MRSA* and *B. subtilis*, compared to MTP/Ag NCs. BTP/Ag-500 had less biocidal effects by 4 and 16 times that of MTP/Ag-500 on *MRSA* and *B. subtilis*, consecutively. This reflected that BTP and AgNPs have less synergistic interactions than MTP. However, BTP/AgNPs had the same bactericidal activity as MTP/AgNPs against *S. mutans* in 100 and 500 dispersions. Noteworthy, MTP and BTP loaded with 1000 mg L^{-1} resulted in a decrease in MICs by 2049 times against *MRSA* while BTP/Ag-1000 showed higher MIC against *S. mutans* and *B. subtilis* by only 1023 and 512 times, respectively (Tables 1–3). Further, ZOI diameters increased towards *MRSA* treated by TP/Ag NCs in all concentrations of 100, 500, and 1000 mg Ag L^{-1}. After AgNPs incorporation, increased ZOI diameters from 28 ± 1.00 to 35 ± 1.00, 44 ± 1.00, and 49 ± 1.50 mm were achieved for MTP with 100, 500, and 1000 mg Ag L^{-1}, successively (Figure S6). Similarly, ZOI values were promoted from 32 ± 0.60 to 36 ± 1.00, 40 ± 0.60, and 52 ± 1.00 mm after treatment with 100, 500, and 1000 BTP/Ag NCs, progressively. Moreover, MTP improved ZOI values against *S. mutans* from 30 ± 1.00 to 36 ± 1.00 (MTP/Ag-100), 38 ± 1.00 (MTP/Ag-500), and 42 ± 1.00 mm for MTP/Ag-1000, respectively. Likewise, ZOIs exhibited a gradual increase from 37 ± 1.00 in BTP to 40 ± 1.00 (BTP/Ag-100), 43 ± 0.60 (BTP/Ag-500), and 49 ± 0.100 mm (BTP/Ag-1000). MTP and BTP gave higher ZOIs with diameters of 35 ± 1.00, 38 ± 1.00, and 40 ± 1.00 mm and 36 ± 1.00, 41 ± 1.00, and 41 ± 1.00 mm, respectively, for *B. subtilis* (Figure 5, Tables 1–3, and Figures S6, S8 and S9). Briefly, MTP/Ag NCs showed dose-effective antibacterial activity against all studied Gram-positive bacterial strains.

Table 1. Antibacterial parameters of developed antibacterial agents—zone of inhibition (mm), minimum bactericidal concentration (MBC), minimum inhibitory concentration (MIC), and MBC/MIC ratio of compounds (mg/mL)—against *MRSA* and *MRSA* (ATCC-43300).

Compounds	ZOI	*MRSA*			*MRSA* (ATCC-43300)		
		MBC	MIC	MBC/MIC	MBC	MIC	MBC/MIC
MTP	28 ± 1.00	1.25	0.625	2(+)	2.5	1.25	2(+)
MTP/Ag-100	35 ± 1.00	0.3125	0.156	2(+)	0.625	0.3125	2(+)
MTP/Ag-500	44 ± 1.00	0.078	0.039	2(+)	0.078	0.039	2(+)
MTP/Ag-1000	49 ± 1.50	0.0006103	0.000305	2(+)	0.0006103	0.000305	2(+)
BTP	32 ± 1.00	0.625	0.3125	2(+)	2.5	1.25	2(+)
BTP/Ag-100	36 ± 1.00	0.3125	0.156	2(+)	0.625	0.3125	2(+)
BTP/Ag-500	40 ± 1.00	0.156	0.0781	2(+)	0.156	0.0781	2(+)
BTP/Ag-1000	52 ± 1.50	0.000305	0.0001525	2(+)	0.001220	0.0006103	2(+)
Ampicillin	14.77 ± 0.60	6.25	3.13	2(+)	6.25	1.56	4(+)
Ciprofloxacin	17.32 ± 0.60	3.13	0.78	4(+)	6.25	3.13	2(+)

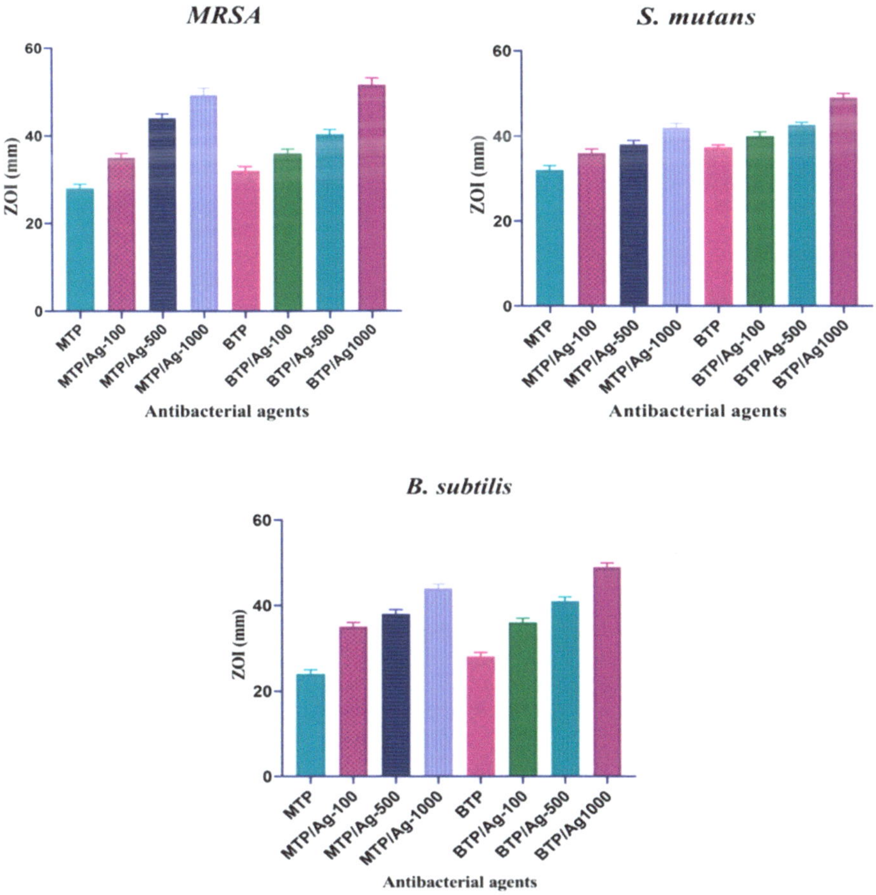

Figure 5. ZOI values of all antibacterial agents towards Gram-positive bacterial strains. The experiments were performed in triplicates.

Table 2. Antibacterial parameters of developed antibacterial agents—zone of inhibition (mm), minimum bactericidal concentration (MBC), minimum inhibitory concentration (MIC), and MBC/MIC ratio of compounds (mg/mL)—against *S. mutans* and *S. mutans* (ATCC-35668).

Compounds	ZOI	*S. mutans*			*S. mutans* (ATCC-35668)		
		MBC	MIC	MBC/MIC	MBC	MIC	MBC/MIC
MTP	30 ± 1.00	0.625	0.3125	2(+)	1.25	0.625	2(+)
MTP/Ag-100	36 ± 1.00	0.156	0.0781	2(+)	0.625	0.3125	2(+)
MTP/Ag-500	38 ± 1.00	0.03906	0.01953	2(+)	0.0781	0.03906	2(+)
MTP/Ag-1000	42 ± 1.00	0.000305	0.0001525	2(+)	0.001220	0.000305	2(+)
BTP	37 ± 0.60	0.3125	0.156	2(+)	0.625	0.3125	2(+)
BTP/Ag-100	40 ± 1.00	0.0781	0.03906	2(+)	0.156	0.0781	2(+)
BTP/Ag-500	43 ± 0.60	0.01953	0.009765	2(+)	0.0781	0.03906	2(+)
BTP/Ag-1000	49 ± 1.00	0.000305	0.0001525	2(+)	0.0006103	0.000305	2(+)
Ampicillin	12 ± 1.00	3.13	1.565	2(+)	6.25	3.13	2(+)
Ciprofloxacin	18.27 ± 0.60	6.25	1.56	4(+)	3.13	1.565	2(+)

Table 3. Antibacterial parameters of developed antibacterial agents—inhibition zone (mm), minimum bactericidal concentration (MBC), minimum inhibitory concentration (MIC) and MBC/MIC ratio of compounds (mg/mL)—against *B. subtilis* and *B. subtilis* (ATCC-6633).

Compounds	ZOI	*B. subtilis*			*B. subtilis* (ATCC-6633)		
		MBC	MIC	MBC/MIC	MBC	MIC	MBC/MIC
MTP	24 ± 1.00	0.625	0.3125	2(+)	1.25	0.625	2(+)
MTP/Ag-100	35 ± 1.00	0.03906	0.01953	2(+)	0.156	0.0781	2(+)
MTP/Ag-500	38 ± 1.00	0.00488	0.00244	2(+)	0.01953	0.009765	2(+)
MTP/Ag-1000	44 ± 1.00	0.0006103	0.000305	2(+)	0.00244	0.001220	2(+)
BTP	28 ± 1.00	0.156	0.0781	2(+)	0.625	0.3125	2(+)
BTP/Ag-100	36 ± 1.00	0.01953	0.009765	2(+)	0.03906	0.01953	2(+)
BTP/Ag-500	41 ± 1.00	0.009765	0.00488	2(+)	0.01953	0.009765	2(+)
BTP/Ag-1000	49 ± 1.00	0.000305	0.0001525	2(+)	0.001220	0.0006103	2(+)
Ampicillin	16.30 ± 0.6	8	4	2(+)	6.25	3.125	2(+)
Ciprofloxacin	18.32 ± 0.60	6.25	1.56	4(+)	3.13	0.78	4(+)

The Killing Action against Gram-Negative Strains

Contrarily, TP analogues had more selective antibacterial properties towards *Pseudomonas aeruginosa* (*P. aeruginosa*), *Salmonella typhi* (*S. typhi*), and *Serratia marcescens* (*S. marcescens*) than previously screened Gram-positive bacteria and reference antibiotics (Figure S13). Towards *P. aeruginosa*, MTP showed a similar MIC value to MRSA at 0.625 mg/mL, which was reduced by 10 and 2.5 times with Ampicillin and Ciprofloxacin references. BTP had an 8-fold lower MIC (=0.078 mg/mL) against *P. aeruginosa* than MTP, indicating higher susceptibility towards Gram-negative strains. Both MTP and BTP compounds had excellent inhibitory properties against *S. typhi* and *S. marcescens*, as their MIC ratio was reduced fourfold. Regarding the Ampicillin and Ciprofloxacin, 5× and 20× MIC reductions by MTP were recorded against *S. typhi*, while 5.0 and 1.2× MIC were dropped with *S. marcescens*. On the contrary, BTP decreased the MICs of Ampicillin and Ciprofloxacin by 20 and 80 times towards *S. typhi*, and to 20 and 5 times against *S. marcescens*, respectively. Furthermore, the selectivity of these TP derivatives was determined against *P. aeruginosa* (ATCC-27853), *S. typhi* (ATCC-6539), and *S. marcescens* (ATCC-13880). Meanwhile, the MICs obtained by inoculating both ATCC isolates of *P. aeruginosa* and *S. marcescens* with MTP were 1.25 mg/mL for *S. typhi* (ATCC-6539). The selectivity of MTP was more effective, affording an MIC value of 0.625 mg/mL. BTP had two lowered MIC values against *P. aeruginosa* (ATCC-27853), *S. typhi* (ATCC-6539), and *S. marcescens*, with 0.3125 mg/mL for *P. aeruginosa* and 0.625 mg/mL for *S. marcescens* (ATCC-13880). On the other hand, ZOI results of MTP and BTP against *P. aeruginosa, S. typhi*, and *S. marcescens* were 28 ± 1.00, 28 ± 1.00, and 35 ± 1.00 mm for MTP, while 33 ± 0.60, 35 ± 1.00, and 38 ± 1.00 mm for BTP, consecutively. Therefore, MBC values ranged from 1.25 to 0.156 mg/mL, resulting in a significant bactericidal efficacy against all bacterial strains with MBC/MIC ratio = 2(+). Notably, AgNPs improved the antibacterial susceptibility of TP cores, lowering MIC values from 0.01953 mg/mL to 7.629×10^{-5} mg/mL. Basically, MTP/Ag-100 minimized the MIC concentration of raw MTP by around 32 times towards *P. aeruginosa*, and 16 times for both *S. typhi* and *S. marcescens*, successively. MTP/Ag-500 reduced MICs by 256 times for *P. aeruginosa* and 128 times for *S. typhi* and *S. marcescens* compared to raw MTP. For MTP/Ag-1000, MTP displayed an elevated antibacterial activity towards *P. aeruginosa, S. typhi*, and *S. marcescens*. Nevertheless, the net antibacterial activity of BTP was higher than MTP, and the combinatorial interactions of AgNPs with MTP were more tunable, unlike BTP. In the meantime, BTP/Ag-100 lessened the MIC ratio to raw BTP by fourfold towards *P. aeruginosa* and eightfold against both *S. typhi* and *S. marcescens*. BTP/Ag-500 had a remarkable bactericidal effect on *S. typhi* up to 128 times. Then, the BTP/Ag-1000 reduced the dose of MIC to 512 times with *P. aeruginosa* and 1023 times with both *S. typhi* and *S. marcescens*, respectively. Pertinently, BTP loaded with AgNPs manifested less powerful bactericidal potency than MTP capped AgNPs (Tables S10–S12). Further, wider ZOI diameters for Gram-negative strains were recorded over Gram-positive strains. In case of MTP after AgNPs dispersion, the ZOIs were increased from 28 ± 1.00 to 34 ± 0.60, 39 ± 1.00, and 43 ± 0.60 mm, whilst BTP/Ag NCs enhanced the gradual enlargement of raw diameter from 33 ± 0.60 (BTP) to 39 ± 1.00, 43 ± 1.00, and 47 ± 1.00 mm in the studied ranges (i.e., 100, 500, and 1000), consecutively. In a dose-dependent manner, *S. typhi* inoculated with MTP/Ag NCs yielded ZOI values of 38 ± 1.00, 41 ± 1.00, and 48 ± 1.00 and 43 ± 1.00, 48 ± 1.00, and 54 ± 1.00 mm for BTP/Ag NCs, sequentially. AgNPs anchoring increased the ZOIs of raw MTP and BTP against *S. marcescens* from 35 ± 1.00 to 41, 45, and 49 ± 1.00 and 38 ± 1.00 to 44, 47, and 54 ± 1.00 mm, consecutively (Figure 6, Tables 4–6, and Figures S10–S12. In summary, the effective synergy between TPs and AgNPs displayed great results with all studied bacterial strains. The presence of TP moiety as a self-biologically active material was effective in comparison to other reported AgNP-based antibacterial agents (Table S4).

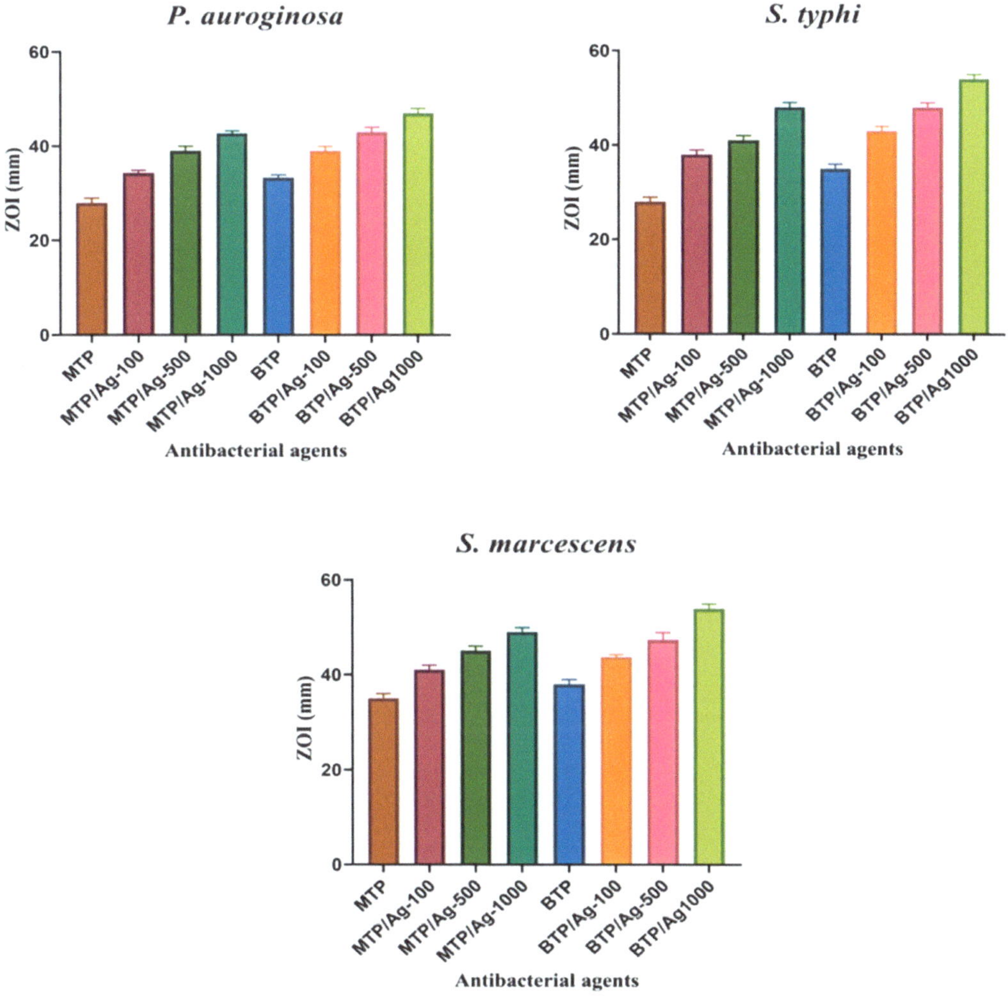

Figure 6. ZOI values of all antibacterial agents towards Gram-negative bacterial strains. The experiments were performed in triplicates.

Table 4. Antibacterial parameters of developed antibacterial agents—zone of inhibition (mm), minimum bactericidal concentration (MBC), minimum inhibitory concentration (MIC) and MBC/MIC ratio of compounds (mg/mL)—against *P. aeruginosa* and *P. aeruginosa* (ATCC-27853).

Compounds	ZOI	*P. aeruginosa*			*P. aeruginosa* (ATCC-27853)		
		MBC	MIC	MBC/MIC	MBC	MIC	MBC/MIC
MTP	28 ± 1.00	1.25	0.625	2(+)	2.5	1.25	2(+)
MTP/Ag-100	34 ± 0.60	0.03906	0.01953	2(+)	0.156	0.0781	2(+)
MTP/Ag-500	39 ± 1.00	0.00488	0.00244	2(+)	0.01953	0.009765	2(+)
MTP/Ag-1000	43 ± 0.60	0.000305	0.0001525	2(+)	0.001220	0.0006103	2(+)
BTP	33 ± 0.60	0.156	0.0781	2(+)	0.625	0.3125	2(+)
BTP/Ag-100	39 ± 1.00	0.03906	0.01953	2(+)	0.156	0.0781	2(+)
BTP/Ag-500	43 ± 1.00	0.00488	0.00244	2(+)	0.01953	0.009765	2(+)
BTP/Ag-1000	47 ± 1.00	0.000305	0.0001525	2(+)	0.001220	0.0006103	2(+)
Ampicillin	8.7 ± 0.60	12.5	6.25	2(+)	6.25	1.56	4(+)
Ciprofloxacin	16.37 ± 0.60	6.25	1.56	4(+)	3.13	0.78	4(+)

Table 5. Antibacterial parameters of developed antibacterial agents—inhibition zone (mm), minimum bactericidal concentration (MBC), minimum inhibitory concentration (MIC) and MBC/MIC ratio of compounds (mg/mL)—against *S. typhi* and *S. typhi* (ATCC-6539).

Compounds	ZOI	*S. typhi*			*S. typhi* (ATCC-6539)		
		MBC	MIC	MBC/MIC	MBC	MIC	MBC/MIC
MTP	28 ± 1.00	0.625	0.3125	2(+)	1.25	0.625	2(+)
MTP/Ag-100	38 ± 1.00	0.03906	0.01953	2(+)	0.156	0.0781	2(+)
MTP/Ag-500	41 ± 1.00	0.00488	0.00244	2(+)	0.01953	0.009765	2(+)
MTP/Ag-1000	48 ± 1.00	0.000305	0.0001525	2(+)	0.001220	0.0006103	2(+)
BTP	35 ± 1.00	0.156	0.0781	2(+)	0.625	0.3125	2(+)
BTP/Ag-100	43 ± 1.00	0.01953	0.009765	2(+)	0.0781	0.03906	2(+)
BTP/Ag-500	48 ± 1.00	0.00244	0.001220	2(+)	0.009765	0.00488	2(+)
BTP/Ag-1000	54 ± 1.00	0.0001525	0.00007629	2(+)	0.0006103	0.000305	2(+)
Ampicillin	14.32 ± 0.60	3.13	1.565	2(+)	6.25	1.56	4(+)
Ciprofloxacin	18.32 ± 0.60	12.5	6.25	2(+)	3.13	0.78	4(+)

Table 6. Antibacterial parameters of developed antibacterial agents—zone of inhibition (mm), minimum bactericidal concentration (MBC), minimum inhibitory concentration (MIC), and MBC/MIC ratio of compounds (mg/mL)—against *S. marcescens* and *S. marcescens* (ATCC-13880).

Compounds	ZOI	*S. marcescens*			*S. marcescens* (ATCC-13880)		
		MBC	MIC	MBC/MIC	MBC	MIC	MBC/MIC
MTP	35 ± 1.00	1.25	0.625	2(+)	2.5	1.25	2(+)
MTP/Ag-100	41 ± 1.00	0.0781	0.03906	2(+)	0.3125	0.156	2(+)
MTP/Ag-500	45 ± 1.00	0.009765	0.00488	2(+)	0.01953	0.009765	2(+)
MTP/Ag-1000	49 ± 1.00	0.001220	0.0006103	2(+)	0.00244	0.00122	2(+)
BTP	38 ± 1.00	0.3125	0.156	2(+)	1.25	0.625	2(+)
BTP/Ag-100	44 ± 0.60	0.03906	0.01953	2(+)	0.156	0.0781	2(+)
BTP/Ag-500	47 ± 1.50	0.00244	0.001220	2(+)	0.01953	0.009765	2(+)
BTP/Ag-1000	54 ± 1.00	0.000305	0.0001525	2(+)	0.002244	0.001220	2(+)
Ampicillin	14.32 ± 0.60	6.25	3.125	2(+)	3.13	1.565	2(+)
Ciprofloxacin	14.50 ± 0.60	3.13	0.78	4(+)	6.25	1.56	4(+)

3.2.2. Time–Kill Assay

This biological test was executed to explore the bactericidal activity of TP derivatives and their AgNPs-based composites towards bacterial growth over a period [63]. When bacterial cells at a concentration of 1×10^8 CFU/mL were incubated with all raw and AgNPs formulations, the *MRSA* growth rate decreased with time compared to the incremental growth of untreated *MRSA*. Interestingly, the viable cells count (CFU/mL) started to dramatically decline after 1 h of treatment (Figure 7). In the meantime, both raw MTP and BTP compounds reduced the number of surviving cells to (2.9 $\log_{10}$) and (1.8 $\log_{10}$) CFU/mL after 18 h of incubation, respectively. However, once *MRSA* was treated with TP/Ag NCs, the picture was changed where the MTP/Ag-100 induced the killing potential with cell count reductions to (2.2 $\log_{10}$) and (0.9 $\log_{10}$) CFU/mL for MTP/Ag-500, consecutively. More significant reductions of the cultural population of *MRSA* were achieved to (1.1 $\log_{10}$) and (0.3 $\log_{10}$) CFU/mL for BTP/Ag-100 and BTP/Ag-500, progressively. Despite the higher killing efficacy of BTP/Ag NCs than MTP/Ag NCs, the combination between AgNPs and MTP brought more bactericidal advantages over BTP, which was observed from the gradual improvement of killing (%) between dose 100 and 500 for both AgNPs formulations. Remarkably, the entire population was reduced and killed within 8 h, for both MTP (BTP)/Ag-1000 composites. Interestingly, the bactericidal rates towards *MRSA* were previously confirmed by both TP/Ag-1000; where both reduced MBC values to the same degree of 2049 times (Table 1). Based on several reported studies, it was interesting to mention that the rapid bactericidal ability of raw TPs (as aminophophonate-based derivatives), could be attributed to their ability to (1) deactivate the potential of cytoplasmic membrane and interfere with DNA nitrogenous bases through aromatic pi-pi bonds. Besides, (2) to generate reactive nitrogen/oxygen species (RNS/ROS) that caused peroxidation of lipid, glutathione (GSH) conversion to glutathione disulfide (GSSG), and thereby cell malfunction followed by death of bacteria, respectively [64,65]. Additionally, AgNPs exhibited a more considerable bactericidal activity which may be due to their toxic effects on bacterial cell wall and cytoplasmic membrane components, resulting in the reduction of cell wall integrity, functionality, defense system, and metabolic activity [18,66]. Thus, the time-dependent kill study revealed that the investigated compounds were time- and dose-effective bactericidal agents.

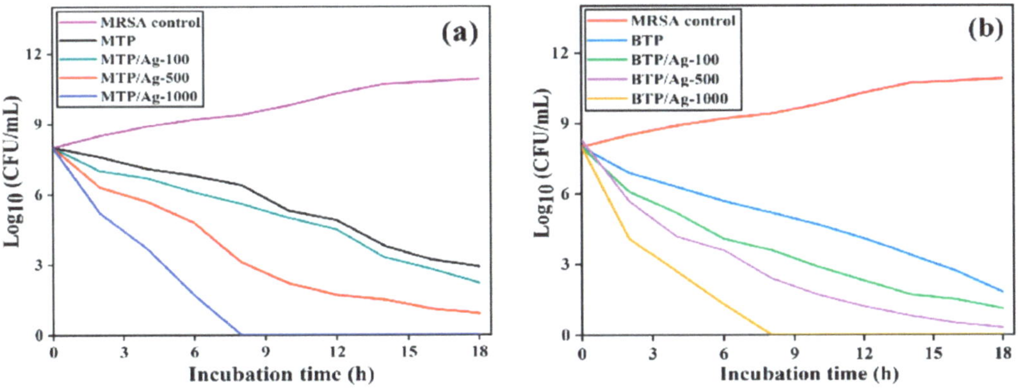

Figure 7. Bactericidal kinetics of (**a**) MTP, and MTP/Ag NCs; and (**b**) BTP, and BTP/Ag NCs against *MRSA*. Untreated *MRSA* cells were employed as a growth control (The experiments were performed with three duplicates).

3.2.3. Antiadhesion Activity

Bacterial adhesion to any object surface is an initial precondition for bacterial growth through biofilm and infection processes. Additionally, there are some crucial parameters controlling the surface tendency for adhesion; these parameters include hydrophobicity, surface energy, and zeta potential charges [67,68]. Hence, fabricating and engineering of novel antiadhesive surfaces with repelling properties against bacteria has become a vital step for investigation (Figure 8). In the current study, all prepared compounds were incubated with high concentration (1×10^6 CFU/mL) of *MRSA* (ATCC-43300) suspensions for 18–24 h, using vancomycin hydrochloride (VAN) as a positive control, and the negative control was tryptic soy broth (TSB). Antiadhesion activity was quantitatively estimated against *MRSA* (ATCC-43300) on the microplate reader at λ_{max} = 570 nm, validating an increase in *MRSA* (ATCC-43300) detachment in a dose-dependent manner within 1.25, 2.5, 5.0, and 10 mg/mL (Figure 9 and Table 7). It was demonstrated that the degree of bacterial adhesion decreased with the increasing hydrophobicity of substrates due to the hydrophilic properties of most strains, such as Gram-positive bacteria. Moreover, there is a direct relation between surface energy and the hydrophobic structure of adhesive surfaces. It has been reported that the higher surface energy stems from the substrates terminated with polar functional groups, such as -NH_2, while those composed of hydrophobic carbon moieties may minimize the surface energy [68]. In conclusion, a higher hydrophobic structure associated with inferior surface energy affords good repelling properties towards bacteria. Accordingly, BTP exhibited higher antiadhesion activity in all utilized concentrations towards *MRSA* (ATCC-43300) than MTP, which could be attributed to its superior hydrophobic characteristics as the non-polar parts (aromatic rings) exceeded the polar ones, based on its molecular formula (M.F), namely, $C_{34}H_{32}N_4O_6P_2S_2$, comparable to MTP with M.F of $C_{21}H_{19}N_2O_4PS$. Moreover, the electrostatic repulsion forces assessed between the negatively charged MTP/Ag NCs and *MRSA* (ATCC-43300) surface played a critical role [69]. As a result, MTP capped AgNPs in 100, 500, and 1000 formulations ascertained more significant increases (relative to raw) in the detachment ability against *MRSA* (ATCC-43300), most notably for 5 and 10 mg/mL. This may originate from the repelling affinity of the negatively charged Ag NCs, e.g., MTP/Ag-1000 with zeta potential = −27.5, mv towards *MRSA* (ATCC-43300). In contrast, inferior repelling rates were estimated for BTP-based AgNPs, especially at 5 and 10 mg/mL, which could be attributed to the tendency of BTP/Ag NCs to form more constrained molecules at high concentrations, thus lowering the contact surface area for repulsion, in addition to their less negative zeta charge like that of BTP/Ag-1000 in −12.4 mv in comparison to that of MTP/Ag-1000 (Figure S14) [70]. Additionally, at 1.25 and 2.5 mg/mL, BTP/Ag NCs displayed more notable repellent properties than that of MTP/Ag NCs at the same concentration. Thus, a greater contact surface area of BTP/Ag NCs could be obtained at lower concentrations, providing more hydrophobic and repelling characteristics. Further, the positive control (VAN) used at (100 mg/mL) showed lower antiadhesion activity (8.9%) compared to TSB as a negative control. The hydrophilic and polycationic characteristics of VAN towards the *MRSA* (ATCC-43300) surface may relate to this weak detachment activity [71]. On this account, the TP/Ag NCs proved to be efficient antifouling surfaces against multidrug-resistant Gram-positive bacteria such as *MRSA* (ATCC-43300).

Table 7. Antiadhesion assay of tested compounds towards *MRSA* (ATCC-43300) based on quadruplicate results with standard deviation, (n = 4).

Concentration	MTP	MTP/Ag-100	MTP/Ag-500	MTP/Ag-1000	BTP	BTP/Ag-100	BTP/Ag-500	BTP/Ag-1000
10 mg/mL	11.8 ± 0.06	33.6 ± 0.11	50.2 ± 0.11	58.8 ± 0.08	25.4 ± 0.05	49.5 ± 0.22	55.4 ± 0.05	67.4 ± 0.11
5 mg/mL	5.3 ± 0.06	28.4 ± 0.08	41.9 ± 0.06	47.5 ± 0.13	19.8 ± 0.08	35.5 ± 0.11	49.8 ± 0.08	54.2 ± 0.11
2.5 mg/mL	3.8 ± 0.07	12.6 ± 0.09	24.7 ± 0.14	32.3 ± 0.12	8.8 ± 0.07	27.3 ± 0.07	33.8 ± 0.07	39.3 ± 0.09
1.25 mg/mL	1.7 ± 0.06	8.8 ± 0.06	16.4 ± 0.09	24.9 ± 0.09	3.4 ± 0.05	18.5 ± 0.07	23.4 ± 0.05	28.5 ± 0.09

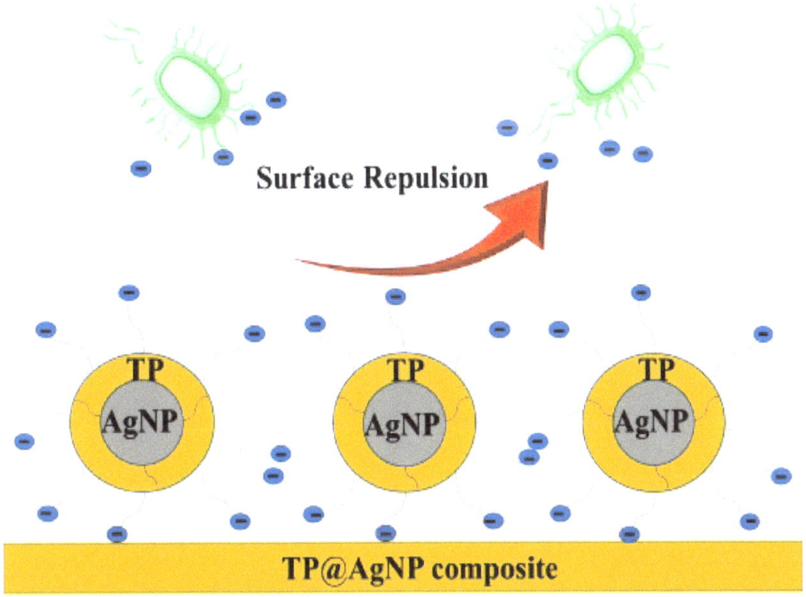

Figure 8. Schematic representation of the surface repulsion of the negatively charged TP/Ag NCs with *MRSA* (ATCC-43300) surface.

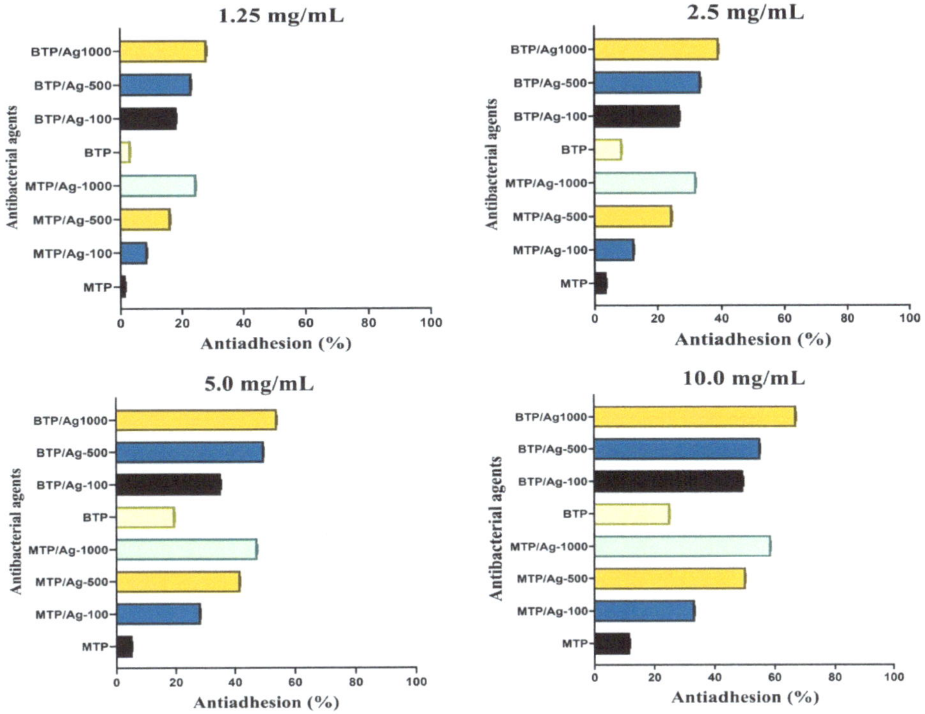

Figure 9. Antiadhesion assay of tested compounds towards *MRSA* (ATCC-43300) based on quadruplicate results with standard deviation, (n = 4).

3.2.4. Antibiofilm Assay

Methicillin-resistant *Staphylococcus aureus* (*MRSA*) is one of the most opportunistic and resistant pathogens, being able to produce an extracellular polymeric substance (EPS) inducing biofilm growth prior to the occurrence of cross infection [72]. The antibiofilm activity of the prepared compounds was tested against *MRSA* (ATCC-43300) as a Gram-positive bacterium with reference to vancomycin hydrochloride (VAN) as a positive control. The biofilm disintegration activity (%) was validated by the microtiter plate assay using a semi-quantitative analysis based on crystal violet staining. Regarding 96-well plates treated with raw MTP and BTP, the biofilm (violet color circle) was slightly eliminated, while the gradual removal was notably viewed by six TP/Ag NCs, (Figures S15 and S16). Therefore, these results suggested the superb antibiofilm potency of TP-wrapped AgNPs composites. Moreover, the decline (%) of biofilm formation was determined through a quantitative analysis appreciated by the photometric microplate reader at $\lambda_{max} \approx 570$ nm with respect to the negative control of tryptic soy broth (TSB). The results showed a significant reduction in biofilm growth when treated with raw TPs, even after 24 h of incubation. The biofilm inhibition (%) was promoted with the gradual increase in the concentrations of tested compounds in the 1.25, 2.5, 5.0, and 10.0 mg/mL (Table 8, Figure 10). Yet, from the economic point of view, the 5.0 mg/mL concentration for all incubated formulations was thought to be the most synergistic and effective dose. The anti-biofilm activity of the positive control (VAN) reached $43 \pm 0.17\%$ when used even at 100 mg/mL, while raw BTP demonstrated higher (58.8%) antibiofilm activity than MTP (41.9%) at 5.0 mg/mL, which could be due to higher number of bio-active groups in BTP. Thus, the antibiofilm assay showed the strong potential of TP conjugates to disrupt biofilm EPS matrices of *MRSA* (ATCC-43300). The studied TP cores (α-aminophosphonate derivatives) are considered structural bio-isosteres of α-amino acids (peptides) with a common amine functional group, but the carboxylic groups in α-amino acids are replaced with related phosphorous-containing moieties such as phosphonic acid. However, the reported data about their antibiofilm mechanism of action towards MRSA biofilm are directed for hybrid α-APs; thus, the inhibitory actions of mentioned α-APs analogues were proposed [65,73]. First, the interference with the quorum sensing (QS) system, which represents a major source of biofilm nutrition and protection, could be a reason [74]. Moreover, the interaction with the extracellular DNA (e-DNA) of biofilm affects its integrity and biological functionality. The generation of reactive oxygen/nitrogen species (ROS/RNS) could cause oxidative stress as reported for based α-AP derivatives [65]. It was assessed that phosphorous-containing groups such as phosphonate compounds tend to inhibit cell wall synthetic enzymes and DNA bases and increase the permeability of bacterial cell membrane [75,76].

After AgNPs functionalization, biofilm inhibition capability (%) was promoted for both MTP and BTP in all studied concentrations (1.25, 2.5, 5.0, and 10.0 mg/mL), consecutively. The most effective and synergistic concentration needed for the disruption of MRSA (ATCC-43300) biofilm was observed at 5.0 mg/mL for both TP/Ag NCs. For 10.0 mg/mL, the biofilm eradicating ability for both MTP(BTP)/Ag-1000 reached maximum values at 79.5 and 83.6%, progressively (Table 8, Figure 10). Nonetheless, higher antibiofilm rates were accomplished for BTP/Ag NCs than that of MTP, the antibacterial effect of AgNPs showed a promising synergy with raw MTP conjugates over that of BTP, exhibiting improved toxicity when compared to TPs alone. Meanwhile, many reports showed that AgNPs affect biofilm integrity; smaller and spherical metal nanoparticles (AgNPs) were related to good biofilm eradication activity. In the current study, the capped AgNPs were spherical, with an average mean size in the range of (5.6–22.6 nm), which could facilitate antibacterial activity and provide more possible interactions with the bacterial surface. Additionally, it was thought that the ability of AgNPs to disrupt biofilm layers could be attributed to their severe inhibition of EPS matrix, deactivating the external protective layers of bacterial cell, as reported in [77]. Furthermore, a pH of the biofilm environment below 7 could change the negatively charged nanocomposites to positive ones, increasing electrostatic interactions with the bacterial surface [78]. Some studies illustrated that AgNPs tend to interact with molecular oxygen in an aqueous environment, thus giving more leached Ag^+ ions and reactive oxygen species (ROS), which increased the toxic effects on the integrity of bacterial cell wall. Additionally, ROS can cause the total impairment of envelope-bound proteins, deoxyribonucleic acid (DNA), respiratory coenzymes, and antioxidants such as glutathione (GSH) [72]. Remarkably, these findings were consistent with the estimated antibiofilm activity (%) and scanning electron microscopy (SEM) images of AgNPs-treated *MRSA* (ATCC-43300) in the next section [79].

Table 8. Anti-biofilm assay of tested compounds towards *MRSA* (ATCC-43300) (experiment evaluated based on quadruplicate results with standard deviation (n = 4)).

Concentration	MTP	MTP/Ag-100	MTP/Ag-500	MTP/Ag-1000	BTP	BTP/Ag-100	BTP/Ag-500	BTP/Ag-1000
10 mg/mL	50.2 ± 0.11	68.3 ± 0.08	72.7 ± 0.06	79.5 ± 0.02	62.9 ± 0.07	71.8 ± 0.06	77.4 ± 0.07	83.6 ± 0.11
5 mg/mL	41.9 ± 0.06	57.3 ± 0.08	68.6 ± 0.08	75.5 ± 0.11	58.8 ± 0.07	65.3 ± 0.06	71.9 ± 0.06	78.4 ± 0.08
2.5 mg/mL	24.7 ± 0.13	43.3 ± 0.05	52.8 ± 0.08	57.3 ± 0.07	43.9 ± 0.07	51.8 ± 0.07	61.4 ± 0.07	68.6 ± 0.09
1.25 mg/mL	16.4 ± 0.09	32.8 ± 0.06	34.7 ± 0.07	38.5 ± 0.07	34.6 ± 0.08	43.7 ± 0.06	46.4 ± 0.07	48.8 ± 0.06

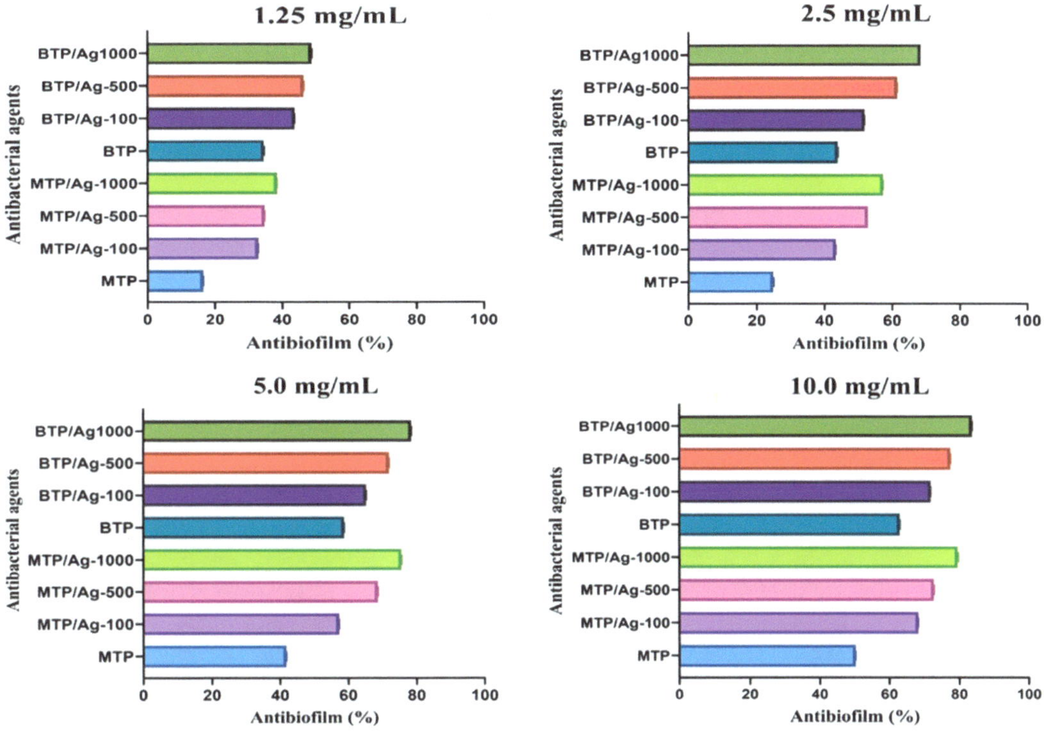

Figure 10. Biofilm eradication ability of tested compounds towards *MRSA* (ATCC-43300) based on quadruplicate results with standard deviation, (n = 4).

3.2.5. Morphological Imaging of Treated *MRSA* (ATCC-43300)

The biofilm inhibition of *MRSA* (ATCC-43300) was also qualitatively verified through scanning electron microscopy (SEM) after incubation by 100 µg/mL of raw compounds and their TP/Ag-1000. The two upper images (Figures 11 and 12) represent the positively controlled (untreated) *MRSA* (ATCC-43300) surface on which aggregating grape-like colonies were developed to form the biofilm. On the contrary, low percentages of biofilm clusters were present on the surfaces of *MRSA* (ATCC-43300) after treatment with raw MTP and BTP, indicating that these compounds could prevent bacterial biofilm formation and induce cell death. Moreover, almost no biofilm matrices could be observed on MRSA treated with MTP and BTP decorated with AgNPs, validating the potent biofilm disintegration ability of TP/Ag NCs. In summary, these observations were in line with antibiofilm investigation results and other studies referring to the ability of synthesized AgNPs to severely interfere with cell wall (biofilm) components, thus hampering metabolic functions, and thereby, MRSA (ATCC-43300) cells are killed [79].

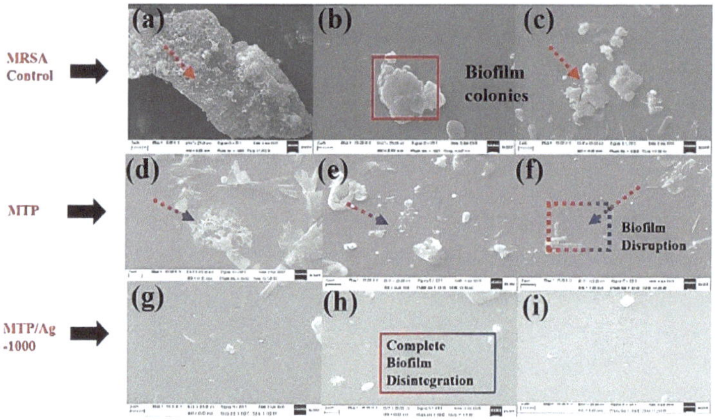

Figure 11. (**a**–**i**) SEM images showing the biofilm reduction of treated *MRSA* (ATCC-43300) by (100 μg/mL) of MTP and MTP/Ag-1000 on plasma-coated titanium surface at different magnifications.

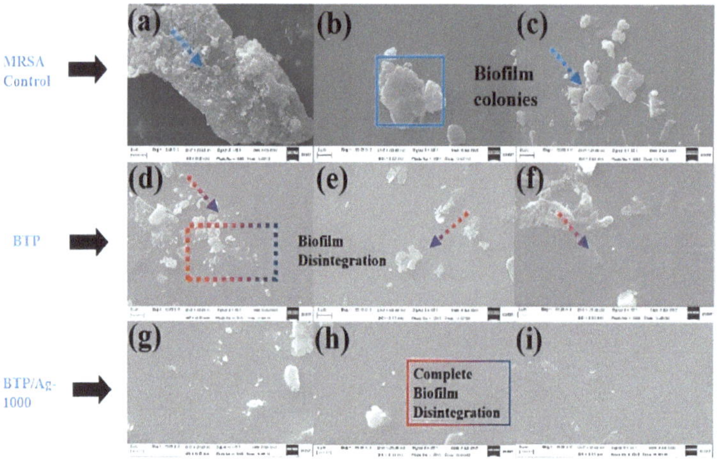

Figure 12. (**a**–**i**) SEM images showing the biofilm reduction of treated *MRSA* (ATCC-43300) by (100 μg/mL) of BTP and BTP/Ag-1000 on plasma-coated titanium surface at different magnification.

3.3. Molecular Docking Study

Molecular docking studies were conducted for the prepared TP compounds to investigate their binding affinity for Gram-positive (*MRSA* and *B. subtilis*) and Gram-negative (*P. aeruginosa* and *S. typhi*) bacterial proteins with respective codes of PDB: 4DKI, 2FQT, 5ZHN, and 3ZQE, in addition to confirming their illegibility as antibacterial agents with the experimental work. Furthermore, the docking results for the prepared raw compounds (MTP and BTP) in all downloaded proteins, along with type of chemical bonding and the amino acids involved in the interaction with the protein, were estimated. Additionally, values recorded for binding affinity and root mean square deviation (RMSD) were tabulated. There are different types of interactions, including hydrogen and hydrophobic H-*pi* interactions, with the binding sites of all the investigated proteins (Table 9). The best binding affinity for BTP was recorded with protein PDB (code: 2FQT) for *B. subtilis*, followed by protein PDB (code: 4DKI) for *MRSA*, with values of −7.9776 kcal/mol and −7.9074 kcal/mol, respectively. Amino acids involved in the interaction between BTP and the B. subtilis protein were GLY127 (H-acceptor, P=O), GLY127 (H-pi, H-Ar), and GLU57 (H-donor, >NH), which are the same amino acids involved in the interaction of the co-crystallized ligand and the protein (Figure 13). MTP also exhibited considerable binding interactions towards protein PDB (code: 4DKI) for MRSA then the 5ZHN of *P. aeruginosa*, with respective binding affinity values of −6.0126 and −5.976 kcal/mol. Moreover, the amino acids participating in the interactions with *MRSA* were MET641 (H-donor, P=O) and TYR446 (H-acceptor, C=S) (Figure 14), while TYR120 (H-donor) and GLU121 (H-donor) were contributed for *P. aeruginosa* interactions, consecutively (Table 9). It was noticed that the binding affinity and RMSD values were more promising for BTP than in MTP, which prompted our interest to incorporate AgNPs and evaluate the nano formulation effect on the antibacterial activity as conducted in the experimental work. Briefly, molecular modeling studies were performed for MTP-capped AgNPs based on the antibacterial progress that the biological results validated. Afterward, a noteworthy improvement against *B. subtilis* protein was observed, recording better binding affinity of −7.6668 kcal/mol, with a perfect fitting at the RMSD value of 1.2593 Å (Figure 15). Interestingly, these results were consistent with the experimental work, implying the considerable inhibition of AgNPs incorporated with MTP. As clearly demonstrated from the docking study, the superior efficacy of AgNPs could be attributed to the following: (a) The MTP/AgNP composites exerted Ag-acceptor bonds with both amino acids (SER80 and GLU57), along with the H-bonding interactions between raw MTP-capping compounds with amino acids of *B. subtilis* proteins (Figure 13). These binding interactions resulted in the formation of an Ag–protein complex, causing severe distortion in the elastic and geometric properties of the protein with several impairments to the biofilm [80]. (b) The inhibition of some biological enzymes, such as the S-ribosyl homocysteinase (LuxS), which is responsible for the communication system between *B. subtilis* cells via quorum sensing (QS) and thereby for biofilm growth [81,82]; thus, the (in silico) approach of TP-based analogues revealed their good stability profiles as potent antibacterial candidates.

Table 9. Docking results of MTP and BTP compounds with four different proteins of Gram-positive and negative bacterial strains.

Compound	Protein		BE (Kcal/mol)	RMSD (Å)	Amino Acid Interactions
	Bacterial Strains	PDB Code			
MTP	*MRSA*	4DKI	−6.0126	1.4454	MET641 (H-donor), TYR446(H-acceptor).
	Bacillus	2FQT	−5.562	1.979	GLU57(H-donor), GLY127(H-acceptor).
	Pseudo	5ZHN	−5.976	2.247	TYR120(H-donor), GLU121(H-donor).
	Typhi	3ZQE	−4.8091	1.7241	ARG58(H-acceptor).
BTP	*MRSA*	4DKI	−7.9074	1.7812	THR600(H-acceptor), HIS583(H-acceptor), ASN464(H-acceptor), GLY640 (H-*pi*).
	Bacillus	2FQT	−7.9776	1.8475	GLY127(H-acceptor), GLY127 (*pi*-H), GLU57 (H-donor)
	Pseudo	5ZHN	−5.7701	1.5838	SER (H-*pi*).
	Typhi	3ZQE	−6.7920	1.8609	ALA229(H-donor), TYR54 (*pi*-H).

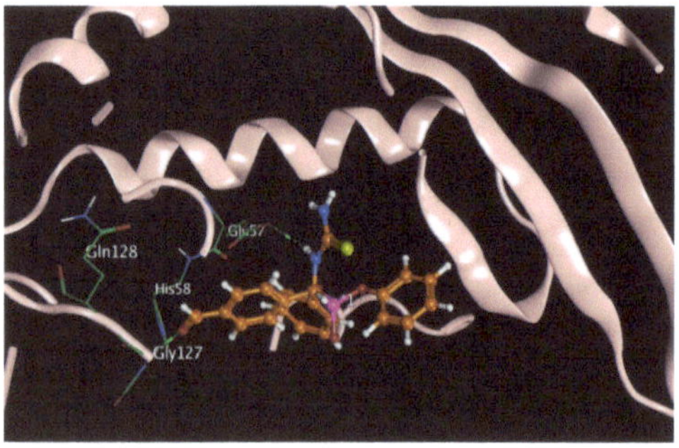

(**a**)

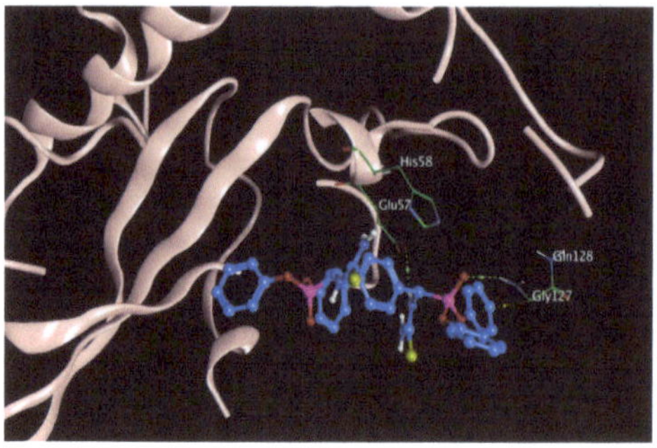

(**b**)

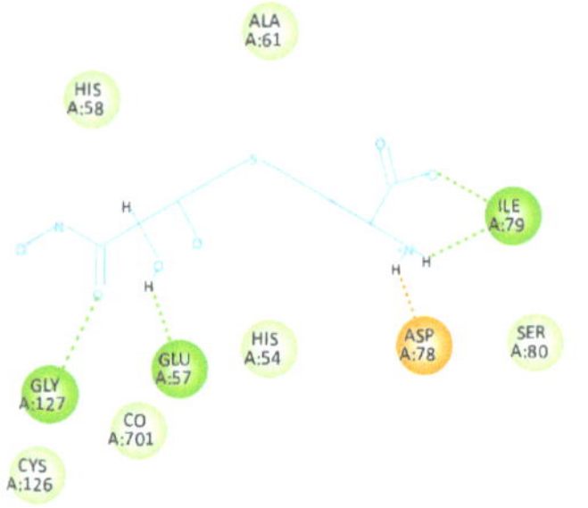

(**c**)

Figure 13. Chemical bonding involved in interaction between *bacillus subtilis* protein active site and (**a**) MTP compound via orange balls and sticks; (**b**) BTP compound in blue balls and sticks (whereas H-bonds have a green color and H-*pi* ones are yellow); and (**c**) the co-crystalized ligand 2D representation of the chemical interactions with the given protein, where H-bonds are in green while hydrophobic bonds are in orange.

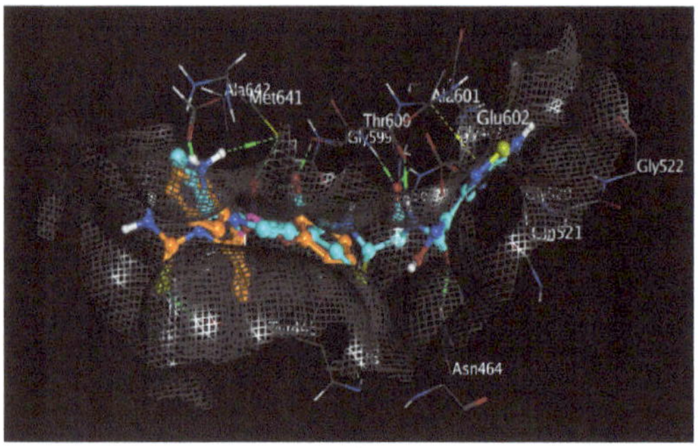

(**a**)

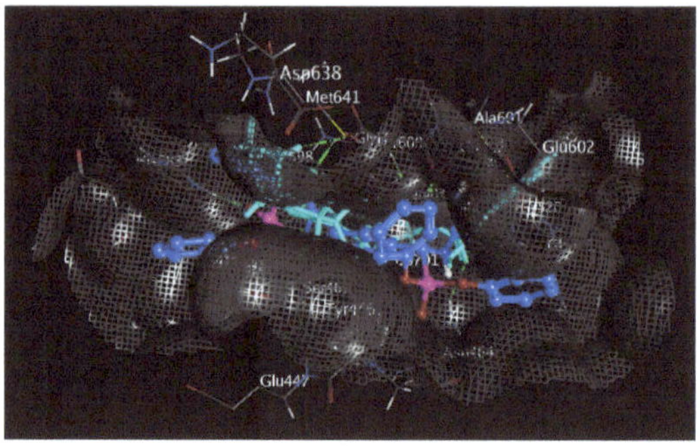

(**b**)

Figure 14. *Cont.*

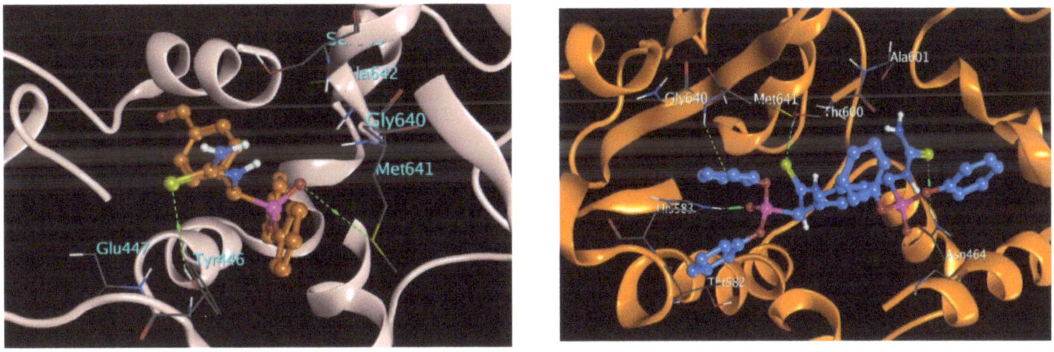

(c) (d)

Figure 14. Surface of interaction at the *MRSA* protein active site showing the co-crystalized ligand in cyan balls and/or sticks complexed with (**a**) MTP compound (orange balls and sticks) and (**b**) BTP compound (blue balls and sticks). Chemical bonding involved in the interaction between the *MRSA* protein active site and (**c**) MTP compound (orange balls and sticks) and (**d**) BTP compound (blue balls and sticks), where H-bonds have a green color and H–pi bonds are yellow color.

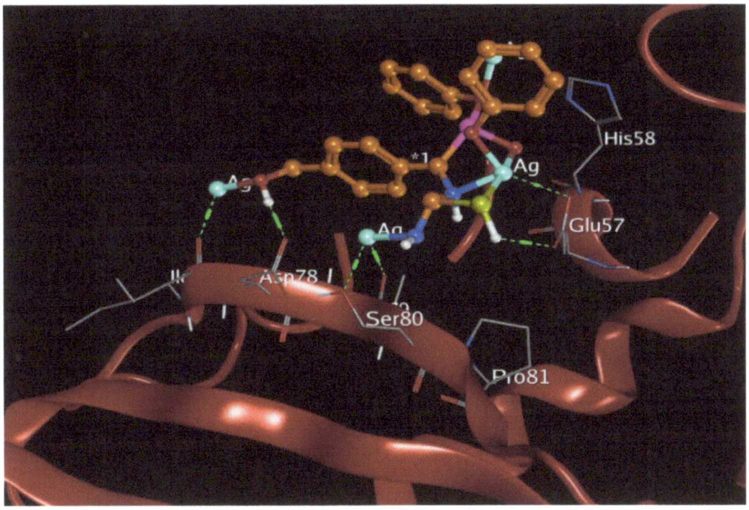

Figure 15. Site view of amino acids involved in interactions of MTP/Ag NC with *Bacillus subtilis* protein PDB-2FQT. *1 is the position of the co-crystalized ligand.

It is pertinent to note that in this study, the structural and functional diversity of raw TP surfaces afforded highly tunable surface interactions and synergy, with AgNPs giving remarkable antibacterial activity. Additionally, the molecular docking studies were in good coherence with most experimental results for TPs and TP/Ag NCs. Based on the above considerations, some structural modifications may be applied in the future to exploit these compounds in various applications such as antibacterial textile fabrics, antibacterial food packaging films, and antibacterial thermoplastic polymer nanocomposites [83–85].

3.4. In Silico Pharmacokinetics Investigation

Absorption, distribution, metabolism, and excretion (ADME) analysis is very helpful in simplifying clinical trials, especially in the early stage of drug design. Intestinal absorption, skin sensitization, and oral bioavailability are absorption parameters considered in drug discovery [86]. An intestinal absorption score >30% indicates perfect absorbance [86,87]. As tabulated in Table 10, both compounds recorded intestinal absorption of more than 30%, with excellent absorbance rates of 92% and 69% achieved for MTP-AgNPs and BTP-AgNPs, respectively. A compound is known to have relatively low skin permeability if it has log $Kp > -2.5$ [86]; however, the prepared TP/silver nanocomposites revealed good skin permeability, with permeability scores around −2.7cm/h. Compounds are considered to have high human colon adenocarcinoma (Caco-2) permeability when they record a Caco-2 value > 0.9 [86]; it measures the ability of a compound to cross a monolayer of Caco-2 cells, which are derived from human colon adenocarcinoma cells and have similar characteristics to small intestine epithelial cells. The currently investigated compounds revealed a moderate Caco2 score of 0.794 for MTP-AgNPs and very low score of −1.021 for BTP-AgNPs, which suggests that the compound may have poor absorption in the human small intestine. To investigate compounds' distribution in silico, volume of distribution (VDss), blood–brain barrier (BBB) membrane permeability, and central nervous system (CNS) permeability, were assessed. VDss values disclosed distribution volumes with −0.573 and −1.411 log L/kg for MTP-AgNPs and BTP-AgNPs, respectively (Table 10). The log BB value for compounds will reflect low BBB if <−1, as reported. MTP-AgNPs expressed −1.404, while BTP-AgNPs disclosed a low permeability of the BBB membrane with a score of −2.836. Log permeability surface (PS) values for CNS permeability were −2.434 and −3.136 for MTP-AgNPs and BTP-AgNPs, respectively, and since low CNS permeability is reported if log PS is <−3 [86], MTP-AgNPs is considered to have promising CNS permeability while BTP-AgNPs shows CNS impermeability. Hepatic and renal clearance were used to examine the overall drug clearance. Total clearance calculates the drug concentration in the body utilizing the elimination rate. A compound's excretion rate is demonstrated in log (mL/min/kg) (Table 10). The anticipated scores for ADME analysis are summarized (Table 10). In drug design, toxicity is a significant criterion which plays a remarkable role in the selection of sufficient drug candidates [88]. Regarding AMES toxicity, a positive test indicates a compound is mutagenic and carcinogenic [86,88]. Compound MTP-AgNPs has mutagen properties and hence the expected cytotoxicity; on the contrary, compound BTP-AgNPs recorded no AMES toxicity; however, both compounds revealed neither predicted hepatotoxicity nor skin allergic response. ERG inhibition (I and II) is a fundamental agent for toxicity analysis, in addition to it also including cardiotoxicity; hERG I was inhibited by both screened compounds. Toxicity against T. Pyriformis protozoa's recorded IGC_{50} value was 0.335 and 0.285log μg/L for MTP-AgNPs and BTP-AgNPs, respectively. The anticipated scores are summarized below.

Table 10. In silico ADMET assessment of the prepared TP/Ag NCs.

Model Name	Predicted Value for MTP-AgNPs	Predicted Value for BTP-AgNPs
Absorption		
Water solubility (log mol/L)	−4.889	−2.945
Caco-2 permeability (log Papp in 10^{-6} cm/s	0.794	−1.021
Intestinal absorption (human) (% Absorbed)	92.615	69.71
Skin Permeability (log Kp)	−2.738	−2.735
Distribution		
VDss (human)	−0.573	−1.411
Fraction unbound (human)	0	0.253
BBB permeability	−1.404	−2.836
CNS permeability	−2.434	−3.136

Table 10. *Cont.*

Model Name	Predicted Value for MTP-AgNPs	Predicted Value for BTP-AgNPs
Metabolism		
CYP2D6 substrate	No	Yes
CYP3A4 substrate	Yes	Yes
CYP1A2 inhibitor	Yes	No
CYP2C19 inhibitor	Yes	Yes
CYP2C9 inhibitor	Yes	Yes
CYP2D6 inhibitor	No	No
CYP3A4 inhibition	Yes	Yes
Excretion		
Total Clearance (log mL/min/kg)	−0.555	−1.316
Renal OCT2 substrate (Yes/No)	No	No
Toxicity		
AMES toxicity	Yes	No
Max. tolerated dose (human) (log mg/kg/day)	0.145	0.412
hERG I inhibitor	No	No
hERG II inhibitor	Yes	Yes
Oral Rat Acute Toxicity (LD50) (mol/kg)	2.532	2.439
Hepatotoxicity	No	No
Skin Sensitization	No	No
T. Pyriformis toxicity (log μg/L)	0.335	0.285

4. Conclusions

Two potent antibacterial agents were facilely synthesized in a one-pot green Kabachnik–Fields reaction and then exploited as reducing/capping surfaces for Ag^+ ions affording TP/Ag NCs, the physicochemical properties of which were thoroughly investigated through FT-IR, (^{1}H, ^{13}C, and ^{31}P)-NMR, elemental analysis, and TEM, XRD, and XPS analyses, respectively. The antibacterial properties of the as-prepared raw cores were studied via tuning different concentrations of silver nitrate, i.e., 100, 500, and 1000 mg L^{-1}. Both raw Mono-TP and Bis-TP analogues proved to be bactericidal towards all isolates. In a dose-increasing manner, time–kill assay results manifested the record-breaking bactericidal effect of both MTP(BTP)/Ag-1000 towards all *MRSA* cells within 8 h. At high concentrations, the antifouling characteristics of evaluated compounds were influenced by the surface electrostatic repulsion with MRSA (ATCC-43300), while hydrophobicity played a critical role at lower concentrations. Targeting the biofilm of *MRSA* (ATCC-43300) was confirmed, with net activity of 79.5 and 83.6% for MTP/Ag-1000 and BTP/Ag-1000, progressively, at highest used concentration. Nonetheless, higher net antibiofilm activity was observed in BTP/Ag NCs; the simpler MTP structure tuned the surface work function with Ag^+ ions, giving better colloidal AgNPs and a gradual improvement in the biofilm disruption % after the nanoloading. The docking results were in line with the experimental work, where the best results were estimated for raw BTP towards *B. subtilis*-2FQT protein, recording binding energy (BE) of −7.9776 Kcal/mol. Interestingly, the progress in BE of MTP/AgNPs to −7.6668 Kcal/mol could stem from the exerted Ag-acceptor bonds with both amino acids (SER80 and GLU57) of *B. subtilis*-2FQT protein. Further, in silico pharmacokinetics assessment was conducted as a step to predict the potential safety and toxicity of the TP/Ag NCs, which revealed AMES toxicity for one of the compounds with neither hepatic toxicity nor skin sensitization. In summary, this study has provided a good design for the synthesis and development of a new generation of nano-based aminophosphonate composites as promising antibacterial candidates, although their safety should be carefully evaluated for each specific application; further studies are needed to fully understand the toxicity mechanisms and the optimal conditions for their pharmaceutical application.

Supplementary Materials: The following supporting information can be downloaded at: https://www.mdpi.com/article/10.3390/pharmaceutics15061666/s1, Figure S1 (a,b) 1H-NMR spectra; (c,d) 13C-NMR spectra; and (e,f) 31P-NMR spectra of MTP and BTP derivatives, respectively, Figure S2. The element percentages of (a) MTP; and (b) BTP derivatives. Figure S3. The structural effect of MTP and BTP on AgNPs loading, Figure S4. Digital photos of MTP, BTP, and their Ag NCs at (100, 500, and 1000) mg L^{-1} displaying gradual changes in color with concentration increase of nanoloading, Figure S5. XPS spectra for (a) C 1s; (b) N 1s; (c) O 1s; (d) S 2p; (e) P 2p; and (f) Ag 3d in MTP/Ag500 with reference to MTP, Figure S6. Digital photos of inhibition zones developed by all antibacterial agents against MRSA compared to positive and negative controls. Figure S7. ZOI diameter percentage for treated MRSA by all studied compounds comparable to both references, Figure S8. Digital photos of inhibition zones developed by all antibacterial agents against S. mutans compared to positive and negative controls, Figure S9. Digital photos of inhibition zones developed by all antibacterial agents against B. subtilis compared to positive and negative controls, Figure S10. Digital photos of inhibition zones developed by all antibacterial agents against P. aeruginosa compared to positive and negative controls, Figure S11. Digital photos of inhibition zones developed by all antibacterial agents against S. typhi compared to positive and negative controls, Figure S12. Digital photos of inhibition zones developed by all antibacterial agents against S. marcescens compared to positive and negative controls, Figure S13. 3D-representation figure for the ZOI values of all antibacterial agents towards the treated Gram positive and negative strains.; Figure S14. The zeta potential of (a) MTP/Ag-1000; and (b) BTP/Ag-10000 respectively, Figure S15. Influence of MTP, and MTP/Ag NCs (100, 500, and 1000 mg Ag L^{-1}) on the viability of MRSA (ATCC-43300) biofilm via crystal violet staining. The experiments were conducted with three duplicates, Figure S16. Influence of BTP, and BTP/Ag NCs (100, 500, and 1000 mg Ag L^{-1}) on the viability of MRSA (ATCC-43300) biofilm via crystal violet staining. The experiments were conducted with three duplicates.; Table S1. The elemental analysis data of MTP and BTP conjugates, Table S2. The FT-IR data of MTP, BTP, and their AgNP dispersions in 100, 500, and 1000 mg Ag L^{-1}, Table S3. XPS data along with the chemical assignments for each functional group in MTP/Ag-500 NC in comparison to AgNPs-free MTP, Table S4. Comparative ZOI and MIC values of studied antibacterial agents with some reported in literature (References [89–101] are cited in the Supplementary Materials).

Author Contributions: Conceptualization, N.F.A., E.I.E. and A.I.E.-T.; methodology, A.I.E.-T., E.I.E. and A.U.S.; software, E.I.E. and A.I.E.-T.; validation, A.I.E.-T., E.I.E., S.M.E., A.A.H.A.A., R.B. and N.F.A.; formal analysis, A.I.E.-T., A.U.S., S.M.E. and N.E.E.; investigation, A.I.E.-T., E.I.E., N.E.E. and N.F.A.; resources, A.I.E.-T., E.I.E., A.A.H.A.A. and W.H.E.; data curation, A.I.E.-T., A.A.H.A.A., S.M.E., W.H.E. and A.U.S.; writing—original draft preparation, A.I.E.-T., E.I.E., A.U.S., N.E.E. and A.A.H.A.A.; writing—review and editing, A.I.E.-T., E.I.E. and N.F.A.; visualization, A.I.E.-T., E.I.E., S.M.E., A.A.H.A.A., R.B. and N.F.A.; supervision, N.F.A. and E.I.E.; funding acquisition, E.I.E. and R.B. All authors have read and agreed to the published version of the manuscript.

Funding: This work was funded by Princess Nourah bint Abdulrahman University Researchers Supporting Project number (PNURSP2023R304).

Institutional Review Board Statement: Not applicable.

Informed Consent Statement: Not applicable.

Data Availability Statement: Not applicable.

Acknowledgments: The authors acknowledge funding for this work by Princess Nourah bint Abdulrahman University Researchers Supporting Project number (PNURSP2023R304), Princess Nourah bint Abdulrahman University, Riyadh, Saudi Arabia.

Conflicts of Interest: The authors declare no conflict of interest.

References

1. Murray, C.J.; Ikuta, K.S.; Sharara, F.; Swetschinski, L.; Aguilar, G.R.; Gray, A.; Han, C.; Bisignano, C.; Rao, P.; Wool, E.J.T.L. Global burden of bacterial antimicrobial resistance in 2019: A systematic analysis. *Lancet* **2022**, *399*, 629–655. [CrossRef] [PubMed]
2. Larsson, D.J.; Flach, C. Antibiotic resistance in the environment. *Nat. Rev. Microbiol.* **2022**, *20*, 257–269. [CrossRef] [PubMed]
3. Yadav, H.; Mahalvar, A.; Pradhan, M.; Yadav, K.; Sahu, K.K.; Yadav, R. Exploring the potential of phytochemicals and nanomaterial: A boon to antimicrobial treatment. *Med. Drug Discov.* **2023**, *17*, 100151. [CrossRef]

4. Mirzaei, R.; Ranjbar, R. Hijacking host components for bacterial biofilm formation: An advanced mechanism. *Int. Immunopharmacol.* **2022**, *103*, 108471. [CrossRef]
5. Goel, N.; Hashmi, Z.; Khan, N.; Ahmad, R.; Khan, W.H. Recent Strategies to Combat Multidrug Resistance. In *Non-Traditional Approaches to Combat Antimicrobial Drug Resistance*; Springer: Berlin/Heidelberg, Germany, 2023; pp. 1–27. [CrossRef]
6. Singh, R.; Dutt, S.; Sharma, P.; Sundramoorthy, A.K.; Dubey, A.; Singh, A.; Arya, S. Future of Nanotechnology in Food Industry: Challenges in Processing, Packaging, and Food Safety. *Glob. Chall.* **2023**, *7*, 2200209. [CrossRef] [PubMed]
7. Sinha, A.; Simnani, F.Z.; Singh, D.; Nandi, A.; Choudhury, A.; Patel, P.; Jha, E.; Kaushik, N.K.; Mishra, Y.K.; Panda, P. The translational paradigm of nanobiomaterials: Biological chemistry to modern applications. *Mater. Today Bio* **2022**, *17*, 100463. [CrossRef]
8. Sun, Y.; Waterhouse, G.I.; Qiao, X.; Xiao, J.; Xu, Z. Determination of chloramphenicol in food using nanomaterial-based electrochemical and optical sensors—A review. *Food Chem.* **2023**, *410*, 135434. [CrossRef]
9. Xia, K.; Yamaguchi, K.; Suzuki, K. Recent Advances in Hybrid Materials of Metal Nanoparticles and Polyoxometalates. *Angew. Chem. Int. Ed. Engl.* **2023**, *62*, e202214506. [CrossRef] [PubMed]
10. Farooq, U.; Ahmad, T.; Naaz, F.; Islam, S. Review on Metals and Metal Oxides in Sustainable Energy Production: Progress and Perspectives. *Energy Fuels* **2023**, *37*, 1577–1632. [CrossRef]
11. Frei, A.; Verderosa, A.D.; Elliott, A.G.; Zuegg, J.; Blaskovich, M. Metals to combat antimicrobial resistance. *Nat. Rev. Chem.* **2023**, *7*, 202–224. [CrossRef] [PubMed]
12. Ali, M.R.; Wu, Y.; El-Sayed, M. Gold-nanoparticle-assisted plasmonic photothermal therapy advances toward clinical application. *Nanomedicine* **2019**, *123*, 15375–15393. [CrossRef]
13. Chandrakala, V.; Aruna, V.; Angajala, G. Review on metal nanoparticles as nanocarriers: Current challenges and perspectives in drug delivery systems. *Emergent Mater.* **2022**, *5*, 1593–1615. [CrossRef] [PubMed]
14. Zhao, R.; Xiang, J.; Wang, B.; Chen, L.; Tan, S. Recent advances in the development of noble metal NPs for cancer therapy. *Bioinorg. Chem. Appl.* **2022**, *2022*, 2444516. [CrossRef] [PubMed]
15. Lu, C.; Zhou, S.; Gao, F.; Lin, J.; Liu, J.; Zheng, J. DNA-mediated growth of noble metal nanomaterials for biosensing applications. *TrAC Trends Anal. Chem.* **2022**, *148*, 116533. [CrossRef]
16. González-Pedroza, M.G.; Benítez, A.R.T.; Navarro-Marchal, S.A.; Martínez-Martínez, E.; Marchal, J.A.; Boulaiz, H.; Morales-Luckie, R. Biogeneration of silver nanoparticles from Cuphea procumbens for biomedical and environmental applications. *Sci. Rep.* **2023**, *13*, 790. [CrossRef]
17. Napagoda, M.; Wijayaratne, G.B.; Witharana, S. Applications of Nanotechnology in Dermatology. In *Nanotechnology in Modern Medicine*; Springer: Berlin/Heidelberg, Germany, 2022; pp. 135–168. [CrossRef]
18. Joshi, A.S.; Singh, P.; Mijakovic, I. Interactions of gold and silver nanoparticles with bacterial biofilms: Molecular interactions behind inhibition and resistance. *Int. J. Mol. Sci.* **2020**, *21*, 7658. [CrossRef]
19. Terzioğlu, E.; Arslan, M.; Balaban, B.G.; Çakar, Z. Microbial silver resistance mechanisms: Recent developments. *World J. Microbiol. Biotechnol.* **2022**, *38*, 158. [CrossRef]
20. Akter, M.; Sikder, M.T.; Rahman, M.M.; Ullah, A.A.; Hossain, K.F.B.; Banik, S.; Hosokawa, T.; Saito, T.; Kurasaki, M. A systematic review on silver nanoparticles-induced cytotoxicity: Physicochemical properties and perspectives. *J. Adv. Res.* **2018**, *9*, 1–16. [CrossRef]
21. Malik, M.; Iqbal, M.A.; Iqbal, Y.; Malik, M.; Bakhsh, S.; Irfan, S.; Ahmad, R.; Pham, P. Biosynthesis of silver nanoparticles for biomedical applications: A mini review. *Inorg. Chem. Commun.* **2022**, *145*, 109980. [CrossRef]
22. Attia, N.F.; Moussa, M.; Sheta, A.M.; Taha, R.; Gamal, H. Synthesis of effective multifunctional textile based on silica nanoparticles. *Prog. Org. Coat.* **2017**, *106*, 41–49. [CrossRef]
23. Attia, N.F.; Eid, A.M.; Soliman, M.A.; Nagy, M. Exfoliation and decoration of graphene sheets with silver nanoparticles and their antibacterial properties. *J. Polym. Environ.* **2018**, *26*, 1072–1077. [CrossRef]
24. Dallas, P.; Sharma, V.K.; Zboril, R. polymeric nanocomposites as advanced antimicrobial agents: Classification, synthetic paths, applications, and perspectives. *Adv. Colloid. Interface Sci.* **2011**, *166*, 119–135. [CrossRef]
25. Li, S.; Mu, B.; Zhang, H.; Kang, Y.; Wang, A. Incorporation of silver nanoparticles/curcumin/clay minerals into chitosan film for enhancing mechanical properties, antioxidant and antibacterial activity. *Int. J. Biol. Macromol.* **2022**, *223*, 779–789. [CrossRef] [PubMed]
26. Mohammed, A.M.; Hassan, K.T.; Hassan, O. Assessment of antimicrobial activity of chitosan/silver nanoparticles hydrogel and cryogel microspheres. *Int. J. Biol. Macromol.* **2023**, *233*, 123580. [CrossRef]
27. Ren, R.; Lim, C.; Li, S.; Wang, Y.; Song, J.; Lin, T.-W.; Muir, B.W.; Hsu, H.-Y.; Shen, H.-H.J.N. Recent Advances in the Development of Lipid-, Metal-, Carbon-, and Polymer-Based Nanomaterials for Antibacterial Applications. *Nanomaterials* **2022**, *12*, 3855. [CrossRef] [PubMed]
28. Yousefi, M.; Ehsani, A.; Jafari, S. Lipid-based nano delivery of antimicrobials to control food-borne bacteria. *Adv. Colloid. Interface Sci.* **2019**, *270*, 263–277. [CrossRef] [PubMed]
29. Shrivastava, V.; Chauhan, P.S.; Tomar, R. Bio-Fabrication of metal nanoparticles: A review. *Int. J. Curr. Res. Life Sci.* **2018**, *7*, 1927–1932.

30. Mao, H.; Zhu, K.; Liu, X.; Yao, C.; Kobayashi, M. Facile synthetic route to Fe_3O_4/silica nanocomposites pillared clay through cationic surfactant-aliphatic acid mixed system and application for magnetically controlled drug release. *Microporous Mesoporous Mater.* **2016**, *225*, 216–223. [CrossRef]
31. Zhou, R.; Gao, H. Cytotoxicity of graphene: Recent advances and future perspective. *Wiley Interdiscip. Rev. Nanomed. Nanobiotechnol.* **2014**, *6*, 452–474. [CrossRef]
32. Wang, Z.; Sun, C.; Yang, K.; Chen, X.; Wang, R. Cucurbituril-Based Supramolecular Polymers for Biomedical Applications. *Angew. Chem. Int. Ed. Engl.* **2022**, *61*, e202206763. [CrossRef]
33. Gurunathan, S.; Kim, J.H. Synthesis, toxicity, biocompatibility, and biomedical applications of graphene and graphene-related materials. *Int. J. Nanomed.* **2016**, *11*, 1927–1945. [CrossRef] [PubMed]
34. Amira, A.; Aouf, Z.; K'tir, H.; Chemam, Y.; Ghodbane, R.; Zerrouki, R.; Aouf, N.-E. Recent Advances in the Synthesis of α-Aminophosphonates: A Review. *ChemistrySelect* **2021**, *6*, 6137–6149. [CrossRef]
35. Keri, R.; Patil, M.; Brahmkhatri, V.P.; Budagumpi, S.; Adimule, V. Copper (II)-β-Cyclodextrin Promoted Kabachnik-Fields Reaction: An Efficient, One-Pot Synthesis of α-Aminophosphonates. *Top. Catal.* **2022**. [CrossRef]
36. Neiber, R.R.; Galhoum, A.A.; El-Tantawy El Sayed, I.; Guibal, E.; Xin, J.; Lu, X. Selective lead (II) sorption using aminophosphonate-based sorbents: Effect of amine linker, characterization and sorption performance. *Chem. Eng. J.* **2022**, *442*, 136300. [CrossRef]
37. Fouda, S.R.; El-Sayed, I.E.; Attia, N.F.; Abdeen, M.M.; Abdel Aleem, A.A.H.; Nassar, I.F.; Mira, H.I.; Gawad, E.A.; Kalam, A.; Al-Ghamdi, A.A.; et al. Mechanistic study of Hg(II) interaction with three different α-aminophosphonate adsorbents: Insights from batch experiments and theoretical calculations. *Chemosphere* **2022**, *304*, 135253. [CrossRef] [PubMed]
38. Galhoum, A.A.; Elshehy, E.A.; Tolan, D.A.; El-Nahas, A.M.; Taketsugu, T.; Nishikiori, K.; Akashi, T.; Morshedy, A.S.; Guibal, E. Synthesis of polyaminophosphonic acid-functionalized poly(glycidyl methacrylate) for the efficient sorption of La(III) and Y(III). *Chem. Eng. J.* **2019**, *375*, 121932. [CrossRef]
39. Imam, E.A.; Hashem, A.I.; Tolba, A.A.; Mahfouz, M.G.; El-Sayed, I.E.-T.; El-Tantawy, A.I.; Galhoum, A.A.; Guibal, E. Effect of mono-vs. bi-functionality of aminophosphonate derivatives on the enhancement of U (VI) sorption: Physicochemical properties and sorption performance. *J. Environ. Chem. Eng.* **2023**, *11*, 109951. [CrossRef]
40. Sipyagina, N.A.; Malkova, A.N.; Straumal, E.A.; Yurkova, L.L.; Baranchikov, A.E.; Ivanov, V.K.; Lermontov, S.A. Novel aminophosphonate ligand for the preparation of catalytically active silica aerogels with finely dispersed palladium. *J. Porous Mater.* **2023**, *30*, 449–457. [CrossRef]
41. Delehedde, C.; Culcasi, M.; Ricquebourg, E.; Cassien, M.; Siri, D.; Blaive, B.; Pietri, S.; Thétiot-Laurent, S. Novel Sterically Crowded and Conformationally Constrained α-Aminophosphonates with a Near-Neutral pKa as Highly Accurate 31P NMR pH Probes. Application to Subtle pH Gradients Determination in Dictyostelium discoideum. *Cells* **2022**, *27*, 4506.
42. Silva, V.B.; Santos, Y.H.; Hellinger, R.; Mansour, S.; Delaune, A.; Legros, J.; Zinoviev, S.; Nogueira, E.S.; Orth, E.S. Organophosphorus chemical security from a peaceful perspective: Sustainable practices in its synthesis, decontamination and detection. *Green. Chem.* **2022**, *24*, 585–613. [CrossRef]
43. Nikitin, E.; Shumatbaev, G.; Terenzhev, D.; Sinyashin, K.O.; Kazimova, K. New α-Aminophosphonates as Corrosion Inhibitors for Oil and Gas Pipelines Protection. *Civ. Eng. J.* **2019**, *5*, 963–970. [CrossRef]
44. Aissa, R.; Guezane-Lakoud, S.; Toffano, M.; Gali, L.; Aribi-Zouioueche, L. Fiaud's Acid, a novel organocatalyst for diastereoselective bis α-aminophosphonates synthesis with in-vitro biological evaluation of antifungal, antioxidant and enzymes inhibition potential. *Bioorganic Med. Chem. Lett.* **2021**, *41*, 128000. [CrossRef]
45. Elsherbiny, D.A.; Abdelgawad, A.M.; El-Naggar, M.E.; El-Sherbiny, R.A.; El-Rafie, M.H.; El-Sayed, I.E.-T. Synthesis, antimicrobial activity, and sustainable release of novel α-aminophosphonate derivatives loaded carrageenan cryogel. *Int. J. Biol. Macromol.* **2020**, *163*, 96–107. [CrossRef] [PubMed]
46. Boshta, N.M.; Elgamal, E.A.; El-Sayed, I.E.T. Bioactive amide and α-aminophosphonate inhibitors for methicillin-resistant Staphylococcus aureus (MRSA). *Monatsh. Chem.* **2018**, *149*, 2349–2358. [CrossRef]
47. Joossens, J.; Ali, O.M.; El-Sayed, I.; Surpateanu, G.; Van der Veken, P.; Lambeir, A.-M.; Setyono-Han, B.; Foekens, J.A.; Schneider, A.; Schmalix, W.; et al. Small, Potent, and Selective Diaryl Phosphonate Inhibitors for Urokinase-Type Plasminogen Activator with In Vivo Antimetastatic Properties. *J. Med. Chem.* **2007**, *50*, 6638–6646. [CrossRef]
48. Saleh, N.M.; Moemen, Y.S.; Mohamed, S.H.; Fathy, G.; Ahmed, A.A.S.; Al-Ghamdi, A.A.; Ullah, S.; El Sayed, I.E. Experimental and Molecular Docking Studies of Cyclic Diphenyl Phosphonates as DNA Gyrase Inhibitors for Fluoroquinolone-Resistant Pathogens. *Antibiotics.* **2022**, *11*, 53. [CrossRef]
49. Sharaf, A.; Ragab, S.S.; Elbarbary, A.A.; Shaban, E.; El Sayed, I.E.T. Synthesis and biological evaluation of some 3H-quinazolin-4-one derivatives. *J. Iran. Chem. Soc.* **2022**, *19*, 291–302. [CrossRef]
50. Attia, N.F.; Morsy, M.S. Facile synthesis of novel nanocomposite as antibacterial and flame retardant material for textile fabrics. *Mater. Chem. Phys.* **2016**, *180*, 364–372. [CrossRef]
51. Alshehri, L.A.; Attia, N.F. Reinforcement and Antibacterial Properties of Hand Embroidery Threads Based on Green Nanocoatings. *Coatings* **2023**, *13*, 747. [CrossRef]
52. Ayad, M.M.; Amer, W.A.; Kotp, M.G.; Minisy, I.M.; Rehab, A.F.; Kopecký, D.; Fitl, P. Synthesis of silver-anchored polyaniline–chitosan magnetic nanocomposite: A smart system for catalysis. *RSC Adv.* **2017**, *7*, 18553–18560. [CrossRef]
53. Vilar, S.; Cozza, G.; Moro, S. Medicinal chemistry and the molecular operating environment (MOE): Application of QSAR and molecular docking to drug discovery. *Curr. Top. Med. Chem.* **2008**, *8*, 1555–1572. [CrossRef] [PubMed]

54. Lovering, A.L.; Gretes, M.C.; Safadi, S.S.; Danel, F.; de Castro, L.; Page, M.G.P.; Strynadka, N.C.J. Structural Insights into the Anti-methicillin-resistant Staphylococcus aureus (MRSA) Activity of Ceftobiprole. *J. Biol. Chem.* **2012**, *287*, 32096–32102. [CrossRef] [PubMed]
55. Shen, G.; Rajan, R.; Zhu, J.; Bell, C.E.; Pei, D. Design and Synthesis of Substrate and Intermediate Analogue Inhibitors of S-Ribosylhomocysteinase. *J. Med. Chem.* **2006**, *49*, 3003–3011. [CrossRef] [PubMed]
56. Zhong, W.; Pasunooti, K.K.; Balamkundu, S.; Wong, Y.H.; Nah, Q.; Gadi, V.; Gnanakalai, S.; Chionh, Y.H.; McBee, M.E.; Gopal, P.; et al. Thienopyrimidinone Derivatives That Inhibit Bacterial tRNA (Guanine37-N(1))-Methyltransferase (TrmD) by Restructuring the Active Site with a Tyrosine-Flipping Mechanism. *J. Med. Chem.* **2019**, *62*, 7788–7805. [CrossRef]
57. Lunelli, M.; Hurwitz, R.; Lambers, J.; Kolbe, M. Crystal structure of PrgI-SipD: Insight into a secretion competent state of the type three secretion system needle tip and its interaction with host ligands. *PLoS Pathog.* **2011**, *7*, e1002163. [CrossRef]
58. Elmongy, E.I.; Altwaijry, N.; Attallah, N.G.M.; AlKahtani, M.M.; Henidi, H.A. In-Silico Screening of Novel Synthesized Thienopyrimidines Targeting Fms Related Receptor Tyrosine Kinase-3 and Their In-Vitro Biological Evaluation. *Pharmaceuticals* **2022**, *15*, 170. [CrossRef]
59. Elmongy, E.I.; Ahmed, A.A.S.; El Sayed, I.E.T.; Fathy, G.; Awad, H.M.; Salman, A.U.; Hamed, M.A. Synthesis, Biocidal and Antibiofilm Activities of New Isatin–Quinoline Conjugates against Multidrug-Resistant Bacterial Pathogens along with Their In Silico Screening. *Antibiotics* **2022**, *11*, 1507. [CrossRef]
60. Attia, N.F.; Lee, S.M.; Kim, H.J.; Geckeler, K.E. Preparation of polypyrrole nanoparticles and their composites: Effect of electronic properties on hydrogen adsorption. *Polym. Int.* **2015**, *64*, 696–703. [CrossRef]
61. Ogundare, S.A.; Muungani, G.; Amaku, J.F.; Ogunmoye, A.O.; Adesetan, T.O.; Olubomehin, O.O.; Ibikunle, A.A.; van Zyl, W.E. *Mangifera indica* L. stem bark used in the bioinspired formation of silver nanoparticles: Catalytic and antibacterial applications. *Chem. Zvesti* **2023**, *77*, 2647–2656. [CrossRef]
62. Eisa, W.H.; Zayed, M.F.; Anis, B.; Abbas, L.M.; Ali, S.S.M.; Mostafa, A.M. Clean production of powdery silver nanoparticles using Zingiber officinale: The structural and catalytic properties. *J. Clean. Prod.* **2019**, *241*, 118398. [CrossRef]
63. Rather, M.A.; Deori, P.J.; Gupta, K.; Daimary, N.; Deka, D.; Qureshi, A.; Dutta, T.K.; Joardar, S.N.; Mandal, M. Ecofriendly phytofabrication of silver nanoparticles using aqueous extract of Cuphea carthagenensis and their antioxidant potential and antibacterial activity against clinically important human pathogens. *Chemosphere* **2022**, *300*, 134497. [CrossRef] [PubMed]
64. Wang, J.; Ansari, M.F.; Lin, J.-M.; Zhou, C.-H. Design and Synthesis of Sulfanilamide Aminophosphonates as Novel Antibacterial Agents towards Escherichia coli. *Chin. J. Chem.* **2021**, *39*, 2251–2263. [CrossRef]
65. Yang, X.-C.; Zeng, C.-M.; Avula, S.R.; Peng, X.-M.; Geng, R.-X.; Zhou, C. Novel coumarin aminophosphonates as potential multitargeting antibacterial agents against Staphylococcus aureus. *Eur. J. Med. Chem.* **2023**, *245*, 114891. [CrossRef] [PubMed]
66. Singh, S.; Mishra, P. Bacitracin and isothiocyanate functionalized silver nanoparticles for synergistic and broad spectrum antibacterial and antibiofilm activity with selective toxicity to bacteria over mammalian cells. *Adv. Biomater.* **2022**, *133*, 112649. [CrossRef] [PubMed]
67. Sánchez-Salcedo, S.; García, A.; González-Jiménez, A.; Vallet-Regí, M.J.A.B. Antibacterial effect of 3D printed mesoporous bioactive glass scaffolds doped with metallic silver nanoparticles. *Acta Biomater.* **2023**, *155*, 654–666. [CrossRef]
68. Oh, J.K.; Yegin, Y.; Yang, F.; Zhang, M.; Li, J.; Huang, S.; Verkhoturov, S.V.; Schweikert, E.A.; Perez-Lewis, K.; Scholar, E. The influence of surface chemistry on the kinetics and thermodynamics of bacterial adhesion. *Sci. Rep.* **2018**, *8*, 17247. [CrossRef]
69. Abu Jarad, N.; Rachwalski, K.; Bayat, F.; Khan, S.; Shakeri, A.; MacLachlan, R.; Villegas, M.; Brown, E.D.; Hosseinidoust, Z.; Didar, T.F.; et al. A Bifunctional Spray Coating Reduces Contamination on Surfaces by Repelling and Killing Pathogens. *ACS Appl. Mater. Interfaces* **2023**, *15*, 16253–16265. [CrossRef]
70. Monserud, J.H.; Schwartz, D.K. Effects of molecular size and surface hydrophobicity on oligonucleotide interfacial dynamics. *Biomacromolecules* **2012**, *13*, 4002–4011. [CrossRef]
71. Cui, Q.; Bian, R.; Xu, F.; Li, Q.; Wang, W.; Bian, Q. Chapter 10—New molecular entities and structure–activity relationships of drugs designed by the natural product derivatization method from 2010 to 2018. In *Studies in Natural Products Chemistry*; Atta ur, R., Ed.; Elsevier: Amsterdam, The Netherlands, 2021; Volume 69, pp. 371–415. [CrossRef]
72. Sahli, C.; Moya, S.E.; Lomas, J.S.; Gravier-Pelletier, C.; Briandet, R.; Hémadi, M. Recent advances in nanotechnology for eradicating bacterial biofilm. *Theranostics* **2022**, *12*, 2383–2405. [CrossRef]
73. Borse, A.; Shinde, N.; Bhosale, S.K. Dipeptide Conjugates: An Important Class of Therapeutic Agents. *Indian J. Pharm. Educ. Res.* **2023**, *57*, 15–21. [CrossRef]
74. Cella, M.A.; Coulson, T.; MacEachern, S.; Badr, S.; Ahmadi, A.; Tabatabaei, M.S.; Labbe, A.; Griffiths, M.W.J.S.R. Probiotic disruption of quorum sensing reduces virulence and increases cefoxitin sensitivity in methicillin-resistant Staphylococcus aureus. *Sci. Rep.* **2023**, *13*, 4373. [CrossRef] [PubMed]
75. Jan, B.; Jan, R.; Afzal, S.; Ayoub, M.; Masoodi, M.H. Treatment Strategies to Combat Multidrug Resistance (MDR) in Bacteria. In *Non-Traditional Approaches to Combat Antimicrobial Drug Resistance*; Springer: Berlin/Heidelberg, Germany, 2023; pp. 79–100. [CrossRef]
76. Li, D.; Bheemanaboina, R.R.Y.; Battini, N.; Tangadanchu, V.K.R.; Fang, X.F.; Zhou, C.H. Novel organophosphorus aminopyrimidines as unique structural DNA-targeting membrane active inhibitors towards drug-resistant methicillin-resistant Staphylococcus aureus. *MedChemComm* **2018**, *9*, 1529–1537. [CrossRef] [PubMed]

77. McNeilly, O.; Mann, R.; Hamidian, M.; Gunawan, C. Emerging Concern for Silver Nanoparticle Resistance in Acinetobacter baumannii and Other Bacteria. *Front. Microbiol.* **2021**, *12*, 652863. [CrossRef]
78. Wu, J.; Li, F.; Hu, X.; Lu, J.; Sun, X.; Gao, J.; Ling, D. Responsive Assembly of Silver Nanoclusters with a Biofilm Locally Amplified Bactericidal Effect to Enhance Treatments against Multi-Drug-Resistant Bacterial Infections. *ACS Cent. Sci.* **2019**, *5*, 1366–1376. [CrossRef]
79. Wang, J.; Li, J.; Guo, G.; Wang, Q.; Tang, J.; Zhao, Y.; Qin, H.; Wahafu, T.; Shen, H.; Liu, X. Silver-nanoparticles-modified biomaterial surface resistant to staphylococcus: New insight into the antimicrobial action of silver. *Sci. Rep.* **2016**, *6*, 32699. [CrossRef] [PubMed]
80. Karthik, C.S.; Chethana, M.H.; Manukumar, H.M.; Ananda, A.P.; Sandeep, S.; Nagashree, S.; Mallesha, L.; Mallu, P.; Jayanth, H.S.; Dayananda, B.P. Synthesis and characterization of chitosan silver nanoparticle decorated with benzodioxane coupled piperazine as an effective anti-biofilm agent against MRSA: A validation of molecular docking and dynamics. *Int. J. Biol. Macromol.* **2021**, *181*, 540–551. [CrossRef]
81. Majumdar, M.; Khan, S.A.; Biswas, S.C.; Roy, D.N.; Panja, A.S.; Misra, T.K. In vitro and in silico investigation of anti-biofilm activity of Citrus macroptera fruit extract mediated silver nanoparticles. *J. Mol. Liq.* **2020**, *302*, 112586. [CrossRef]
82. Duanis-Assaf, D.; Steinberg, D.; Chai, Y.; Shemesh, M. The LuxS Based Quorum Sensing Governs Lactose Induced Biofilm Formation by Bacillus subtilis. *Front. Microbiol.* **2015**, *6*, 1517. [CrossRef]
83. Attia, N.F.; Mohamed, A.; Hussein, A.; El-Demerdash, A.-G.M.; Kandil, S. Bio-inspired one-dimensional based textile fabric coating for integrating high flame retardancy, antibacterial, toxic gases suppression, antiviral and reinforcement properties. *Polym. Degrad. Stab.* **2022**, *205*, 110152. [CrossRef]
84. Sharma, C.; Dhiman, R.; Rokana, N.; Panwar, H. Nanotechnology: An untapped resource for food packaging. *Front. Microbiol.* **2017**, *8*, 1735. [CrossRef]
85. Attia, N. Nanoporous carbon doped with metal oxide microsphere as renewable flame retardant for integrating high flame retardancy and antibacterial properties of thermoplastic polymer composites. *J. Therm. Anal. Calorim.* **2023**, *148*, 5335–5346. [CrossRef]
86. Pires, D.E.; Blundell, T.L.; Ascher, D. pkCSM: Predicting small-molecule pharmacokinetic and toxicity properties using graph-based signatures. *J. Med. Chem.* **2015**, *58*, 4066–4072. [CrossRef] [PubMed]
87. Dahlgren, D.; Lennernäs, H. Intestinal permeability and drug absorption: Predictive experimental, computational and in vivo approaches. *Pharmaceutics* **2019**, *11*, 411. [CrossRef] [PubMed]
88. Han, Y.; Zhang, J.; Hu, C.Q.; Zhang, X.; Ma, B.; Zhang, P. In silico ADME and toxicity prediction of ceftazidime and its impurities. *Front. Pharmacol.* **2019**, *10*, 434. [CrossRef]
89. Daoud, A.; Malika, D.; Bakari, S.; Hfaiedh, N.; Mnafgui, K.; Kadri, A.; Gharsallah, N. Assessment of polyphenol composition, antioxidant and antimicrobial properties of various extracts of Date Palm Pollen (DPP) from two Tunisian cultivars. *Arab. J. Chem.* **2019**, *12*, 3075–3086. [CrossRef]
90. Eloff, J.N. A Sensitive and Quick Microplate Method to Determine the Minimal Inhibitory Concentration of Plant Extracts for Bacteria. *Planta Medica* **1998**, *64*, 711–713. [CrossRef]
91. Ozturk, S.; Ercisli, S. Chemical composition and in vitro antibacterial activity of Seseli libanotis. *World J. Microbiol. Biotechnol.* **2006**, *22*, 261–265. [CrossRef]
92. Poonacha, N.; Nair, S.; Desai, S.; Tuppad, D.; Hiremath, D.; Mohan, T.; Vipra, A.; Sharma, U. Efficient Killing of Planktonic and Biofilm-Embedded Coagulase-Negative Staphylococci by Bactericidal Protein P128. *Antimicrob. Agents Chemother.* **2017**, *61*, e00457-17. [CrossRef]
93. Kemung, H.M.; Tan, L.T.-H.; Khaw, K.Y.; Ong, Y.S.; Chan, C.K.; Low, D.Y.S.; Tang, S.Y.; Goh, B.-H. An Optimized Anti-adherence and Anti-biofilm Assay: Case Study of Zinc Oxide Nanoparticles versus MRSA Biofilm. *Prog. Microbes Mol. Biol.* **2020**, *3*. [CrossRef]
94. O'Toole, G.A. Microtiter dish biofilm formation assay. *J. Vis. Exp.* **2011**, e2437.
95. Badger-Emeka, L.I.; Emeka, P.M.; Ibrahim, H.I.M. A Molecular Insight into the Synergistic Mechanism of *Nigella sativa* (Black Cumin) with β-Lactam Antibiotics against Clinical Isolates of Methicillin-Resistant *Staphylococcus aureus*. *Appl. Sci.* **2021**, *11*, 3206. [CrossRef]
96. Sebastian, D. Characterization of Green Synthesized Antibacterial Silver Nanoparticles from *Amaranthus spinosus* L. Extract. *BioNanoScience* **2022**, *12*, 502–511.
97. Ramzan, M.; Karobari, M.I.; Heboyan, A.; Mohamed, R.N.; Mustafa, M.; Basheer, S.N.; Desai, V.; Batool, S.; Ahmed, N.; Zeshan, B. Synthesis of Silver Nanoparticles from Extracts of Wild Ginger (*Zingiber zerumbet*) with Antibacterial Activity against Selective Multidrug Resistant Oral Bacteria. *Molecules* **2022**, *27*, 2007. [CrossRef]
98. Bezza, F.A.; Tichapondwa, S.M.; Chirwa, E.M. Synthesis of biosurfactant stabilized silver nanoparticles, characterization and their potential application for bactericidal purposes. *J. Hazard. Mater.* **2020**, *393*, 122319. [CrossRef] [PubMed]
99. Alsakhawy, S.A.; Baghdadi, H.H.; El-Shenawy, M.A.; El-Hosseiny, L.S. Antibacterial Activity of Silver Nanoparticles Phytosynthesized by Citrus Fruit Peel Extracts. *BioNanoScience* **2022**, *12*, 1106–1115. [CrossRef]

100. Hamida, R.S.; Ali, M.A.; A Goda, D.; Al-Zaban, M.I. Lethal Mechanisms of Nostoc-Synthesized Silver Nanoparticles Against Different Pathogenic Bacteria. *Int. J. Nanomed.* **2020**, *15*, 10499–10517. [CrossRef]
101. Kumar, M.; Wangoo, N.; Gondil, V.S.; Pandey, S.K.; Lalhall, A.; Sharma, R.K.; Chhibber, S. Glycolic acid functionalized silver nanoparticles: A novel approach towards generation of effective antibacterial agent against skin infections. *J. Drug Deliv. Sci. Technol.* **2020**, *60*, 102074. [CrossRef]

pharmaceutics

MDPI

Article

Characterization of the Antimicrobial Activities of *Trichoplusia ni* Cecropin A as a High-Potency Therapeutic against Colistin-Resistant *Escherichia coli*

Hyeju Lee [1], Byeongkwon Kim [1], Minju Kim [1], Seoyeong Yoo [1], Jinkyeong Lee [1], Eunha Hwang [2] and Yangmee Kim [1,*]

[1] Department of Bioscience and Biotechnology, Konkuk University, Seoul 05029, Republic of Korea; hju0814@konkuk.ac.kr (H.L.); matt97@konkuk.ac.kr (B.K.); alswn7074@konkuk.ac.kr (M.K.); leejk809@konkuk.ac.kr (J.L.)

[2] Center for Research Equipment, Korea Basic Science Institute, Cheongju 28119, Republic of Korea; hwang0131@kbsi.re.kr

* Correspondence: ymkim@konkuk.ac.kr; Tel.: +82-2-450-3421

Abstract: The spread of colistin-resistant bacteria is a serious threat to public health. As an alternative to traditional antibiotics, antimicrobial peptides (AMPs) show promise against multidrug resistance. In this study, we investigated the activity of the insect AMP *Tricoplusia ni* cecropin A (*T. ni* cecropin) against colistin-resistant bacteria. *T. ni* cecropin exhibited significant antibacterial and antibiofilm activities against colistin-resistant *Escherichia coli* (ColREC) with low cytotoxicity against mammalian cells in vitro. Results of permeabilization of the ColREC outer membrane as monitored through 1-N-phenylnaphthylamine uptake, scanning electron microscopy, lipopolysaccharide (LPS) neutralization, and LPS-binding interaction revealed that *T. ni* cecropin manifested antibacterial activity by targeting the outer membrane of *E. coli* with strong interaction with LPS. *T. ni* cecropin specifically targeted toll-like receptor 4 (TLR4) and showed anti-inflammatory activities with a significant reduction of inflammatory cytokines in macrophages stimulated with either LPS or ColREC via blockade of TLR4-mediated inflammatory signaling. Moreover, *T. ni* cecropin exhibited anti-septic effects in an LPS-induced endotoxemia mouse model, confirming its LPS-neutralizing activity, immunosuppressive effect, and recovery of organ damage in vivo. These findings demonstrate that *T. ni* cecropin exerts strong antimicrobial activities against ColREC and could serve as a foundation for the development of AMP therapeutics.

Keywords: antimicrobial peptide; colistin-resistant *Escherichia coli*; lipopolysaccharide; *Trichoplusia ni* cecropin

Citation: Lee, H.; Kim, B.; Kim, M.; Yoo, S.; Lee, J.; Hwang, E.; Kim, Y. Characterization of the Antimicrobial Activities of *Trichoplusia ni* Cecropin A as a High-Potency Therapeutic against Colistin-Resistant *Escherichia coli*. *Pharmaceutics* **2023**, *15*, 1752. https://doi.org/10.3390/pharmaceutics15061752

Academic Editors: Aura Rusu and Valentina Uivarosi

Received: 28 May 2023
Revised: 13 June 2023
Accepted: 13 June 2023
Published: 16 June 2023

1. Introduction

Gram-negative bacterial infections constitute a serious public health concern because they can cause extensive infections such as pneumonia, urinary tract infections, and bloodstream infections [1]. *Escherichia coli* (*E. coli*), a major cause of bacterial nosocomial infections, is treated with a variety of antibiotics and has acquired resistance to them. The production of extended-spectrum β-lactamase (ESBL) is a prominent resistance that interferes with the treatment of infections caused by *E. coli*. ESBL-producing *E. coli* acquires antibiotic resistance by hydrolyzing β-lactam antibiotics. There are various families of ESBLs, including temoniera (TEM), sulphydryl variable (SHV), and cefotaximase-Munich (CTX-M) types [2]. Carbapenems were chosen to treat ESBL-producing *E. coli*, which also developed resistance to carbapenems by producing carbapenemase [3]. *E. coli* have adapted to antibiotic environmental pressure, rendering them difficult to treat and often requiring the use of antibiotics of last resort such as colistin (polymyxin E), thereby posing a major global threat [4]. Polymyxins are polycationic antibiotics, first discovered in the 1940s, that exhibit potent activity against Gram-negative bacteria, including many that were resistant to other antibiotics [5]. However, despite their potent antibacterial activity, the use of polymyxins has been limited by their potential toxicity, including nephrotoxicity, neurotoxicity, and other adverse effects [6]. Owing to these concerns, the use of polymyxins declined in the 1980s, but with the emergence of multidrug-resistant bacteria, colistin was reconsidered as a treatment option [7].

Polymyxin B and colistin, the two types of polymyxins used in clinical practice, are polypeptides consisting of a heptapeptide ring connected to an N-terminal acylated tripeptide. The amino acids comprising the ring include D-Phe for polymyxin B, whereas colistin includes D-Leu in position 6 [8]. The mechanism of action of polymyxins involves binding to the negatively charged lipopolysaccharides (LPS) that are a component of the outer membrane of Gram-negative bacteria. LPS is composed of three domains: O-antigen, core oligosaccharide, and lipid A [9]. Polymyxins interact with LPS by binding to its lipid A portion, which is responsible for the endotoxic activity of LPS [10]. The hydrophilic part of polymyxins, which includes the cationic L-2,4-diaminobutyric acid (Dab), interacts with the negatively charged phosphate groups in the lipid A part of LPS [11]. This electrostatic interaction initially temporarily stabilizes the complex, allowing the N-terminal fatty acyl chain of the polymyxins to approach the outer membrane [12]. The hydrophobic tail of polymyxin inserts into the lipid A fatty acyl chain, eventually disrupting the integrity of the bacterial membrane. Hydrogen bonding interactions between the hydrophilic amino acids in polymyxins and the sugar moieties in LPS also contribute to the stability of the colistin–LPS complex [13]. Furthermore, the divalent cations (Ca^{2+}, Mg^{2+}) that provide additional stability to the outer membrane are substituted by colistin, leading to displacement of the cations by electrostatic interaction and resulting in disorganization of the bacterial membrane through the release of LPS [14]. Binding to LPS is essential for the antibacterial activity of polymyxins, which disrupts the integrity of the outer membrane of Gram-negative bacteria and ultimately leads to cell death [15].

Colistin is widely used clinically for the treatment of patients with Gram-negative bacterial infections; however, the emergence of colistin-resistant bacteria constitutes a growing threat, exacerbated by the lack of significant advances in the development of alternatives against bacterial infection. One of the main mechanisms by which Gram-negative bacteria develop colistin resistance is by modifying the composition of their outer membrane, mediated by bacterial adaptation to exposure to this antibiotic. This involves the alteration of LPS via cationic modification by adding a positively charged phosphoethanolamine moiety together with 4-amino-4-deoxy-L-arabinose to the 4′- and/or 1-phosphate of the lipid A part, resulting in a reduction in the electronegativity of the cell membrane. Further modifications of lipid A also include its acylation or deacylation [16]. In turn, the binding affinity of polymyxins toward LPS in colistin-resistant bacteria significantly decreases, resulting in the loss of their bactericidal activity [17,18]. Additionally, some bacteria can overexpress efflux pump systems that excrete colistin [19]. These mechanisms of resistance can emerge through spontaneous genetic mutations or be acquired through the transfer of resistance genes between bacteria [20]. Numerous studies are currently being conducted with the aim of restoring the activity of polymyxins against resistant strains by designing polymyxin derivatives. FADDI series derivatives, in which hydrophobicity was modified through the replacement of amino acids at residues 6 and 7 or by the substitution of an acyl chain, were developed by researchers at Monash University. These derivatives have been shown to exhibit improved binding to lipid A, resulting in increased activity relative to those of polymyxin B and colistin in polymyxin-resistant strains [21,22]. Ongoing clinical trials for various derivatives of polymyxin B, including SPR 206 (NCT number: NCT04868292), QPX9003 (NCT number: NCT04808414), and MRX-8 (NCT number: NCT04649541), are focused on reducing nephrotoxicity and improving pharmacokinetic properties to enhance clinical efficacy [23–25]. As such, developing alternative agents to counter colistin resistance constitutes an essential public health challenge.

Antimicrobial peptides (AMPs), which comprise innate immune molecules that combat microbials in various organisms, have come under the spotlight as an alternative potential tool to overcome the problem of antibiotic resistance [26]. AMPs typically function by disrupting bacterial membranes, leading to cell lysis and death [27]. This mechanism differs from that of conventional antibiotics, which typically target specific intracellular targets such as bacterial enzymes or proteins; AMPs also have immunomodulatory effects [28,29]. Insects in particular produce AMPs to strengthen their innate immune systems, countering their constant exposure to pathogens as a result of living in the wild; this results in high resistance to microbial infections. The first insect defense antimicrobial peptide, cecropin A (KWKLFKKIEKVGQNIRDGIIKAGPAVAVVGQATQIAK-NH 2), was isolated from the hemolymph of the moth *Hyalophora cecropia* and is classified as an α-helical AMP [30]. Subsequently, various cecropins have been isolated from insects such as the silk moth *Bombyx mori*, wax moth *Galleria mellonella*, Chinese oak silkmoth *Antheraea pernyi*, and Asian swallowtail *Papilio xuthus* [31–34]. Insect cecropins display potent antibacterial, antifungal, anticancer, and anti-septic activities [35–41]. We have determined the structure of an insect cecropin, papiliocin, containing a cationic amphipathic α-helix at the N-terminus and hydrophobic C-terminal helix connected by a hinge region, which are critical for bacterial membrane permeabilization as well as LPS interactions [42,43]. These structural components are generally conserved in insect cecropins [42,44,45].

The structural component composition involving separate amphipathic and hydrophobic parts of insect cecropins is similar to that of colistin. Consistent with this, we found that insect cecropins show antibacterial activity against Gram-negative bacteria and binding affinity to LPS comparable to those of polymyxin B and colistin; moreover, they also exhibit antibacterial activity against multidrug-resistant Gram-negative bacteria [37,46,47]. Here we further hypothesize that unlike for polymyxins, whose LPS-binding affinity is highly sensitive to the modified outer membrane LPS lipids in colistin-resistant Gram-negative bacteria, the antimicrobial activities of insect cecropins might not be disrupted by such LPS modifications as a consequence of their own evolutionary adaptation. Therefore, cecropins may represent potent candidates as new types of antibiotics against colistin-resistant Gram-negative bacteria.

In particular, the expression of *Trichoplusia ni* cecropin A (*T. ni* cecropin), a 38-mer AMP (RWKFFKKIEKVGQNIRDGIIKAGPAVAVVGQAASITGK-NH2) first isolated and sequenced by Kang et al. through differential display [48], is increased in *T. ni* larvae upon bacterial infection [49], suggesting its potential antimicrobial functionality. Notably, *T. ni* cecropin is unique among all known insect cecropins as it contains an additional Phe at the N-terminus, which might be important for its antibacterial activity. However, compared with those of other cecropins, the potential benefits of *T. ni* cecropin as an antimicrobial peptide remain to be elucidated. Because *colistin resistance* is most frequently observed in *E. coli* among various Gram-negative bacteria [50], in this study we investigated the antibacterial and anti-inflammatory activities of *T. ni* cecropin against colistin-resistant *E. coli* (ColREC). Furthermore, we elucidated the underlying antimicrobial mechanism of action through the analysis of LPS-neutralizing activities together with the evaluation of anti-septic activities in an in vivo mouse endotoxemia model. Together, our findings highlight the potential of *T. ni* cecropin in the fight against Gram-negative antibiotic-resistant bacteria.

2. Materials and Methods

2.1. Peptide Synthesis

All peptides (*T. ni* cecropin, cecropin A from *H. cecropia*, polymyxin B, colistin, LL-37, and melittin) were solid-phase synthesized using fluorenylmethoxycarbonyl (Fmoc) chemistry at Anygen Co., Ltd. (Gwangju, Republic of Korea). They were purified to >95% purity using high-performance liquid chromatography using a C18 column and characterized using matrix-assisted laser-desorption ionization-time-of-flight mass spectrometry (Figure S1).

2.2. Bacteria Strains

E. coli (KCTC 1682) was obtained from the Korean Collection for Type Cultures (KCTC, Jeongeup, Republic of Korea), and *Acinetobacter baumannii* (KCCM 40203) and *Pseudomonas aeruginosa* (KCCM 11328) from the Korea Culture Center of Microorganisms (KCCM, Seoul, Republic of Korea). *Klebsiella pneumoniae* (NCCP 16054), colistin-resistant *E. coli* NMA 1557 (ColREC 1557), NMS 12 (ColREC 12), and colistin-resistant *A. baumannii* NMS 1915 (ColRAB 1915), as well as colistin-resistant *K. pneumoniae* NMS 139 (ColRKP 139), were obtained from the National Institute of Health Multidrug Resistant Bacteria Specialized Pathogen Resources Bank (Osong, Republic of Korea).

2.3. Minimum Inhibitory Concentration (MIC)

The antibacterial abilities of the peptides (*T. ni* cecropin, cecropin A, polymyxin B, colistin, and melittin) were determined using the broth dilution method as previously reported [51]. The peptides dissolved at 10 mg/mL in deionized water were serially diluted from 64 μM to 0.5 μM in 96-well plates using Mueller–Hinton (MH) broth, and bacteria cultured to exponential growth were added at 2×10^5 cells/mL. The group of bacteria that grew untreated in the broth was set as the positive control, and the uninoculated broth as the negative control. Dissolved peptides are colorless and equal to the OD value of the medium only. After 16 h incubation at 37 °C, the absorbance at 600 nm was measured using a SpectraMAX microplate reader (Molecular Devices, San Jose, CA, USA). Each optical density (OD) value was expressed as a percentage, with 100% growth for the positive control and 0% growth for the negative control, and the concentration that showed >95% killing was indicated as a MIC value.

2.4. Cytotoxicity

Murine macrophage RAW 264.7 cells and mouse fibroblast L-929 cells were used for research and were purchased from the Korea Cell Line Bank (Seoul, Republic of Korea). Both cells were cultured in Dulbecco's Modified Eagle's Medium (DMEM; Welgene, Gyeongsan, Republic of Korea) supplemented with 10% fetal bovine serum and 1% antibiotics (penicillin/streptomycin) at 37 °C in the presence of 5% CO_2. To measure the cytotoxicities of peptides against RAW 264.7 cells and L-929 cells, both cell lines were seeded at a density of 1×10^5 cells/well in a 96-well plate, to which each concentration of peptide solution (from 1.6 μM to 100 μM) was added, followed by incubation for 22 h. Subsequently, WST-8 (Biomax Co., Ltd., Guri, Republic of Korea) was added at 10% volume of the final solution, and the mixture was incubated for an additional 2 h. Absorbance was measured at 450 nm. Percentages were calculated based on untreated cells.

2.5. Hemolysis

Sheep red blood cells (sRBCs; KisanBio, Seoul, Republic of Korea) were added to three volumes of phosphate-buffered saline (PBS; 35 mM phosphate buffer containing 150 mM NaCl, pH 7.4) and centrifuged five times at 4 °C, 1000× *g* for 5 min, followed by a final suspension in PBS at 4% (*w*/*v*). Peptides serially diluted from 100 μM to 3.1 μM in PBS at 100 μL in a 96-well plate were prepared, and an equal volume of blood solution was added. After incubation at 37 °C for 1 h, the plates were centrifuged for 5 min at 4 °C, 1000× *g*. The absorbance of the supernatant was measured at 405 nm. The 100% hemolysis control was 0.1% Triton-X 100 added to the blood solution; the negative control was blood solution added to PBS.

2.6. Biofilm Inhibition Assay

To quantify the biofilm inhibitory activity of each peptide, ColREC 1557 and ColREC 12 were cultured in Luria–Bertani (LB) broth overnight and then sub-cultured in MH broth. Different concentrations of peptide (from 1 μM to 64 μM) were prepared in 96-well plates using MH broth (containing 0.2% glucose) and incubated with bacteria (2×10^5 cells/mL) at 37 °C for 16 h. After incubation, the culture medium was removed and methanol was added as a fixative for 15 min. The completely dried plates were stained for 2 h by adding 100 μL of staining solution (0.1% (*w*/*v*) crystal violet in 0.25% (*v*/*v*) acetic acid). The residual staining solution was gently rinsed off three times using distilled water. Subsequently, 90% ethanol was used to dissolve the dye, and absorbance was measured at 600 nm. The untreated bacterial group was used as a control to compare biofilm production rates.

2.7. Bacteria Outer Membrane Permeability Test

The bacteria were grown to OD 0.6, washed three times with wash buffer (5 mM HEPES, 20 mM glucose, pH 7.4), and resuspended to OD 0.05 in the same buffer. To examine the permeability of the bacterial outer membrane by the peptide, 5 μM 1-N-phenylnaphthylamine (NPN) was added to 2 mL of bacteria suspension and monitored until the fluorescence intensity stabilized. This stabilized value was used as a control. Fluorescence was measured using a fluorescence spectrophotometer (Shimadzu Scientific Instruments, Kyoto, Japan) at excitation and emission wavelengths of 350 and 420 nm, respectively; the fluorescence intensity was checked by gradually increasing the peptide concentration (1, 2, 4, 6, and 8 μM). Fluorescence intensity data were analyzed after subtracting the fluorescence background level of NPN alone.

2.8. Circular Dichroism (CD) Analysis

To study the secondary structure of peptides, CD spectra of the peptides were collected using a J-810 spectropolarimeter (Jasco, Tokyo, Japan). Peptides (50 μM) in aqueous solution, 50 mM dodecylphosphorcholine (DPC), and 100 mm sodium dodecyl sulfate (SDS) micelles in a 1 mm path length cell were scanned three times with 0.1 nm intervals and recorded at 190 to 250 nm. Data were converted to mean residue ellipticity (θ) in $deg{\cdot}cm^2{\cdot}dmol^{-1}$ units as previously described [52].

2.9. Antimicrobial Activity Time-Course Assay

To determine the antibacterial activity of peptides over time, a 2 mL bacterial suspension was treated with *T. ni* cecropin at different concentrations (2 μM, 4 μM) and incubated at 37 °C. At each time point (5, 10, 15, 30, 45, 60, and 120 min), 100 μL of culture medium was smeared on LB agar plates; colonies were counted after 12 h of incubation at 37 °C.

2.10. Bacteria Morphology Imaging

Field emission-scanning electron microscopy (SU8020; Hitachi, Tokyo, Japan) was used to analyze changes in bacterial membrane morphology. Bacteria cultured to exponential growth were treated with peptides at 4 μM for 4 h, washed by PBS, fixed with 2.5% (*w*/*v*) glutaraldehyde overnight at 4 °C, further fixed with 1% osmium tetroxide, and dehydrated with progressively increasing concentrations of 50, 60, 70, 80, 90, and 100% ethanol solutions. The dehydration process was then extended by varying the volume ratio of ethanol to isoamyl acetate to 2:1, 1:1, and 1:2, followed by incubation in hexamethyldisilane for an additional 30 min. The dehydrated samples were then coated with platinum and imaged by scanning electron microscopy.

2.11. Limulus Amebocyte Lysate (LAL) Assay

To investigate the LPS-neutralizing activity, LAL assays were performed according to the protocol provided in the LAL assay kit (ToxinSensor™ Chromogenic LAL Endotoxin Assay Kit; GenScript, Piscataway, NJ, USA). Briefly, peptides diluted from 50 μM to 1.6 μM in LAL reagent water were incubated with LPS (2 ng/mL) for 10 min at 37 °C. LAL enzyme was then added and incubated under the same conditions. Substrate was added to react, after which three kinds of stop solutions were added in order. Absorbance (545 nm) was measured and quantified using an endotoxin standard graph.

2.12. BODIPY-TR-Cadaverine (BC) Displacement Assay

To measure the binding ability of peptides and LPS by concentration, fluorescent dye was prepared in 50 mM Tris buffer (pH 7.4) containing 50 μg/mL of LPS from *E. coli* O55:B5 (Sigma-Aldrich, St Louis, MO, USA) and 5 μg/mL of BC (ThermoFisher Scientific Inc., Waltham, MA, USA) and incubated for 6 h. Peptides were diluted from 50 μM to 1.6 μM using 50 mM tris buffer in a black 96-well plate, and an equal volume of fluorescent dye was added. After 30 min incubation, the activity was measured using a spectrofluorometer (Spectra Max Gemini; Molecular Devices) with an excitation wavelength of 580 nm and an emission wavelength of 620 nm.

2.13. Isothermal Titration Calorimetry (ITC)

To measure the binding affinity of a peptide to LPS, ITC experiments were performed using a MicroCal AutoiTC200 (Malvern Panalytical, Malvern, UK) at the Korea Basic Science Institute (KBSI, Ochang, Republic of Korea). *T. ni* cecropin (0.1 mM) was injected into 370 μL of 25 μM LPS (*E. coli* O111:B4, Sigma-Aldrich) in Dulbecco's phosphate-buffered saline (DPBS, pH 7.0; Welgene) at 2.5 s intervals for 98 s at 37 °C for 38 injections. LPS was pretreated with 15 min vortex, 5 min heating at 60 °C, followed by 5 min sonication. The data were analyzed for binding affinity using MicroCal Origin software (MicroCal Origin, Northhampton, MA, USA).

2.14. Saturation Transfer Difference (STD)-Nuclear Magnetic Resonance (NMR)

To investigate the interaction between a peptide (0.5 mM) and LPS (O111:B4, 25 μM), STD-NMR spectra were obtained using a Bruker 700 MHz spectrometer (Bruker Biospin, Rheinstetten, Germany) at KBSI. Sample was dissolved in 20 mM sodium phosphate buffer (pH 5.9). Spectra were provided at −3.0 ppm with saturation of the LPS resonance selectively, and a reference spectrum at 40 ppm. STD-NMR data were acquired by subtracting off-resonances from the on-resonance spectrum with a cascade of 40 Gaussian-shaped pulses of 50 ms duration (total saturation time was 2 s) to obtain a difference spectrum. ^{1}H chemical shifts of aromatic residues were assigned using NOESY (mixing time of 250, 350 ms) and TOCSY (mixing time of 70 ms) experiments.

2.15. Suppression of LPS-Induced Inflammatory Cytokines

Murine macrophage RAW 264.7 cells were used to measure the anti-inflammatory activities of peptides. Culture plates (96-well) were seeded at a density of 1×10^5 cells/well and stimulated with 20 ng/mL LPS (O111:B4; Sigma-Aldrich) for 16 h after 1 h pretreatment with each concentration of peptide (0.6 to 10 μM). The control is an untreated cell. The culture supernatant was added to an equal volume of Griess reagent (Sigma-Aldrich), and the absorbance was measured at 540 nm. Nitrite production was quantified using a standard curve constructed using $NaNO_2$.

Interleukin-6 (IL-6)-specific enzyme-linked immunosorbent assays (ELISA; R&D Systems, Minneapolis, MN, USA) were performed according to the method specified by the manufacturer. Briefly, cell culture supernatants were added to immune plates treated with the capture antibody, followed by the detection antibody and streptavidin-horseradish peroxidase. For each step, the plates were washed twice with PBS containing 0.05% Tween 20. The plates were incubated with tetramethylbenzidine substrate (Invitrogen, Carlsbad, CA, USA), and the reaction was stopped with 2 N H_2SO_4 to measure absorbance at 450 nm. A standard graph of each marker was plotted and quantified.

2.16. Suppression of Colistin-Resistant Bacteria-Induced Inflammatory Cytokines

To investigate the inflammatory response induced by ColREC 1557, RAW 264.7 cells (1×10^5 cells/well) were treated with various concentrations of peptide (0.6 to 10 μM) 1 h before bacterial infection. The control was an untreated cell. ColREC 1557 that had been cultured in LB broth overnight and sub-cultured to the exponential phase were harvested, suspended in DMEM, and used to infect RAW 264.7 cells to a final concentration of

1×10^5 cells/well. Subsequent nitrite and IL-6 detection was performed as described in Section 2.15.

2.17. Inhibition of Nitric Oxide (NO) Production by T. ni Cecropin in Response to Various Toll-like Receptors (TLRs)

RAW 264.7 cells, which express various TLRs, were used to investigate the inflammatory response to specific TLRs. Experiments were performed as previously described [53]. RAW 264.7 cells were seeded at 1×10^5 cells/well in 96-well plates and stimulated with agonists of various TLRs after 1 h pretreatment with *T. ni* cecropin at each concentration. Agonists were purchased from Invivogen (San Diego, CA, USA), including Pam_2CSK_4 (TLR2/6), Pam_3CSK_4 (TLR1/2), LPS (O111:B4) (TLR4), imiquimod (TLR7), and ODN1826 (TLR9). NO production measurements were performed using a Griess reagent.

2.18. Secreted Embryonic Alkaline Phosphatase (SEAP) Assay

Human embryonic kidney (HEK)-Blue^{TM} hTLR4 (Invivogen) cells were prepared in HEK-Blue detection medium (Invivogen) to enable real-time detection of SEAP. The SEAP assay was performed as previously described [54]. Briefly, peptides were prepared by concentration in 96-well plates, and cells were added at 2.5×10^4 cells/well. After 1 h, they were stimulated with LPS (O111:B4) (20 ng/mL), followed by 16 h incubation, and the 620 nm absorbance was measured.

2.19. Surface Plasmon Resonance (SPR)

Binding affinity measurements of the peptide to TLR4/myeloid differentiation factor 2 (MD-2) protein (R&D Systems) were performed on a Biacore T200 instrument (GE Healthcare, Danderyd, Sweden). The receptor was covalently bound to the carboxymethylated sensor chip surface using standard NHS/EDC coupling procedures. The sensor chip (Sensor Chip CM5; Cytiva, MA, USA) was loaded with 30 μg/mL of protein in sodium acetate buffer (pH 4.0) to a resonance value of 2500. Measurements were performed at a flow rate of 30 μL/min with increasing concentrations of peptide dissolved in PBS containing 0.05% Tween 20 at 25 °C. Analysis was performed using Biacore T200 Evaluation Software 3.0 (GE Healthcare, Chicago, IL, USA).

2.20. Flow Cytometry

Cell surface receptor and peptide interactions were investigated by flow cytometry. RAW 264.7 cells were pretreated with 10 μM *T. ni* cecropin, treated with LPS (O111:B4, 50 ng/mL) 30 min later, and incubated for 24 h. Harvested cells were blocked with 0.5% bovine serum albumin for 1 h. They were then incubated with anti-TLR4 antibody (ab13556, Abcam, Cambridge, MA, USA; 0.5 μg/1×10^6 cells) for 20 min, followed by incubation with Alexa Fluor 546-conjugated secondary antibody (A-10040, Invitrogen; 1:200 dilution) for 20 min. Cold PBS washes were performed between each step. Cells were then suspended in 1% paraformaldehyde and analyzed using a CytoFlex flow cytometry analyzer (Beckman Coulter, Brea, CA, USA).

2.21. Animal Study Information

ICR mice (female, 6-week-old) were purchased from Orient Bio (Seongnam, Republic of Korea). All mice were housed in specific pathogen-free conditions with controlled temperature and humidity. All procedures were approved by the Institutional Animal Care and Use Committee (IACUC) of Konkuk University, Seoul, Korea (IACUC number: KU22174).

2.22. Mouse Model of LPS-Induced Endotoxemia

ICR mice were randomly divided into four groups (three mice per group). Mock-treated "normal" animals were i.p. injected with PBS alone. The peptide control group was injected with *T. ni* cecropin (1 mg/kg); the LPS control group received LPS O127:B8 (18 mg/kg; Sigma-Aldrich). In the peptide treatment group, *T. ni* cecropin was injected

1 h prior to LPS injection. At 16 h post-injection, mice were euthanized, and serum was obtained for measurement of the levels of inflammatory cytokines IL-6 using ELISA kits (R&D Systems). The aspartate aminotransferase (AST), alanine aminotransferase (ALT), and blood urea nitrogen (BUN) levels in the serum were measured using standard kits from Asan Pharmaceutical (Seoul, Republic of Korea), as described previously [55].

2.23. Histological Analysis of Lung Tissue

Lungs were obtained after the euthanasia of mice in four groups, as described in Section 2.22. After obtaining tissue, it was washed twice in PBS, fixed in 4% (v/v) paraformaldehyde, and prepared as paraffin blocks for sectioning. After sectioning at a thickness of 6 mm, paraffin was deparaffinized with xylene. They were rehydrated with an ethanol concentration gradient and stained with hematoxylin and eosin. Lung sections were prepared on microscope slides and imaged with a light microscope (Eclipse Ni; Nikon, Tokyo, Japan).

2.24. Data Analysis

Data from experiments performed at least three times are presented as the mean ± standard error of the mean (SEM) of independent experiments. One-way and two-way analysis of variance (ANOVA) and Dunnett's test were performed using GraphPad Prism software (GraphPad Software Inc., La Jolla, CA, USA). Values of $p < 0.05$ (*), $p < 0.01$ (**), $p < 0.001$ (***) were considered to represent statistically significant differences.

3. Results

3.1. Antibacterial Activities of T. ni Cecropin

The MIC of *T. ni* cecropin was examined to verify its antibacterial activities compared with those of cecropin A from *H. cecropia*, two polymyxins (polymyxin B and colistin), and melittin, a peptide that exhibits high antibacterial activity against Gram-negative bacteria [56]. Various standard Gram-negative bacteria (*E. coli*, *A. baumannii*, *P. aeruginosa*, and *K. pneumoniae*) and colistin-resistant bacteria (ColREC 1557, ColREC 12, ColRAB 1915, and ColRKP 139) were used for the measurement. MIC values are given in Table 1. *T. ni* cecropin possessed potent antibacterial activities. For all bacteria, *T. ni* cecropin showed superior antibacterial activities to those of melittin. Moreover, peptide activity was maintained regardless of antibiotic resistance. In addition, polymyxin B and colistin showed poor antibacterial activities against all ColREC, ColRAB, and ColRKP strains that acquired colistin resistance, whereas *T. ni* cecropin retained bactericidal activities against all colistin-resistant bacteria. Using the geometric mean (GM) value of the averaged MIC across all strains to assess bactericidal activity, *T. ni* cecropin had the best performance among the comparators with a mean MIC of 1.63, followed by cecropin A (2.25), melittin (14.25), polymyxin B (17.88), and colistin (33.72) (Table 1).

Table 1. Minimum inhibitory concentration (MIC) of antimicrobial peptides against various microorganism.

	Minimal Inhibitory Concentration (μM)				
Microorganism	**Cecropin A**	***T. ni* Cecropin**	**Polymyxin B**	**Colistin**	**Melittin**
E. coli	2	2	0.25	0.25	8
A. baumannii	2	1	0.5	0.25	4
P. aeruginosa	8	4	2	1	32
K. pneumoniae	1	1	0.25	0.25	32
ColREC 1557	1	1	8	8	2
ColREC 12	1	1	4	4	2
ColRAB 1915	1	1	64	>64	2
ColRKP 139	2	2	64	>64	32

Table 1. *Cont.*

Microorganism	Minimal Inhibitory Concentration (μM)				
	Cecropin A	*T. ni* Cecropin	Polymyxin B	Colistin	Melittin
GM *	2.25	1.63	17.88	33.72	14.25
HC_{10} †	200	200	200	200	3.1
Relative selective Index **	88.89	123.08	11.19	5.93	0.22

* Geometric mean (GM) represents the average MIC value of all bacterial strains. † Hemolysis concentration $(HC)_{10}$ is the concentration that causes 10% hemolysis in sheep red blood cells. ** Relative selective index was calculated as HC_{10}/GM. For the calculation, 200 μM was applied to the formula if no hemolysis was observed at 100 μM. For MIC values above 64 μM, 128 μM was used in the calculations. Higher relative selective index values indicate higher cell selectivity. ColREC: colistin-resistant *Escherichia coli (E. coli)*; ColRAB: colistin-resistant *Acinetobacter baumannii (A. baumannii)*; ColRKP: colistin-resistant *Klebsiella pneumoniae (K. pneumonia)*.

3.2. Toxicity of *T. ni* Cecropin to Mammalian Cells

To evaluate the potential use of *T. ni* cecropin as a drug, we obtained toxicity measurements in mammalian cells (murine macrophage RAW 264.7 cells and mouse fibroblast L-929 cells). In RAW 264.7 cells, melittin showed 3.1% cell viability at 12.5 μM (Figure 1a). Conversely, cells exposed to colistin and polymyxin B at a high concentration (100 μM) showed 70.1 and 31.3% viability, respectively, with *T. ni* cecropin exhibiting an outstanding survival rate of 93.6%. Similarly, in L-929 cells, the survival rate following melittin treatment was below 5% even at a concentration of 1.6 μM, whereas *T. ni* cecropin maintained 95% viability up to 100 μM (Figure 1b). Colistin (95.0%) and polymyxin B (96.0%) also showed similar survival rates. These results confirmed the safety of *T. ni* cecropin and indicated that melittin, which showed strong antimicrobial activity, is highly toxic to mammalian cells.

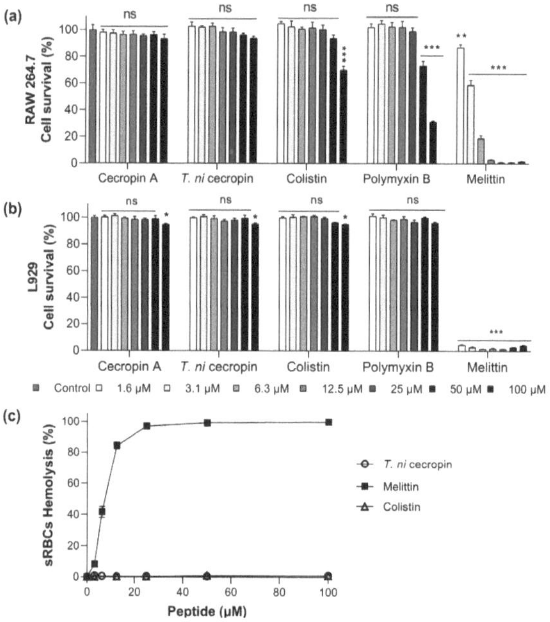

Figure 1. Cytotoxicity of peptides against (**a**) RAW 264.7 cells, (**b**) L929, and (**c**) sheep red blood cells (sRBCs). Data are presented as the mean ± SEM from triplicate experiments. * $p < 0.05$, ** $p < 0.01$, *** $p < 0.001$; and ns, nonsignificant compared to that in the non-treatment group (two-way analysis of variance).

To further evaluate the toxicity of the peptides to mammalian cells, we investigated their hemolytic activity against sRBCs. Melittin showed substantial hemolytic activity (8.2%) at 3.1 μM and 84.3% at 12.5 μM, whereas *T. ni* cecropin and colistin showed no hemolytic activity even at 100 μM (Figure 1c). Together, the results of these toxicity studies confirmed the biocompatibility of *T. ni* cecropin with mammals. The relative selective index value was highest for *T. ni* cecropin (123.08), which was significantly higher than that for colistin (5.93) (Table 1).

3.3. *T. ni Cecropin Inhibits ColREC Biofilm Formation*

Biofilms create a growth environment for bacteria and are a cause of antibiotic resistance. To determine the effectiveness of the peptides against ColREC, biofilm formation inhibition was measured. The cecropins were superior to the polymyxins in antibiofilm activity. For ColREC 1557, *T. ni* cecropin showed 75.3% inhibition even at 2 μM and over 90% inhibition at 4 μM. In contrast, colistin prevented only 58.6% of the biofilm formation of ColREC 1557 at 16 μM (Figure 2a). Moreover, whereas 2 μM of colistin inhibited 28.9% of the biofilm formation in ColREC 12, the same concentration of *T. ni* cecropin and cecropin A had a higher inhibition rate of 82.5% and 80.8%, respectively (Figure 2b). This showed that *T. ni* cecropin as well as cecropin A interfere with the growth environment of colistin-resistant bacteria.

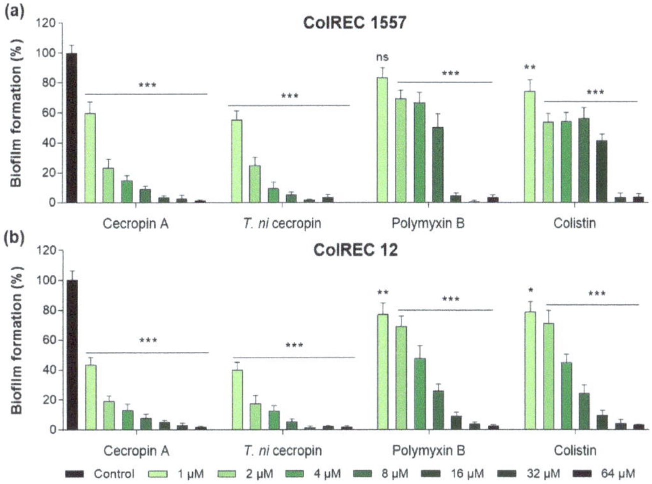

Figure 2. Inhibitory effects of peptides in biofilm assays performed in (**a**) ColREC 1557 and (**b**) ColREC 12. Data are presented as the mean ± SEM from triplicate experiments. * $p < 0.05$, ** $p < 0.01$, *** $p < 0.001$; and ns, nonsignificant compared to that in the non-treatment group (two-way ANOVA).

3.4. *Antibacterial Mechanisms of T. ni Cecropin against Gram-Negative Bacteria*

3.4.1. LPS-Neutralizing Capacity of *T. ni* Cecropin

As the peptide forms a strong bond with LPS, it can suppress endotoxin toxicity caused by bacterial infection and lower the incidence of disease. The ability of the peptide to neutralize LPS was measured by quantifying the colorimetric reaction, indicating that LPS catalyzes proenzyme activation in LAL. LL-37, a strong LPS-neutralizing peptide, was used as a control [26]. The LAL test showed that *T. ni* cecropin and cecropin A reacted with LPS in a concentration-dependent manner, with 50 μM of the peptide nearly neutralizing 10 enzyme units (EU) of LPS (Figure 3a), as compared with the 12.5 μM required for LL-37.

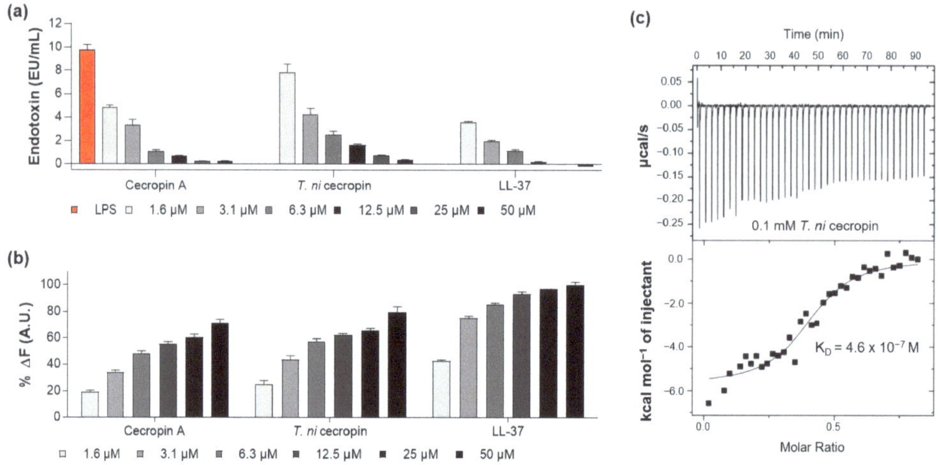

Figure 3. Measurement of interaction between lipopolysaccharide (LPS) and peptides. (**a**) Limulus amebocyte lysate assay showing the LPS neutralization capacities of peptides. (**b**) BODIPY-TR-cadaverine displacement from LPS after treatment with peptides. (**c**) Isothermal titration calorimetry measurement showing the binding affinity of *Trichoplusia ni* cecropin (*T. ni* cecropin) (0.1 mM) to 0.025 mM LPS. Data are presented as the mean ± SEM from triplicate experiments. The concentration of the peptides at each x-axis is indicated at the bottom of (**a**,**b**) by the color notation.

The BC displacement assay was used to measure the ability of peptides to interact with LPS. BC fluorescent dyes quench when bound to cell-free LPS and emit fluorescence when LPS binds to the peptide. As shown in Figure 3b, *T. ni* cecropin induced concentration-dependent BC displacement. Based on a 100% displacement rate for 50 μM of LL-37, that for 50 μM of *T. ni* cecropin and cecropin A was 79.7% and 71.3%, respectively. These results demonstrate that both cecropins exhibit similar LPS neutralization and binding interactions as those of LL-37.

ITC analysis revealed that the binding affinity of *T. ni* cecropin to LPS was as high as 4.6×10^{-7} M, indicating an exothermic process with strong electrostatic interactions (Figure 3c). These results showed that *T. ni* cecropin directly interacts with LPS and neutralizes LPS, contributing to its antibacterial activity against Gram-negative bacteria.

3.4.2. Membrane Depolarization Ability of *T. ni* Cecropin against *E. coli*

As we found that *T. ni* cecropin strongly interacted with LPS, we used the NPN uptake assay to measure the ability of the peptides to depolarize the outer membranes of *E. coli* and ColREC. NPN is a hydrophobic fluorescent probe that fluoresces in a hydrophobic environment and is used as an indicator of partitioning of the outer membrane. As shown in Figure 4, a dose-dependent increase in fluorescence intensity was observed upon treating each bacterium with various concentrations of peptide. For *E. coli*, colistin and *T. ni* cecropin showed similar permeation rates, whereas in resistant bacteria, *T. ni* cecropin permeated the membrane more efficiently than colistin. This provides evidence that *T. ni* cecropin can overcome resistance mechanisms by disrupting the integrity of the outer membrane of colistin-resistant bacteria.

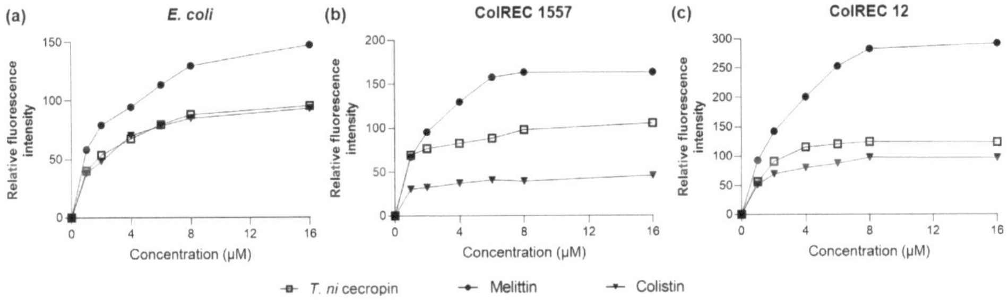

Figure 4. Fluorescence intensity as measured via peptide-induced membrane disruption. Relative fluorescence intensities in (**a**) *E. coli*, (**b**) ColREC 1557, and (**c**) ColREC 12 as measured using 1-N-phenylnaphthylamine uptake.

3.4.3. *T. ni* Cecropin Induces *E. coli* Cell Membrane Damage

The optimal duration of peptide exposure to *E. coli* was determined by considering the killing rate of the bacteria over time. For *T. ni* cecropin at 2 μM (1 × MIC) and 4 μM (2 × MIC), live bacteria were completely eradicated by 2 h incubation (Figure 5a). As shown in Figure 5b, exposure of *E. coli* to 4 μM of *T. ni* cecropin for 4 h caused substantial bacterial membrane damage. The control bacteria maintained a smooth and plump shape (Figure 5b) whereas those exposed to the peptide showed a distorted shape and obvious changes such as membrane contraction (Figure 5c). These data visually demonstrated that the peptides cause damage to the membrane and the presumed leakage of internal substances. Peptides may allow the efflux of internal cytoplasmic components through disruption of cytoplasmic membrane integrity, eventually leading to cell death. These results confirmed that *T. ni* cecropin shows antibacterial activity via a membrane disruption mechanism to resist microorganisms.

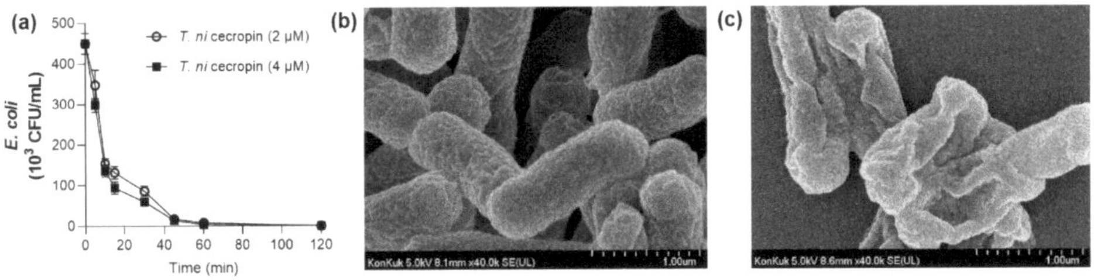

Figure 5. (**a**) Time-dependent killing activity of *T. ni* cecropin. Field emission-scanning electron microscopy images showing the morphology of *E. coli* treated with *T. ni* cecropin. (**b**) Untreated *E. coli* with intact morphology, and (**c**) after incubation for 4 h with *T. ni* cecropin at 4 μM (2 × MIC). Data are presented as the mean ± SEM from triplicate experiments.

3.4.4. *T. ni* Cecropin Directly Interacts with LPS

STD-NMR analysis was performed to specify the residues that interact with LPS. Peptide (0.5 mM) was reacted with 15 μM LPS. Notably, despite its high sequence homology with other cecropins, *T. ni* cecropin uniquely harbors an additional Phe at the fourth residue, substituting for Leu; thus, *T. ni* cecropin contains one Trp and two Phe residues. This difference may induce a strong interaction between *T. ni* cecropin and the bacterial membrane. The top spectrum in Figure 6 shows the reference spectrum of the free peptide, whereas the spectrum at the bottom shows the STD effect of the peptide bound to LPS (Figure 6 bottom). STD-NMR data showed that aromatic and amide protons, as well as aliphatic protons, contribute to the LPS interaction. Especially strong STD effects were identified at 7.0–7.7 ppm, corresponding to the aromatic ring protons of the Trp2, Phe4, and

Phe5 shown in Figure 6, implying that these aromatic residues are important for interaction with LPS and the antibacterial activities of *T. ni* cecropin.

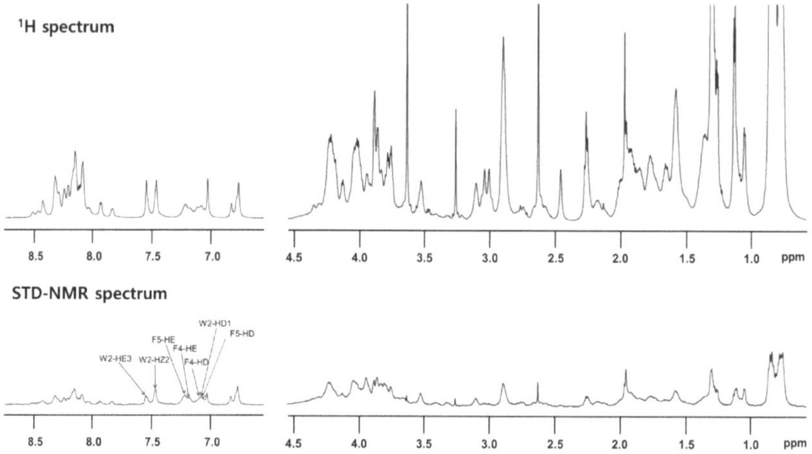

Figure 6. Reference one-dimensional nuclear magnetic resonance (NMR) spectrum for *T. ni* cecropin (**top**) and saturation transfer difference (STD) NMR spectrum obtained through interaction with LPS (**bottom**) dissolved in 20 mM sodium phosphate buffer (pH 5.9). Two regions corresponding to amide protons and aromatic ring protons (left side from 6.5 ppm to 9 ppm) and aliphatic protons (right side from 0.5 ppm to 4.5 ppm) are shown.

3.4.5. Secondary Structure of *T. ni* Cecropin

To determine the environment-dependent structure of the peptide, CD spectrum analysis was performed. *T. ni* cecropin was not structured in aqueous solution (Figure 7). However, in SDS micelles, which mimic negatively charged bacterial cells, or in DPC micelles, which mimic zwitterionic cell membranes, it was observed to adopt a helical structure with strong positive values at 192 nm and double minima at 208 and 222 nm, equivalent to the characteristics of the α-helical structures of cecropin A [57].

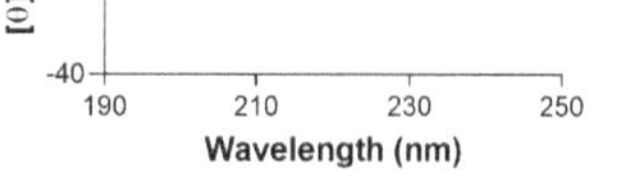

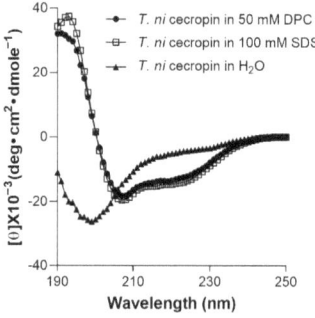

Figure 7. Secondary structures of *T. ni* cecropin in membrane-mimetic environments as observed via circular dichroism spectroscopy. DPC: dodecylphosphorcholine; SDS: sodium dodecyl sulfate.

3.5. Inhibition of Cytokine Production in RAW 264.7 Cells Stimulated by LPS or ColREC

LPS is a key virulence molecule of Gram-negative bacteria that stimulates an inflammatory cascade in macrophages. As part of the inflammatory response, stimulated cells secrete cytokines such as NO and IL-6 to regulate the inflammatory response. To evaluate whether *T. ni* cecropin, which we demonstrated to bind directly to LPS, has anti-inflammatory properties against LPS-induced inflammation, we measured its ability to inhibit cytokine production. The anti-inflammatory ability of colistin was evaluated in parallel. NO production was measured using the Griess assay to detect NO_2^-, whereas IL-6 was quantified using a sandwich ELISA. The untreated cells used as controls showed little cytokine release. NO was inhibited by 80.1% in LPS-stimulated RAW 264.7 cells upon the addition of 5 μM of *T. ni* cecropin (Figure 8a). At the same concentration, IL-6 secretion was reduced by 86.5% (Figure 8a,b). Cecropin A (5 μM) yielded similar outcomes as *T. ni* cecropin, with 81.2% and 91.0% inhibition of NO and IL-6, respectively. At the same concentration, colistin showed over 90% inhibition of both cytokines.

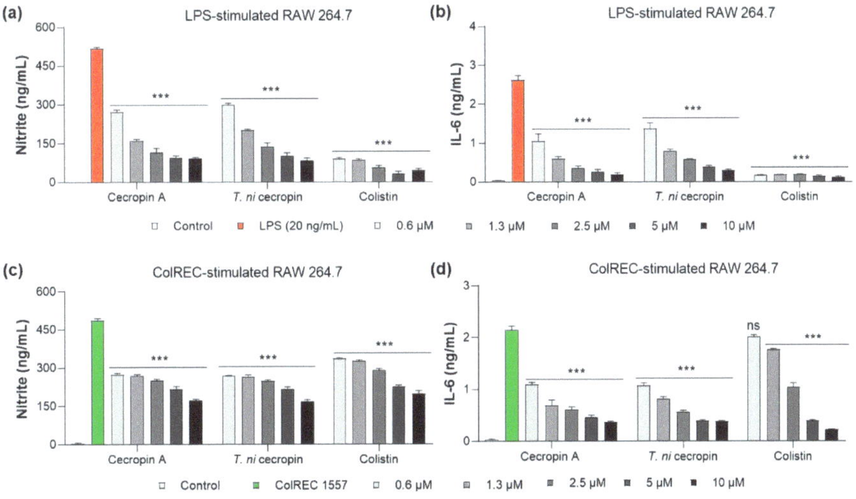

Figure 8. Anti-inflammatory effect in RAW 264.7 cells induced by stimulants. Graphs show the dose-dependent nitrite and interleukin-6 (IL-6) inhibitory effects of the peptide (**a**,**b**) on LPS stimulation and (**c**,**d**) ColREC stimulation. Data are presented as the mean ± SEM from triplicate experiments. *** $p < 0.001$ and ns, nonsignificant compared to that in the LPS or ColREC 1557 treatment group (two-way ANOVA).

Moreover, *T. ni* cecropin showed superior activity with regard to antibacterial activity against ColREC, the direct cause of the infection, compared with that of colistin. Therefore, we aimed to identify differences in activity in the inflammatory response in macrophages infected with ColREC. RAW 264.7 cells were stimulated with ColREC, and the effect on cytokine production was measured using ELISA. Overall, cecropins showed enhanced anti-inflammatory activity compared with that of colistin, with predominant activity at lower concentrations (Figure 8c,d). NO and IL-6 were inhibited by 46.2 and 63.0%, respectively, upon the addition of 1.3 μM *T. ni* cecropin, whereas colistin showed much lower inhibition rates of 24.7 and 18.4% (Figure 8c,d). These results confirmed that *T. ni* cecropin can effectively counteract the inflammatory response induced by colistin-resistant bacteria even at concentrations as low as 0.6 μM.

3.6. T. ni Cecropin Selectively Targets the TLR4-Inflammatory Signaling Pathway

To understand the mechanism by which *T. ni* cecropin inhibits inflammation, we applied agonists for various TLRs to macrophage RAW 264.7 cells and evaluated their specificity against TLR proteins. Pam_3CSK_4, Pam_2CSK_4, LPS, imiquimod, and ODN 1826 were used as agonists for TLR2/1, TLR2/6, TLR4, TLR7, and TLR9, respectively. Only the group stimulated by LPS, an agonist for TLR4, showed cecropin-induced inhibition of inflammation (Figure 9a). *T. ni* cecropin had no effect on stimulation by other agonists, indicating that *T. ni* cecropin specifically targets TLR4.

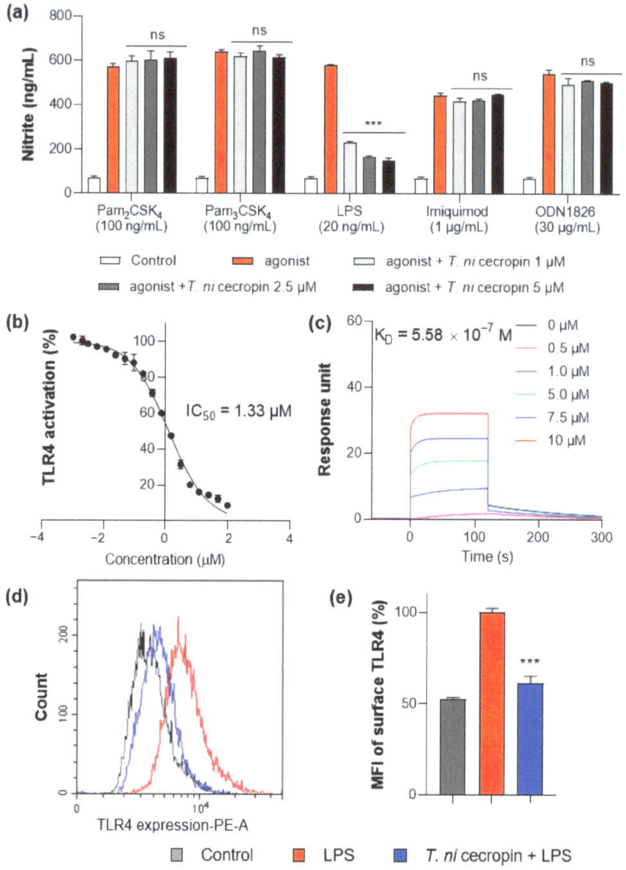

Figure 9. Measurement of interaction between Toll-like receptor 4 (TLR4) and peptides. (**a**) Specific agonist treatment for each TLR receptor shows TLR4 selectivity of *T. ni* cecropin. (**b**) Results of secreted embryonic alkaline phosphatase assay show the TLR4 inactivating effect of *T. ni* cecropin on LPS-stimulated human embryonic kidney-Blue hTLR4 cells. (**c**) Surface plasmon resonance sensorgrams of TLR4/MD-2 complex protein interaction with varying concentrations of *T. ni* cecropin. (**d**) Flow cytometry results showing the effect of *T. ni* cecropin on preventing TLR4 expression in LPS-stimulated cells and (**e**) indicating the mean fluorescence intensity (MFI) (%). Data are presented as the mean ± SEM from triplicate experiments. *** $p < 0.001$ and ns, nonsignificant compared to that in the agonist treatment group (**a**) (one-way ANOVA); *** $p < 0.001$ compared to that in the LPS group (**e**) (two-way ANOVA).

To determine the specific action of *T. ni* cecropin on TLR4, we utilized HEK-Blue hTLR4 cells, which express the NF-κB-inducible SEAP reporter gene upon stimulation with LPS. Following 20 ng/mL LPS stimulation, *T. ni* cecropin treatment significantly reduced TLR4-mediated SEAP gene expression with a low half-maximal inhibitory concentration (IC_{50}) of 1.33 μM (Figure 9b). This supports the model that *T. ni* cecropin specifically targets TLR4 signaling.

We next investigated the interaction between the TLR4/MD-2 complex and *T. ni* cecropin by performing SPR (Figure 9c). The protein complex was coated on a sensor chip and probed with various concentrations of peptide. *T. ni* cecropin bound to TLR4/MD2 in a concentration-dependent manner with high affinity, having an equilibrium constant (K_D) of 5.58×10^{-7} M.

We next used flow cytometry to examine whether the expression level of the TLR4 receptor presented on the surface of RAW 264.7 macrophages was changed by *T. ni* cecropin (Figure 9d). The fluorescence of LPS-stimulated compared with LPS-untreated RAW 264.7 cells was measured using a fluorescent antibody attached to an anti-TLR4 antibody. Cells stimulated with LPS (red) expressed TLR4 on their surface and showed higher fluorescence compared to that of unstimulated control cells (gray). Cells co-treated with *T. ni* cecropin and LPS (blue) showed a significant decrease in TLR4 expression compared with that from LPS treatment alone, as confirmed by evaluating relative expression (61.4%) in LPS/*T. ni* cecropin-co-treated cells based on normalizing the fluorescence intensity from LPS-stimulated cells to 100% ($p < 0.001$). These results suggest that *T. ni* cecropin interferes with LPS binding to TLR4 and may blunt TLR4 surface presentation on macrophages.

3.7. T. ni Cecropin Significantly Attenuates LPS-Induced Endotoxemia in a Mouse Model

We investigated the ability of *T. ni* cecropin to attenuate LPS-induced endotoxemia. *T. ni* cecropin treatment significantly reduced the endotoxin levels in an LPS-induced endotoxemia model, which agrees well with its LPS-neutralizing activities as shown via the in vitro LAL assay (Figures 3a and 10a). Next, we tested the ability of *T. ni* cecropin to suppress pro-inflammatory cytokine production in the serum. Whereas LPS induced a marked increase in cytokines, pretreatment with *T. ni* cecropin downregulated LPS-induced cytokine levels by 46.1% for IL-6, which agrees well with its in vitro anti-inflammatory effects in LPS or ColREC-stimulated RAW 264.7 cells (Figures 8b,d and 10b). Furthermore, we investigated the ability of *T. ni* cecropin to reduce LPS-induced organ damage as measured by serum AST, ALT, and BUN levels. An increase in AST and ALT levels induced by LPS detected in the serum indicates liver damage, while an elevation of BUN levels induced by LPS indicates kidney damage. *T. ni* cecropin elicited significant suppression of LPS-induced AST, ALT, and BUN levels, showing reductions of 49.5, 54.2, and 66.7%, respectively (Figure 10c–e). In the lungs, the administration effect of *T. ni* cecropin was observed by microscopy of tissue stained with hematoxylin and eosin. As shown in Figure 10f, alveolar structure destruction, hemorrhage, and neutrophilic infiltration were observed in LPS-injected mice. These damages were not observed in the other groups. The results suggest that *T. ni* cecropin reduces LPS-induced lung inflammation.

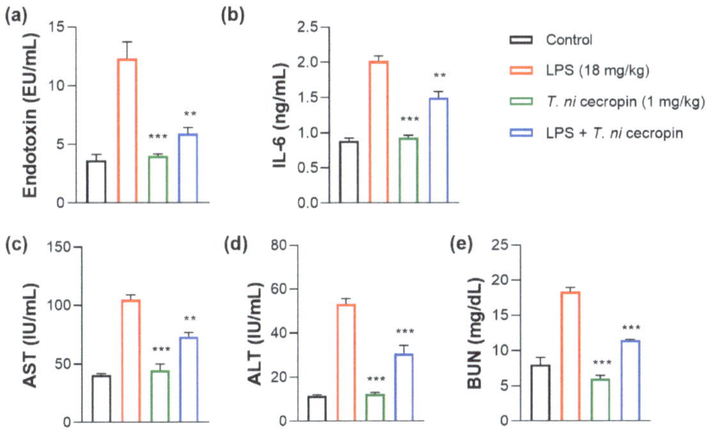

Figure 10. *Cont.*

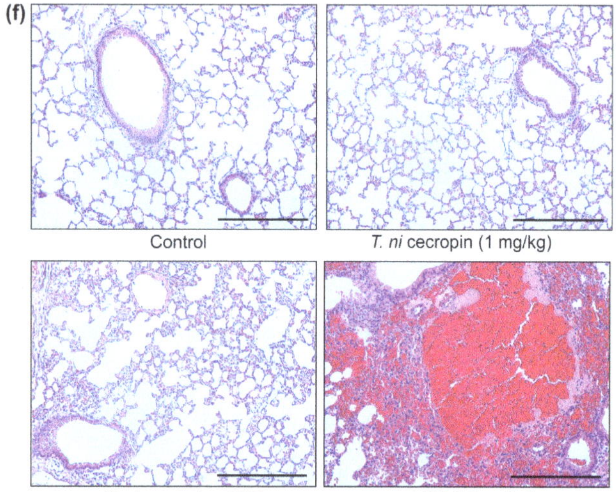

Figure 10. Anti-septic effects of *T. ni* cecropin in an LPS-induced endotoxemia septic shock mouse model. Suppressive effects on circulating serum (**a**) endotoxin levels and (**b**) IL-6 in the endotoxemia mouse model. (**c–e**) Recovery of aspartate aminotransferase (AST), alanine aminotransferase (ALT), and blood urea nitrogen (BUN) levels in the serum of the LPS-stimulated endotoxemia mouse model following treatment with *T. ni* cecropin. Data are presented as the mean ± SEM (n = 3 per group). ** $p < 0.01$ and *** $p < 0.001$ compared to that in the control group (one-way ANOVA). (**f**) Micrograph of lung histology for control, *T. ni* cecropin, LPS, and pre-treatment *T. ni* cecropin groups (clockwise) as indicated at the bottom of each photograph. Bars: 100 μm; 20× magnification.

4. Discussion

Overuse of antibiotics has been attributed as a primary factor underlying the emergence and persistence of multidrug-resistant bacteria, promoting their rapid evolution. Particularly, Gram-negative bacteria represent a serious clinical as well as global public health problem, with infections with colistin-resistant Gram-negative bacteria at the top of the World Health Organization priority list as targets for the development of new types of antibiotics [58]. Toward this end, the aim of the present study was to ultimately resolve the problems associated with infection by colistin-resistant bacteria by proposing a new peptide antibiotic. Specifically, we evaluated the potency of *T. ni* cecropin against Gram-negative bacteria, focusing on colistin-resistant bacteria. The results showed that compared with colistin, *T. ni* cecropin exhibited superior activity against colistin-resistant bacteria owing to strong binding interactions with LPS, confirming its therapeutic potential as a peptide antibiotic. To our knowledge, this represents the first report investigating the efficacy of any cecropin against colistin-resistant bacteria and the underlying antimicrobial mechanism of action.

Various attempts have been made to develop peptide antibiotics derived from natural cecropin peptides. Peptides with a short length are more cost effective for therapeutic applications. In particular, 12-meric Pap12-6 peptides designed from the N-terminal 12 amino acids of the insect cecropin papiliocin have demonstrated anti-sepsis activity against *E. coli*-infected mice [55]. Another strategy is to hybridize known peptides with cecropins to improve antibacterial activity while maintaining low cytotoxicity. In this regard, W-BP100 and CAME, conjugated peptides of cecropin and melittin, have the characteristics of active peptides with improved bactericidal power in vitro and in a sepsis animal model [59]. A cecropin A–melittin hybrid peptide has been shown to exhibit antimicrobial activity against multidrug-resistant bacteria in insects in vivo [60]. A hybrid of cecropin A and magainin 2 (CAMA) has demonstrated anti-septic activity with low toxicity [61] and antifungal activity [62]. Finally, PapMA-3, derived from papiliocin and magainin 2, showed outstanding synergistic effects with antibiotics [63].

In this study, *T. ni* cecropin showed promising potency compared to that of cecropin A, polymyxin B, colistin, and melittin against colistin-resistant bacteria, exhibiting the highest relative selectivity index value among all tested peptides. Moreover, *T. ni* cecropin demonstrated superior bactericidal activity against four colistin-resistant bacteria and also inhibited the biofilm formation of ColREC more potently than colistin. Biofilms provide an environment for bacteria to survive and even become adaptable to the medical environment, which is one of the reasons bacteria become resistant to antibiotics [64]. Therefore, blocking biofilm formation is a therapeutic approach to Gram-negative infections. Overall, our data confirmed the superior selectivity of *T. ni* cecropin over that of colistin against colistin-resistant bacteria, with low cytotoxicity against mammalian cells.

In patients with Gram-negative bacterial infection, the presence of circulating LPS induces the excessive production of inflammatory cytokines, which causes serious septic shock. To support its potential as an anti-endotoxin agent, the interaction of the *T. ni* cecropin peptide with LPS was characterized using LAL, BC displacement assays, STD NMR, and ITC measurements. The results showed that *T. ni* cecropin exhibits comparable LPS binding to that of LL-37, a known LPS-binding peptide. As shown in CD spectra, the formation of α-helical structures in membrane-mimetic environments, which constitute important characteristics for the membrane-disrupting properties of AMP [65], may facilitate *T. ni* cecropin permeabilization of the outer membrane of colistin-resistant bacteria. Moreover, the cationic N-terminal helices as well as the hydrophobic C-terminal helix of *T. ni* cecropin may allow it to permeate the ColREC membrane more efficiently than colistin. FE-SEM findings also suggested the membrane-targeting lethality mechanism as being due to bacterial membrane penetration and the resulting death from intracellular fluid efflux. Three-dimensional structural studies using NMR spectroscopy are currently underway. As *T. ni* cecropin uniquely possesses an additional Phe at the fourth position of its N-terminal helix compared to other cecropins, knowledge of the structure–activity relationships will shed light on understanding the mechanism of action and help to develop short novel peptide antibiotic derivatives based on structure–activity relationships.

We found that *T. ni* cecropin significantly inhibited the release of nitrite and IL-6 in murine macrophage RAW 264.7 cells stimulated with LPS as well as in ColREC-infected murine macrophages. Furthermore, by stimulating macrophages with agonists for various TLRs, we demonstrated that *T. ni* cecropin specifically regulates TLR4 downstream signaling, which is activated by LPS stimulation. Inhibition of TLR4-mediated inflammatory signaling by *T. ni* cecropin was further confirmed by the inhibition of SEAP activity as well as macrophage presentation of TLR4 receptors as determined using flow cytometry. In addition, SPR measurements revealed the micromolar binding affinity of *T. ni* cecropin for the TLR4/MD2 protein complex. Together, these results imply that *T. ni* cecropin not only inhibits cell surface expression of TLR4 as well as the LPS-induced TLR4 signaling cascade by directly binding to LPS but may also inhibit LPS binding to TLR4/MD2 by direct interactions with the TLR4/MD2 complex. Analysis of the downstream TLR4 signaling pathway should be further elucidated to understand the detailed mechanism using immunoblotting or reverse transcription polymerase chain reaction.

The results of evaluating *T. ni* cecropin toxicity against mammalian cells demonstrated the biocompatibility of this peptide, thereby addressing potential safety concerns regarding the future therapeutic application of *T. ni* cecropin in the clinic. Moreover, *T. ni* cecropin neutralized LPS and efficiently suppressed inflammatory cytokine levels in the serum of an endotoxemia mouse model, confirming its therapeutic potential to treat Gram-negative sepsis. Additionally, reduced levels of AST, ALT, and BUN confirmed *T. ni* cecropin's ability to alleviate liver and kidney damage. Furthermore, *T. ni* cecropin alleviated LPS-induced inflammation in the lungs. These findings are consistent with those of *Aedes aegypti* cecropin, which suppressed the inflammatory response in mice infected with *E. coli* or *P. aeruginosa* and exhibited anti-sepsis activity with organ protection [40]. Papiliocin showed anti-septic effects in an *E. coli* K1-septic mouse model, alleviating the inflammatory response and organ damage [37]. Nevertheless, prior to therapeutic and clinical application, the in vivo therapeutic potency of *T. ni* cecropin needs to be further confirmed by establishing an animal model of infection induced by a colistin-resistant pathogen.

5. Conclusions

Our study suggested a basis for the development of peptide antibiotics against colistin-resistant bacteria. *T. ni* cecropin demonstrated good antibacterial and antibiofilm activity against Gram-negative bacteria, showing that it fulfills the requirements of a peptide antibiotic. It exhibited strong membrane permeability and potent antibacterial activity even against colistin-resistant bacteria by targeting the outer membrane of Gram-negative bacteria via strong binding to LPS. In addition, *T. ni* cecropin exerts anti-inflammatory effects, inhibiting inflammatory responses to LPS and ColREC stimulation. This effect was found to be based on the inhibition of TLR4-mediated inflammatory signaling. Notably, *T. ni* cecropin also exhibited LPS-neutralizing and immunosuppressive activities in an endotoxemia mouse model, implying that *T. ni* cecropin has considerable potential as a potent anti-septic peptide. Taken together, our results support the idea that *T. ni* cecropin may be a promising starting point for the development of novel peptide antibiotic alternatives to polymyxins for the treatment of colistin-resistant Gram-negative infections.

Supplementary Materials: The following supporting information can be downloaded at: https://www.mdpi.com/article/10.3390/pharmaceutics15061752/s1, Figure S1. Characterization of synthesized *T. ni* cecropin by high-performance liquid chromatography (HPLC) and mass spectrometry (MS).

Author Contributions: Conceptualization, Y.K.; investigation, H.L., B.K., M.K., S.Y., J.L. and E.H.; data curation, H.L.; writing—original draft preparation, review and editing, H.L., B.K. and Y.K.; visualization, H.L. and B.K.; supervision, Y.K.; funding acquisition, Y.K. All authors have read and agreed to the published version of the manuscript.

Funding: This work was supported by a National Research Foundation of Korea (NRF) grant funded by the Korean government (MSIT) (No. RS-2023-00207959) and by research fund No. 2022-ER2204-01 from the Korea Disease Control and Prevention Agency.

Institutional Review Board Statement: Not applicable.

Informed Consent Statement: Not applicable.

Data Availability Statement: The data presented in the manuscript are available on request from the corresponding author.

Acknowledgments: The pathogen resources (NCCP 16054, NMS 1557, NMS 12, NMS 1915, and NMS 139) for this study were provided by the National Institute of Health Multidrug Resistant Bacteria Specialized Pathogen Resources Bank in Korea.

Conflicts of Interest: The authors declare no conflict of interest.

References

1. Holmes, C.L.; Anderson, M.T.; Mobley, H.L.T.; Bachman, M.A. Pathogenesis of Gram-Negative Bacteremia. *Clin. Microbiol. Rev.* **2021**, *34*, e00234-20. [CrossRef] [PubMed]
2. Castanheira, M.; Simner, P.J.; Bradford, P.A. Extended-spectrum beta-lactamases: An update on their characteristics, epidemiology and detection. *JAC Antimicrob. Resist.* **2021**, *3*, dlab092. [CrossRef] [PubMed]
3. Walas, N.; Slown, S.; Amato, H.K.; Lloyd, T.; Bender, M.; Varghese, V.; Pandori, M.; Graham, J.P. The role of plasmids in carbapenem resistant E. coli in Alameda County, California. *BMC Microbiol.* **2023**, *23*, 147. [CrossRef] [PubMed]
4. Bassetti, M.; Peghin, M.; Vena, A.; Giacobbe, D.R. Treatment of Infections Due to MDR Gram-Negative Bacteria. *Front. Med.* **2019**, *6*, 74. [CrossRef] [PubMed]
5. Benedict, R.G.; Langlykke, A.F. Antibiotic activity of Bacillus polymyxa. *J. Bacteriol.* **1947**, *54*, 24. [PubMed]
6. Sisay, M.; Hagos, B.; Edessa, D.; Tadiwos, Y.; Mekuria, A.N. Polymyxin-induced nephrotoxicity and its predictors: A systematic review and meta-analysis of studies conducted using RIFLE criteria of acute kidney injury. *Pharmacol. Res.* **2021**, *163*, 105328. [CrossRef]

7. Mohapatra, S.S.; Dwibedy, S.K.; Padhy, I. Polymyxins, the last-resort antibiotics: Mode of action, resistance emergence, and potential solutions. *J. Biosci.* **2021**, *46*, 85. [CrossRef]
8. Poirel, L.; Jayol, A.; Nordmann, P. Polymyxins: Antibacterial Activity, Susceptibility Testing, and Resistance Mechanisms Encoded by Plasmids or Chromosomes. *Clin. Microbiol. Rev.* **2017**, *30*, 557–596. [CrossRef]
9. Ayoub Moubareck, C. Polymyxins and Bacterial Membranes: A Review of Antibacterial Activity and Mechanisms of Resistance. *Membranes* **2020**, *10*, 181. [CrossRef]
10. Velkov, T.; Roberts, K.D.; Nation, R.L.; Thompson, P.E.; Li, J. Pharmacology of polymyxins: New insights into an 'old' class of antibiotics. *Future Microbiol.* **2013**, *8*, 711–724. [CrossRef]
11. Domingues, M.M.; Inacio, R.G.; Raimundo, J.M.; Martins, M.; Castanho, M.A.; Santos, N.C. Biophysical characterization of polymyxin B interaction with LPS aggregates and membrane model systems. *Biopolymers* **2012**, *98*, 338–344. [CrossRef] [PubMed]
12. Gallardo-Godoy, A.; Hansford, K.A.; Muldoon, C.; Becker, B.; Elliott, A.G.; Huang, J.X.; Pelingon, R.; Butler, M.S.; Blaskovich, M.A.T.; Cooper, M.A. Structure-Function Studies of Polymyxin B Lipononapeptides. *Molecules* **2019**, *24*, 553. [CrossRef] [PubMed]
13. Velkov, T.; Thompson, P.E.; Nation, R.L.; Li, J. Structure-activity relationships of polymyxin antibiotics. *J. Med. Chem.* **2010**, *53*, 1898–1916. [CrossRef] [PubMed]
14. Fu, L.; Wan, M.; Zhang, S.; Gao, L.; Fang, W. Polymyxin B Loosens Lipopolysaccharide Bilayer but Stiffens Phospholipid Bilayer. *Biophys. J.* **2020**, *118*, 138–150. [CrossRef] [PubMed]
15. Goode, A.; Yeh, V.; Bonev, B.B. Interactions of polymyxin B with lipopolysaccharide-containing membranes. *Faraday Discuss.* **2021**, *232*, 317–329. [CrossRef] [PubMed]
16. Zhang, H.; Srinivas, S.; Xu, Y.; Wei, W.; Feng, Y. Genetic and Biochemical Mechanisms for Bacterial Lipid A Modifiers Associated with Polymyxin Resistance. *Trends Biochem. Sci.* **2019**, *44*, 973–988. [CrossRef]
17. Hamel, M.; Rolain, J.M.; Baron, S.A. The History of Colistin Resistance Mechanisms in Bacteria: Progress and Challenges. *Microorganisms* **2021**, *9*, 442. [CrossRef]
18. Olaitan, A.O.; Morand, S.; Rolain, J.M. Mechanisms of polymyxin resistance: Acquired and intrinsic resistance in bacteria. *Front. Microbiol.* **2014**, *5*, 643. [CrossRef]
19. Srinivasan, V.B.; Rajamohan, G. KpnEF, a new member of the Klebsiella pneumoniae cell envelope stress response regulon, is an SMR-type efflux pump involved in broad-spectrum antimicrobial resistance. *Antimicrob. Agents Chemother.* **2013**, *57*, 4449–4462. [CrossRef]
20. Son, S.J.; Huang, R.; Squire, C.J.; Leung, I.K.H. MCR-1: A promising target for structure-based design of inhibitors to tackle polymyxin resistance. *Drug. Discov. Today* **2019**, *24*, 206–216. [CrossRef]
21. Velkov, T.; Roberts, K.D.; Nation, R.L.; Wang, J.; Thompson, P.E.; Li, J. Teaching 'old' polymyxins new tricks: New-generation lipopeptides targeting gram-negative 'superbugs'. *ACS Chem. Biol.* **2014**, *9*, 1172–1177. [CrossRef] [PubMed]
22. Jiang, X.; Han, M.; Tran, K.; Patil, N.A.; Ma, W.; Roberts, K.D.; Xiao, M.; Sommer, B.; Schreiber, F.; Wang, L.; et al. An Intelligent Strategy with All-Atom Molecular Dynamics Simulations for the Design of Lipopeptides against Multidrug-Resistant Pseudomonas aeruginosa. *J. Med. Chem.* **2022**, *65*, 10001–10013. [CrossRef] [PubMed]
23. Rodvold, K.A.; Bader, J.; Gupta, V.K.; Lister, T.; Srivastava, P.; Bruss, J. 625. SPR206 Pharmacokinetics (PK) in Plasma, Epithelial Lining Fluid (ELF), and Alveolar Macrophages (AM) in Healthy Adult Subjects. *Open Forum Infect. Dis.* **2022**, *9*. [CrossRef]
24. Griffith, D.; Carmeli, Y.; Gehrke, S.; Morgan, E.; Dudley, M.; Loutit, J. 217. A Phase 1 Study of the Safety, Tolerability, and Pharmacokinetics of Multiple Doses of the Lipopeptide QPX9003 in Healthy Adult Subjects. *Open Forum Infect. Dis.* **2022**, *9*. [CrossRef]
25. Lepak, A.J.; Wang, W.; Andes, D.R. Pharmacodynamic Evaluation of MRX-8, a Novel Polymyxin, in the Neutropenic Mouse Thigh and Lung Infection Models against Gram-Negative Pathogens. *Antimicrob. Agents Chemother.* **2020**, *64*, e01517-20. [CrossRef] [PubMed]
26. Mookherjee, N.; Anderson, M.A.; Haagsman, H.P.; Davidson, D.J. Antimicrobial host defence peptides: Functions and clinical potential. *Nat. Rev. Drug. Discov.* **2020**, *19*, 311–332. [CrossRef] [PubMed]
27. Raheem, N.; Straus, S.K. Mechanisms of Action for Antimicrobial Peptides With Antibacterial and Antibiofilm Functions. *Front. Microbiol.* **2019**, *10*, 2866. [CrossRef]
28. Uddin, T.M.; Chakraborty, A.J.; Khusro, A.; Zidan, B.R.M.; Mitra, S.; Emran, T.B.; Dhama, K.; Ripon, M.K.H.; Gajdacs, M.; Sahibzada, M.U.K.; et al. Antibiotic resistance in microbes: History, mechanisms, therapeutic strategies and future prospects. *J. Infect. Public Health* **2021**, *14*, 1750–1766. [CrossRef]
29. Mahlapuu, M.; Björn, C.; Ekblom, J.J. Antimicrobial peptides as therapeutic agents: Opportunities and challenges. *Crit. Rev. Biotechnol.* **2020**, *40*, 978–992. [CrossRef]
30. Steiner, H.; Hultmark, D.; Engstrom, A.; Bennich, H.; Boman, H.G. Sequence and specificity of two antibacterial proteins involved in insect immunity. *Nature* **1981**, *292*, 246–248. [CrossRef]
31. Morishima, I.; Suginaka, S.; Ueno, T.; Hirano, H. Isolation and structure of cecropins, inducible antibacterial peptides, from the silkworm, Bombyx mori. *Comp. Biochem. Physiol. B* **1990**, *95*, 551–554. [CrossRef] [PubMed]
32. Kim, S.R.; Hong, M.Y.; Park, S.W.; Choi, K.H.; Yun, E.Y.; Goo, T.W.; Kang, S.W.; Suh, H.J.; Kim, I.; Hwang, J.S. Characterization and cDNA cloning of a cecropin-like antimicrobial peptide, papiliocin, from the swallowtail butterfly, Papilio xuthus. *Mol. Cells* **2010**, *29*, 419–423. [CrossRef] [PubMed]

33. Kim, C.H.; Lee, J.H.; Kim, I.; Seo, S.J.; Son, S.M.; Lee, K.Y.; Lee, I.H. Purification and cDNA cloning of a cecropin-like peptide from the great wax moth, Galleria mellonella. *Mol. Cells* **2004**, *17*, 262–266. [PubMed]
34. Qu, Z.; Steiner, H.; Engstrom, A.; Bennich, H.; Boman, H.G. Insect immunity: Isolation and structure of cecropins B and D from pupae of the Chinese oak silk moth, Antheraea pernyi. *Eur. J. Biochem.* **1982**, *127*, 219–224. [CrossRef] [PubMed]
35. Ramos-Martin, F.; Herrera-Leon, C.; D'Amelio, N. Bombyx mori Cecropin D could trigger cancer cell apoptosis by interacting with mitochondrial cardiolipin. *Biochim. Biophys. Acta Biomembr.* **2022**, *1864*, 184003. [CrossRef]
36. Kalsy, M.; Tonk, M.; Hardt, M.; Dobrindt, U.; Zdybicka-Barabas, A.; Cytrynska, M.; Vilcinskas, A.; Mukherjee, K. The insect antimicrobial peptide cecropin A disrupts uropathogenic Escherichia coli biofilms. *NPJ Biofilms Microbiomes* **2020**, *6*, 6. [CrossRef]
37. Krishnan, M.; Choi, J.; Jang, A.; Choi, S.; Yeon, J.; Jang, M.; Lee, Y.; Son, K.; Shin, S.Y.; Jeong, M.S.; et al. Molecular mechanism underlying the TLR4 antagonistic and antiseptic activities of papiliocin, an insect innate immune response molecule. *Proc. Natl. Acad. Sci. USA* **2022**, *119*, e2115669119. [CrossRef]
38. Peng, C.; Liu, Y.; Shui, L.; Zhao, Z.; Mao, X.; Liu, Z. Mechanisms of Action of the Antimicrobial Peptide Cecropin in the Killing of Candida albicans. *Life* **2022**, *12*, 1581. [CrossRef]
39. Mikonranta, L.; Dickel, F.; Mappes, J.; Freitak, D. Lepidopteran species have a variety of defence strategies against bacterial infections. *J. Invertebr. Pathol.* **2017**, *144*, 88–96. [CrossRef]
40. Wei, L.; Yang, Y.; Zhou, Y.; Li, M.; Yang, H.; Mu, L.; Qian, Q.; Wu, J.; Xu, W. Anti-inflammatory activities of Aedes aegypti cecropins and their protection against murine endotoxin shock. *Parasit. Vectors* **2018**, *11*, 470. [CrossRef]
41. Lee, E.; Shin, A.; Kim, Y. Anti-inflammatory activities of cecropin A and its mechanism of action. *Arch. Insect Biochem. Physiol.* **2015**, *88*, 31–44. [CrossRef] [PubMed]
42. Kim, J.K.; Lee, E.; Shin, S.; Jeong, K.W.; Lee, J.Y.; Bae, S.Y.; Kim, S.H.; Lee, J.; Kim, S.R.; Lee, D.G.; et al. Structure and function of papiliocin with antimicrobial and anti-inflammatory activities isolated from the swallowtail butterfly, Papilio xuthus. *J. Biol. Chem.* **2011**, *286*, 41296–41311. [CrossRef] [PubMed]
43. Lee, E.; Kim, J.K.; Jeon, D.; Jeong, K.W.; Shin, A.; Kim, Y. Functional Roles of Aromatic Residues and Helices of Papiliocin in its Antimicrobial and Anti-inflammatory Activities. *Sci. Rep.* **2015**, *5*, 12048. [CrossRef] [PubMed]
44. Holak, T.A.; Engstrom, A.; Kraulis, P.J.; Lindeberg, G.; Bennich, H.; Jones, T.A.; Gronenborn, A.M.; Clore, G.M. The solution conformation of the antibacterial peptide cecropin A: A nuclear magnetic resonance and dynamical simulated annealing study. *Biochemistry* **1988**, *27*, 7620–7629. [CrossRef]
45. Ramos-Martin, F.; Herrera-Leon, C.; D'Amelio, N. Molecular basis of the anticancer, apoptotic and antibacterial activities of Bombyx mori Cecropin A. *Arch. Biochem. Biophys.* **2022**, *715*, 109095. [CrossRef]
46. Zheng, Z.; Tharmalingam, N.; Liu, Q.; Jayamani, E.; Kim, W.; Fuchs, B.B.; Zhang, R.; Vilcinskas, A.; Mylonakis, E. Synergistic Efficacy of Aedes aegypti Antimicrobial Peptide Cecropin A2 and Tetracycline against Pseudomonas aeruginosa. *Antimicrob. Agents Chemother.* **2017**, *61*, e00686-17. [CrossRef]
47. Brady, D.; Grapputo, A.; Romoli, O.; Sandrelli, F. Insect Cecropins, Antimicrobial Peptides with Potential Therapeutic Applications. *Int. J. Mol. Sci.* **2019**, *20*, 5862. [CrossRef]
48. Kang, D.; Liu, G.; Gunne, H.; Steiner, H. PCR differential display of immune gene expression in Trichoplusia ni. *Insect Biochem. Mol. Biol.* **1996**, *26*, 177–184. [CrossRef]
49. Freitak, D.; Wheat, C.W.; Heckel, D.G.; Vogel, H. Immune system responses and fitness costs associated with consumption of bacteria in larvae of Trichoplusia ni. *BMC Biol.* **2007**, *5*, 56. [CrossRef]
50. Yamaguchi, T.; Kawahara, R.; Hamamoto, K.; Hirai, I.; Khong, D.T.; Nguyen, T.N.; Tran, H.T.; Motooka, D.; Nakamura, S.; Yamamoto, Y. High Prevalence of Colistin-Resistant Escherichia coli with Chromosomally Carried mcr-1 in Healthy Residents in Vietnam. *mSphere* **2020**, *5*, e00117-20. [CrossRef]
51. Wiegand, I.; Hilpert, K.; Hancock, R.E. Agar and broth dilution methods to determine the minimal inhibitory concentration (MIC) of antimicrobial substances. *Nat. Protoc.* **2008**, *3*, 163–175. [CrossRef] [PubMed]
52. Krishnan, M.; Choi, J.; Jang, A.; Kim, Y. A Novel Peptide Antibiotic, Pro10-1D, Designed from Insect Defensin Shows Antibacterial and Anti-Inflammatory Activities in Sepsis Models. *Int. J. Mol. Sci.* **2020**, *21*, 6216. [CrossRef] [PubMed]
53. Kim, J.; Durai, P.; Jeon, D.; Jung, I.D.; Lee, S.J.; Park, Y.M.; Kim, Y. Phloretin as a Potent Natural TLR2/1 Inhibitor Suppresses TLR2-Induced Inflammation. *Nutrients* **2018**, *10*, 868. [CrossRef] [PubMed]
54. Cheon, D.; Kim, J.; Jeon, D.; Shin, H.C.; Kim, Y. Target Proteins of Phloretin for Its Anti-Inflammatory and Antibacterial Activities Against Propionibacterium acnes-Induced Skin Infection. *Molecules* **2019**, *24*, 1319. [CrossRef] [PubMed]
55. Kim, J.; Jacob, B.; Jang, M.; Kwak, C.; Lee, Y.; Son, K.; Lee, S.; Jung, I.D.; Jeong, M.S.; Kwon, S.H.; et al. Development of a novel short 12-meric papiliocin-derived peptide that is effective against Gram-negative sepsis. *Sci. Rep.* **2019**, *9*, 3817. [CrossRef] [PubMed]
56. Manniello, M.D.; Moretta, A.; Salvia, R.; Scieuzo, C.; Lucchetti, D.; Vogel, H.; Sgambato, A.; Falabella, P. Insect antimicrobial peptides: Potential weapons to counteract the antibiotic resistance. *Cell Mol. Life Sci.* **2021**, *78*, 4259–4282. [CrossRef]
57. Lee, E.; Jeong, K.W.; Lee, J.; Shin, A.; Kim, J.K.; Lee, J.; Lee, D.G.; Kim, Y. Structure-activity relationships of cecropin-like peptides and their interactions with phospholipid membrane. *BMB Rep.* **2013**, *46*, 282–287. [CrossRef]
58. World Health Organization. *Global Antimicrobial Resistance Surveillance System (GLASS): The Detection and Reporting of Colistin Resistance*; World Health Organization: Geneva, Switzerland, 2018.

59. Ferreira, A.R.; Teixeira, C.; Sousa, C.F.; Bessa, L.J.; Gomes, P.; Gameiro, P. How Insertion of a Single Tryptophan in the N-Terminus of a Cecropin A-Melittin Hybrid Peptide Changes Its Antimicrobial and Biophysical Profile. *Membranes* **2021**, *11*, 48. [CrossRef]
60. Vergis, J.; Malik, S.V.S.; Pathak, R.; Kumar, M.; Kurkure, N.V.; Barbuddhe, S.B.; Rawool, D.B. Exploring Galleria mellonella larval model to evaluate antibacterial efficacy of Cecropin A (1-7)-Melittin against multi-drug resistant enteroaggregative Escherichia coli. *Pathog. Dis.* **2021**, *79*, ftab010. [CrossRef]
61. Lee, J.K.; Seo, C.H.; Luchian, T.; Park, Y. Antimicrobial Peptide CMA3 Derived from the CA-MA Hybrid Peptide: Antibacterial and Anti-inflammatory Activities with Low Cytotoxicity and Mechanism of Action in Escherichia coli. *Antimicrob. Agents Chemother.* **2016**, *60*, 495–506. [CrossRef]
62. Namvar Erbani, S.; Madanchi, H.; Ajodani Far, H.; Rostamian, M.; Rahmati, S.; Shabani, A.A. First report of antifungal activity of CecropinA-Magenin2 (CE-MA) hybrid peptide and its truncated derivatives. *Biochem. Biophys. Res. Commun.* **2021**, *549*, 157–163. [CrossRef] [PubMed]
63. Choi, J.; Jang, A.; Yoon, Y.K.; Kim, Y. Development of Novel Peptides for the Antimicrobial Combination Therapy against Carbapenem-Resistant Acinetobacter baumannii Infection. *Pharmaceutics* **2021**, *13*, 1800. [CrossRef] [PubMed]
64. Jamal, M.; Ahmad, W.; Andleeb, S.; Jalil, F.; Imran, M.; Nawaz, M.A.; Hussain, T.; Ali, M.; Rafiq, M.; Kamil, M.A. Bacterial biofilm and associated infections. *J. Chin. Med. Assoc.* **2018**, *81*, 7–11. [CrossRef] [PubMed]
65. Li, S.; Wang, Y.; Xue, Z.; Jia, Y.; Li, R.; He, C.; Chen, H. The structure-mechanism relationship and mode of actions of antimicrobial peptides: A review. *Trends Food Sci. Technol.* **2021**, *109*, 103–115. [CrossRef]

pharmaceutics

MDPI

Article

Effects of Dimerization, Dendrimerization, and Chirality in p-BthTX-I Peptide Analogs on the Antibacterial Activity and Enzymatic Inhibition of the SARS-CoV-2 PL^{pro} Protein

Natália Vitória Bitencourt [1], Gabriela Marinho Righetto [2], Ilana Lopes Baratella Cunha Camargo [2], Mariana Ortiz de Godoy [2], Rafael Victorio Carvalho Guido [2], Glaucius Oliva [2], Norival Alves Santos-Filho [1,*] and Eduardo Maffud Cilli [1,*]

1 Department of Biochemistry and Organic Chemistry, Institute of Chemistry, São Paulo State University (UNESP), Araraquara 14800-060, SP, Brazil
2 São Carlos Institute of Physics, University of São Paulo, São Carlos 13563-120, SP, Brazil
* Correspondence: norival.santos-filho@unesp.br (N.A.S.-F.); eduardo.cilli@unesp.br (E.M.C.)

Abstract: Recent studies have shown that the peptide [des-Cys^{11},Lys^{12},Lys^{13}-(p-BthTX-I)$_2$K] (p-Bth) is a p-BthTX-I analog that shows enhanced antimicrobial activity, stability and hemolytic activity, and is easy to obtain compared to the wild-type sequence. This molecule also inhibits SARS-CoV-2 viral infection in Vero cells, acting on SARS-CoV-2 PL^{pro} enzymatic activity. Thus, the present study aimed to assess the effects of structural modifications to p-Bth, such as dimerization, dendrimerization and chirality, on the antibacterial activity and inhibitory properties of PL^{pro}. The results showed that the dimerization or dendrimerization of p-Bth was essential for antibacterial activity, as the monomeric structure led to a total loss of, or significant reduction in, bacterial activities. The dimers and tetramers obtained using branched lysine proved to be prominent compounds with antibacterial activity against Gram-positive and Gram-negative bacteria. In addition, hemolysis rates were below 10% at the corresponding concentrations. Conversely, the inhibitory activity of the PL^{pro} of SARS-CoV-2 was similar in the monomeric, dimeric and tetrameric forms of p-Bth. Our findings indicate the importance of the dimerization and dendrimerization of this important class of antimicrobial peptides, which shows great potential for antimicrobial and antiviral drug-discovery campaigns.

Keywords: p-BthTX-I; p-Bth; multidrug-resistant bacteria; antimicrobial peptide; dendrimers; PL^{pro}; SARS-CoV-2; COVID-19

Citation: Bitencourt, N.V.; Righetto, G.M.; Camargo, I.L.B.C.; de Godoy, M.O.; Guido, R.V.C.; Oliva, G.; Santos-Filho, N.A.; Cilli, E.M. Effects of Dimerization, Dendrimerization, and Chirality in p-BthTX-I Peptide Analogs on the Antibacterial Activity and Enzymatic Inhibition of the SARS-CoV-2 PL^{pro} Protein. *Pharmaceutics* **2023**, *15*, 436. https://doi.org/10.3390/pharmaceutics15020436

Academic Editor: Aura Rusu

Received: 21 December 2022
Revised: 18 January 2023
Accepted: 25 January 2023
Published: 28 January 2023

1. Introduction

The growing bacterial resistance, combined with the decline in the discovery of new antibiotics, makes the post-antibiotic era, in which minor injuries can result in death, increasingly possible [1,2]. One of the ways to circumvent the situation triggered by bacterial resistance is to invest in research and development focusing on new molecules with antibacterial potential, among which antimicrobial peptides (AMPs) stand out. These molecules are constituents of the defense systems of several organisms, are widely distributed in nature, and act against various pathogens, including bacteria, fungi, *Leishmania*, and viruses [3,4]. AMPs are promising novel antibiotics that kill multidrug-resistant bacteria and show activity against some bacteria that are considered a priority by the WHO [5]. Their sequence normally has from 10 to 50 amino acids and is modulated by structure–function relationships [6]. The charge, amphipathicity, hydrophobicity and helicity of peptides are fundamental to their biological activity [7]. Although promising, AMPs face challenges regarding their therapeutic application, such as poor pharmacokinetic properties, including low absorption and stability, due to their rapid proteolytic degradation, in addition to their high production cost [8]. Strategies to address these issues include structural modifications, such as dendrimerization and chirality modifications [9]. Many studies have shown that the complete replacement of L with D-amino acids in the peptide sequence to obtain D-enantiomers leads to conservation or increased antimicrobial activity, in addition to increased resistance to proteolytic degradation [10].

Dendrimeric antimicrobial peptides (DMPAs) are commonly obtained from poly-L-lysine nuclei, in which lysine units are used as branch points with the growth of identical peptide chains of linear AMPs in their α and ε amino groups [7,11,12]. This strategy leads to the production of peptides with enhanced antimicrobial activity compared to their monomers. The enhanced activity is due to multivalence; that is, a greater number of peptide chains, leading to greater local concentration and enhanced proteolytic stability due to steric hindrance, and thereby decreasing susceptibility to proteases [13].

Recently, a cationic peptide, named p-BthTX-I, was designed based on the sequence between residues 115-129 of the C-terminal region of Bothropstoxin I (BthTX-I). The peptide p-BthTX-I was previously studied by our research group and showed high antibacterial potential, especially in its dimeric form, linked through disulfide bonds between cysteine residues in KKYRYHLKPFCKK $(p\text{-BthTX-I})_2$. In the monomeric form, the peptide undergoes oxidation and forms a dimer in solution and culture medium, showing that the dimeric form is responsible for the antibacterial activity of the p-BthTX-I peptide. Moreover, this peptide did not show activity against *Candida albicans* or cytotoxicity against macrophages, erythrocytes, and epithelial cells, indicating promising selective toxicity [14].

The dimeric peptide $(p\text{-BthTX-I})_2$ was subjected to stability tests in serum and its stable by-product [des-Lys^{12},Lys^{13}-$(p\text{-BthTX-I})_2$] showed similar antibacterial potential and, in some cases, was superior to the original molecule [15]. Furthermore, this peptide showed different mechanisms of action against Gram-positive and negative bacteria [16]. To avoid the oxidation step and make the peptide more stable, our group promoted dimerization using a lysine residue as a branch point. The analog [des-Cys^{11},Lys^{12},Lys^{13}-$(p\text{-BthTX-I})_2K$], of sequence $(KKYRYHLKPF)_2K$ (p-Bth), was the most potent analog of the series [17].

Antimicrobial peptides were also reported as potential antiviral compounds [18]; thus, we assessed the p-Bth and analogs' inhibitory activities against SARS-CoV-2 infection in Vero cells. These molecules showed a potent inhibition of viral infection, acting on the inhibition of PL^{pro} from SARS-CoV-2, a key enzyme in the viral replication process and innate immunity inhibition [19]. Moreover, p-Bth demonstrated antithrombotic activity, possibly due to kallikrein inhibition, suggesting its strong biotechnological potential [20].

Thus, this study aimed to assess and compare L- and D-p-Bth analogs (monomer, dimer and tetramer) regarding their antibacterial activity and inhibition of PL^{pro} of SARS-CoV-2.

2. Materials and Methods

2.1. Peptides Synthesis

Peptides were manually synthesized through solid-phase peptide synthesis (SPPS) using the methodology described by Merrifield, 1963 [21]. To obtain dimers and tetramers, the amino acid Fmoc-Lys(Fmoc)-OH was used at the beginning of the synthesis as a branch point, allowing for the growth of peptide chains from the α-amino and ε-amino groups of lysine, as described by Lorenzón et al., 2012 and Santos-Filho et al., 2021 [7,17]. After synthesis, the peptides were purified by semi-preparative HPLC using a Shimadzu chromatograph (Tokyo, Japan) equipped with a C18 Jupiter column of 25 × 1 cm, with a particle size of 10 µm. The purity contents (<95%) of the obtained materials were determined by analytical HPLC in a Shimadzu chromatograph (Kyoto, Japan) column (0.46 × 15 cm) of reverse-phase C18, with a particle size of 5 µm (Agilent, Santa Clara, CA, USA). Confirmations that the desired materials were obtained were evaluated by mass spectrometry, using an Ion Trap MS mass spectrometer (Bruker), direct injection and positive detection mode.

2.2. Determination of the Minimum Inhibitory Concentration and Minimum Bactericidal Concentration

Bacterial isolates from the American Type Culture Collection (ATCC) were obtained from the Collection of Reference Bacteria on Health Surveillance, Oswaldo Cruz Foundation (FIOCRUZ) after phenotypic and molecular quality control and were registered at SISGEN under the number ADB556B. The minimum inhibitory concentration (MIC) was determined as previously described by Santos-Filho et al., 2021 [17], using the broth microdilution method. The MIC was the lowest concentration that inhibited microbial growth. A total of 100 μL from each well, without growth from the MIC assay, was subcultured on CA-MH agar plates and incubated at 37 °C for 24 h to determine the minimum bactericidal concentration (MBC). MBC was defined as the lowest peptide concentration with no visible growth on the plate. An MBC/MIC ratio >4 suggests bacteriostatic activity in a peptide [22]. The assay was performed in triplicate, and the values represent the mode of the obtained results.

2.3. Hemolysis Assay

Peptide hemolytic activity was determined as previously described[15]. Peptides were incubated with erythrocytes in the range from 512 μg/mL to 0.06 μg/mL for 1 h at 37 °C. Triton X-100 1% was used as a positive control for hemolysis. Assays were performed in duplicate. The Research Ethics Committee approved this project under the number 90291518.4.0000.5426.

2.4. Circular Dichroism Spectroscopy

Circular dichroism spectra were obtained using a Jasco J-815 spectrophotometer (Tokyo, Japan). The wavelength range in which the analyses were recorded ranged from 190 to 260 nm, at a temperature of 25 °C, with three accumulations. To analyze the secondary structure of the CD spectra, analogs were obtained with the peptide at a concentration of 30 μM in aqueous solution (PBS Buffer, pH = 7) and in the well-known structuring solvents trifluoroethanol (TFE—60%), lysophosphatidylcholine micelles (LPC) and sodium dodecyl sulfate (SDS), which were used at concentrations of 10 mM, above the critical micelle concentration (CMC). Furthermore, to analyze the interactions between peptides and bacterial cell components, lipopolysaccharide (LPS) from *E. coli*—Sigma Aldrich® (Sigma-Aldrich, St. Louis, MO, USA) and total lipid extract of *E. coli* (Avanti Polar Lipids, Alabaster, AL, USA) were added to peptides at concentrations of 1, 5 and 10% at 30 μM in buffer solution (PBS, pH = 7). The spectra of LPS and total lipid extract of *E. coli* were used as negative controls and subtracted from the spectra containing peptides.

2.5. Permeability in Different Vesicle Compositions

The permeabilization of lipid vesicles containing carboxyfluorescein was carried out using a spectrofluorometer model Fluorolog-3 FL3-122 from Horiba Jobin Yvon (Newark, NJ, USA) (dimers and tetramers) or in a spectrofluorometer model RF-1501 Shimadzu (Kyoto, Japan) (monomer). For RF-1501, the quantification of the fluorescence intensity was performed every 20 s. Two vesicle compositions were used: (1) 80% 1-palmitoyl-2-oleoyl-sn-glycero-3-phosphoethanolamine (POPE) and 20% 1-palmitoyl-2-oleoyl-sn-glycero- 3-phospho-(10-rac-glycerol) (POPG); and (2) 95% 1-palmitoyl-2-oleoyl-sn-glycero-3-phosphocholine (POPC) and 5% POPG. The percentage of leakage was obtained through the following equation:

$$\% \text{ release} = (F_{measured} - F_{initial})/(F_{final} - F_{initial}) \times 100,$$

where F_{final} is the average fluorescence value obtained after the addition of Triton, $F_{initial}$ is the average of the initial values of the run before the addition of the peptide, and $F_{measured}$ are the fluorescence values obtained at each point of the experiment.

2.6. PL^{pro} Inhibition

Both the methodology of the enzyme inhibition assay and the cloning, expression and purification of the SARS-CoV-2 PL^{pro} protease were carried out in accordance with the article by Freire et al., 2021 [19].

3. Results and Discussion

3.1. Peptide Synthesis

All p-Bth analogs were synthesized with D-amino or L-amino acids to evaluate the effect of the chirality on their activities (Figure 1). L- and D-monomers (Figure 1A,B) of sequence KKYRYHLKPF were obtained to understand the impact of dimerization on the antibacterial effects and the ability to inhibit the enzymatic activity of PL^{pro} of SARS-CoV-2. The dimer (Figure 1C,D) and tetramer (Figure 1E,F) analogs (L and D isomers) were obtained using the previously described strategy, using one or three Fmoc-Lys(Fmoc)-OH in the C-terminal region [17]. The chains were grown in α- and ε-amino groups, obtaining homodimers. Chromatographic profiles and mass spectra are presented in the Supplementary Material (Figures S1–S6 and Table S1).

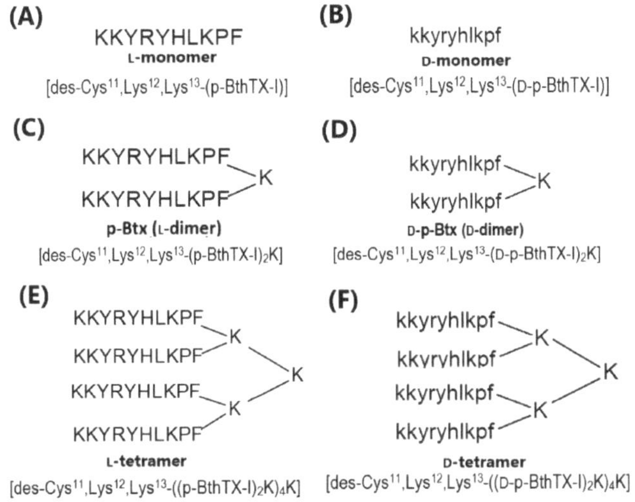

Figure 1. p-Bth peptide analogs, structure, codes and sequences. (**A**) L-monomer, (**B**) D-monomer, (**C**) L-dimer, (**D**) D-dimer, (**E**) L-tetramer, and (**F**) D-tetramer.

3.2. Biological Activity

In 2017, the World Health Organization (WHO) published a list of pathogens for which the development of new antimicrobial agents is urgent due to the severe therapeutic limitations. *Enterococcus faecium*, *Staphylococcus aureus*, *Klebsiella pneumoniae*, *Acinetobacter baumannii*, *Pseudomonas aeruginosa*, and *Enterobacter* spp. (ESKAPE) bacteria are microorganisms capable of escaping the action of antibiotics, and are part of the WHO list as high priorities in the development of therapeutic options [1].

Thus, to assess the relevance of the antimicrobial effect of p-Bth analogs, their Minimum Inhibitory Concentration (MIC) and Minimum Bactericidal Concentration (MBC) were analyzed against relevant bacteria. The evaluated strains were the Gram-positives: *S. aureus* ATCC 25923, *S. epidermidis* ATCC 35984, *E. faecalis* ATCC 29212, and *E. faecium* ATCC 70022 (Table 1); and the Gram-negatives: *K. pneumoniae* ATCC 700603, *E. coli* ATCC 25922, *A. baumannii* ATCC 19606, and *P. aeruginosa* ATCC 27853 (Table 2).

Table 1. Minimal inhibitory, bactericidal concentration and antibacterial activity of p-BthTX-I analogs against Gram-positive bacteria.

Peptides	*S. aureus* ATCC 25923				*S. epidermidis* ATCC 35984				*E. faecalis* ATCC 29212				*E. faecium* ATCC 700221			
	MIC µg/mL	MIC µM	MBC µg/mL	Act	MIC µg/mL	MIC µM	MBC µg/mL	Act	MIC µg/mL	MIC µM	MBC µg/mL	Act	MIC µg/mL	MIC µM	MBC µg/mL	Act
L-monomer	>512	>371	>512	ND	>512	>371	>512	ND	>512	>371	>512	ND	>512	>371	>512	ND
D-monomer	>512	>371	>512	ND	>512	>371	>512	ND	>512	>371	>512	ND	>512	>371	>512	ND
L-dimer	32	11	128	Bc	8	2	16	Bc	64	22	128	Bc	16	5	>64	Bs
D-dimer	256	89	>512	ND	16	5	16	Bc	512	178	512	Bc	64	22	>256	Bs
L-tetramer	64	10	256	Bc	16	2	32	Bc	64	10	128	Bc	16	2	32	Bc
D-tetramer	64	10	64	Bc	16	2	16	Bc	32	5	32	Bc	16	2	16	Bc

Abbreviations: MIC, minimum inhibitory concentration; MBC, minimum bactericidal concentration; Act, antibacterial activity; ND, not determined; Bc, bactericidal, Bs, bacteriostatic.

Table 2. Minimal inhibitory, bactericidal concentration and antibacterial activity of p-BthTX-I analogs against Gram-negative bacteria.

Peptides	*K. pneumoniae* ATCC 700603				*E. coli* ATCC 25922				*A. baumannii* ATCC 19606				*P. aeruginosa* ATCC 27853			
	MIC µg/mL	MIC µM	MBC µg/mL	Act	MIC µg/mL	MIC µM	MBC µg/mL	Act	MIC µg/mL	MIC µM	MBC µg/mL	Act	MIC µg/mL	MIC µM	MBC µg/mL	Act
L-monomer	>512	>371	>512	ND	>512	>371	>512	ND	>512	>371	>512	ND	>512	>371	>512	ND
D-monomer	512	371	512	Bc	256	185	256	Bc	>512	>371	>512	ND	>512	>371	>512	ND
L-dimer	>128	>44	ND	ND	32	11	64	Bc	256	89	>512	ND	>512	>178	ND	ND
D-dimer	64	22	128	Bc	32	11	32	Bc	16	5	64	Bc	256	89	512	Bc
L-tetramer	32	5	>128	Bs	32	5	>128	Bs	32	5	64	Bc	32	5	64	Bc
D-tetramer	32	5	32	Bc	32	5	>128	Bs	32	5	32	Bc	32	5	64	Bc

Abbreviations: MIC, minimum inhibitory concentration; MBC, minimum bactericidal concentration; Act, antibacterial activity; ND, not determined; Bc, bactericidal, Bs, bacteriostatic.

MIC values of the peptides are presented in μM and μg/mL. A data analysis of the two measurement units is necessary to adequately compare the biological activity of monomers, dimers, and tetramers with respect to the number of chains. As the monomers have a molecular mass of 1378.67 g/mol, the dimers have a mass of 2868.5 g/mol and the tetramers a mass of 5848.06 g/mol, the results in μg/mL are more correct than those in μM when comparing the molecules, considering the same number of monomeric chains.

Neither the D- nor the L-monomer showed significant antimicrobial activity against Gram-positive (Table 1) and -negative (Table 2) strains at all tested concentrations. These findings agree with Santos-Filho's hypothesis that the antimicrobial action of the p-BthTX-I peptide relies on its dimeric form, either due to disulfide bonds between cysteine or single or poly-L-lysines [17]. However, the D-monomer showed low bactericidal action against *K. pneumoniae* and *E. coli* at 512 and 256 μg/mL concentrations, respectively.

When comparing the results of the biological activity of the dimer enantiomers against Gram-positive bacterial strains, we observed that the L-dimer showed enhanced antibacterial activity compared to the D-dimer for all tested bacteria. Nevertheless, when comparing the activities of the different dimer enantiomers in Gram-negative bacteria, the D-peptide showed better biological activity than the L-peptide against all bacterial species. Thus, this shows that modifying the dimer's chirality alters its biological activity in the different tested bacterial species. This finding suggested that the mechanism of action of the peptide p-Bth is different in Gram-negative and Gram-positive bacteria, as found in the peptide (p-BthTX-I)$_2$ [16]. Santos-Filho concluded that, in Gram-positive bacteria, (p-BthTX-I)$_2$ showed direct action on the bacterial surface, while in Gram-negative bacteria, the peptide was internalized and acted on a specific target. Therefore, the enhanced activity of the D-enantiomeric form in Gram-negative bacteria could be explained by its interactions with specific targets (e.g., proteins and DNA) or by the greater stability of D-enantiomer against proteases [23].

In the case of a peptide analog with four chains, the difference in chirality did not affect the antimicrobial activity once the MIC values were the same among the two enantiomeric tetramer pairs (32 μg/mL or 5 μM) against *K. pneumoniae* and *A. baumannii*.

The increase in the monomeric units of the peptide from two to four did not enhance the antibacterial activity. Exceptions were found for *K. pneumoniae* and *P. aeruginosa* bacteria, in which the tetramers were more active than dimers, suggesting that the inhibitory activity is directed towards a specific target. Peptides presenting the same monomeric chain number have similar activity.

When the MIC values in μM were analyzed, both tetramers showed the same value as the L-dimer against the tested *Staphylococcus*. Furthermore, tetramers were the most potent p-Bth analogs in Gram-negative bacteria, with an MIC value of 5 μM against all strains. These findings showed that, with the same peptide concentration, the tetramerization increases the MIC.

Thus, the D-tetramer was shown to be the most potent analog against both Gram-positive and Gram-negative bacteria. Therefore, the combined strategies of the structural modification of peptides by dendrimerization and chirality changes delivered the best analog in the study.

3.3. Hemolysis Assay

Antimicrobial peptides have attracted increasing attention as a promising treatment option. In 2019, approximately 10,000 articles were published on AMPs, with 3000 antimicrobial peptides listed in the Antimicrobial Peptide Database 3 (APD3) [24]. However, AMPs have limitations, and one of them is their toxicity. Thus, hemolytic activity studies were carried out to analyze the potential application of these molecules [25]. The results regarding the hemolytic activity of the p-Bth analogs peptides are shown in Figure 2. Both monomers (Figure 2A,B) and dimeric (Figure 2C,D) peptides showed low hemolytic activity (below 10%) at all evaluated concentrated. The tetramers (Figure 2E,F) showed a slight increase in hemolytic activity compared to the other analogs, with the D-tetramer being more hemolytic.

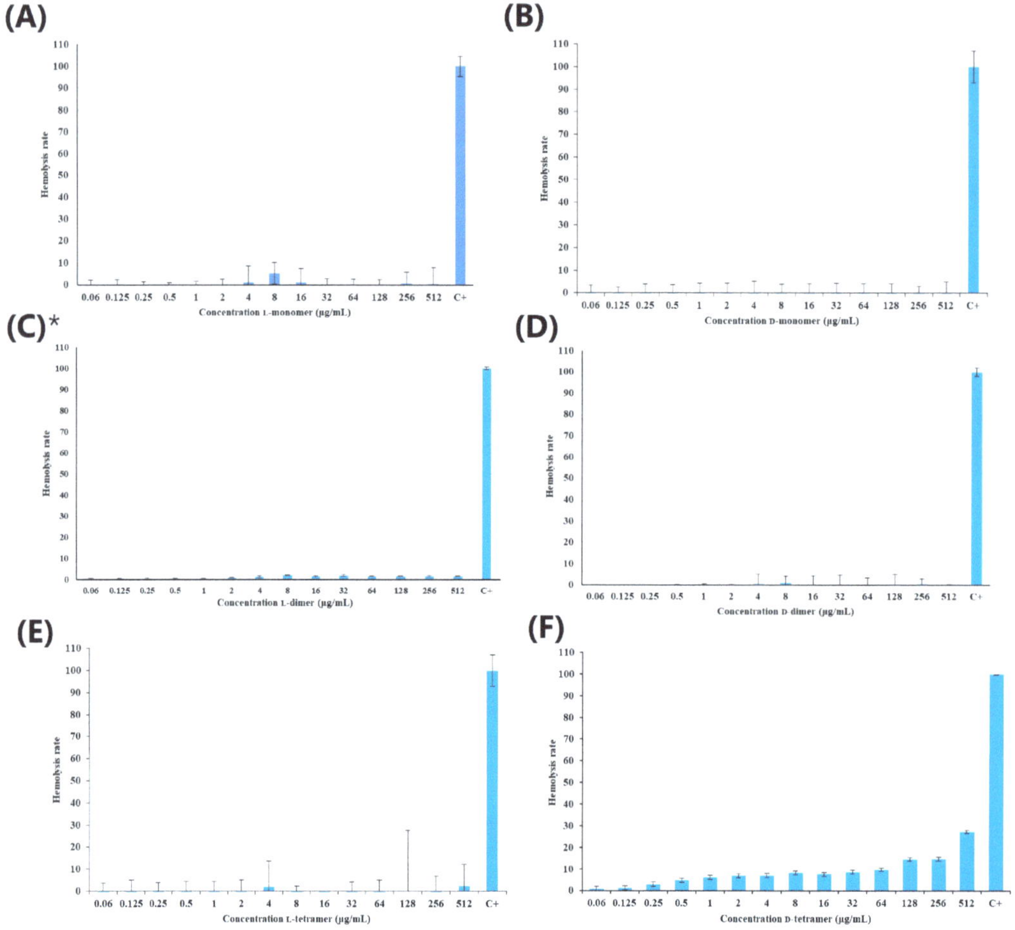

Figure 2. Hemolytic activity of peptides: (**A**) L-monomer, (**B**) D-monomer, (**C**) L-dimer, (**D**) D-dimer, (**E**) L-tetramer, and (**F**) D-tetramer at hemolytic rate (%) as a function of the peptide concentration μg/mL. Results provided in the article by Santos-Filho et al., 2021 [17].

Then, p-Bth analogs were shown to be extremely promising; they have potent antibacterial activity and a low hemolytic rate at the same concentration. The MIC values of the tetramers ranged from 16 to 64 μg/mL and, at these concentrations, peptides presented 10% hemolysis, similar to those observed for the CAMEL peptide [26]. It is important to emphasize that dendrimerization appears to increase the hemolytic activity of the analogs, as the monomers and dimers maintain a hemolysis percentage below 10%, even at 512 μg/mL, and the D-tetramer reaches 28% hemolysis at this concentration. These results confirmed what was observed with the L-dimer [des-Cys^{11},Lys^{12},Lys^{13}-(p-BthTX-I)$_2$K] and the eight analogs synthesized through the alanine scanning conducted by Santos-Filho et al. in 2021: a hemolysis rate below 5%, even at a concentration of 512 μg/mL [17]. None of the peptides obtained from the C-terminal region of the homologous PLA_2 showed hemolytic activity, as this depends on the quaternary structure of the protein [14]. These results indicated that the peptide analogs are promising, with low hemolytic activity and selective toxicity against procaryotes.

3.4. Circular Dichroism

The peptide structures are influenced by the environment and directly affect the mechanism of action [27]. The circular dichroism technique is a spectroscopic tool used to determine the secondary structures of peptides [28,29]. Compounds structured in α-helix present a minimum negative at 208 and 216 nm and a positive maximum at 195 nm. β-sheet-structured peptides have a minimum at negative 218 nm and a maximum peak at positive 196 nm. However, proteins and peptides with a random structure have an ellipsis with a minimum peak at 195 nm and a maximum positive peak at 218 nm [30]. CD was also used to investigate interactions between peptides and cellular components, aiming to better understand the mechanism of action of antimicrobial peptides, as such peptides can present structural changes when interacting with cellular components, membrane mimetic environments, and different solutions [30–32].

The secondary structure of p-Bth analogs peptides (Figure 3) was obtained at a peptide concentration of 30 μM in an aqueous solution (Buffer PBS, pH = 7.4), with known structuring solvent trifluoroethanol (TFE 60%) and micelles of lysophosphatidylcholine (LPC) and sodium dodecyl sulfate (SDS) at 10 mM, above the critical micelle concentration (CMC), forming the membranes' mimetic environments.

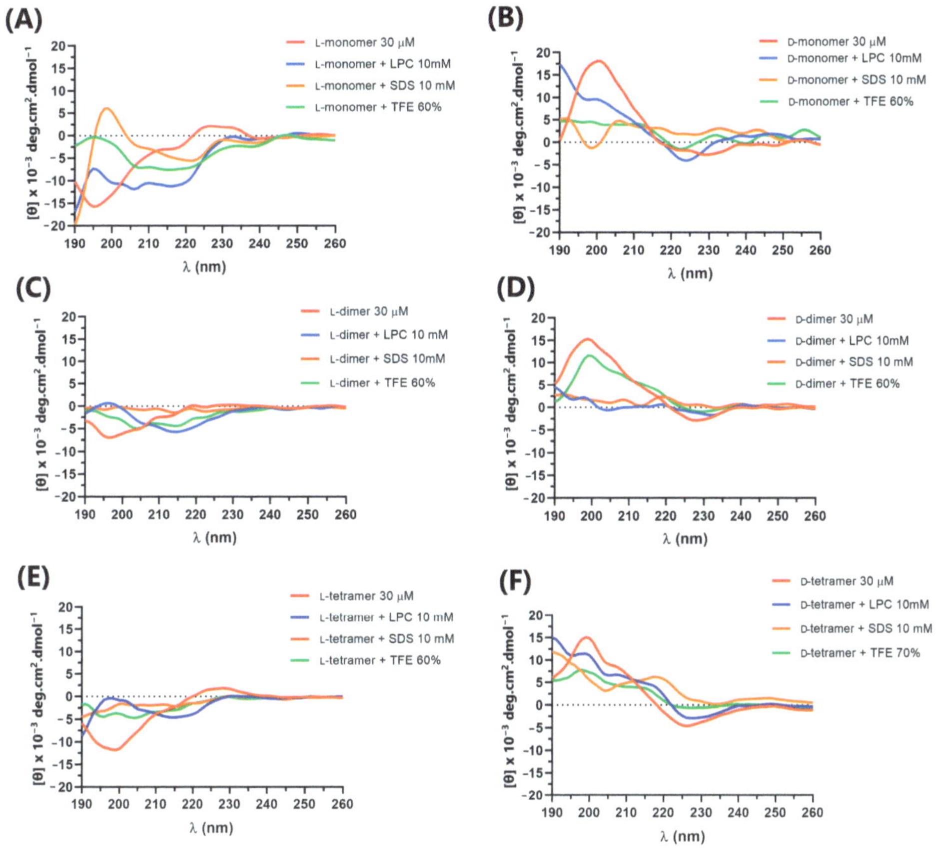

Figure 3. Circular dichroism of peptides: (**A**) L-monomer, (**B**) D-monomer, (**C**) L-dimer, (**D**) D-dimer, (**E**) L-tetramer, and (**F**) D-tetramer at 30 μM in PBS, LPC, SDS and TFE.

In an aqueous solution, the L-peptides did not present defined secondary structures. They showed the spectra characteristics of random structures, with negative bands ranging from 195 to 200 nm and a positive band close to 220 [30]. D-peptides in an aqueous solution also showed characteristic spectra of a random structure, with opposite peaks to those observed for L-peptides, bands close to 195–200 nm and a negative band close to 220 nm. This result was expected as the CD of an enantiomeric pair must be the mirror image of the other [33]. In TFE and SDS, the peptide spectra became less characteristic of a random structure, but without bands indicating defined secondary structures. The only exception was the monomer peptide with L-amino acids, which, in SDS, showed a positive maximum at 195 nm and a negative band near 222 nm, characterizing the low content of the α-helix structure [30]. In LPC, all peptides seemed to undergo a slight conformational change, without showing a well-defined structure.

In addition, to evaluate the interaction with cell-wall components in addition to the cell membrane, the CD spectra of the peptides were obtained in the presence of *E. coli* lipopolysaccharide (LPS) Sigma Aldrich® and *E. coli* total lipid extract (Avanti®) at concentrations of 1, 5 and 10% (Figures 4 and 5) in relation to the peptide quantity. The interaction between the peptides and cellular components can lead to structural variations that directly impact the mechanism of action of antimicrobial peptides, such as cecropin A and magainin 2, which, in solution, have a random structure, but acquire α-helix secondary structure in the presence of LPS, vesicles or micelles [34].

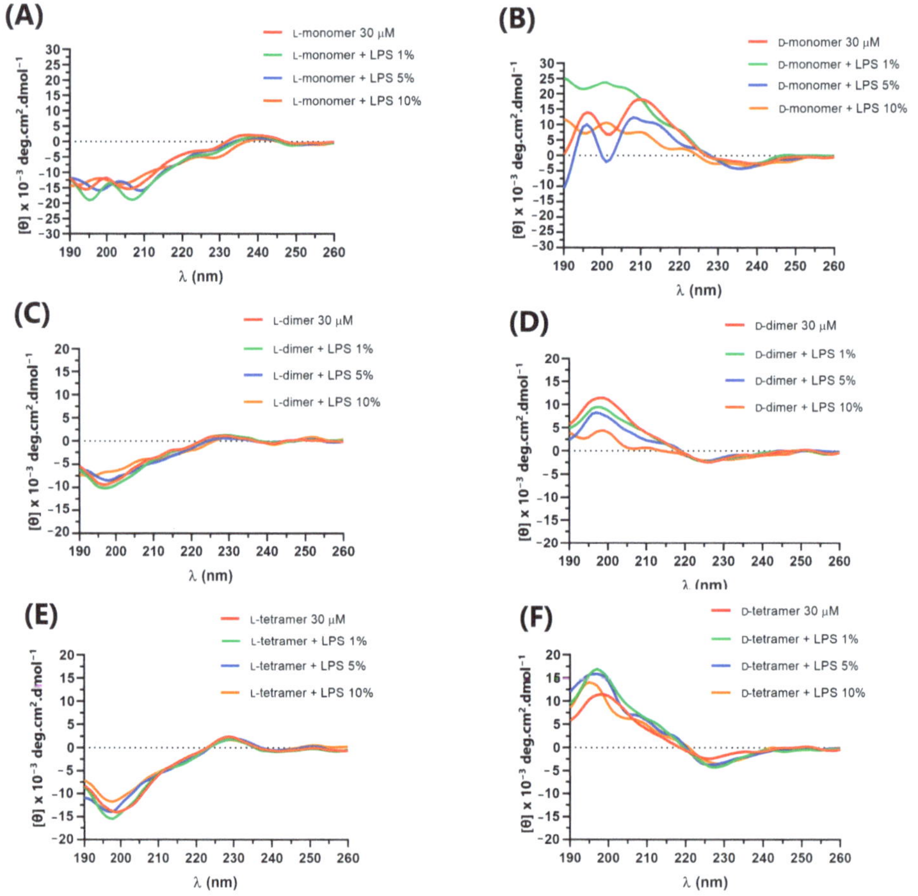

Figure 4. Circular dichroism of peptides: (**A**) L-monomer, (**B**) D-monomer, (**C**) L-dimer, (**D**) D-dimer, (**E**) L-tetramer, and (**F**) D-tetramer at 30 µM in PBS and in the presence of 1, 5 and 10% LPS.

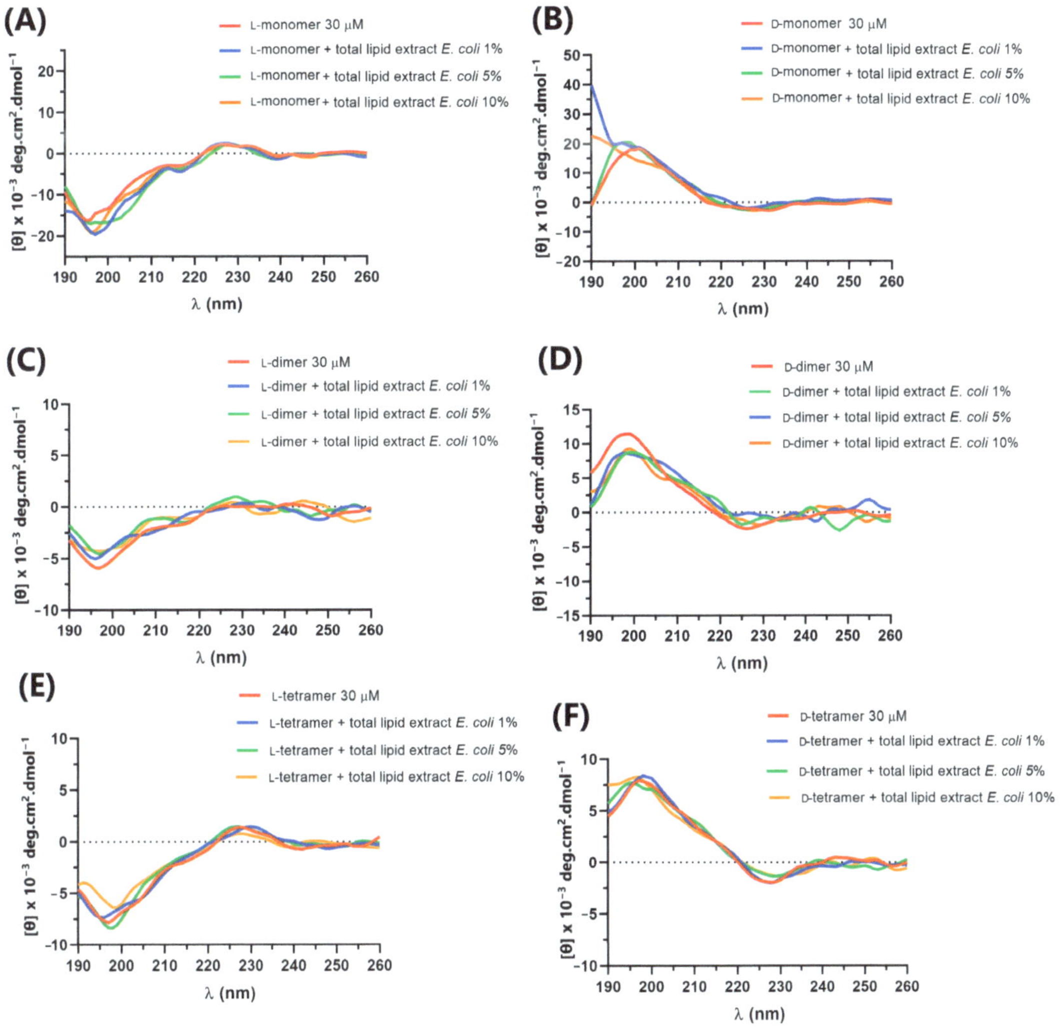

Figure 5. Circular dichroism of peptides: (**A**) L-monomer, (**B**) D-monomer, (**C**) L-dimer, (**D**) D-dimer, (**E**) L-tetramer, and (**F**) D-tetramer at 30 μM in PBS and in the presence of 1, 5 and 10% *E. coli* total lipid extract.

The L-peptides (Figure 4A,C,E) showed no variation in the CD spectra in the presence of different concentrations of LPS, indicating no interaction with the lipopolysaccharides. However, the D-dimer enantiomer showed a small variation in the CD spectra (Figure 4B,D,F), which suggested that such molecules interact with the component present in the outer membrane of the Gram-negative bacteria. As the D-dimer was more active against Gram-negative bacteria than the L-dimer, this result may be related to the possible interaction between such peptides and the lipopolysaccharide, and the greater specificity of such enantiomers.

In the presence of *E. coli* total lipid extract, as shown in Figure 5, the peptides did not show prominent variations compared to their spectrum in solution, indicating no interaction with lipids.

3.5. Vesicle Permeabilization

Peptides that act through mechanisms that lead to membrane damage, such as pore formation (barrel-stave or toroidal) and/or destabilization of the lipid bilayer (carpet-like), are called permeabilizing peptides [35]. The membranes of organisms serve as protective barriers and, therefore, are treated as biological targets for drugs (as antimicrobial peptides) [35]. Other action mechanisms involving metabolic dysfunctions, such as the inhibition of proteins, DNA synthesis and other enzymatic pathways, must also be considered [36].

The vesicle permeabilization assay is used to investigate the mechanism of action of peptides by analyzing the interaction between such molecules and unilamellar vesicles and obtain insights into the sequence–structure–function relationships of membrane-active peptides [35].

Here, we evaluated two systems of membrane mimetics, including vesicles with a composition of 80% POPE and 20% POPG, and another with 95% POPC and 5% POPG. The first is widely used as a model of bacterial membranes, specifically of *E. coli* membrane [37]. Membranes constituting POPC and POPG were used to mimic mammalian membranes due to the presence of choline-containing lipids in animal membranes [14].

Carboxyfluorescein release data in the vesicle of composition 80% POPE and 20% POPG (Figure 6) showed that all analogs, in both enantiomeric forms, have less leakage, with a maximum percentage of 15% reached by the monomers and L-dimer at a concentration of 50 μM. These results showed that the peptides did not have the formation of pores or destabilization of the plasma membrane as their main mechanism of action. Most peptides have an MIC value below 50 μM (Tables 1 and 2). This observation was made with the peptide p-BthTX-I and $(p\text{-BthTX-I})_2$ by Santos-Filho et al. (2015) [14], where the p-BthTX-I and $(p\text{-BthTX-I})_2$ peptides did not show fluorophore release in vesicles of the same lipid composition. The results indicated that peptides derived from the homologous PLA_2 protein BthTX-I and analogs show antimicrobial action that is promoted by the action on specific targets, either on the membrane or in the intracellular medium. To confirm this hypothesis, more complex and elucidative studies are needed.

The leakage of CF in 95% POPC and 5% POPG vesicles (Figure 7) was greater than that in 80% POPE/20% POPG, but did not exceed the value of 40%. This indicated that dimerization or/and dendrimerization using poly-L-lysine increases the interaction between peptides and vesicles. The monomers led to low leakage values, while the dimers and tetramers significantly increased permeabilization [14]. However, this interaction is small compared to other peptides, such as the W^6-Hy-a1 peptide studied by Crusca Jr (2011) [38], which, at a concentration of 4 μM, showed about 90% leakage in the studied LUVs. The D-dimer analog at 50 μM is less active than the peptide used in 4 μM, and only 20% of CF leakage was found.

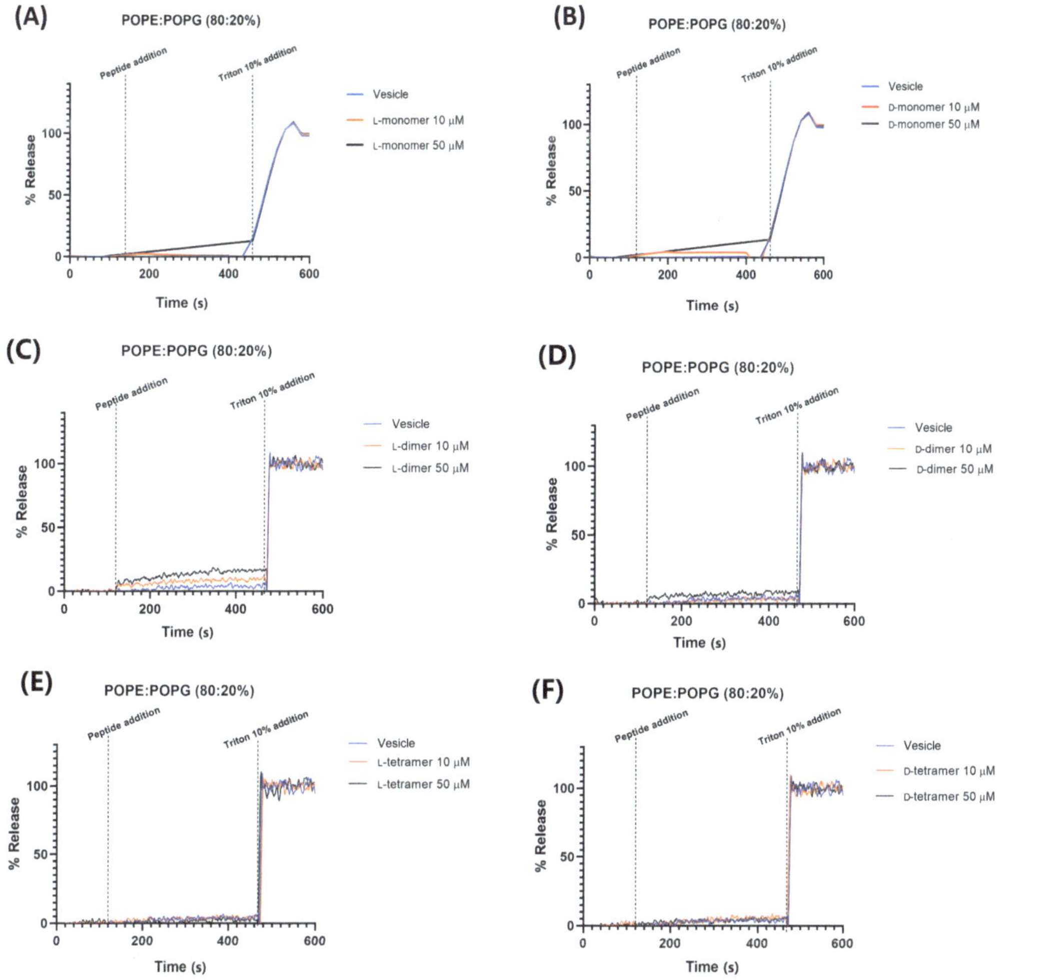

Figure 6. Permeabilization in 80% POPE and 20% POPG vesicles of the peptides: (**A**) L-monomer, (**B**) D-monomer, (**C**) L-dimer, (**D**) D-dimer, (**E**) L-tetramer, and (**F**) D-tetramer at concentrations of 10 and 50 μM.

The D-peptides in 95% POPC and 5% POPG vesicles showed 15, 20, and 35% fluorescein leakages for the monomer, dimer, and tetramer, respectively. These results agree with those obtained in the hemolysis assay of the peptides, where the most hemolytic peptide was the tetramer analog. The red blood cell contains a higher quantity of the POPC in its membrane. Gogoi et al. (2021) also showed that the hemolytic activity increased with the branching of the peptide [39].

In addition, dimeric peptides showed a concentration-dependent relationship with CF leakage; at 50 μM, the observed leakage was greater than that at 10 μM. These results could indicate a hybrid leakage model [35], where most permeabilization of the fluorescein occurs immediately after the addition of peptides to vesicles (burst of leakage), followed by a dramatic slowing of leakage over a short period of time. This slight fluorescein leakage could indicate that peptides may induce small and transient apertures in the target membrane, as observed with magainin 2, which forms pores that are not as stable, but are transient structures [40]. When the transient pores are closed, the peptide chains translocate across the bilayer and could be adsorbed in the head group region in the cell or act on other action targets, such as enzymes and DNA.

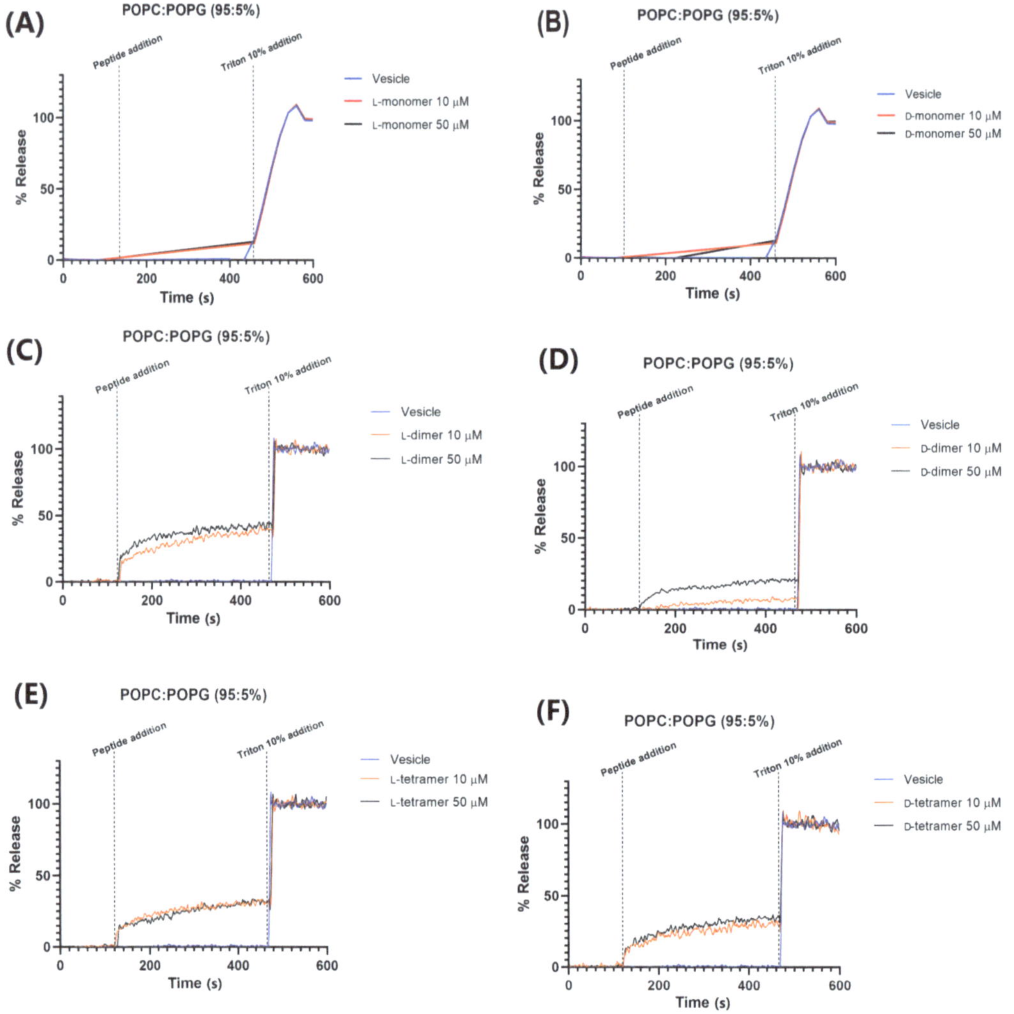

Figure 7. Permeabilization in 95% POPC and 5% POPG vesicles of the peptides: (**A**) L-monomer, (**B**) D-monomer, (**C**) L-dimer, (**D**) D-dimer, (**E**) L-tetramer, and (**F**) D-tetramer at concentrations of 10 and 50 µM.

This hypothesis is confirmed by antimicrobial data, where dendrimeric analogs show small leakage in the membrane model but potent antimicrobial activity.

3.6. Inhibition of SARS-CoV-2 PL^{pro} Enzymatic Activity

In December 2019, the first case of viral infection with a new coronavirus was reported in China, which was later named severe acute respiratory syndrome coronavirus 2 (SARS-CoV-2), and the disease caused by this was named coronavirus-2019 or COVID-19 by the WHO. This disease has taken on great proportions, causing a pandemic scenario and great global concern. Even with the improvements in disease control, there is still a need for new, specific antiviral therapeutic options [41]. As antimicrobial peptides also have antiviral action [18], the L-dimer, D-dimer and L-tetramer, in addition to other p-Bth analogs obtained through alanine scanning studies, were evaluated regardinng their ability to inhibit SARS-CoV-2 infection, showing percentage inhibitions of infection of 27, 69 and 54%, respectively [19]. These data were published in a previous study that showed that modifications of chirality more than doubled the dimer's ability to inhibit SARS-CoV-2 infection, and the tetramer led to significantly improved inhibition activity. The antiviral activity of p-Bth analogs was attributed to the peptide's ability to inhibit the enzymatic activity of papain-like cysteine protease (PL^{pro}), which is important in the cleavage and processing of polyproteins that are part of the viral replication complex and affects the innate immune responses. Thus, by inhibiting PL^{pro}, the peptides derived from p-BthTX-I promote dysfunction in the replication and viral propagation of SARS-CoV-2.

Aiming to understand the need for the dimeric or tetrameric forms of the peptide in the enzymatic inhibition of the papain-like cysteine protease, we assessed the enzymatic inhibition of PL^{pro} by the L- and D-monomers. Moreover, to obtain better molecules by joining the dendrimerization and D-compounds in the same molecule, we also assessed the enzymatic inhibition promoted by the D-tetramer.

The inhibition of PL^{pro} of SARS-CoV-2 at 10 μM of the p-BthTX-I analog peptides was maintained when the peptides were in monomer form, showing only a slight reduction, which was more significant for the D-monomer (Table 3). The IC_{50} values of the peptide analogs showed comparable inhibition values (Table 3) and profiles. This is a strong indication that the antiviral activity of the peptide did not depend on its dimeric or tetrameric form. These findings contrast with the observed antibacterial activity, which showed a drastic reduction in potency when the analogs occurred in the form of monomers. This phenomenon can be explained by the vast differences between the structures, components and physiology of bacteria and viruses and, consequently, the different targets in which the peptides perform their antibacterial and antiviral action. A preliminary structure–activity relationship (SAR), which modeled the peptide binding to PL^{pro} from SARS-CoV-2, suggested that the L-dimer is in close contact with key amino acids involved in the enzymatic catalysis [19].

Table 3. PL^{pro} activity by peptide analogs of p-BThTX-I at the concentration of 10 μM and IC_{50} values. Representative concentration–response inhibition curves against PL^{pro} from SARS-CoV-2 are presented in the Supplementary Material (Figure S7).

Peptide	Inhibition (%) at 10 μM	IC_{50} μM
L-monomer	93.30 ± 0.00	2.1 ± 0.1
D-monomer	85.00 ± 3.00	3.0 ± 1
L-dimer *	98.05 ± 1.62	2.4 ± 0.1
D-dimer *	96.35 ± 0.91	1.30 ± 0.03
L-tetramer *	98.40 ± 0.00	1.40 ± 0.02
D-tetramer	94.00 ± 3.00	2.7 ± 0.5

* Results provided in the article by Freire et al., 2021 [19].

Differing from what was expected, the combination of the two structural modification strategies in the D-tetramer did not lead to an increase in the percentage of inhibition of the enzymatic activity of PL^{pro}. However, all the peptides in the work, except for the D-monomer, led to PL^{pro} inhibition percentages close to 100% and were interesting molecules, whose antiviral actions against SARS-CoV-2 should be studied in more depth.

4. Conclusions

The evaluation of the antibacterial activity of such molecules led to the confirmation of the hypothesis that the antimicrobial action of p-Bth analog peptides relies on their dimeric or dendrimeric form.

By contrast, the inhibition of the enzymatic activity of the PL^{pro} of SARS-CoV-2 was maintained when the peptides were in monomer form. Therefore, the studied peptides led to interesting inhibition percentages of the enzymatic activity of PL^{pro} (85 to 98% at 10 μM), and stand out as molecules whose antiviral actions against SARS-CoV-2 should be studied in more depth.

The peptides' p-Bth analogs had high antibacterial potency and an increased ability to inhibit the PL^{pro} enzyme of SARS-CoV-2, proving to be promising for the development of new drugs.

Supplementary Materials: The supporting information can be downloaded at: https://www.mdpi.com/article/10.3390/pharmaceutics15020436/s1. The synthesis and characterization of the peptides and PL^{pro} inhibition assays are available online.

Author Contributions: Conceptualization, N.V.B., N.A.S.-F. and E.M.C.; Validation, R.V.C.G.; Formal analysis, N.V.B. and E.M.C.; Investigation, N.V.B., G.M.R. and M.O.d.G.; Resources, I.L.B.C.C., R.V.C.G., G.O. and E.M.C.; Data curation, I.L.B.C.C.; Writing—original draft, N.V.B., N.A.S.-F. and E.M.C.; Writing—review & editing, I.L.B.C.C., R.V.C.G., N.A.S.-F. and E.M.C.; Supervision, I.L.B.C.C., R.V.C.G., N.A.S.-F. and E.M.C.; Project administration, E.M.C.; Funding acquisition, G.O. and E.M.C. All authors have read and agreed to the published version of the manuscript.

Funding: São Paulo Research Foundation (FAPESP grant #2013/07600-3; #2014/50926-0; #2020/12904-5), the Coordination for the Improvement of Higher Education Personnel (CAPES), and the National Council of Technological and Scientific Development (CNPq).

Institutional Review Board Statement: Not applicable.

Informed Consent Statement: Not applicable.

Data Availability Statement: Not applicable.

Acknowledgments: The authors are grateful to the São Paulo Research Foundation (FAPESP), the Coordination for the Improvement of Higher Education Personnel (CAPES), and the National Council of Technological and Scientific Development (CNPq) for financial support. The EMC is a senior researcher at CNPq (304739/2021-9). NASF received a post-doctoral fellowship from FAPESP (#2014/05538-1). GMR received a Ph.D. fellowship (grant #2018/15887-4, São Paulo Research Foundation (FAPESP)). ILBCC is a CNPq Research Productivity Fellow—Level 2 (304325/2021-0).

Conflicts of Interest: The authors declare no conflict of interest.

References

1. Oliveira, D.M.; Forde, B.M.; Kidd, T.J.; Harris, P.N.; Schembri, M.A.; Beatson, S.A.; Paterson, D.L.; Walker, M.J. Antimicrobial Resistance in ESKAPE Pathogens. *Clin. Microbiol. Rev.* **2020**, *33*, e00181-19. [CrossRef] [PubMed]
2. Yadav, S.; Kapley, A. Antibiotic resistance: Global health crisis and metagenomics. *Biotechnol. Rep.* **2021**, *29*, e00604. [CrossRef] [PubMed]
3. Dijksteel, G.S.; Ulrich, M.M.; Middelkoop, E.; Boekema, B.K. Lessons learned from clinical trials using antimicrobial peptides (AMPs). *Front. Microbiol.* **2021**, *12*, 616979. [CrossRef] [PubMed]
4. Costa, N.C.S.; Piccoli, J.P.; Santos-Filho, N.A.; Clementino, L.C.; Fusco-Almeida, A.M.; De Annunzio, S.R.; Cilli, E.M. Antimicrobial activity of RP-1 peptide conjugate with ferrocene group. *PLoS ONE* **2020**, *15*, e0228740. [CrossRef] [PubMed]
5. Roque-Borda, C.A.; Silva, P.B.; Rodrigues, M.C.; Filippo, L.D.; Duarte, J.L.; Chorilli, M.; Vicente, E.F.; Garrido, S.S.; Pavan, F.R. Antimicrobial peptides as potential new drugs against WHO list of critical, high, and medium priority bacteria. *Pharm. Nanotechnol. Eur. J. Med. Chem.* **2022**, *241*, 114640. [CrossRef] [PubMed]
6. Hassan, M.; Flanagan, T.W.; Kharouf, N.; Bertsch, C.; Mancino, D.; Haikel, Y. Antimicrobial Proteins: Structure, Molecular Action, and Therapeutic Potential. *Pharmaceutics* **2023**, *15*, 72. [CrossRef]
7. Lorenzón, E.N.; Piccoli, J.P.; Santos-Filho, N.A.; Cilli, E.M. Dimerization of antimicrobial peptides: A promising strategy to enhance antimicrobial peptide activity. *Protein Pept. Lett.* **2019**, *26*, 98–107. [CrossRef]
8. Liu, Y.S.; Jingru, T.Z.; Jia, Y.Y.; Bingqing, W.Z. The revitalization of antimicrobial peptides in the resistance era. *Pharmacol. Res.* **2021**, *163*, 1043–6618. [CrossRef]
9. Rezende, S.B.; Oshiro, K.G.; Júnior, N.G.; Franco, O.L.; Cardoso, M.H. Advances on chemically modified antimicrobial peptides for generating peptide antibiotics. *Chem. Commun.* **2021**, *57*, 11578–11590. [CrossRef]
10. Gan, B.G.J.; Rowe, S.M.; Deingruber, T.; Spring, D.R. The multifaceted nature of antimicrobial peptides: Current synthetic chemistry approaches and future directions. *Chem. Soc. Rev.* **2021**, *50*, 7820–7880. [CrossRef]

11. Lorenzón, E.N.; Cespedes, G.F.; Vicente, E.F.; Nogueira, L.G.; Bauab, T.M.; Cilli, E.M.; Castro, M.S. Effects of Dimerization on the Structure and Biological Activity of Antimicrobial Peptide Ctx-Ha. *Antimicrob. Agents Chemother.* **2012**, *56*, 3004–3010. [CrossRef] [PubMed]
12. Mirakabad, F.S.T.; Khoramgah, M.S.; Keshavarz, K.; Tabarzad, M.; Ranjbari, J. Peptide dendrimers as valuable biomaterials in medical sciences. *Life Sci.* **2019**, *233*, 116754. [CrossRef] [PubMed]
13. Giuliani, A.R.; Andrea, C. Beyond natural antimicrobial peptides: Multimeric peptides and other peptidomimetic approaches. *Cell. Mol. Life Sci.* **2011**, *68*, 2255–2266. [CrossRef] [PubMed]
14. Santos-Filho, N.A.; Ramos, M.A.; Santos, C.T.; Piccoli, J.P.; Bauab, T.M.; Fusco-Almeida, A.M.; Cilli, E.M. Synthesis and characterization of an antibacterial and non-toxic dimeric peptide derived from the C-terminal region of Bothropstoxin-I. *Toxicon* **2015**, *103*, 160–168. [CrossRef] [PubMed]
15. Santos-Filho, N.A.; Fernandes, R.S.; Sgardioli, B.F.; Ramos, M.A.S.; Piccoli, J.P.; Camargo, I.L.B.C.; Bauab, T.M.; Cilli, E.M. Antibacterial Activity of the Non-Cytotoxic Peptide (p-BthTX-I)$_2$ and Its Serum Degradation Product against Multidrug-Resistant Bacteria. *Molecules* **2017**, *22*, 1898. [CrossRef]
16. Santos-Filho, N.A.; De Freitas, L.M.; Dos Santos, C.T.; Piccoli, J.P.; Fontana, C.R.; Fusco-Almeida, A.M.; Cilli, E.M. Understanding the mechanism of action of peptide (p-BthTX-I)2 derived from C-terminal region of phospholipase A2 (PLA2)-like bothropstoxin-I on Gram-positive and Gram-negative bacteria. *Toxicon* **2021**, *196*, 44–55. [CrossRef]
17. Santos-Filho, N.A.; Righetto, G.M.; Pereira, M.R.; Piccoli, J.P.; Almeida, L.M.T.; Leal, T.C.; Camargo, I.L.B.C.; Cilli, E.M. Effect of C-terminal and N-terminal dimerization and alanine scanning on antibacterial activity of the analogs of the peptide p-BthTX-I. *Pept. Sci.* **2021**, *114*, e24243. [CrossRef]
18. Vilas Boas, L.C.P.; Campos, M.L.; Berlanda, R.L.A.; De Carvalho Neves, N.; Franco, O.L. Antiviral peptides as promising therapeutic drugs. *Cell. Mol. Life Sci.* **2019**, *76*, 3525–3542. [CrossRef]
19. Freire, M.C.; Noske, G.D.; Bitencourt, N.V.; Sanches, P.R.; Santos-Filho, N.A.; Gawriljuk, V.O.; Souza, E.P.; Nogueira, V.H.R.; Godoy, M.O.; Nakamura, A.M.; et al. Non-Toxic Dimeric Peptides Derived from the Bothropstoxin-I Are Potent SARS-CoV-2 and Papain-like Protease Inhibitors. *Molecules* **2021**, *26*, 4896. [CrossRef]
20. Nogueira, R.S.; Salu, B.R.; Nardelli, V.G.; Bonturi, C.R.; Pereira, M.R.; Maffei, F.H.A.; Cilli, E.M.; Oliva, M.L.V. A snake venom-analog peptide that inhibits SARS-CoV-2 and papain-like protease displays antithrombotic activity in mice arterial thrombosis model, without interfering with bleeding time. *Thromb. J.* **2023**, *21*, 3–10. [CrossRef]
21. Merrifield, R.B. Solid Phase Peptide Synthesis. I. The Synthesis of a Tetrapeptide. *J. Am. Chem. Soc.* **1963**, *85*, 2149–2154. [CrossRef]
22. Pankey, G.A.; Sabath, L.D. Clinical relevance of bacteriostatic versus bactericidal mechanisms of action in the treatment of Gram-positive bacterial infections. *Clin. Infect. Dis.* **2004**, *38*, 864–870. [CrossRef] [PubMed]
23. Bobone, S.; Stella, L. Selectivity of Antimicrobial Peptides: A Complex Interplay of Multiple Equilibria. *Antimicrob. Pept.* **2019**, *1117*, 175–214.
24. Wang, Y.; Chang, R.Y.K.; Britton, W.J.; Chan, H.K. Advances in the development of antimicrobial peptides and proteins for inhaled therapy. *Adv. Drug Deliv. Rev.* **2022**, *180*, 114066. [CrossRef] [PubMed]
25. Greco, I.; Molchanova, N.; Holmedal, E.; Jenssen, H.; Hummel, B.D.; Watts, J.L.; Håkansson, J.; Hansen, P.R.; Svenson, J. Correlation between hemolytic activity, cytotoxicity and systemic in vivo toxicity of synthetic antimicrobial peptides. *Sci. Rep.* **2020**, *10*, 13206. [CrossRef] [PubMed]
26. Neubauer, D.; Jaśkiewicz, M.; Migoń, D.; Bauer, M.; Sikora, K.; Sikorska, E.; Kamysz, E.; Kamysz, W. Retro analog concept: Comparative study on physico-chemical and biological properties of selected antimicrobial peptides. *Amino Acids* **2017**, *49*, 1755–1771. [CrossRef]
27. Pathania, A.R. Circular dichroism and its uses in biomolecular research. *E3S Web Conf.* **2021**, *309*, 01095.
28. Keiderling, T.A. Structure of Condensed Phase Peptides: Insights from Vibrational Circular Dichroism and Raman Optical Activity Techniques. *Chem. Rev.* **2020**, *120*, 3381–3419. [CrossRef]
29. Woody, R.W. Circular dichroism of peptides. In *The Peptides*; Hruby, V.J., Ed.; Academic Press: New York, NY, USA, 1985; Volume 7, pp. 15–114.
30. Harada, T.; Moriyama, H. *Solid-State Circular Dichroism Spectroscopy. Encyclopedia of Polymer Science and Technology*; John Wiley & Sons: Hoboken, NJ, USA, 2002.
31. Ding, L.; Yang, L.; Weiss, T.M.; Waring, A.J.; Lehrer, R.I.; Huang, H.W. Interaction of Antimicrobial Peptides with Lipopolysaccharides. *Biochemistry* **2003**, *42*, 12251–12259. [CrossRef]
32. Torcato, I.M.; Castanho, M.A.R.B.; Henriques, S.T. The Application of Biophysical Techniques to Study Antimicrobial Peptides. *Spectrosc. Int. J.* **2012**, *27*, 541–549. [CrossRef]
33. Zhou, N.; Luo, Z.; Luo, J.; Fan, X.; Cayabyab, M.; Hiraoka, M.; Huang, Z. Exploring the Stereochemistry of CXCR4-Peptide Recognition and Inhibiting HIV-1 Entry with d-Peptides Derived from Chemokines. *J. Biol. Chem.* **2002**, *277*, 17476–17485. [CrossRef] [PubMed]
34. Avitabile, C.; D'andrea, L.D.; Romanelli, A. Circular Dichroism studies on the interactions of antimicrobial peptides with bacterial cells. *Sci. Rep.* **2014**, *4*, 4293. [CrossRef]
35. Wimley, W.C.; Hristova, K. The mechanism of membrane permeabilization by peptides: Still an enigma. *Aust. J. Chem.* **2019**, *73*, 96–103. [CrossRef] [PubMed]

36. Corrêa, J.A.F.; Evangelista, A.G.; De Melo Nazareth, T.; Luciano, F.B. Fundamentals on the molecular mechanism of action of antimicrobial peptides. *Materialia* **2019**, *8*, 100494. [CrossRef]
37. Lopes, S.C.; Ribeiro, C.; Gameiro, P. A New Approach to Counteract Bacteria Resistance: A Comparative Study Between Moxifloxacin and a New Moxifloxacin Derivative in Different Model Systems of Bacterial Membrane. *Chem. Biol. Drug Des.* **2013**, *81*, 265–274. [CrossRef] [PubMed]
38. Crusca, E., Jr.; Rezende, A.A.; Marchetto, R.; Mendes-Giannini, M.J.; Fontes, W.; Castro, M.S.; Cilli, E.M. Influence of N-terminus modifications on the biological activity, membrane interaction, and secondary structure of the antimicrobial peptide hylin-a1. *Pept. Sci.* **2011**, *96*, 41–48. [CrossRef] [PubMed]
39. Gogoi, P.; Shrivastava, S.; Shah, P.; Saxena, S.; Srivastava, S.; Gaur, G.K. Linear and branched forms of short antimicrobial peptide-IRK inhibit growth of multi drug resistant Staphylococcus aureus isolates from mastitic cow milk. *Int. J. Pept. Res. Ther.* **2021**, *27*, 2149–2159. [CrossRef]
40. Ludtke, S.J.; He, K.; Heller, W.T.; Harroun, T.A.; Yang, L.; Huang, H.W. Membrane pores induced by magainin. *Biochemistry* **1996**, *35*, 13723–13728. [CrossRef]
41. Zhu, Y.; Li, J.; Pang, Z. Recent insights for the emerging COVID-19: Drug discovery, therapeutic options and vaccine development. *Asian J. Pharm. Sci.* **2021**, *16*, 4–23. [CrossRef]

MDPI AG
Grosspeteranlage 5
4052 Basel
Switzerland
Tel.: +41 61 683 77 34

Pharmaceutics Editorial Office
E-mail: pharmaceutics@mdpi.com
www.mdpi.com/journal/pharmaceutics

www.ingramcontent.com/pod-product-compliance
Lightning Source LLC
LaVergne TN
LVHW072322090526
838202LV00019B/2335